Family Health Care Nursing
Theory, Practice, and Research

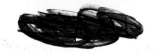

The University of Lethbridge

School of Health Sciences

Family Health Care Nursing
Theory, Practice, and Research

Third Edition

Shirley Mae Harmon Hanson, PMHNP, PhD, RN, FAAN, CFLE, LMFT
Professor Emerita
Oregon Health & Sciences University
School of Nursing
Portland, Oregon

Vivian Gedaly-Duff, MS, DNSc, RN
Associate Professor
Oregon Health & Sciences University
School of Nursing
Portland, Oregon

Joanna Rowe Kaakinen, PhD, RN
Associate Professor
University of Portland
Portland, Oregon

F.A. DAVIS • Philadelphia

F.A. Davis Company
1915 Arch Street
Philadelphia, PA 19103
www.fadavis.com

Copyright © 2005 by F.A. Davis Company

Printed in the United States of America

Last digit indicates print number: 10 9 8 7 6 5 4 3 2 1

Acquisitions Editor: Joanne P. DaCunha, RN, MSN
Developmental Editor: Caryn Abramowitz

As new scientific information becomes available through basic and clinical research, recommended treatments and drug therapies undergo changes. The author(s) and publisher have done everything possible to make this book accurate, up to date, and in accord with accepted standards at the time of publication. The author(s), editors, and publisher are not responsible for errors or omissions or for consequences from application of the book, and make no warranty, expressed or implied, in regard to the contents of the book. Any practice described in this book should be applied by the reader in accordance with professional standards of care used in regard to the unique circumstances that may apply in each situation. The reader is advised always to check product information (package inserts) for changes and new information regarding dose and contraindications before administering any drug. Caution is especially urged when using new or infrequently ordered drugs.

Library of Congress Cataloging-in-Publication Data

Family health care nursing : theory, practice, and research / [edited]
by Shirley May Harmon Hanson, Vivian Gedaly-Duff & Joanna Rowe Kaakinen.— 3rd ed.
    p. ; cm.
  Includes bibliographical references and index.
  ISBN 0-8036-1202-8 (alk. paper)
  1. Family nursing. 2. Family—Health and hygiene.
  [DNLM: 1. Family Nursing. WY 159.5 F1985 2005] I. Hanson, Shirley
M. H., 1938- II. Gedaly-Duff, Vivian, 1948- III. Kaakinen, Joanna Rowe,
1951-
  RT120.F34F35 2005
  610.73—dc22

2005007496

Cover: "Scratched, Fretted, Worked" by Marcia Hindman

I dedicate this book to my parents and siblings from my family of origin and to my children and grandchildren from my family of procreation. They have been a source of love and constancy during the good times and not so good times in my life. I also appreciate the many children, couples, and families from whom I learned during 45 years of professional service as a nurse and therapist. Finally, I dedicate this book to the students of nursing and child/family therapy who stand on my shoulders in service to families across the world.

SHIRLEY MAY HARMON HANSON

My family, who traveled and lived in several countries during my growing-up years, helped me learn the many meanings and diversity of family life. Although travel opened the way to experience many things, it was the stability of my family that facilitated the curiosity and thirst to learn more. A special dedication goes to my parents, Hazel and Al Gedaly, who created the adventure, and to my husband, Robert W. Duff, whose laughter, love, and support continue to energize our life together. Working on this textbook renewed the significance of family for me, particularly during times of illness and end-of-life.

VIVIAN GEDALY-DUFF

I would like to dedicate this to my father, Robert A. Rowe, who believed in me and was always in my corner but also said that life teaches us much and we must listen to the lessons. Because of the love and support of my husband John and son Thomas, I was able to dedicate the time and energy that this project required. I also want to thank my mother and my sister for being a loving family who guided me and supported my endeavors in pursuing nursing. I would like to thank Dr. Patricia Chadwick, Dean of the University of Portland in 1989, who placed a new faculty member with no teaching experience in the new family nursing course. This chance assignment changed my view and practice of nursing.

JOANNA ROWE KAAKINEN

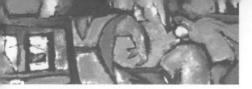

ACKNOWLEDGMENTS

We would like to thank the new and continuing contributors for this third edition. All authors dedicated serious time to create or update their particular specialty area of family nursing. They spent many hours making their work current, theory-guided, and evidence-based. Without their diligence and commitment to the nursing of families, this edition would not be possible.

We had an excellent editorial team at F.A. Davis Publishing. Joanne DaCunha, nursing acquisitions editor, graciously headed the F.A. Davis team again for this third edition. Our developmental editor, Caryn Abramowitz, put in countless hours of detailed work and pulled the book together so that it spoke with one voice. Kristin Kern, our project editor, did an excellent job in helping this edition be readable and artistic. We thank you all at F.A. Davis.

Two assistants played important roles in the development of this edition. Erin Leben provided clerical responsibilities during the initial organizational phase of the project. Vicki Montag provided technical assistance later in the project. Both deserve a very special thank-you and recognition. Both women helped us meet deadlines and produced quality work.

SMHH, VGD, & JRK

I am grateful to all the wonderful people who have played a role in three successful editions of this textbook. If it takes a community to raise a child, it clearly takes many communities to give birth to a book. It has been a privilege to have made so many professional friends and colleagues from around the world as a result of this textbook. This international community joined me in the belief that "nurses care about people and have passion and compassion for their work."

I am eternally grateful that Joanna and Vivian came on as coeditors for this third edition. Their warm friendship and highest level of professionalism have made this third edition the most satisfying of all editions. I will be forever indebted for their gift to family nursing and to me personally. I know this important textbook will be in good hands as it moves into future editions and as I move toward retirement.

SMHH

Shirley Hanson is a dedicated crusader for the plight of families and an adamant family mental health nurse practitioner. She is a gracious teacher, and she took time to mentor both of us. Both of us, from deep in our hearts, thank Shirley for sharing her lifework in the nursing of families and guiding us on this journey. Shirley's humor and passion about family nursing guided us in producing this book. Shirley, you are truly special!

JRK & VGD

FOREWORD

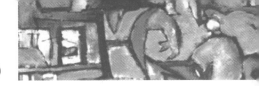

A current knowledge of family nursing theory, practice, and research is indispensable in addressing the burgeoning and complex health care needs of our increasingly diverse and aging population. Nurses with family preparation and orientation possess the perspective necessary to address the nursing care of individuals and families across the life span. *Family Health Care Nursing: Theory, Practice, and Research* provides the critical foundation in the nursing of families for baccalaureate- and master's-level students, as well as for practicing registered nurses. This book portrays family nursing perspectives in theory, practice, and research, and it thoroughly applies this perspective to specific populations. Shirley Hanson has provided continuity of leadership and expertise as editor and contributor in three editions of this classic text. Two new coeditors, Vivian Gedaly-Duff and Joanna Kaakinen, have added their voices to this third edition. Collectively, the three editors melded their theoretical orientation, practice backgrounds, and research knowledge to ensure that each chapter reflects the current state of the science and art of family health care nursing.

Contributors to this book include some of the most prominent practitioners, educators, and researchers in family nursing. This collaboration resulted in an exceptional text that links family theory and research to practice in specific populations, with attention to different issues throughout the life span. The authors of clinical chapters use a common organizing framework for the population-specific chapters, which includes the following: health promotion; acute and chronic illness; end-of-life care; theory, practice, and research; and implications for nursing education. This framework is useful to readers when linking and comparing concepts and information from one chapter to another. The editors have intentionally structured the book to foster the application of theory and research to practice and policy.

Both previous editions have been popular and comprehensive textbooks for nursing students and practicing nurses who are learning family nursing. The textbook is now being used around the world. The third edition of the book has not only updated and streamlined the work of previous editions but also added additional chapters of importance to modern-day family nursing and an online instructor's guide.

Four new chapters featured in this new edition help to make this book one of the most current and comprehensive in the family nursing arena. "Family and Health Demographics" educates nurses about the makeup of the types of families they will actually see in practice. Information about demographics and health priorities and the nation's stance in relation to these priorities is critical in the arsenal of knowledge for family nurses.

Burgeoning information in the area of genomics renders Chapter 17 a must-read for all nurses working with families. "Genomics, Family Nursing, and Families across the Life Span" teaches learners to help families manage genetic information so that they can promote healthy family functioning.

People are living longer with chronic illness, and families are their primary caregivers. Nurses need to understand their multifaceted roles and find ways to meet family expectations amid increasingly complex caregiving situations. "Families with Chronic Illness" focuses on family issues across the life span. The evidence base for chronic illness across the life span reflected in this third edition echoes the substantive contributions of family nursing scholars in theory development, research, and practice in this area. A case in point is the body of knowledge regarding families who are caring for family members with chronic conditions.

The chapter titled "International Family Nursing" is also a welcome addition that illustrates how family health theory and research can be applied to nursing practice in a global community. This chapter builds on the generation of international knowledge among family nurse scholars that developed through educational experiences, faculty/student exchange, research collaboration, and forums, such as the International Family Nursing Conferences (IFNC).

Accompanying these new chapters, and another welcome addition to this edition of the book, is an online instructor's guide. The guide offers chapter-by-chapter study and test questions; case studies for discussion; substantive, chapter-specific PowerPoint presentations for use and adaptation by faculty teaching family nursing courses; and a variety of other learning tools and ideas that instructors will find useful in creating lesson plans.

Because the primary responsibility for health promotion and the burden of caregiving frequently falls on families and community, it is incumbent that nurse educators prepare students in the areas of family assessment and nursing interventions. By addressing family systems as a whole and recognizing the reality of family roles today, nurses enhance the health and quality of life of individuals and their families. For example, by equipping individuals and their family caregivers with the knowledge, skills, and resources needed to manage chronic conditions, nurses ensure that ill family members receive the care and support needed while minimizing negative consequences for the family caregivers themselves. Delivering nursing care from a standpoint of promoting family health helps nurses actuate families' abilities to attend to health and developmental needs and prevent secondary disabilities.

A family nursing orientation reflects the way that families across the life span manage health and illness. Families are dealing concurrently with a variety of health and illness issues for members at different developmental stages. Nurses need the educational acumen to tailor their practice interventions to families managing health and illness in today's society. *Family Health Care Nursing: Theory, Practice, and Research* is exactly the resource nurses need to support them as they develop and test the efficacy and cost-effectiveness of intergenerational models of family health promotion and care delivery.

Ann Williams Garwick PhD, RN, LP, LMFT, FAAN
Professor and Director of the Center for Child & Family Health Promotion
School of Nursing, University of Minnesota

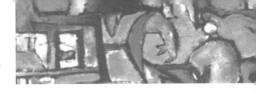

INTERNATIONAL FAMILY NURSING: THE VIEW FROM JAPAN

As diversity of families and issues regarding families have increased and have gotten more and more complicated throughout the world, the need for family nursing has grown rapidly. For this reason, I would like to celebrate the publication of the third edition of *Family Health Care Nursing: Theory, Practice, and Research*. As a scholar who studied at Oregon Health Sciences University in Portland, Oregon, and as one of the individuals who translated the first edition of this book into Japanese, I feel very honored and privileged to have this opportunity to contribute this foreword to its third edition.

In order to present an international perspective, I would like to offer some background on the development of family nursing in Japan and how the translation of the first edition of *Family Health Care Nursing* has influenced nursing in Japan.

DEVELOPMENT OF FAMILY NURSING IN JAPAN

We have a long nursing history of assisting families in Japan, but the modern idea of caring for a family as one unit of care began in the 1990s. Since that time, family nursing has become one of the special fields in nursing, with an evolving and developing role.

The systematic approach toward family nursing began in 1994 and 1995 when two seminal events occurred: the founding of the Japanese Association for Research in Family Nursing (1994) and the publication of the *Japanese Journal of Research in Family Nursing* (1995). More recently, the Japanese Nursing Association launched a new biyearly journal, *Family Nursing*, in 2003. Through these major events, family nursing in Japan has made a great advancement, facilitating the collaboration among researchers, practitioners, and health care organizations and the linkage between research and practice.

As family nursing recently has been incorporated into the general curriculum of nursing education in Japan, Japanese nursing students now have an opportunity to study family nursing as a part of a fundamental nursing education. Some graduate schools offer a course specializing in family nursing, and family nursing also has been included in the Japanese clinical nurse specialist program. Two universities currently offer a course for clinical nurse specialists (CNSs) in family nursing, so we will soon have nurses certified in family nursing.

The following factors account, at least in part, for the recent development of family nursing in Japan: low birth rate; rapidly aging population; diversified values in the society; changes in families; changes in disease structures; changes in health care systems; social needs accompanying the development of home health care; needs for family nursing due to various difficulties that family members face, such as raising children and taking care of aging parents; a sense of responsibility in nursing for these needs; quality improvement in nursing; and a desire to establish an academic structure of family nursing. Furthermore, several other factors have contributed to the development of family nursing in Japan. These include the development and advancement of family nursing overseas, especially in the United States and Canada; the introduction to Japan of relevant overseas achievements through translation of works, seminars, and lectures by established scholars in the field; Japanese nurses increasing their knowledge base by studying abroad and attending international seminars and conferences in family nursing; and Japanese nurses exchanging information and research results with scholars abroad.

SIGNIFICANCE AND CONTRIBUTION OF FAMILY HEALTH CARE NURSING: THEORY, PRACTICE, AND RESEARCH IN JAPAN

Next, I would like to describe how the first edition of *Family Health Care Nursing: Theory, Practice, and Research* translated into Japanese has been considered and used in Japan. When I introduced the first edition of this book to a Japanese publisher several years ago, I firmly believed (and still believe) the following:

1. The book helps nurses understand comprehensively how, in a specific cultural background, family nursing is structured, how it is applied to clinical situations and policy making, and how it contributes to improving health of families.

2. As the title suggests, the book brings together the theory, research, and practice of family nursing, presents a model as to how theory and research can be applied to various practice settings in which family nursing takes place, and acknowledges that family nursing can be practiced across the family life cycle.

3. The book would facilitate ideas for research and practice in family nursing in Japan and assist Japanese nurses with construction and development of family nursing structures, based on Japanese culture and family characteristics observed in Japan.

The translation of the first edition was introduced in the book review section of *Kango* ("Nursing" in English), the official journal of the Japanese Nursing Association, in 2002. The review described the book as very helpful for studying family nursing and for clinical applications. The book has been read by those nurses and nursing students who are interested in family nursing. I recommend that my graduate students read the translated first edition, along with the second edition in English. The book has been cited frequently and listed as reference material in Japanese books and papers.

Japanese family nursing now stands at the starting point for its second stage of development. Our goal at this point in time is to entrench family nursing further to meet the needs of our culture, time, and society and to contribute even more to the health and welfare of families. The Japanese Association for Research in Family Nursing holds an annual conference every year. Dr. Shirley Hanson, the editor of this book, was a keynote speaker at the 11th conference where the theme was "Facilitation of Family Nursing Research: Systematic Development of Knowledge and Improvement of Family Health."

I firmly believe that the third edition of *Family Health Care Nursing: Theory, Practice, and Research* will lead the world with a further refined model for family nursing. It will provide significant implications to those who theorize, practice, conduct research, or teach family nursing, working hard together to bring better health to families in communities throughout the world.

Keiko Murata, RN, PhD
Professor, Department of Nursing
Kobe University
Kobe, Japan
Translated by Masako Hayano

PREFACE

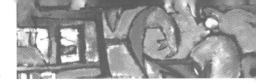

Family health care nursing is here to stay. Health care professionals are keenly aware of the importance of the interaction that exists among individuals, families, and their health status. We have long interacted within the therapeutic triangle of individuals, families, and the health care team. Yet, as we are now in the third generation of family nursing scholars, much has evolved in family nursing since thinkers and writers started 20 years ago. We are grateful for the exchange of ideas and for what we have learned from the work of early family nurses, including Florence Nightingale, and other contemporary family nursing colleagues. A few of these authors include the following: Rinda Alexander, Kathryn Barnard, Janice Bell, Perri Bomar, Vicky Bowden, Marion Broome, Martha Crafting-Rosenberg, Carol Danielson, Janice Denehy, Sharon Denham, Suzanne Feetham, Marilyn Friedman, Marie-Luise Friedemann, Catherine Gillis, Brenda Hamel-Bissell, Elaine Jones, Mary Ann Johnson, Kathleen Knafl, Maureen Leahey, Judy Malone, Marilyn McCubbin, Susan Meister, Karen Pridham, Wendy Watson, Gail Wegner, Patricia Winstead-Fry, Lorraine Wright, Beth Vaughan-Cole, and B. Lee Walker.

The first edition of *Family Health Care Nursing: Theory, Practice, and Research* came out in 1996, and it was extremely well received. It also was translated into Japanese. The second edition of the book, prepared for the new millennium, was published in 2001, and its influence surpassed that of the first edition. The third edition of the textbook has 19 chapters (a change from 16 in the first edition and 17 in the second), all of which have been thoroughly revised and updated. There are four brand-new chapters and subjects in this edition: Chapter 2, Family and Health Demographics; Chapter 16, Families and Chronic Illness across the Life Span; Chapter 17, Genomics, Family Nursing, and Families across the Life Span; and Chapter 18, International Family Nursing. A completely new feature accompanying this book is the Instructor's Manual, which is online through F.A. Davis Publishers at www.FADAVIS.com and which is available to all faculty who adapt this textbook for their classrooms.

The purpose of this book is to provide a foundation in the concepts of family health care nursing, to learn how these concepts and theories are practiced in the traditional specialties within the nursing profession, and to see how these concepts play out in the theory, practice, research, education, and social policy arena of family nursing and what this may mean for families and nurses in the future. It is our belief that family nursing is no longer just another evolving specialty in nursing, but rather family nursing is THE UMBRELLA under which all specialties would/could/should practice. For example, child-rearing family nursing draws on different theories and research than does gerontological family nursing, but they are both "family nursing." Family nursing focuses on the family, specifically how a family and all its members respond to a health concern, whereas nursing, in general, looks for the response of the individual to a health issue, with family clearly in the background of care. To be able to practice family nursing, it appears to be a matter of whether nurses have been educated in the family nursing paradigm as part of their formal undergraduate/graduate education or are self-taught by experience. We believe this book promotes "the art and the science of family nursing" into the first and second decade of this new millennium by integrating the theory, practice, research (TPR), education, and social policy of family nursing. This book makes the connection between assessment and intervention strategies. It was created to be a theory- and research-guided textbook to be used by students and practitioners at all levels and across a spectrum of clinical professions.

Family Health Care Nursing is organized so that it can be used in its entirety from cover to cover for a course in family nursing. An alternative approach for the use of this text is to teach Section I, pertaining to the Foundations of Family Health Care Nursing, early in the nursing curriculum. Then students can be exposed to the specialty chapters in Section II related to Family Nursing Practice while they are going through the various clinical rotations in their curriculum. Section III on Futures of Families and Family Nursing could be addressed during the latter part of the year. Another alternative is to use this book as a reference text or as an adjunct to other textbooks that address specific specialties such as maternity, pediatrics, geriatrics, or community health. There is something in this book for all levels of students and for all levels and specialties of practicing nurses.

People who are sound theoreticians, practitioners, researchers, and academicians from a variety of settings across the country were recruited as contributors for this book. A few people who wrote for the first two editions dropped away for a variety of reasons, but most stayed with the project. A few mentors turned their chapter revisions over to the next generation of scholars. We found all contributors responsible, articulate, and committed. The third edition of the book was easier to develop because of electronic-age technology. We had an excellent working team among the editors of the book and the publishing company. No single person has the knowledge and skills to single-handedly author any textbook in today's world. Congratulations to these contributors for their tenacity in this 2-year process and for their commitment to families and nursing!

Two forewords are included in the front matter of the book. Ann Garwick, PhD, RN, from the University of Minnesota, was selected to write the main foreword to the book. She summarizes the value of this book within the larger context of family nursing scholarship. Keiko Murata, PhD, RN, from the University of Kobe in Japan, was asked to comment on international family nursing and provide a view from Japan. This textbook has been translated and is used throughout Japan. We are grateful to have such high endorsement from these family scholars.

The main body of the book is divided into three sections: Unit I—**Foundations of Family Health Care Nursing;** Unit II—**Family Nursing Practice;** and Unit III—**Futures of Families and Family Nursing.** There are nine chapters in Unit I, nine chapters in Unit II, and one chapter in Unit III.

Chapter 1, Family Health Care Nursing: An Introduction, was written by Shirley Hanson, PhD, RN, Professor Emeritus from Oregon Health & Science University School of Nursing. This chapter lays a foundation by introducing family health care nursing. Definitions of "family," "family health," and "family nursing" are presented along with the reasons for learning about family nursing. Critical concepts include the following: health of individuals affect all members of families; health and illness are family events; and families influence the process and outcome of health care. Although "family" is defined in many ways, the most salient definition to guide family nurses is "the family is who they say they are." Other

concepts discussed include the history of families, history of family nursing, approaches to family nursing, variables influencing family nursing, family nursing roles, obstacles influencing family nursing practice, and concepts for family health care. This is a chapter to be read by all students, as it lays the foundation for other theoretical or practice chapters that follow.

Chapter 2, Family and Health Demographics, was coauthored by two individuals: Lynne Casper, PhD, from the National Institute of Child Health and Human Development, and John Haaga, PhD, from the National Institute on Aging. Both are experts in statistics and demographics of families across the life span. In this new chapter, the authors highlight the profound changes in families and households and the ethnic diversity and age composition of the American population that sets the social context in which health care is provided. The aging and growing diversity of the American population, combined with shifts in the economy and changing norms, values, and laws, are altering the context of family health care nursing. Implications for family nursing conclude this chapter.

Chapter 3, Theoretical Foundations for the Nursing of Families, was developed by Shirley Hanson, PhD, RN, Professor Emeritus from Oregon Health & Science University School of Nursing, and Joanna Kaakinen, PhD, RN, from the University of Portland School of Nursing. They shared their insights about theories and models that provide nurses with various options to shape how they approach caring for families. The authors stress that nurses who use only one theoretical approach to working with families limit their professional capabilities to help families. Questions such as "What is theory?" "What are the functions of theory?" and "What are the criteria for evaluating theory?" are answered in this chapter. The chapter summarizes selected theories from family social science, family therapy, and nursing science that help frame research and practice in family nursing. This chapter lays the foundation for theory discussions within each of the practice chapters in **Unit II.**

Chapter 4, Research in Families and Family Nursing, was penned by Gail Houck, PhD, RN, Sheila Kodadek, PhD, RN, and Catherine Samson, MPH, RN, from Oregon Health & Science University. This chapter has been significantly updated in this edition to address the important issues of theory-guided evidence-based research as it pertains to the nursing of families. It covers issues important to conducting family nursing research, such as asking the right research question, selecting the appropriate research method (qualitative and quantitative approaches), and evaluating family nursing research. This chapter would complement any nursing research course and serves as a primer to review the research reviewed in Unit II of the text.

Chapter 5, Family Structure, Function, and Process, was completely rewritten by family scholar Sharon Denham, DSN, RN, of Ohio University School of Nursing. This chapter summarizes basic core issues pertaining to families. This important foundational information is needed by nurses to analyze family structure, family function, and family processes and to understand how these concepts relate to health care of families. Family structure is described in terms of family types, membership, and context. Functions of families include affective, reproductive, economic, and health. Roles, communication, power, decision making, coping strategies, and marital satisfaction are the family processes or interactions through which members accomplish instrumental and expressive tasks. Family nurses practice in ways that affect families' structure, functions, and processes and intervene in ways that promote health and wellness, prevent illness risks, treat disease conditions, and manage rehabilitative care needs.

Chapter 6, Families, Nursing, and Social Policy, was updated by Kristine Gebbie, PhD, RN, from Columbia University School of Nursing and Eileen Gebbie, MA, from the Metropolitan Alliance for the Common Good in Portland, Oregon. These authors look at the practice of family nursing within the social and political structure of society. This chapter discusses some of the dominant ways that public social policy (governmental policy decisions such as legal relationships, support systems, and financing of care) affects families, particularly family health. Included in this chapter are different definitions of "family," discussion of policies that affect the ability to parent and provide care to the young and the old, and policies that influence work, welfare, and education. The chapter also presents policies specifically related to health and wellness care.

Chapter 7, Sociocultural Influences on Family Health, was written by Eleanor Ferguson-Marshalleck, PhD, RN, and Jung Kim Miller, PhD, RN, from California State University Department of Nursing (Los Angeles). The authors point out that ethnicity and social class are two primary holders of family values, family behaviors, and family structure during times of health and illness. In addition, the authors note the increasing disparity between social classes in the United States and health services and care. This chapter examines the extent to which health beliefs and practice influence family health. An exploration of social class structure as a decisive factor in family health is included. The chapter reviews implications for family nursing practice, such as ways to enhance cultural sensitivity and competency.

Chapter 8, Family Nursing Assessment and Intervention, was written by Joanna Kaakinen, PhD, RN, from the University of Portland School of Nursing, and Shirley Hanson, PhD, RN, Professor Emeritus from Oregon Health & Science University. They discuss the reasoning that nurses use to make skilled judgments and develop collaborative processes to help families when they experience health problems. Nurses determine whether the health problem will be addressed from the perspective of family-as-context, family-as-client, family-as-system, or family-as-community. The authors expand on the concept of assessment as the first and essential ingredient to provide comprehensive family health care. They share strategies to help families develop realistic outcomes that are based on the strengths of the family. One section covers how to select appropriate measurement instruments, and another describes three family nursing assessment models that were developed by and for family nurses.

Chapter 9, Family Health Promotion, was written by Perri Bomar, PhD, RN, from the University of North Carolina School of Nursing at Wilmington. This chapter on family health promotion presents ways that nurses can work with families to empower them to achieve healthier lives for each member and for the family as a whole. A new model of family health promotion is presented, along with intervention strategies that promote family health. The chapter also connects family health promotion to the Healthy People 2010 program. The information in this chapter is essential, as much of nursing education is focused in the acute care arena. This chapter discusses family health promotion across settings and in different family situations. Finally, the implications for practice, education, family policy, and research are discussed in relation to family health promotion.

Unit II of this book addresses **Family Nursing Practice** and consists of nine chapters focused on the practice of family nursing in some major clinical areas. **Chapter 10, Family Nursing with Childbearing Families,** was written by Louise Martell, PhD, RN, retired faculty from the University of Washington School of Nursing. The emphasis of this chapter is on family relationships and health promotion in childbearing families. New to this edition is information on parenting, adoption, postpartum depression, and threats to childbearing. Family systems, transition, and family development theories are presented to assist nurses in developing care plans for the childbearing family. The chapter concludes with suggestions for practice, policy development, and education.

Chapter 11, Family Child Health Nursing, was authored by Vivian Gedaly-Duff, DNSc, RN, Marsha Heims, EdD, RN, and Ann Nielsen, MN, RN, from Oregon Health & Science University School of Nursing. The Family Interaction Model is used to connect theory and practice of families with children. Issues of family health promotion germane to families with children, such as parenting, grandparenting, child care, and after-school activities, are discussed. New content includes the issues of end-of-life. The chapter addresses child abuse, violence, obesity, and pediatric mental health issues. It presents family-centered care and nursing actions specific to family well-being and children's health. The chapter concludes with suggestions for research, education, and health policy specific to family child health.

Chapter 12, Family-Focused Medical-Surgical Nursing, was created by Nancy Artinian, PhD, RN, from Wayne State University College of Nursing. Artinian reviews structural-functional, family systems, and family resilience theories as they apply to patients and family members experiencing the stressors of foreign hospital environments during illness and end-of-life. According to this chapter, nursing actions focus on providing assurance, enhancing the proximity of patient and family, managing information, facilitating comfort, and reinforcing support. Common family concerns in chronic illness, such as guilt, fear, uncertainty, anger, and lack of knowledge about the illness, care requirements, or resources, may require interventions. At end-of-life, interventions are directed toward helping families move through the phases of adaptation in response to the fatal illness of a family member. Families need help dealing with other end-of-life issues such as making decisions regarding withdrawal of life support or organ donation and witnessing cardiopulmonary resuscitation efforts. Implications for family nursing conclude this chapter.

Chapter 13, Family Mental Health Nursing, was written by returning contributor, Helene Moriarty,

PhD, RN, from Philadelphia Veterans Affairs Medical Center, and Suzanne Brennan, PhD, RN, from Contextual Therapy Associates in Philadelphia. This chapter describes how mental health nurses practice family-centered care in a variety of settings. New to this edition of the chapter is information pertaining to domestic and family abuse. An overview of common theoretical perspectives in family mental health nursing provides important background information on ideas shaping contemporary family mental health nursing. Using realistic case examples from inpatient and outpatient settings, the chapter addresses family mental health nursing in health promotion, acute illness, chronic illness, and end-of-life care. After illustrating multiple roles for the family mental health nurse, the chapter concludes with implications of family mental health nursing for practice, education, research, and health policy.

Chapter 14, Gerontological Family Nursing, was written by Mary LuAnne Lilly, PhD, RN, from Indiana University School of Nursing. In this chapter, the focus is for nurses to learn ways to assist elderly individuals and their families. These interventions include the application of specialized knowledge related to aging individuals and family development, health maintenance, acute and chronic illness, family caregiving dynamics, interpersonal communication, referral resources, and evidence-based interventions. The issues of aging families are explored via the systems model and the Family Resiliency Model. New in this chapter is coverage of end-of-life care for the aging family and a section on elder abuse. The chapter concludes with specific issues on social policy, nursing education, and research for aging families.

Chapter 15, Families and Community/Public Health Nursing, was coauthored by Debra Anderson, PhD, RN, and Kacy Allen-Bryant, BS, RN, both from the University of Kentucky College of Nursing. This chapter has been updated to address public health nursing, as well as community nursing, from a family nursing perspective. The concepts of community-based and community nursing are explored. The theoretical lens used is the Family Caregiving Model for Public Health Nursing. Health promotion as disease prevention, community as client, secondary prevention in families with acute and chronic illness, and end-of-life community nursing are new sections in this updated edition.

Chapter 16, Families with Chronic Illness. Jane Kurz, PhD, RN, and Margaret Shepard, PhD, RN, from Temple University in Philadelphia coauthored this new chapter. The chapter discusses the principles of chronic illness using Rolland's Family Systems and Illness Model. Chronic illnesses are challenges to families throughout the life span and render families particularly vulnerable at times of transitions. Nurses help families manage chronic illnesses and aid them to anticipate losses and ambiguous situations at all stages of the family life cycle. Implications for family nursing theory, research, social policy, and education conclude this chapter.

Chapter 17, Genomics, Family Nursing, and Families across the Life Span, was written by Janet Williams, PhD, RN, from the University of Iowa, along with an international scholar, Heather Skirton, PhD, RN, from the University of Plymouth, United Kingdom. This new chapter was added to bring family nursing science up to date with the explosion of genetics and health care information that came about as a result of the Human Genome Project. Although genetic nursing is not new, the breadth and depth of genetic knowledge and its applications in family nursing practice are rapidly changing. The purpose of this chapter is to describe the relevance of genetic information within families, especially when there is a question about genetic aspects of health or disease of family members. The authors describe situations throughout the life span of family members, where nursing knowledge of genetic concerns is necessary for nurses to provide comprehensive assessment, interventions, and evaluation of nursing care. Implications for education, practice, research, and health care policy conclude the chapter.

Chapter 18, International Family Nursing. Susan Elliott, PhD, RN, from Azusa Pacific University wrote this new chapter that reflects the global nature of family nursing. The purpose of this chapter is to introduce issues common to providing family nursing care in culturally diverse international settings, to discuss issues that affect global health and well-being, and to discuss community-based health care as a proven international family nursing practice model. International issues are explored when applying family theories in international environments. There is a section, with examples, on cultural awareness, cultural sensitivity, cultural adaptation, and culture shock. A global family care model is used as the theoretical perspective. Implications for family nursing end this chapter.

Unit III focuses on **Futures of Families and Family Nursing. Chapter 19, The Futures of Families, Health, and Family Nursing,** is the last chapter of the book, and it was authored by Shirley Hanson, PhD, RN, Professor Emeritus from Oregon Health & Science University School of Nursing. The purpose of this chapter is to look at what the future means for family nursing. It summarizes general patterns of changing families, future demographics of American families, and glimpses of world demographic trends. It also discusses the health of American families (trends, morbidity, and mortality) and selected factors such as terrorism/war, health care workforce, health care reform, aging, religion, sexuality, health care technology, and ethnic diversity, as well as how these factors play a role in the nation's health and in family nursing. The future of and implications for family nursing theory, practice, research, education, and social policy conclude this chapter.

An **Instructor's Manual** was developed by Deborah Coehlo, PhD, RN, faculty at Oregon State University and Oregon Health & Science University School of Nursing. This is a new and important feature for this edition of the textbook. We believe that it will be immensely helpful to both new and experienced faculty who teach family nursing. The Instructor's Manual resides online at F.A. Davis Publishers' Website and is available to faculty who adopt this textbook. It is designed for faculty to take students through the process of learning and understanding new information, applying that information in a variety of learning activities, including examination and review questions and other learning activities, and synthesizing newly applied information through application in case studies and reflection activities. Each chapter contains these sections: key concepts, key terms, examination questions, learning activities, and case studies. Each chapter also contains a PowerPoint presentation that can be used to present the material to audiences. These slides support both on-site and online courses in family nursing. Finally, each chapter offers suggested references for students.

As editors of this edition and authors of some of the chapters in this textbook, we are joyful that this 2-year project has been completed successfully. We encourage anyone to write us with your critiques, your counterpoints, and your ideas so that we may incorporate them in the next edition of this textbook. This book was not meant to be a template but rather a catalyst to move the art and science of family nursing forward.

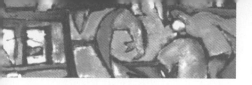

CONTRIBUTORS

Kacy Allen-Bryant, RN, BSN
Graduate Research Assistant
University of Kentucky, College of Nursing
Lexington, Kentucky

Debra Gay Anderson, PhD, RNC
Associate Professor
University of Kentucky, College of Nursing
Lexington, Kentucky

Nancy Trygar Artinian, PhD, RN, BC
Associate Professor
Wayne State University, College of Nursing
Detroit, Michigan

Suzanne Marie Brennan, Phd, RN
Contextual Therapy Associates in Philadelphia
Philadelphia, Pennsylvania

Perri J. Bomar, PhD, RN
Professor and Associate Dean for Research and
Community Partnership
University of North Carolina School of Nursing at
Wilmington
Wilmington, North Carolina

Lynne M. Casper, BA, AM, PhD
Health Scientist Administrator and Demographer
Demographic and Behavioral Sciences Branch
Center for Population Research
National Institute of Child Health and Human
Development
Bethesda, Maryland

Deborah Padgett Coehlo, PhD, RN, C-PNP
Assistant Professor
Oregon State University
Bend, Oregon
Oregon Health & Science University
School of Nursing
Portland, Oregon

Sharon A. Denham, DSN, RN
Professor

Ohio University School of Nursing
Athens, Ohio

Susan E. Elliot, PhD, RN, FNP, WHNP
Assistant Professor of Nursing
Coordinator, International Health Family Nurse
Practitioner Program
California State University, Los Angeles
Los Angeles, California

Eleanor Ferguson-Marshalleck, MPH, PhD, RN
Professor, School of Nursing
Acting Associate Dean, College of Health and Human
Services
California State University, Los Angeles
Los Angeles, California

Eileen Gebbie, MA
Independent Scholar
Metropolitan Alliance for the Common Good
Portland, Oregon

Kristine M. Gebbie, DrPH, RN
Elizabeth Standish Gill Associate Professor of
Nursing
Columbia University School of Nursing
New York, New York

Vivian Gedaly-Duff, MS, DNSc, RN
Associate Professor
Oregon Health & Science University
School of Nursing
Portland, Oregon

John G. Haaga, PhD
Deputy Associate Director
Behavioral and Social Research
National Institute on Aging
Bethesda Maryland

Shirley Mae Harmon Hanson, PMHNP, PhD, RN,
FAAN, CFLE, LMFT
Professor Emerita
Oregon Health & Science University

School of Nursing
Portland, Oregon

Marsha L. Heims, EdD, RN
Associate Profoessor
Oregon Health & Science University
School of Nursing
Portland, Oregon

Gail M. Houck, PhD, RN
Professor
Oregon Health & Science University
School of Nursing
Portland, Oregon

Joanna Rowe Kaakinen, PhD, RN
Associate Professor
University of Portland
Portland, Oregon

Sheila M. Kodadek, PhD, RN
Professor, Child, Adolescent and Family Nursing
Oregon Health & Science University
School of Nursing
Portland, Oregon

Jane M. Kurz, PhD, RN
Associate Professor and Director of Graduate Studies
Temple University
Philadelphia, Pennsylvania

Mary LuAnne Lilly, PhD, RN,CS
Assistant Professor of Nursing and Clinical Psychiatry
Indiana University–Purdue University
School of Nursing
Indianapolis, Indiana

Louise Martell, PhD, RN
Retired Nursing Faculty
University of Washington
School of Nursing
Seattle, Washington

Jung Kim Miller, PhD, RN
Professor, School of Nursing
Associate Director of Education, The Roybai Institute
for Applied Gerontology
California State University, Los Angeles
Los Angeles, California

Helene J. Moriarty, PhD, RN, CS
Nurse Researcher
Philadelphia Veterans Affairs Medical Center
Philadelphia, Pennsylvania

Ann Nielsen, MN, RN
Instructor and Faculty in Residence
Oregon Health & Science University
School of Nursing
Portland, Oregon

Margaret P. Shepard, PhD, RN
Assistant Professor
Temple University
Philadelphia, Pennsylvania

Heather Skirton, PhD, MSc, RGN, Dip
Nurse Consultant in Clinical Genetics
Clinical Genetics Unit
Taunton and Somerset NHS Trust
Taunton, Somerset, UK
Reader in Health Genetics
Faculty of Health and Social Work
University of Plymouth
United Kingdom

Janet Karen D. Williams, PhD, RN, PNP, CGC, FAAN
Professor of Nursing
Director of Post-doctoral Clinical Genetics Research
Training
The University of Iowa

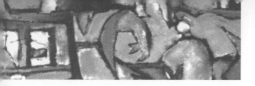

REVIEWERS

Ellen G. Christian, MS, RN-C
Professor
Institutional Nursing
BSN Program
University of Massachusetts
North Dartmouth, Massachusetts

Ruth P. Cox, PhD, LMFT, CRNP, ARNP
Assistant Professor
BSN & MSN Programs
University of Alabama
School of Nursing
Birmingham, Alabama

JoAnn K. Gottlieb, ARNP, CS, MS
Assistant Professor
BSN & MSN-NP Programs
Barry University
North Miami, Florida

Elizabeth S. Tiechler, MSN, PhD(c), RN-C, FNP
Senior Instructor
MSN-NP Program
University of Colorado Health Sciences Center
Denver, Colorado

Lynette Leeseberg Stamler, PhD, RN
Assistant Professor
BSN & MSN Programs
University of Windsor
School of Nursing
Windsor, Ontario, Canada

Nancy Symmes, BSN, MAEd(c), RN
Faculty
College of New Caledonia
Prince George, British Columbia, Canada

CONTENTS

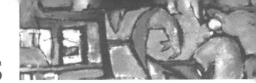

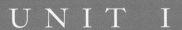

UNIT I

Foundations of Family Health Care Nursing

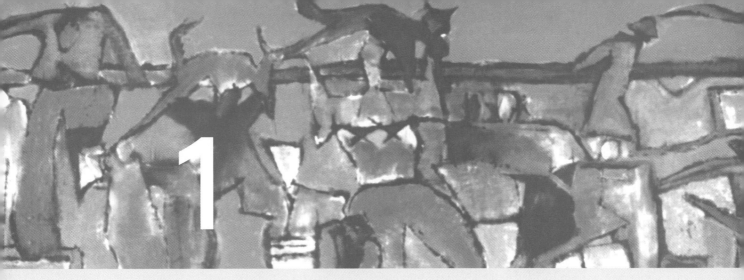

Family Health Care Nursing: An Introduction

Shirley May Harmon Hanson, RN, PMHNP, PhD, FAAN, CFLE, LMFT

CRITICAL CONCEPTS

- It is important to embrace a family focus in nursing practice because health of individuals affects all members of families, health and illness are family events, and families influence the process and outcome of health care.

- Family health care nursing knowledge and skills are important for nurses who practice in generalized as well as specialized settings.

- The term "family" is defined in many ways, but the most salient definition is "the family is who they say they are."

- There are four different approaches or views to the

- nursing care of families and they are all considered family nursing.

- The demographics of American families are changing and have an effect on family nursing.

- The history of families and family nursing impact the nursing of families today.

- Family functions have been constant over history, although there are more expectations of families today than there were previously.

- Family nursing can be practiced in a number of different settings and in many kinds of roles.

INTRODUCTION TO FAMILY HEALTH CARE NURSING

Traditionally, the focus of most nursing education has been on the practice of nursing with individual patients. All patients are members of families, and families are the basic unit of every society. By making a systematic study of the many kinds of families in various health settings, nurses are better prepared to work with families as a whole and families as the context.

Family health care nursing is an art and a science that has evolved over the last 20 years as a way of thinking about and working with families. Family nursing comprises a philosophy and a way of interacting with clients that affects how nurses collect information, intervene with patients, advocate for patients, and approach spiritual care with families. This philosophy and practice incorporates the assumption that health affects all members of families, that health and illness are family events, and that families influence the process and outcome of health care. All health care attitudes, beliefs, behaviors, and decisions are made within the context of larger family and societal systems. It is important that concepts and principles of family health care become part of nurses' value systems and knowledge base as they embark on a generalized or specialized practice in nursing. After all, all nursing practice involves families.

> ❝Family health care nursing is an art and a science that has evolved as a way of thinking about and working with families.❞

Much nursing talent and effort during the last 10 years has gone into elevating family health care nursing to where it is today. Family nursing as a specialty body of knowledge in nursing has evolved over the last 20 years as demonstrated by the following:

1. The growing number of textbooks focusing on family theory, practice, research, and social policy
2. The proliferation of family-related articles written by nurses and published in an array of scientific journals within and outside of nursing
3. Increasing research in families and health being carried out by nurses and family social science professionals
4. Family nursing as a philosophy becoming acknowledged all over the world
5. Family nursing content being incorporated and integrated in undergraduate and graduate nursing curricula
6. National and international family nursing conferences being held around the globe
7. The increasing numbers of national and international nursing journals as well as other journals focused on the family

Box 1–1 lists the many professional journals that explore themes related to families and nursing.

Although the specialty of family nursing has come a long way, continuing efforts are necessary to achieve the following goals: (1) to conceptualize and further delineate the phenomena of family health care nursing, (2) to build a nursing science through further family research that is cumulative and hypothesis building, and (3) to further develop and test theories evolving out of clinical practice that help improve nursing and family interaction in health and illness.

The overall goal of this book is to enhance nurses' knowledge and skills that pertain to the theory, practice, research, and social policy that are important for the nursing care of families. This chapter provides a broad overview of family health care nursing and why it is important to teach nurses about family health care. It begins with an exploration of the definition of family health care nursing and a discussion of where the profession of nursing is in relationship to nursing care of families. It reviews the concepts for family health care, such as the family health/illness cycle and the role of the nurse in the therapeutic triangle. This chapter provides context by discussing the history of families, the functions of families, and some of the changing family demographics. The chapter also covers the history of family nursing and current trends in family nursing practice, research, and education.

WHY TEACH NURSES ABOUT FAMILY NURSING?

Many people assume they are "experts in families," having had individual personal experiences with their own families. So why teach nurses about families? Based on their own personal family history, belief system, and limited experiences with other families, nurses are liable to make assumptions and judgments about families with whom they work. When nurses operate from a personal experience perspective, they are limited in their view. Nurses' individual socialization, culture, and value systems do and should affect the way they work with families. But personal experience should not be their only guide.

Family nursing is a scientific discipline based in theory. Universally, families are basic social units in all

Box 1–1 **JOURNALS RELATED TO FAMILIES AND FAMILY NURSING**

American Journal of Family Therapy
Community and Family Health
Family and Child Mental Health Journal
Journal of the Jewish Board of Family and Children's Services
Families in Society: The Journal of Contemporary Human Services
Family and Community Behavior
Family and Community Health
Family Behavior
Family Health
Family Medicine
Family Planning Digest
Family Planning Perspectives
Family Planning/Population Reporter
Family Process
Family Relations (previous title: Family Coordinator)
Family Science Review
Family Studies Review Yearbook
Family Systems Medicine
Family Therapy Collections
Family Therapy Networker
Family Therapy News
Health and Social Work
Health Care for Women International
Inventory of Marriage and Family Literature
Journal of Adolescent Research
Journal of Child and Family Nursing
Journal of Comparative Family Studies
Journal of Divorce
Journal of Family History
Journal of Family Issues
Journal of Family Nursing
Journal of Family Practice
Journal of Family Psychology
Journal of Marital and Family Therapy
Journal of Marriage and the Family
Marriage and Family Review
Maternal-Child Health
Merrill-Palmer Quarterly of Behavior and Development
Social Forces
Social Problems
Social Work
Social Work and Health Care
Sociology of Health & Illness
The Family Journal: Counseling and Therapy for Couples and Families
Women and Health
Women and Health Care
Youth and Society

societies. Nurses can combine their personal experience with their knowledge of this theory to practice effectively with families. Families vary in structure and function. Families even vary within a given culture, as all families have their own unique culture. People who come from the same family of origin create different families over time. Nurses should learn about family nursing so that they can provide client-centered holistic nursing care. Nurses need to be knowledgeable in the theory of families and the structure, function, and processes of families in order to assist families in achieving or maintaining a state of health.

> 66 Family nursing is a scientific discipline based in theory. 99

The centrality of the family in health care delivery is emphasized by the American Nurses Association (ANA) in its recent publication, *Nursing's Social Policy Statement* (ANA, 2003a). Additionally, ANA's statement on the scope and standards of nursing practice mandate nurses to provide family care (ANA, 2003b). New challenges in health care, such as changing health care policies and health care economics, new technology, shorter hospital stays, and health care moving from the hospital to the community and/or family home, are prompting the change from the individual paradigm of nursing to a family paradigm. This paradigm shift is affecting the development of family theory, practice, research, social policy, and education, and it is critical for nurses to be knowledgeable about and at the forefront of this shift.

DIMENSIONS OF FAMILY NURSING

What are the components of family nursing? In this section, three components are discussed: (1) how we define "family," (2) how we define "family health," and (3) what constitutes a "healthy family."

What Is the Family?

There is no generally agreed-upon definition of "family." "Family" is a word that conjures up different images for every individual and group, and the word has evolved in its meaning over time. Definitions differ by discipline, as shown in the following examples:

* Legal: relationships through blood ties, adoption, guardianship, or marriage
* Biological: genetic biological networks among people
* Sociological: groups of people living together
* Psychological: groups with strong emotional ties

Early family social science theorists (Burgess & Locke, 1953, pp. 7–8) adopted the following traditional definition in their writing:

> 66 The family is a group of persons united by ties of marriage, blood, or adoption, constituting a single household; interacting and communicating with each other in their respective social roles of husband and wife, mother and father, son and daughter, brother and sister; and creating and maintaining a common culture. 99

Presently, the U.S. Census Bureau defines "family" as two or more people living together who are related by birth, marriage, or adoption (Seccombe & Warner, 2004, p. 6). This traditional definition continues to be the basis for the implementation of many social programs and policies. This definition is not very satisfying because it excludes many diverse groups who

---

Box 1–2	**FAMILY FOCUS IN NURSING**

Why is this family focus important for nursing? According to Hanson (2001a, 2001b), the research literature generally concludes the following: (1) Health promotion, health maintenance, and the restoration of the health of families are important to the survival of all societies. (2) Health and illness beliefs and behaviors are learned within the context of family. (3) Family units are affected when one or more members experience health problems, and families are a significant factor in the health care and well-being of their individual members. (4) Conversely, families as a whole also impact how individual members resolve health problems that arise, and each individual member's health events and health practices affect the family as a whole. (5) Health care effectiveness is improved when emphasis is placed on the family, rather than just on the individual.

consider themselves families. Are cohabiting couples families? What about gay and lesbian couples? Do foster parents and the children for whom they are responsible constitute families? What about groups living in a communal setting where child care is shared among unrelated adults? Some groups under the Census Bureau's definition are considered families even though some observers might disagree (Greenstein, 2001). For example, should we define two elderly siblings living together as a family? Are childless married couples families?

Several studies demonstrate the changing public perception of how families are defined. A national poll by the Roper Organization in the 1990s found that although all respondents (98 percent) defined a married couple with children as a family, more than three-quarters also considered other people groupings as families (cohabiting couples, single parents, and so forth), demonstrating that more and more people are accepting other possible definitions of "family" (Greenstein, 2001). Ford (1994) also explored peoples' perceptions of "family." Young college students defined "family" as shifting to include a greater variety of possibilities, such as cohabiting couples without children, same-gender partners, and certain extended groups. Females were more likely to consider alternative scenarios as families than were male students. Ford concluded that there will be even more alternative family forms in the future and that professionals must explore their own perceptions and definitions of "family" to enhance their work with alternative family structures. A 2001 study based on five large national data sources found increasing tolerance of family diversity since the 1960s whereby definitions are reflecting the reality of the rich diversity of family life in society today (Thornton & Young-DeMarcho, 2001). Many more family forms are acceptable in today's world than in yesteryear's.

The definition of "family" adopted by this textbook is as follows:

> ❝*"Family" refers to two or more individuals who depend on one another for emotional, physical, and economical support. The members of the family are self-defined.* ❞

Nurses working with families should find out whom clients consider members of their family and should include those persons in health care planning. The family may range from traditional notions of the family (Dad, Mom, child, grandparents, uncles, aunts,

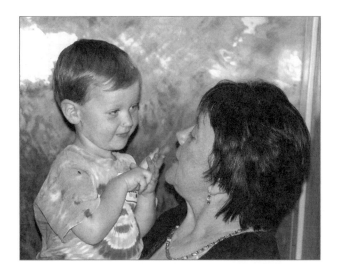

cousins) to such "postmodern" family structures as single-parent families, stepfamilies, and same-gender families.

What Is Family Health?

The construct of family health lacks consensus and precision. Anderson and Tomlinson (1992) suggested that the analysis of family health must include simultaneously both health and illness, as well as the individual and the collective. They underscore the growing evidence that the stress of a family member's serious illness exerts a powerful influence on family function and health, and that families' behavior patterns or reactions to the illness influence the individual family members.

The World Health Organization defines "health" as a state of complete physical, mental, and social well-being and not merely the absence of disease and infirmity. This definition applies to individuals as well as to families. The term "family health" is often used interchangeably with the terms "family functioning," "healthy families," or "familial health." To some, family health is the composite of individual family members' physical health, because it is impossible to make a single statement about the whole family's physical health.

The definition of "family health" adopted in this textbook is as follows:

> ❝*"Family health" is a dynamic changing state of well-being, which includes the biological, psychological, spiritual, sociological, and cultural factors of individual members and the whole family system.* ❞

Thus, this definition and approach combines the biological, psychological, social, cultural, and spiritual aspects of life for individual members as well as for the whole family. An individual's health (on the wellness-to-illness continuum) affects the entire family's functioning, and in turn, the family's ability to function affects each individual member's health. Assessment of family health involves simultaneous data collection on individual family members and the whole family system.

66 *"Family health" refers to the biological, psychological, social, cultural, and spiritual aspects of life for individual members as well as for the whole family.* 99

What Are Healthy Families?

It is possible to define "family health," but what about "healthy families"? Characteristics used to describe healthy families or family strengths have varied throughout time in the literature (Hanson, 2001b). Otto (1963), the first scholar to develop psychosocial criteria for assessing family strengths, emphasized the need to focus on positive family attributes instead of the pathological approach that accentuates family problems and weaknesses. Pratt (1976) introduced the idea of the "energized family" as one whose structure encourages and supports persons to develop their capacities for full functioning and independent action, thus contributing to family health. Stinnett, Chesser, and DeFrain (1979) described characteristics of family strengths. Their work led to research conducted by Curran. Curran (1983, 1985) investigated not only family stressors but also traits of healthy families, incorporating moral and task focus into traditional family functioning (see Box 1–3). Beavers and Hampson (1993), scholars who developed the Beavers Systems Model, characterized "healthy families" or optimally functioning families as families that do the following:

- Consistently demonstrate high degrees of capable negotiation skills in dealing with problems
- Are clear, open, and spontaneous in their expression of a wide range of feelings, beliefs, and differences
- Are respectful of members' feelings
- Encourage autonomy of their members
- Expect members to take personal responsibility for their actions

- Demonstrate closeness and warmth toward each other, with parents taking the leadership
- Express optimism and enjoyment with each other

Furthermore, according to Becvar and Becvar (2000), Gladding (1998), and Stinnett and DeFrain (1985), healthy families have a number of characteristics in common:

- A legitimate source of authority, established and supported over time
- A stable rule system established and consistently acted on
- Stable and consistent sharing of nurturing behavior
- Effective and stable child-rearing and marriage-maintenance practices
- A set of goals toward which the family and each individual work
- Sufficient flexibility and adaptability to accommodate normal developmental challenges as well as unexpected crisis
- Commitment to the family and its individuals
- Appreciation for each other (i.e., a social connection)
- Willingness to spend time together
- Effective communication patterns
- A high degree of religious/spiritual orientation
- Ability to deal with crisis in a positive manner (i.e., adaptability)
- Encouragement of individuals
- Clear roles

Thus, healthy families are both an ideal and a reality. There are still ongoing debates and disagreements as to the qualities of healthy families. Most scholars agree that health is more than the absence of pathology but rather an interactive process associated with positive relationships and outcomes (Gladding, 1998).

66 Most scholars agree that health is more than the absence of pathology but rather an interactive process associated with positive relationships and outcomes (Gladding, 1998). 99

FAMILY HEALTH CARE NURSING DEFINED

The specialty area of family health care nursing has been evolving over the last couple of decades. For some, there is blurring of lines as to how family health

Box 1–3 TRAITS OF HEALTHY FAMILIES

- Communicates and listens
- Fosters table time and conversation
- Affirms and supports each member
- Teaches respect for others
- Develops a sense of trust
- Has a sense of play and humor
- Has a balance of interaction among members
- Shares leisure time
- Exhibits a sense of shared responsibility
- Teaches a sense of right and wrong
- Abounds in rituals and traditions
- Shares a religious core
- Respects the privacy of each member
- Values service to others
- Admits to problems and seeks help

Source: Hanson, S. M. H. (2001b). Family health care nursing: An introduction. In S. M. H. Hanson (Ed.), *Family health care nursing: Theory, practice, and research* (pp. 2–35). Philadelphia: FA Davis. (Adapted from Curran, D. [1983]. *Traits of a healthy family.* Minneapolis: Winston Press Harper and Row.)

care nursing is distinctive from other specialties that involve families, such as maternal-child health nursing, community health nursing, and mental health nursing.

Family health care nursing is defined as follows:

> ❝Family health care nursing is the process of providing for the health care needs of families that are within the scope of nursing practice. This nursing care can be aimed toward the family as context, the family as a whole, the family as a system, or the family as a component of society. ❞

Family nursing takes into consideration all four approaches to viewing families and, at the same time, cuts across the individual, family, and community for the purpose of promoting, maintaining, and restoring the health of families. This framework shows the intersecting concepts of the individual, the family, nursing, and society (see Figure 1–1). Another model for viewing family nursing practice, where family nursing is seen conceptually as the confluence of theories and strategies from nursing, family therapy, and family social science, is depicted in Figure 1–2. Family nursing continues to incorporate ideas from family therapy and family social science. In fact, many nurses

pursue advanced preparation in those disciplines. See Chapter 3, Theoretical Foundation for the Nursing of Families, for more discussion about these theories.

> ❝Family nursing continues to incorporate ideas from family therapy and family social science. ❞

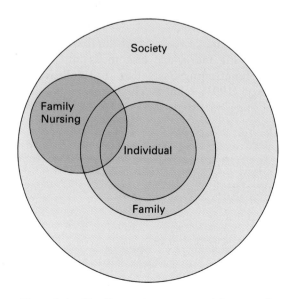

Figure 1–1 Family nursing conceptual framework.

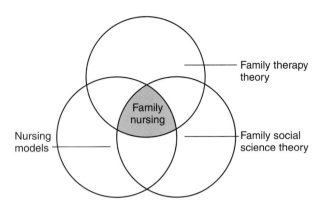

Figure 1–2 Family nursing practice.

Several family scholars have written about levels of family health care nursing practice. For example, Wright and Leahey (1994) differentiated among several levels of knowledge and skill that family nurses need for a generalist versus specialist practice, and they defined the role of higher education for the two different levels of practice. They proposed that nurses receive a generalist or basic level of knowledge and skill in family nursing during their undergraduate work and advanced specialization in family nursing or family therapy at the graduate level. They recognized that advanced specialists in family nursing have a narrower focus than generalists; however, they purported that family assessment is an important skill for all nurses practicing with families. Building on this previous work, Bomar (2004) further delineated five different levels of family health care nursing practice. Table 1–1 shows how the two levels of generalist and advanced practice were further delineated with levels of education and types of clients and relates them to Benner's paradigm of novice to expert (Benner, 2001).

Nature of Interventions in Family Nursing

There are 10 distinctive interventions for family nursing that emphasize the multivariate nature of the relationship between family health and the health of individual members (Gilliss, Roberts, Highley, & Martinson, 1989). In describing the nature of interventions in family nursing, the following points were determined:

Table 1–1 LEVELS OF FAMILY NURSING PRACTICE

LEVEL OF PRACTICE	GENERALIST/SPECIALIST	EDUCATION	CLIENT
Expert	Advanced Specialist	Doctoral degree	All levels Family nursing theory development Family nursing research
Proficient	Advanced Specialist	Master's degree with added experience	All levels Beginning family nursing research
Competent	Beginning Specialist	Master's degree	Individual in the family context Interpersonal family nursing Family unit Family aggregates
Advanced beginner	Generalist	Bachelor's degree with experience	Individual in the family context Interpersonal family nursing (family systems nursing) Family unit
Novice	Generalist	Bachelor's degree	Individual in the family context

Source: Bomar, P. J. (Ed.) (2004). *Promoting health in families: Applying family research and theory to nursing practice* (p. 19). Philadelphia: Saunders/Elsevier.

1. Family care is concerned with the experience of the family over time. It considers both the history and the future of the family group.
2. Family nursing considers the community and cultural context of the group. The family is encouraged to receive from and give to community resources.
3. Family nursing considers the relationships between and among family members and recognizes that, in some instances, all individual members and the family group will not achieve maximum health simultaneously.
4. Family nursing is directed at families whose members are both healthy and ill. Family health is not indexed by the degree of individual health or illness.
5. Family nursing is often offered in settings in which individuals present with physiologic or psychological problems. Along with being competent in treatment of individual health problems, family nurses must recognize the reciprocity between individual family members' health and collective health within the family.
6. The family system is influenced by any change in its members; therefore, when caring for individuals in health and illness, the nurse must elect whether to attend to the family. Both individual health and collective health are intertwined and will be influenced by any nursing care given.
7. Family nursing requires that the nurse manipulate the environment to increase the likelihood of family interaction; however, the absence of family members does not preclude the nurse from offering family care.
8. The family nurse recognizes that which person in a family is the most symptomatic may change over time; this means that the focus of the nurse's attention will also change over time.
9. Family nursing focuses on the strengths of individual family members and the family group to promote their mutual support and growth as it is possible.
10. Family nurses must define with the family which persons constitute the family and where they will place their therapeutic energies.

These are the distinctive intervention statements specific to family nursing that appear continuously in the care and study of families in nursing, regardless of the theoretical model in use.

Approaches to Family Nursing

There are four different approaches to care inherent in family nursing: (1) family as the context for individual development, (2) family as a client, (3) family as a system, and (4) family as a component of society. Figure 1–3 illustrates these approaches to the nursing of families. Each approach derived its foundations from different nursing specialties: maternal-child nursing, primary care nursing, psychiatric/mental health nursing, and community health nursing, respectively (Hanson, 2001a). All four approaches have legitimate implications for nursing assessment and intervention. The approach that nurses use is determined by many factors, including the health care setting, family circumstances, and nurse resources. Figure 1–4 shows how a nurse can view all four approaches to families through just one set of eyes. It is important to keep all four perspectives in mind when working with any given family.

Family as Context

The first approach to family nursing care focuses on the assessment and care of an individual client in which the family is the context. This is the traditional nursing focus, in which the individual is foreground and the family is background. The family serves as context for the individual as either a resource or a stressor to their health and illness. Most existing nursing theories or models were originally conceptualized using the individual as a focus. Alternative labels for this approach are "family-centered" or "family-focused." This approach is rooted in the specialty of maternal-child nursing and underlies the philosophy of many maternity and pediatric health care settings. A nurse using this focus might say to an individual client: "Who in your family will help you with your nightly medication?" "How will you cover your child care issues when you have your back surgery?" "It is wonderful for you that your wife takes such an interest in your diabetes and has changed all the food preparation to match your dietary needs."

Family as Client

The second approach to family nursing care centers on the assessment of all individual family members; the family as client is the focus of care. In this approach, all the individuals in the family are in the foreground and individuals are not mutually exclusive of the whole. The family is seen as the sum of individual family members, and the focus is concentrated on

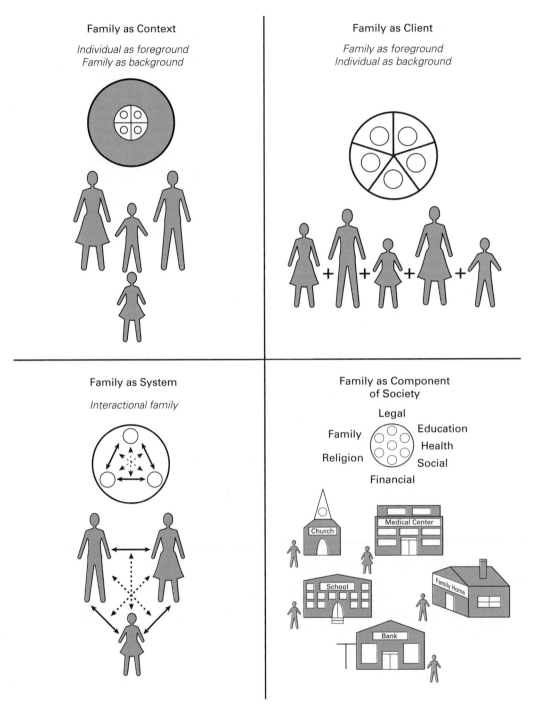

Figure 1–3 Approaches to family nursing.

each individual. Each person is assessed, and health care is provided for all family members. However, the family unit is not necessarily the primary consideration in providing care. General practitioner physicians and family care physicians provided the impetus for this approach to family care in community settings, but nurses and nurse practitioners are also involved with this approach. This approach is typically seen in primary care clinics in the community in which primary care physicians (PCP) or nurse practitioners provide care over time to all individuals in a given family. From this perspective, a nurse might ask a

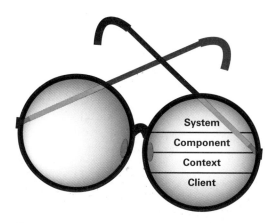

Figure 1–4 Four views of family through a lens.

family member who has just become ill: "How has your diagnosis of juvenile diabetes affected the other individuals in your family?" "Will your nightly need for medication be a problem for your family?" "Who in your family is having the most difficult time with your diagnosis?" "How is the family adjusting to your new medication regimen?"

Family as a System

The third approach to care focuses on the family as a system. The focus is on the family as client, and the family is viewed as an interactional system in which the whole is more than the sum of its parts. In other words, the interactions between family members become the target for nursing interventions that result from the nursing assessment. The family nursing system approach focuses on the individual and family simultaneously. The emphasis is on the interactions between family members—for example, the direct interactions between the parental dyad or the indirect interaction between the parental dyad and the child. The more children there are in a family, the more complex these interactions become.

This interactional model had its start with the specialty of psychiatric and mental health nursing. The system approach always implies that when something happens to one part of the system, the other parts of the system are affected. So, if one family member becomes ill, it affects all other members of the family. Questions that nurses ask in a system approach may be "What has changed between you and your spouse since your child was diagnosed with juvenile diabetes?" or "How has the diagnosis of juvenile diabetes affected the ways in which your family is functioning and getting along with each other?"

Family as a Component of Society

The fourth approach to care views the family as a component of society, in which the family is viewed as one of many institutions in society, similar to the health, educational, religious, or economic institutions. The family is a basic or primary unit of society and is a part of the larger system of society (Figure 1–5). The family as a whole interacts with other institutions to receive, exchange, or give communication and services. Family social science first used this approach in its study of families in society. The approach uses a structural, functional, and exchange theory point of view. Community health nursing has drawn many of its tenets from this perspective as it focuses on the interface between families and community agencies. Questions nurses may ask in this approach include "What issues has the family been experiencing since you made the school aware of your son's diagnosis of HIV?" and "Have you considered joining a support group for families with mothers who have breast cancer? Other families have found this to be an excellent resource and stress reduction strategy."

VARIABLES INFLUENCING FAMILY HEALTH CARE NURSING

The evolution of family health care nursing has been influenced by many variables that are derived from both historical and present events within society and the profession of nursing. Examples include changing

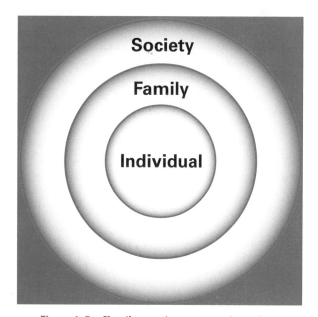

Figure 1–5 Family as primary group in society.

nursing theory, practice, education, and research; new knowledge derived from family social sciences and the health sciences; national and state health care policies; changing health care behavior and attitudes; and national and international political events. Detailed discussions of some of these areas are contained elsewhere in this text (see Chapters 6 and 7 in this book).

> 66 *The evolution of family health care nursing has been influenced by many variables that are derived from both historical and present events within society and the profession of nursing.* 99

Figure 1–6 shows how many variables influence contemporary family health nursing, making the point that the status of family nursing is dependent on what is occurring in the wider society—family as community. A recent example of this point is that health practices and policy changes are under way because of the recognition that current costs of health care are escalating and, at the same time, greater numbers of people are underinsured or uninsured and have lost access to health care. The goal of this health care reform is to make access and treatment available for all at an affordable cost. That will require a major shift in priorities, funding, and services. A major movement toward health promotion and family care in the community will greatly affect the evolution of family nursing.

FAMILY NURSING ROLES

The roles of family health care nurses are evolving along with the specialty. Figure 1–7 shows the many roles that nurses can assume with families as the focus. This figure was constructed from some of the first family nursing literature that appeared and is a composite of what various scholars believe to be some of the roles of nurses today (Bomar, 2004; Friedman et al., 2003; Hanson, 2001b). Each health care setting affects roles that nurses assume with families, and many of these roles may occur in the same setting as well.

1. Health teacher. The family nurse teaches about family wellness, illness, relations, and parenting, to name a few. The teacher-educator function is ongoing in all settings in both formal and informal ways. Examples include teaching new parents how to care for their infant and giving instruction about

diabetes to a newly diagnosed adolescent boy and his family members.

2. Coordinator, collaborator, and liaison. The family nurse coordinates the care that families receive, collaborating with the family to plan care. For example, if a family member has been in a traumatic accident, the nurse would be a key person in helping families to access resources—from inpatient care, outpatient care, home health care, and social services to rehabilitation. The nurse may serve as the liaison among these services.

3. Deliverer and supervisor of care and technical expert. The family nurse either delivers or supervises the care that families receive in various settings. To do this, the nurse must be a technical expert in terms of both knowledge and skill. For example, the nurse may be the person going into the family home on a daily basis to consult with the family and help take care of a child on a respirator.

4. Family advocate. The family nurse advocates for families with whom they work; the nurse empowers family members to speak with their own voice or the nurse speaks out for the family. An example is the nurse who is advocating for family safety by supporting legislation that requires wearing seat belts in motor vehicles.

5. Consultant. The family nurse serves as a consultant to families whenever asked or whenever necessary. In some instances, he or she consults with agencies to facilitate family-centered care. For example, a clinical nurse specialist in a hospital may be asked to assist the family in finding the appropriate long-term care setting for their sick grandmother. The nurse comes into the family system by request for a short period of time and for a specific purpose.

6. Counselor. The family nurse plays a therapeutic role in helping individuals and families solve problems or change behavior. An example from the mental health arena is a family that requires help with coping with a long-term chronic condition, such as when a family member has been diagnosed with schizophrenia.

7. Case finder and epidemiologist. The family nurse gets involved in case finding and becomes a tracker of disease. For example, consider the situation in which a family

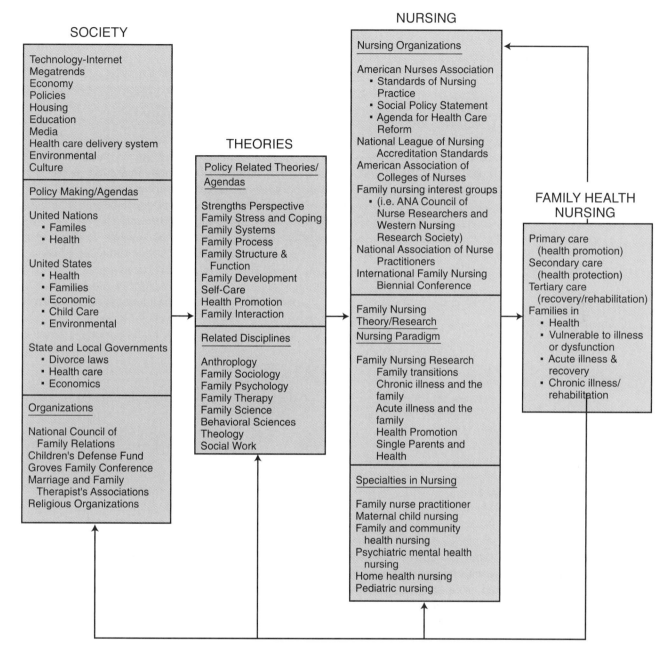

Figure 1–6 Variables influencing contemporary family health nursing. (From Bomar, P. J. [2004]. *Promoting health in families: Applying family research and theory to nursing practice* [3rd ed., p. 17]. Philadelphia: Saunders/Elsevier. With permission.)

member has been recently diagnosed with a sexually transmitted disease. The nurse would engage in sleuthing out the sources of the transmission and in helping to get other sexual contacts in for treatment. Screening of families and subsequent referral of the family members may be a part of this role.

8. Environmental modifier. The family nurse

consults with families and other health care professionals to modify the environment. For example, if a man with paraplegia is about to be discharged from the hospital to home, the nurse assists the family in modifying the home environment so that the patient can move around in a wheelchair and engage in self-care.

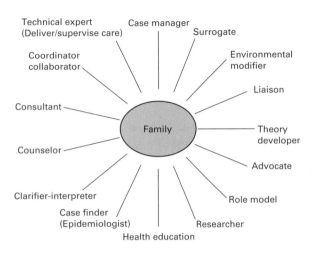

Figure 1–7 Family nursing roles.

9. Clarifier and interpreter. The family nurse clarifies and interprets data to families in all settings. For example, if a child in the family has a complex disease, such as leukemia, the nurse clarifies and interprets information pertaining to diagnosis, treatment, and prognosis of the condition to parents and extended family members.

10. Surrogate. The family nurse serves as a surrogate by substituting for another person. For example, the nurse may stand in temporarily as a loving parent to an adolescent who is giving birth to a child by herself in the labor and delivery room.

11. Researcher. The family nurse should identify practice problems and find the best solution for dealing with these problems through the process of scientific investigation. An example might be collaborating with a colleague to find a better intervention for helping families cope with incontinent elders living in the home.

12. Role model. The family nurse is continually serving as a role model to other people through his or her activities. A school nurse who demonstrates the right kind of health in personal self-care serves as a role model to parents and children alike.

13. Case manager. Although case manager is a contemporary name for this role, it involves coordination and collaboration between a family and the health care system. The case

manager has been formally empowered to be in charge of a case. For example, a family nurse working with seniors in the community may become assigned to be the case manager for a patient with Alzheimer's disease.

OBSTACLES TO FAMILY NURSING PRACTICE

Why has family nursing been practiced only in recent history? A number of reasons exist. First, there is a vast amount of literature on the family, but there was little on the family in nursing curricula until the past decade or two. The majority of practicing nurses have not had exposure to family concepts during their undergraduate education and continue to practice using the individualist medical paradigm.

Moreover, there has been a lack of valid and reliable comprehensive family assessment models, instruments, and strategies in nursing. More scholars are developing ideas and material in this arena; the chapter on family assessment and intervention presents three of the better-known models.

Furthermore, some students and nurses may believe that the study of family and family nursing is "common sense" and therefore does not belong formally in nursing curricula, either in theory or in practice. Nursing also has strong historical ties with the medical model, which has traditionally focused on the individual as client, not the family. At best, families have been viewed in context, and many times, families were considered a nuisance in health care settings—an obstacle to overcome in order to provide care to the individual.

Another obstacle is the fact that the traditional charting system in health care has been oriented to the individual. For example, charting by exception focuses on the physical care of the individual and does not address the whole family or members of families. Likewise, the medical and nursing diagnostic systems used in health care are disease-centered, and diseases are focused on individuals. The *International Classification of Diseases* (ICD) (AMA, 2003), the *Diagnostic and Statistical Manual of Mental Disorders* (DSM-IV) (APA, 2000), the North American Nursing Diagnosis Association (NANDA, 1999), and *The Omaha System: Applications for Community Health Nursing* (Martin & Scheet, 1992) have limited diagnostic codes that pertain to the family as a whole.

To complicate matters further, most insurance companies require that there be one identified patient, with a diagnostic code drawn from an individual disease perspective. Thus, even if health care providers are intervening with entire families, companies require providers to choose one person in the family group as the identified patient and to give that person a physical or mental diagnosis, even though the client is the whole family. There is a need for better family diagnostic codes that are accepted by vendors as legitimate reasons for reimbursement.

The established hours during which health care systems provide services pose another obstacle to focusing on families. Traditionally, office hours take place during the day, when family members cannot accompany other family members. Recently, some urgent care centers and other outpatient settings have incorporated evening and weekend hours into their schedules, making it possible for family members to come in together. However, many clinics and physician offices still operate on traditional Monday through Friday, 9:00 A.M. to 5:00 P.M. schedules. These obstacles to family-focused nursing practice are slowly changing; nurses can continue to lobby for changes that are more conducive to caring for the family as a whole.

SELECTED THEORETICAL PERSPECTIVES

Theorists from other family social sciences have been involved in developing some important ideas about family health care that are pertinent for family nursing. Four of these ideas are presented hereafter: the family health and illness cycle, levels of family care,

when to assemble the family in health care, and the therapeutic triangle in health care (Doherty, 2002; Doherty, 1985; Doherty & McCubbin, 1985; Doherty & Campbell, 1988; Hanson, 2001a).

The Family Health and Illness Cycle

The family health and illness cycle (Figure 1–8) represents an outline of a series of temporal phases in the family's efforts to reduce the risks of illness, to manage the initial onset of illness, and to adapt to death or illness. There is no unilateral direction in the model, but rather each phase in the cycle represents a different aspect of health and illness. Moreover, each phase of the cycle represents an arena around which a body of theory, research, and clinical observations has been built. The function of the model is to show how different topics pertaining to family and health research, theory building, and practice are interrelated.

One area of the cycle in which family nurses work is in *family health promotion and risk reduction*. This area emphasizes the environmental, social, psychological, and interpersonal factors surrounding the family that help promote health and reduce health risk. These factors include family beliefs and activities that help family members maintain good health by avoiding behaviors that increase their likelihood of becoming ill, such as poor diet, lack of exercise, or smoking. Nurses can do a lot to promote family health and to reduce risk.

Another part of the cycle that involves nurses is *family vulnerability and illness onset*. This part includes

Family Health and Illness Cycle

Phase 1. Family health promotion and risk reduction

Phase 2. Family vulnerability and disease onset/relapse

Phase 3. Family illness appraisal

Phase 4. Family acute response

Phase 5. Adaption to illness and recovery

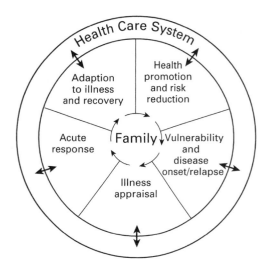

Figure 1–8 Family health and illness cycle. (Adapted from Doherty, W. J., & McCubbin, H. I. [1985]. Families and health care: An emerging arena of theory, research, and clinical intervention, *Family Relations, 34,* 5–11.)

life events and experiences that render family members susceptible to new illness or relapses of chronic illness. For example, nurses work with family stress responses related to relapses or exacerbations of chronic disorders (e.g., diabetes, multiple sclerosis, or schizophrenia). The development of support groups would be one nursing strategy for dealing with family members who have chronic illness.

The third part of the cycle pertinent to family nurses is the *family illness appraisal*, which refers to the family's beliefs about illness and family decisions about health care. An example of a strategy that nurses may use to help families cope with a situation before the situation becomes more acute is identifying teens who are at high risk for depression and suicide and encouraging the family to place their adolescent into a therapy group for depressed adolescents.

The *family acute response* refers to the immediate aftermath of illness and is an important area of intervention. The acute response occurs after an extraordinary event, such as a heart attack or a diagnosis of cancer. Families go through disorganization for a while, and family nurses can intervene by helping them cope with the crisis.

The *family adaptation to illness* portion of the cycle refers to the long-term effects of illness on the family and the role of families in facilitating recovery of individual members. Families must adapt to the demands of the chronic condition; thus, a whole body of information has evolved around family coping and family compliance with medical regimens. How do families promote the recovery of ill members while preserving their energy to nurture other family members and perform other family functions? An example of an appropriate intervention would be to help families find respite care for family caregivers so that caregivers do not "burn out."

Finally, the *family and health care system* part of the cycle refers to the family's decision to seek outside help for the illness or handle it within the family. This family help-seeking behavior can take place at any phase of the family health and illness cycle, and the resources sought can include everything from Western medical protocols to nontraditional New Age health care providers.

Levels of Family Care

The second concept derived from family social scientists and useful for family nursing is levels of family care as described by Doherty (1985). He proposed a continuum of health provider involvement when caring for families.

Level 1: Minimal emphasis on the family involves contacting families only when necessary for practical or legal reasons. Nurses require little knowledge or skill to handle this level of care. An example might be a hospital intensive care nurse contacting the family to get a code or no code signed.

Level 2: Ongoing medical information and advice is given by generalist family nurses to families through regular contact. The nurse may be answering questions or advising families on care management. An example might be a clinic nurse working with a family on diabetic foot care of an elderly patient.

Level 3: Providing support and addressing feelings takes place in families based on knowledge about normal family development and the ways in which families react to stress. The family nurse encourages family members to discuss their reactions and supports them in their coping efforts. Care is more individualized to that particular family. For example, a community health nurse may make a home visit to a newly discharged paraplegic patient who is going home for the first time.

Level 4: A systematic way of assessing families and planning interventions involves a good understanding of family systems and awareness of the nurse's own family systems and the larger systems in which families and health care providers operate. More knowledge and skill are required for this level of activity, and it usually involves graduate training in a specialty that incorporates family into the paradigm of care. An example would be a clinical nurse specialist who is coordinating care for a trauma patient with multiple injuries in a tertiary setting and translating the events to the family members.

Level 5: This level of care requires a high level of knowledge and skill with family systems and patterns of dysfunctional interaction. The nurse prepared to work at this level is a specialist in psychiatric mental health nursing, family therapy, or both. The generalist nurse either refers a family to or consults with a psychiatric mental health liaison nurse who is a clinical nurse specialist or nurse practitioner in this area. For example, a specialist nurse is consulted concerning a difficult and complex family structure in which some members of the family want resuscitation of a dying family member and other members do not. This situation would require organizing a family conference, assessing the function of the family, and mediating a decision.

When to Assemble the Family in Health Care

The third concept that is derived from family social science and is useful for family nursing is Doherty's (1985) guidelines to assist health providers in knowing when to involve whole families while providing care. Figure 1–9 shows a two-sided continuum. The upper half of the continuum pictures the individual patient being seen alone and ranges through organization of whole-family conferences. The bottom half of the continuum speaks to the kind of health care problem being addressed and ranges from minor acute problems (minor suturing) to a serious acute illness (heart attack). The benefit of this idea is that it assists nurses in making decisions about the level or degree of family involvement for any given situation and reassures nurses that "family nursing" can take place even when the whole family is not assembled.

The Therapeutic Triangle in Health Care

The fourth concept of importance to nurses in providing family care is the notion of the therapeutic triangle (Figure 1–10). It is a concept derived from family systems theory, but it applies to all approaches in health care.

In the provision of health care, there are three main actors in the therapeutic triangle: the identified patient, the health care professional, and the family of the identified patient. Relationships exist primarily between the dyads in the triangle with the third party in the triangle in the background. Triangulated relationships are those in which a third party becomes involved to stabilize tensions that exist in the dyadic relationship. The third party distracts from the anxiety level that is based in the dyad. As the given dyad changes, so does the third party; for example, a patient and family dyad may involve the health care professional as the third party in the triangle, or a health care professional and identified patient dyad may include the family as the third party. It is not uncommon for the patient and family to be upset at the physician because of the perceived "withholding of information," thus forming a triangle. Many times, nurses become involved as a third party, with the nursing intervening with patient teaching. Chapter 2 (Theoretical Foundations for the Nursing of Families) and Chapter 13 (Family Mental Health Nursing) both discuss the concept of triangulation in more detail.

Situations occur in which there is difficulty in a nurse-patient relationship and the patient engages his or her family to communicate with the nurse instead of directly confronting the nurse. Or perhaps the health care provider provides a listening ear to a disgruntled patient complaining about his or her family's caregiving ability. Often, health care providers find themselves positioned between family members.

HISTORY OF FAMILY NURSING

Family health nursing has roots in society from prehistoric times. The historical role of women has been inextricably interwoven with the family, for it was the responsibility of women to care for family members who fell ill and to seek herbs or remedies for the illness. In addition, through "proper" housekeeping, women made efforts to provide clean and safe environments for the maintenance of health and wellness for their families (Bomar, 2004; Ham & Chamings, 1983; Whall, 1993).

During the Nightingale era, the historical development of families and nursing became more explicit. Florence Nightingale influenced both the establishment of district nursing of the sick and poor and the work of "health missionaries" through "health-

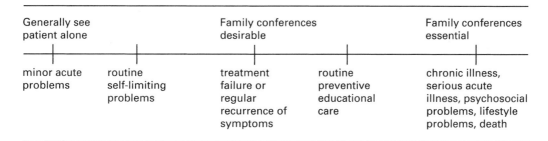

Figure 1–9 When to assemble the family in health care. (Adapted from Doherty, W. [1985]. Family intervention in health care. *Family Relations, 34,* 129–137.)

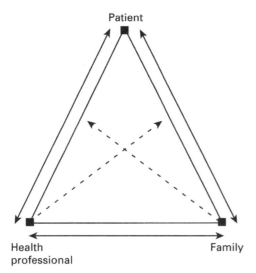

Figure 1–10 The therapeutic triangle in health care. (Adapted from Broderick, C. B. [1983]. *The therapeutic triangle.* Beverly Hills: Sage Publications.)

at-home" teaching. She believed that cleanliness in the home could eradicate high infant mortality and morbidity. She encouraged family members of the fighting troops to come into the hospitals during the Crimean War to take care of their loved ones. Nightingale supported helping women and children toward good health by promoting both nurse midwifery and home-based health services. In 1876, in a document titled *Training Nurses for the Sick Poor*, Nightingale encouraged nurses to serve in nursing both sick and healthy families in the home environment. She appears to have given both home-health nurses and maternal-child nurses the mandate to carry out nursing practice with the whole family as the unit of service (Nightingale, 1979).

In colonial America, women continued the centuries-old traditions of women who nurtured and sustained the wellness of their families and cared for the ill. During the Revolutionary War, women called "camp followers" provided nursing care. These untrained nurses performed many functions for the troops.

During the Civil War (1861 to 1865), nursing of the wounded solders became more organized. Women formed Ladies Aid Societies, groups who met regularly to sew, prepare food and medicines, and gather other items needed by the soldiers. Dorothea Dix was named the Superintendent of Women Nurses of the U.S. Army. Hundreds of women received a month's training to prepare them for military nursing work.

During the industrial revolution of the late 18th century, family members began to work outside the home. Immigrants, in particular, were in need of income, so they went to work for the early hospitals. This was the real beginning of public health and school nursing. The nurses involved in the beginning of the labor movement were concerned with the health of workers, immigrants, and their families. Concepts of maternal child and family care were incorporated into basic curriculums of nursing schools.

Maternity nursing, nurse midwifery, and community nursing historically focused on the quality of family health. Margaret Sanger fought for family planning. Mary Breckenridge formed the famous Frontier Nursing Service (midwifery) to provide training for nurses to meet health needs of mountain families.

There was a concerted expansion of public health nursing during the Depression to work with families. However, before and during World War II, nursing became more focused on the individual, and care became centered in institutional and hospital settings, where it remained until recently.

Since the 1950s, at least 19 disciplines had studied the family and, through research, produced family assessment techniques, conceptual frameworks, theories, and other family material. Recently, this interdisciplinary work has become known as "family social science." Family social science has greatly influenced family nursing in the United States, largely because of the organization called the National Council of Family Relations and their large number of family publications. Many family nurses have become active in this organization. In addition, many nurses are now receiving advanced degrees in family social science departments around the country.

Nursing theorists started in the 1960s to systematize nursing practice. Scholars began to articulate the philosophy and goals of nursing care. Initially theorists were concerned only with individuals, but gradually individuals became viewed as part of a larger social system. See Chapter 3 for nursing theories that contribute to family nursing.

In the 1960s, the nurse practitioner movement began espousing the family as a primary unit of care in their practice. In the 1970s, only one theorist included families as part of the assessment in her system for nursing practice. Other theorists developed models that did not speak specifically to families, but families could be the identified client in some of these theories (Orem, 1995; Roy & Andrews, 1999; Neuman, 1995).

During the 1980s, the refocusing on families as a unit of care was evident in America. Small numbers of people from throughout the country gathered together at their personal expense to discuss and share family nursing concepts (e.g., Wingspread in Racine, Wisconsin). Family nurses started defining the scope of practice, family concepts, and how to teach this information to the next generation of nurses. Family nursing is both old and new—long traditions and new definitions. Family nursing is now beyond youth, more like a young person, but it is still in a state of becoming. Table 1–2 provides a composite of historical factors contributing to the development of family health as a focus in nursing.

> ❝Family nursing is both old and new, but it is still in a state of becoming.❞

HISTORY OF FAMILIES

A brief macroanalytical history of families is important for understanding family nursing. The past helps make the present realities of family life more understandable, because the influence of the past is evident in the present. This historical approach provides a means of conceptualizing family over time and within all of society. Finally, history helps dispel preferences for family forms that are only personally familiar and broaden nurses' view of the world of families.

Prehistoric Family Life

Archaeologists and anthropologists have found evidence of prehistoric family life, that is, family life that existed before the time of written historical sources. These family forms varied from present-day forms, but the functions of the family have remained somewhat constant over time. Families were then and are now a part of the larger community and constitute the basic unit of society.

Family structure, process, and function were a response to everyday needs. As communities grew, families and communities became more institutionalized and homogeneous as civilization progressed. Family culture was that aspect of life derived from membership in a particular group and shared by others. Family culture was composed of values and attitudes that allowed early families to behave in a predictable fashion.

The earliest human matings tended toward permanence and monogamy. Man and woman dyads are the oldest and most tenacious unit in history, which is

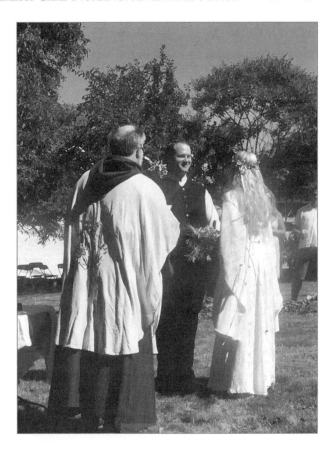

perhaps why the "nuclear" family dominates modern experience. Biologically, human children need care and protection longer than other animals' offspring. This necessity led humans to marriage and permanent relationships; it did not dictate family structure, but it was essential for the activity of parenting.

Economic pairing was not always the same as reproductive pairing, but it was a by-product of reproductive pairing. A variety of skills was needed for living, and no single person possessed all skills, so male and female role differentiation began to be more clearly defined. Early in history, children were part of the economic unit. In most societies, reproductive pairing merged also with the nurturing pair and the economic unit, as well as into respective gender role differentiation, and ultimately into socialization (education). As small groups of conjugal families formed communities, the complexity of the social order increased. This, in turn, changed the definition of the family.

European History

Many Americans are of European ancestry and come out of the family structure that was present there.

Table 1–2 HISTORICAL FACTORS CONTRIBUTING TO THE DEVELOPMENT OF FAMILY HEALTH AS A FOCUS IN NURSING

TIME PERIOD	EVENTS
Pre-Nightingale era	Revolutionary War "camp followers" were an example of family health focus before Florence Nightingale's influence.
Mid-1800s	Nightingale influences district nurses and health missionaries to maintain clean environment for patient's homes and families. Family members provide for soldiers' needs during Civil War through Ladies Aid Societies and Women's Central Association for Relief.
Late 1880s	Industrial Revolution and immigration influence focus of public health nursing on prevention of illness, health education, and care of the sick for both families and communities. Lillian Wald establishes Henry Street Visiting Nurse Service (1893). Focus on family during childbearing by maternal-child nurses and midwives.
Early 1900s	School nursing established in New York City (1903). First White House Conference on Children occurs (1909). Red Cross Town and Country Nursing Service was founded (1912). Margaret Sanger opens first birth control clinic (1916). Family planning and quality care become available for families. Mary Breckinridge forms Frontier Nursing Service (1925). Nurses are assigned to families. Red Cross Public Health Nursing Service meets rural health needs after stock market crash (1929). Federal Emergency Relief Act passed (1933). Social Security Act passed (1935). Psychiatry and mental health disciplines begin family therapy focus (late 1930s).
1960s	Concept of family as a unit of care is introduced into basic nursing curriculum. National League for Nursing (NLN) requires emphasis on families and communities in nursing curriculum. Family-centered approach in maternal-child nursing and midwifery programs is begun. Nurse-practitioner movement—programs to provide primary care to children are begun (1965). Shift from public health nursing to community health nursing occurs. Family studies and research produce family theories.
1970s	Changing health care system focuses on maintaining health and returning emphasis to family health. Development and refinement of nursing conceptual models that consider the family as a unit of analysis or care occur (e.g., King, Newman, Orem, Rogers, and Roy). Many specialties focus on the family (e.g., hospice, oncology, geriatrics, school health, psychiatry, mental health, occupational health, and home health). Master's and doctoral programs focus on the family (e.g., family health nursing, community health nursing, psychiatry, mental health, and family counseling and therapy).

(continued on page 23)

TIME PERIOD	EVENTS
	ANA Standards of Nursing Practice are implemented (1973).
	Surgeon General's Report (1979).
1980s	ANA Social Policy Statement (1980).
	White House Conference on Families.
	Greater emphasis is put on health from very young to very old.
	Increasing emphasis is placed on obesity, stress, chemical dependency, and parenting skills.
	Graduate level specialization is begun with emphasis on primary care outside of acute care settings, health teaching, and client self-care.
	Use of wellness and nursing models in providing care increases.
	Promoting Health/Preventing Disease: Objectives for the Nation (1980) is released by U.S. Department of Health and Human Services.
	Family science develops as a discipline.
	Family nursing research increases.
	National Center for Nursing Research is founded, with a Health Promotion and Prevention Research section.
	First International Family Nursing Conference occurs (1988).
1990s	*Healthy People 2000: National Health Promotion and Disease Prevention Objectives* (1990) is released by U.S. Department of Health and Human Services.
	Nursing's Agenda for Health Care Reform is developed (ANA, 1991).
	Family leave legislation is passed (1991).
	Journal of Family Nursing is born (1995).

Source: Bomar, P. J.(Ed.). (2004). *Promoting health in families: Applying family research and theory to nursing practice* (pp.12–13). Philadelphia: Saunders/Elsevier.

Social organizations called families emphasized consanguineous (genetic) bonds. The tendency toward authority was concentrated in a few individuals at the top of the hierarchical structure (kings, lords, fathers). The heads of families were males.

Property of family transferred through the male line. Females left home to join their husbands' families. A mother did not establish a strong bond with her daughter because the daughter eventually left her home of origin to join her husband's family of origin.

Women and children were property to be transferred. Marriage was a contract between families, not individuals. Extended patriarchal family characteristics prevailed until the advent of industrialism.

Industrialization

There was great stability within family systems until the Industrial Revolution. The revolution first appeared in England around 1750 and spread to Western Europe and North America. Some believe that the nuclear family idea started with the Industrial Revolution. Extended families had always been the norm until families left farms and moved into the cities, where men left home to work in the factories. This left women at home maintaining the home and caring for the children. Extended families were left behind. There is some evidence that English families were nuclear from the 1600s, because family size has stayed constant at 4.75 people per family ever since.

Out of the religious Reformation came a strong movement for individuation, in which the Protestant ethic promoted the idea that the family unit was no longer paramount, but rather the individual within the family. This paradigm shift had a lot to do with the message of personal salvation of the Reformation and Protestantism.

When factories of the Industrial Revolution started to be built, people began moving about. The state had begun to provide services that families previously had performed for their members. Informal contractual arrangements between public and state power and nuclear families took place, in which the state gave fathers the power and authority over their families in exchange for males giving the state their loyalty and service. This may be one of the ways in which families became controlled by patriarchy.

Women were not expected to love husbands but to obey them. Some feminists believe that the introduction of love into human consciousness was done as a purposeful and powerful force to limit female activity and that it is hard to separate love and submission. This notion is very controversial.

Society today is still living with bequests of patriarchal family life. Women are still struggling to get out from under the rules and expectations of the state and of men. The women's movement and the National Organization for Women (NOW) are two of the forces that have improved the level of equality of women in modern society. A lot more work needs to be done on the issues of equality for all Americans, including gender differences.

In recent years, men have also begun identifying the bondage they experience. They cannot meet all of the needs of families and feel inadequate for failing to do so. This is especially true of men who cannot access the resources of money, occupation, and occupational status through education. There is a men's movement afoot that is promoting male causes, although this movement is not as dynamic as it may be in the future. One of the organizations supporting this work is the National Congress for Men.

American Families

American society and families were molded from the beginning by economic logic rather than consanguineous logic. America does not have the history of Europe's preindustrial age. English patriarchy was not transplanted in its pure form to America.

Women as well as men had to labor in the New World. This gave women new power. In addition, the United States had an ethic of achieved status rather than inherited status through familial lines. Female suffrage was easier to obtain on the frontier, as is evidenced by Wyoming being one of the first states to give women the vote.

Children were also experiencing a changing status in American families. Originally, they were part of the economic unit and worked on farms. Then, with the great immigration of the early 1900s, the expectation shifted to parents creating a better world for their children than they themselves had. To do this, children had to become more educated to deal with the developing society. Each generation of children obtained more education and income than their

parents had; they left the family farms and moved to distant cities. As a result of this change, parents lost assurance that their children would take care of them during their old age. This phenomenon is occurring in developing countries today. For example, the city of Seoul, Korea, has grown from 2 to 14 million people in one decade, largely due to young people coming into the cities for work and education.

In addition, the functions of families were changing greatly in earlier American society. The traditional roles that families played were being displaced by the growing numbers and kinds of social institutions. Families have been increasingly surrendering to public agencies many of the socialization functions they previously had performed.

Historically, adolescents worked on the family farms. With the burgeoning of cities in the industrialized world, adolescents lost their productive function on the farm. Teenagers could not be kept from jobs in the cities. The public school system was largely created to help keep adolescents off streets. The concept of the generation gap occurred when the family economic and social functions no longer merged.

Families Today

Today, families cannot be separated from the larger system of which they are a part, nor can they be separated from their historical past. Some people argue that families are in terrible shape, like a rudderless ship in the dark. Other people hail the changes that continue to occur in families and approve the diversity and options that address modern needs. Idealizing past family arrangements and decrying change has become commonplace in the media. Just as some families of both the past and present engaged in behaviors that are destructive to individuals and other social institutions, there are families of the past and present that provide healthy environments. Certainly, the sphere of activity for families is diminishing the strength of the family and lessening their ability to both influence and react to the direction of social change.

If nurses believe that the family as an institution is essential to individuals and society, they can become anxious that the family's traditional tasks are co-opted by other institutions. Many of these institutions (churches, schools, social agencies) actually exert further strain on families even as they attempt to strengthen families. For example, employers (military or business) move families around for the sake of opti-

mizing production. This results in frequent relocations and loss of social support and security, creating a
circumstance in which people in families can turn only
to each other instead of feeling a part of the larger
family or community. These circumstances promote
the intensity of familial interaction that results in
unrealistic expectations of each other. Isolation is one
of the contributing factors to the high incidence of
abuse among military families.

The structure, function, and processes of families
have changed, but the family unit will continue to
survive. It is, in fact, the most tenacious unit in society
and the last stronghold over which families have some
control. More discussion about the future of families
occurs in Chapter 19, The Futures of Families,
Health, and Family Nursing.

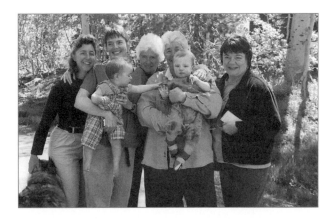

❝The structure, function, and processes of families have changed, but the family unit will continue to survive.❞

Functions of Traditional Families

Throughout history, families have performed a
number of traditional functions (Hanson, 2001b). Six
functions are summarized hereafter; they are not
necessarily listed in order of importance.

Families existed *to achieve economic survival.* Fathers
were breadwinners, going out into the world to "bring
home the bacon," either by self-employment or by
working for others. Mothers were helpmates, homemakers, and nurturers of children. Families had many
children for economic reasons—more children meant
more wealth, an opportunity to work more land, or
care for their parents into old age. Children of earlier
centuries did not experience what we now know as
the teen years. Instead, they worked in the family business as mini-adults and stayed home until they
married. The family was an economic unit to which
all members contributed and from which everyone
benefited.

Families existed *to reproduce the species.* In earlier
times, parents traditionally married before having sex
and children. If women became pregnant outside of
marriage, they were stigmatized and sent away to
homes for unwed mothers. Not many people elected
to stay childless; instead most had children or adopted
children.

Providing protection from hostile forces was an
important family function. Family members protected
other members who could not protect themselves, such
as the very young, the very old, and disabled individ-

uals. Indeed, family groups immigrated together to
avoid facing hostile cultures alone and formed ethnic
blankets (ghettos) in which an "us against them" world
prevailed.

Passing along the religious faith (culture) represented
another important function for families. Families were
the primary medium for passing on religious stories,
doctrines, traditions, and values. Only candidates for
ordination or rich children received formalized religious training. Significant family events were ritualized,
such as births, baptisms, marriages, and deaths. Faith
was an integral part of daily family life.

Families also existed *to educate and socialize their
young.* Boys worked with their fathers to learn trades
or take over family farms. Girls worked with their
mothers, learning homemaking and parenting. Children were largely homeschooled by their parents;
they learned to read from religious books—the Bible
and *Pilgrim's Progress.* The Bible and the gun were
important family tools in young America. The Bible
buttressed faith and staved off ignorance, and the gun
was used to kill game animals and protect the family.

Families served another function—*conferring status.*
A person *was* the family name. It was difficult to
change status in society. If a person's father was a
respected blacksmith, the son was expected to become
the same. If the father was the town drunk, however,
the son had little chance to become something else.
An untarnished family name was especially important
in a nonmobile society. Many people immigrated to
America to seek new opportunities (as well as riches)
that their family names could not provide in the Old
Country.

If families met all of these six functions, they were
considered healthy, or good. A "good family" was one
that was self-sufficient, did not ask for help from
others, supported its community institutions, was
untainted with failure, and met "good family" criteria

as determined by community and church. In other words, the family looked good from the outside. People paid little attention to what went on inside the family. Society was not concerned about good communication, emotional support, or trusting relationships. There was more concern about meeting visible family standards set by the community, such as married parents, religious affiliation, affluence, home ownership, and community respect.

Functions of Contemporary Families

In contemporary times, historical functions of families have changed. Some functions have changed more than others have, and new ones have been added to the list.

The *economic function* of families has changed dramatically. Family members do not need each other as they did in the past to stay financially afloat. Government aid, such as Medicare, Social Security, aid for dependent children, and welfare, helps subsidize families economically. Women do not need to stay married to a man for food, shelter, or respectability, nor do men marry to have someone cook and clean for them. The spinster aunt was replaced by the career woman.

More than 50 percent of women with young children are now working outside of the home, carrying their own weight in the workplace (Lamanna & Riedmann, 2003). Children are no longer viewed as economic assets but as costly luxuries. Children do not need parents to survive economically, as the United States has expansive foster care and welfare programs. Some social reformers are even promoting a guaranteed income for all people. Thus, families are no longer a necessity for economic security.

The *reproductive function* of families has diversified, allowing people many options to have children without marriage and family. For example, one-third of live births in the United States today occur to women who are not married (Lamanna & Riedmann, 2003). Women who were infertile in the past have benefited from in vitro technology and infertility drugs. Sexual activity is more common among all age groups with a whole complement of birth control measures available. Thus, the function of reproduction does not necessarily take place within the boundaries of the traditional family any longer, and family is no longer necessary for reproduction to take place.

Protective functions of families are no longer as important as they used to be. Social, welfare, and law enforcement agencies have largely taken on this activity for the safety and protection of society. Not all families are willing or able to provide these functions for their offspring. For example, if parents are suspected of child abuse, society removes their children from the home, serving as surrogate parents. Another example is the recent mandate for immunization for children, which occurred because not all families protect their children against these diseases.

The *religious (cultural) function* of families has also evolved over time. Instead of families assuming the chief responsibility for passing on the religious faith to the next generation, this responsibility has been taken on by the churches and synagogues. Children attend religious and Sunday schools in order to learn about their religion. As the citizenry has become more secular, fewer religious and cultural values have been passed to the younger generation. Thus, the family structure no longer serves this function in the same way it did in the past.

The *educational and socialization function* of families has been transferred in part to the public and private school system. In fact, educators complain that too much burden has been placed in the hands of teachers and that families are delinquent in their responsibility to and accountability for educating their children. Homeschooling has become slightly more popular with some young parents today, but the majority of mothers are working outside of the home, placing their children in day care centers and preschool. Moreover, any residual teaching that has traditionally taken place in the home is being eroded by television and computers.

The family is usually no longer needed to *confer status.* If you are a Rockefeller or Kennedy, your family name may be helpful, but for the majority of Americans, family heritage is not essential for success. Status today is gained primarily through education, occupation, income, and address. The United States as a country is valued for its "rags to riches" possibilities.

On the other hand, the *relationship function* of families has become important in contemporary families, although it was not considered critical for families in the past. People marry so that they can love and be loved, instead of for basic needs. Couples join in a search for intimacy, not protection. Parents have children to connect to posterity rather than to be taken care of in their old age.

Maslow (1970) wrote that the members of this generation of people are sufficiently beyond basic sustenance needs to be able to focus on the quality of their relationships. Families are self-defining, using criteria based on relationships rather than genes or law. If our deepest relationship needs are not met in our families, we search elsewhere. If we are lonely or unhappy in our relationships, we seek alternatives through divorce, infidelity, overwork, volunteerism, chemical dependency, teen alienation, depression, and suicide. The focus on relationships has become paramount in contemporary families.

The *health function* of families also has been highlighted in contemporary times. Researchers in family health have noted the importance of the interactive effects of the health of individual family members and the health of family. The family can keep its members well by passing along attitudes, beliefs, habits, health promotion, and care of the ill. The family is the genesis of physical and mental health for a lifetime.

Changing Demographics of American Families

Major changes are taking place in American families today that are exerting dramatic influences on family life and family health (Hanson, 2001b). The U.S. Bureau of the Census (Fields, 2001a, 2001b, 2001c; U.S. Census Bureau, 2001) and the National Center for Health Statistics (National Center for Health Statistics, 2003) reported that increases in divorce, remarriage, higher age at first marriage, labor force participation of women, and delays and declines in childbearing are among the more notable trends

today. These individual and collective developments, in the span of just one generation, have altered the structure, process, and function of American families. In comparison to 20 years ago, today's families are smaller and more likely to be maintained by a single parent, have multiple wage earners, require child care assistance, and contain stepchildren. Individual and family life trajectories involve many more transitions today as people form, dissolve, and re-form families.

Families in the past were more homogeneous than they are today. Table 1–3 lists the many current variations of family types. Whereas the past norm was a two-parent family (traditional nuclear family) living together with their biological children, many other family forms are acknowledged and recognized today. It is also important to note that the average person born today will experience many family forms during his or her lifetime. Figure 1–11 depicts the many familial forms that the average person lives through today. It is clear that life is not as simple as it used to be and that practicing nurses are experiencing this proliferation of variation not only in their own personal lives but also with the patients with whom they work in health care settings.

Lamanna and Riedmann (2003, p. 9) summarized what U.S. marriages and families look like today (see Box 1–4). These demographic generalizations are just that, generalizations. The caveat for the following thumbnail sketch is that statistics do not tell the whole story. Readers are referred to Chapter 2—Family and Health Demographics—for a more detailed analysis of

---

Table 1–3 VARIATIONS OF FAMILY AND HOUSEHOLD STRUCTURES

FAMILY TYPE	COMPOSITION
Nuclear dyad	Married couple, no children
Nuclear	Husband, wife, children (may or may not be legally married)
Binuclear	Two post-divorce families with children as members of both
Extended	Nuclear family plus blood relatives
Blended	Husband, wife, and children of previous relationships
Single parent	One parent and child(ren)
Commune	Group of men, women, and children
Cohabitation (domestic partners)	Unmarried man and woman sharing a household
Homosexual	Same-gender couple
Single person (adult)	One person in a household

Source: Kaakinen, J. R., & Hanson, S. M. H. (2004). Family development and family nursing assessment. In M. Stanhope & J. Lancaster (Eds.), *Community & public health nursing* (6th ed., p. 569), St. Louis: Mosby.

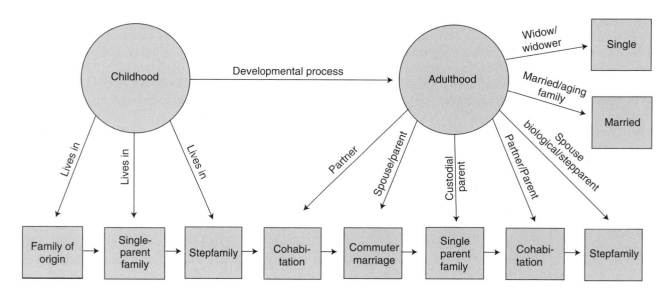

Figure 1–11 An individual's potential family life experiences. (Adapted from Kaakinen, J. R., Hanson, S. M. H., & Birenbaum, L. K. [2004]. Family development and family nursing assessment. In M. Stanhope & J. Lancaster [Eds.], *Community and public health nursing.* St. Louis, MO: Mosby.)

Box 1–4 SUMMARY OF FACTS ABOUT FAMILIES IN THE UNITED STATES

1. *People have been postponing marriage in recent years.* In 2000, the median age at first marriage was 25.1 for women and 26.8 for men, compared with 20.8 for women and 23.2 for men in 1970 and slightly lower than that in the 1950s. Still, over 90 percent of Americans eventually marry.
2. *Fewer people are currently married.* Only 52 percent of households contained a married couple in 2000, compared with 78 percent in 1950. Among adults 18 and over, 60 percent are currently married.
3. *Cohabitation has emerged as a lifestyle intermediate between marriage and singlehood.* From 1990 to 2000, married-couple households increased only 7 percent, while there was a 71 percent increase in the number of unmarried-couple households. Unmarried-couple families still represent only 5 percent of households at any one time, but over 50 percent of marriages were preceded by cohabitation.

    Two-fifths of cohabiting couples lived with children under 18 in 2000. These might be children of the couple or children from a previous marriage or relationship of one or both of the partners.
4. *The number of people living alone is substantial.* Single-person households now represent a quarter of American households. Delayed marriage is a contributing factor, as well as the comparatively good health and economic situation of older persons, enabling unmarried seniors to choose to live independently.

    Because of the increased number of people living alone and because of the smaller number of children per family, the average size of a U.S. household has dropped from 3.14 people in 1970 to 2.59 in 2000.
5. *There are more single-parent households than there were 10 years ago, including a big increase in the number of single fathers.* Single-father households grew 62 percent in the last decade. The increase in single-mother households from 1990 to 2000 was less dramatic but was still five times greater than the increase in households composed of married couples with children. Single-father families still make up only 2.1 percent of all households; single-mother families make up 7 percent.

    The census category "single-parent family household" obscures the fact that there may be other adults present in that household—grandparents or other relatives, for example. Moreover, some unmarried mothers and fathers live with their children in another person's household.

(continued on page 29)

6. *Some cohabitants maintain gay and lesbian domestic partnerships.* Not all cohabiting couples are heterosexual. In the 2000 census, almost 600,000 same-sex couple households were reported, slightly more than one-half of 1 percent of all households. This represents a substantial increase over 1990. The increase may be due to a major change in the census procedure for tallying same-sex households. Or it may represent a real increase in gay and lesbian households or a willingness of gay/lesbian partners to report their relationship to the Census Bureau. Keep in mind that Census Bureau figures concern household composition, not the sexual orientation of individuals or the existence of same-sex relationships in which the parties do not live together.

7. *Many adult children live with their parents.* Of young adults ages 18 to 24, 57 percent of men and 47 percent of women lived with parents in 2000. Men are more likely than women to reside with their parents, and this pattern occurs for somewhat older adults as well.

8. *Parenthood is increasingly postponed, and fertility has declined.* From a high point of 3.7 children per woman in 1957, the *total fertility rate* dropped to 1.7 in 1976. It then rose and has been around two children per woman for two decades.

   Childlessness has increased in recent decades. Of women aged 40 to 44 in 1998, 19 percent had not borne children. Rates of childlessness seem to be leveling off now, though, rather than increasing.

   A more common pattern is delayed childbearing. The 20s are still the most fertile ages for women, but a striking shift toward first and later births in older age groups has occurred. Along with this, we see more frequent multiple births, more common among older mothers and those who have employed fertility drugs.

9. *Most parents are working parents.* In 1999, only 7 percent of households were married-couple households with children *in which only the father was employed.* In fact, 91.3 percent of all parents with children under 6 were employed in that year.

   Furthermore, 60.7 percent of married mothers with children under 6 were employed in 1999, including a majority of those with children less than 1 year old. However, only 35 percent of married mothers of preschoolers worked full-time year-round. Female single-family heads who are mothers of children under 6 have high rates of employment also—68.1 percent and 77 percent, respectively, in 1999.

   And fathers? Some 94.3 percent of married fathers and 88.5 percent of male single-family heads were employed in 1999.

10. *More births are to unmarried mothers than in the past.* But nonmarital childbearing has not continued to grow in the late 1990s. One reason for the increase in single-parent households has been the striking rise in nonmarital births in recent decades. In 1999, 33.0 percent of total births were to unmarried women, whereas in 1940, only 3.8 percent of births were. Unmarried birth rates increased sixfold from 1940 to 1990, growing especially rapidly in the 1970s and 1980s. Estimates are that 54 percent of first births to women aged 15 to 29 were conceived out of wedlock in the early 1990s.

    However, the trend toward nonmarital births seems to have leveled off; in fact, the nonmarital birth rate declined from 1994 to 1999. Pregnancy and birth rates of teen women declined in the 1990s. Approximately 40 percent of unwed births occur to cohabiting couples. Such couples are often living together or involved enough to consider themselves families, at least at the point of birth.

11. *Divorce rates have stabilized, although they remain at high levels. Remarriage rates have decreased, but remain high.* Many people now "know" that approximately half of marriages end in divorce. What is less well known is that the divorce rate [has] been in decline for more than two decades. The divorce rate, which had risen slowly from the 19th century onward, doubled from 1965 to the end of the 1970s. Then it began to drop, falling almost 20 percent between 1981 and 1998.

    Three-quarters of divorced women remarry within 10 years—81 percent of younger women and 68 percent of those who are over 25 when they divorce. Remarriage rates of men are even higher. But remarriage rates have been declining for some time.

(continued on page 30)

Box 1–4 **SUMMARY OF FACTS ABOUT FAMILIES IN THE UNITED STATES** *(Continued)*

12. *A majority of children live in two-parent households.* Despite the visibility of divorce, nonmarital births, and single-parent households, the majority of children live with two parents. A 1996 Census Bureau study (which provides the most recent detailed data on children's living arrangements) found that 62 percent of children lived with two biological parents in an intact marital family. All in all, 71 percent of children under 18 lived with two parents (3 percent were unmarried), 25 percent lived in single-parent households, and the other 4 percent did not live with a parent. Of those not living with any parent, the majority were cared for by relatives, whereas others were in foster care.

13. *But there is considerable variation in children's living arrangements.* First of all, a snapshot taken at one time does not fully capture the variability of family settings experienced by a child, who may live in an intact two-parent family, a single-parent household, and a remarried family in sequence. An earlier study estimated that half of children would live in a single-parent household at some point in their lives.

    Moreover, two-parent families vary considerably in their composition. Just to consider all two-parent families regardless of race or ethnicity, the 1996 study found 88 percent of children living with their biological parents (some unmarried), 7 percent with biological mother and stepfather, 2 percent with biological father and stepmother, 1 percent with adoptive father and biological mother, and smaller numbers yet with an adoptive mother and biological father or an adoptive parent and a stepparent. Blended families are very likely to contain children who are not full biological siblings; they may be step-siblings or half-siblings born to the new couple.

14. *Children are more likely to live with a grandparent today than in the recent past.* In 1970, 3 percent of children lived with a grandparent, but by 1996 that rate had more than doubled, to 7.5 percent. In a quarter of the cases, grandparents had sole responsibility for raising the child; neither parent was in the household. But many households containing grandparents are *extended-family* households, which include other relatives besides parents and children. Many involve single mothers who live with their parents.

15. *Children are more likely than the general population or the elderly to be living in poverty.* We will discuss the economic circumstances of families more generally in the next chapter. But in focusing on children, it seems important to note this point. In 1998 the poverty rate of children stood at 18.9 percent, whereas that of the general population was 12.7 percent and that of the elderly was 10.5 percent. The poverty rate of children has increased 23 percent since 1970.

Source: Lamanna, M. A., & Riedmann, A. C. (2003). Issues for thought: Some facts about families in the United States today. In M. A. Lamanna & A. C. Riedmann (Eds.), *Marriages and families: Making choices in a diverse society* (8th ed., pp. 9–11). Belmont, CA: Thomson/Wadsworth.

family and health demographics and their implications for family nursing.

IMPLICATIONS FOR FAMILY NURSING

This next section will discuss the state of the art and science of family nursing practice, research, and education. Where is the specialty of family nursing at this time in history and what are the implications for the future? See Chapter 6 (Families, Nursing, and Social Policy) for the implications of social policy for family nursing. Chapter 19 (The Future of Families, Health, and Family Nursing) discusses the future of all of these areas: family nursing practice, research, education, and social policy.

Family Nursing Practice

Family nursing practice is still developing and evolving. Earlier in the chapter, we discussed the four approaches to practicing family nursing: family as context, family as client, family as system, and family as a component of society.

Friedemann (1995) also espouses the position that there are multiple ways to practice family nursing. She wrote that family nursing can be practiced at three levels: (1) the individual level, with the family seen as the context of the individual; (2) the interpersonal level, with the family consisting of dyads, triads, and larger units; and (3) the systems level, in which the family is a system with its own structural and functional components and interacts with environmental systems and its own subsystems. A family nurse who practices a higher level (systems level) also includes the levels below (individual and interpersonal levels).

According to Friedemann (1995), the goal for practice on the *individual level* is physical health and personal well-being of family members; interpersonal change and system change are by-products. Family nursing at the *interpersonal level* has as its main goal mutual understanding and support of the family members. It anticipates personal change and understands and includes in the nursing plan interaction between personal and interpersonal factors. Advanced practitioners anticipate system change to avoid harmful situations. This coincides with two of the approaches to family nursing discussed earlier: family as context and family as client. Examples might be a pediatric nurse caring for a hospitalized child (the family is there but the focus is on the child) and a family nurse practitioner seeing all the individuals in a family unit and treating them separately but being mindful that they are part of a whole family unit. The goal for nurses who practice at the *systems level* is change in the family system as a whole and increased harmony between system and subsystems, as well as between system and environment. Changes at all systems levels are carefully predicted, monitored, and corrected, if the need arises. Practicing at the systems level includes the other two approaches: family as a system and family as a unit in society. Examples might include a psychiatric mental health nurse counseling a family where there is marital conflict and the focus is on the interaction between two or more people, and a community health nurse helping the family as a unit coordinate with other agencies in the community.

Friedemann (1995) believes that family nursing can and should be practiced at three levels by all nurses. Nurse generalists (bachelor's degree) are equipped to care for relatively well-functioning families at the individual level and the interpersonal level. Family systems nursing and advanced interpersonal nursing of families with dysfunctions are reserved for advanced nursing specialties (master's degree) that have knowledge and skills in family theory and practice.

Nursing practice at the systems level is focused on family health and strengths, is holistic in character, and requires knowledge of complex interactions of a multitude of family factors at all systems levels. The reciprocal relationship between health problems and family functioning is well-known to clinicians and theoreticians and is well-documented. Health problems influence family perceptions and behaviors; like-wise, family perceptions and behaviors influence health outcomes.

Wright and Leahey (2000) name the systems level "family systems nursing," which they defined as focusing on the whole family as a unit of care. There is simultaneous concentration on both the individual and the family; it is inclusive rather than exclusive. The focus is always on the interaction and reciprocity of the family. Family systems nursing is the integration of nursing, systems, cybernetics, and family therapy theories. Wright and Leahey hypothesize that the future trend in family nursing will be toward increased diversity in clinical practice with families and that more nurses will be involved with families in health care, no matter what type of practice settings nurses choose. Families will be invited in more often for interviews, and more intervention will take place at a systems level. Finally, more one-way mirrors will be used in health care settings to enhance interdisciplinary collaboration and practice.

After four regional continuing education workshops on family nursing, 201 nurses responded to a survey in which they were asked to relate "successes" in family-centered nursing interventions (Kirschling et al., 1994). Using a qualitative approach, the surveys identified five themes as successful outcomes, with commensurate examples of changes in family behavior as a result of family nursing intervention:

1. Families were able to seek help or identify a problem as demonstrated by calling the nurse when experiencing stressors in family members' lives.
2. Families and family members behaved differently as a result of family nursing interventions, such as encouraging an asthmatic family member to stop smoking to provide a smoke-free environment for their child.
3. Family members experienced a change of feelings as a result of such family nursing interventions, such as feeling satisfied with their ability to solve their own problems.
4. Family members increased their knowledge of health terminology, family process, and the beliefs and understanding of other family members as a result of family nursing interventions. For example, nurses may educate all members of a family to work as a team in caring for a high-risk infant at home.
5. Family and individual development continued in spite of illness as a result of family nursing interventions that assisted families to allow

children to lead normal (versus protected) lives, even when they had a chronic illness such as diabetes.

In summary, nurses who considered themselves to be practicing family nursing described family nursing interventions that involved families and family members—including assessment and intervention as well as support, education, and exploration of feelings—as common occurrences.

Family Nursing Research

Although families have been growing in importance in family nursing practice, they have been neglected in nursing research. Most nursing research has focused on the individual; the culture of individualism supersedes commitment to social groups such as the family. Recently nursing has awakened to the connection between family dynamics and health and illness (see Box 1–5). Nonetheless, research pertaining to family and mental health is further advanced than research on family and physical health (Hanson, 2001b).

“Most nursing research has focused on the individual; the culture of individualism supersedes commitment to social groups such as the family.**”**

Studies on the family's effect on physical health of family members predominantly stem from a social and epidemiologic view. For example, researchers have examined family interactions in studies of diabetes and hypertension. Poor diabetic control and hypertension have been associated with unresolved marital conflicts. Marital status has been shown to influence the overall mortality and morbidity of cardiovascular disease. Studies have shown that patients respond more to their family's response to their illness than to the illness itself. In other words, what families believe or perceive about a condition becomes more salient than what is really going on with the individual (Gilliss & Davis, 1993).

The following are three major agenda items for future family nursing research (Wright & Leahey, 2000):

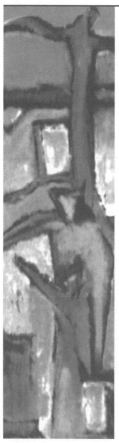

RESEARCH BRIEF

Changes in Western family history have occurred in all aspects of family life and relationships. Of central importance is the shift of many aspects of social organizations from the family to numerous organizations and relationships that are not kinship-based. Increasingly, activities, authority, and relationships have been relocated from the family to schools, factories, and other bureaucratic nonfamilial organizations. Marriage has become less central in organizing and controlling life course transitions, individual identities, intimate relations, living arrangements, and childbearing and child rearing.

Purpose of Study

This study investigated trends of family attitudes and values from the 1960s through the 1990s. Attitudes and values concerning the roles of women and men, marriage, divorce, childlessness, premarital sex, extramarital sex, nonmarital cohabitation, and out-of-wedlock childbearing were examined.

Methods

The Survey Research Center of the University of Michigan has conducted the "Monitoring the Future Study" every year since 1976. Five data sets were used in this particular study: Monitoring the Future, General Social Survey, International Social Science Project, Intergenerational Panel Study of Parents and Children, and the National Survey of Families and Households. As a group, these studies provide a wide and diverse set of indicators of change in attitudes and values concerning American family life. This research was supported by the National Institute of Child Health and Human Development and the Alfred P. Sloan Foundation's Center for the Ethnography of Everyday Life at the University of Michigan.

(continued on page 33)

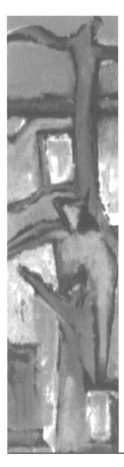

Results

There have been substantial and persistent long-term trends toward the endorsement of general equality in families, which may have plateaued at very high levels in recent years. There have also been high levels of trends toward individual autonomy and tolerance toward a diversity of personal and family behaviors, as reflected in increased acceptance of divorce, premarital sex, unmarried cohabitation, remaining single, and choosing to be childless. At the same time, marriage and family life remain important in the cultural ethos, with a lot of young people embracing marriage and family life as important.

Nursing Implications

Findings underscore the need for family health care nurses to understand the following:

1. Family social science research contributes to the knowledge that family nurses need to embrace in their evolving practice.
2. Families as a unit continue to evolve and solidify in new directions, and at the same time, American culture continues to value marriage and family life.
3. People must choose among the principles of equality, freedom, and family commitment when these highly valued goods become mutually exclusive rather than mutually reinforcing options.
4. Families take advantage of the freedom to pursue their own individual goals and aspirations while at the same time maintaining family commitments and responsibilities.
5. Different priorities and balancing become issues for public debate and policy. Given the different ways in which various people integrate and choose among the principles of family commitment, freedom, and equality, these central issues will continue to be important dimensions of public debate in the years to come.

Source: Thornton, A., & Young-DeMarcho, L. (2001, November). Four decades of trends in attitudes toward family issue in the United States: The 1960s through the 1990s. *Journal of Marriage and Family,*

---

1. Family assessment techniques must be further developed.
2. Research on the reciprocal relationship between family functioning and the course and treatment of illness needs to gain prominence.
3. The efficacy of family treatment will become paramount as the type of health services for specific situations are determined.

Chapter 3 (Theoretical Foundations for the Nursing of Families) and Chapter 4 (Research in Families and Family Nursing) provide additional information on family nursing theory and research. Moreover, most chapters in this textbook contain an example of family nursing research pertinent to the topic of the chapter.

Family Nursing Education

Family nursing education has come of age in the United States and Canada. A research study from the late 1980s examined the status of family nursing

education in all schools of nursing in the United States (Hanson & Heims, 1992). A Canadian study was modeled after the American study (Wright & Bell, 1989). The following list represents findings and recommendations from these studies for family nursing education:

- In general, more family content is being included in undergraduate and graduate nursing curricula, but it could be made more explicit. These clinical courses should be both family-specific and integrated into other coursework.
- Educators are taking an eclectic approach to family assessment, rather than using specific models. Nurses need to learn several models and assessment strategies to be more systematic and thorough in family assessment.
- Clinical practicums in a variety of settings are still focused on individuals rather than on families as a whole. Family systems experiences that focus on relationships and interactions must be developed by faculty.

- The methods of supervision for students are primarily through case discussion and process recordings. The use of audiotapes and videotapes for reviewing case material is becoming more common in nursing. There is a need for more direct and live supervision through the use of one-way mirrors.
- There appears to be a deficit of advanced knowledge and skill level in faculty members responsible for advanced family nursing practice courses. More faculty members need to seek graduate work in family nursing, as well as the family social sciences, family therapy, sociology, and psychology, to fill this gap.
- Schools are better at teaching family assessment than family intervention strategies, which explains the fact that family nursing intervention strategies are still in the early stages of development. More emphasis and resources should be focused on nursing intervention strategies with families.
- Faculty members who teach family nursing originate from varied backgrounds, including maternal-child, community, and psychiatric and mental health nursing. There are a growing number of trained and identified professionals with expertise in teaching family nursing. These faculty members need to be teaching the family content, regardless of the territorial traditions of the specialties.
- Schools of nursing across the different regions of the country do not vary significantly in terms of the amount of family-oriented content in their curricula, nor were there differences in what was being taught in family nursing between schools that had undergraduate programs only and those that also had graduate programs.

Educational Preparation to Practice Family Nursing

Education for family nursing begins during undergraduate nursing education and may continue through postdoctoral training. The question is whether family curriculum should comprise specific courses in the curriculum or whether it should be integrated in all the other coursework that students take. Another question is whether family nursing education should be geared toward undergraduate education (generalist) or toward graduate education (specialist). The American Nurses Association (ANA, 2003b) stated that nurse generalists practice with a comprehensive approach to health care and can meet the diversified health concerns of individuals, families, and communities, whereas nurse specialists are expert in providing care focused on specific clusters of phenomena representing a refinement of interests. In the area of general versus specialist, Gilliss and Davis (1993) wrote that a nurse who views the family in context could be a generalist in family nursing and a specialist in another field of practice. For example, a maternity nurse specializes in a discrete body of knowledge related to prenatal to postnatal nursing care but may work generally with other family members. Conversely, those nurses who practice family nursing are specialists in family care and generalists in other areas of practice. For example, a family community health nurse knows a lot about family care but may not be a specialist in a particular clinical area such as medical-surgical nursing.

Gilliss and Davis (1993, p. 36) and others have proposed a schema to conceptualize the levels of preparation for family nursing education (see Figure 1–12). At the baccalaureate level, students should receive preparation for working with the family as context and the family as a component of society. This is consistent with the generalist orientation of undergraduate nursing education. This approach is more commonly addressed in undergraduate nursing courses that deal with children's, women's, or community health issues. However, family content to prepare nurses to work with families in all areas of practice should be included in other coursework as well.

Master's level preparation is required for specialty practice in family nursing, such as working with the family as a client or the family as a system. This preparation consists of courses pertaining to family theory, nursing intervention with families, advanced practice,

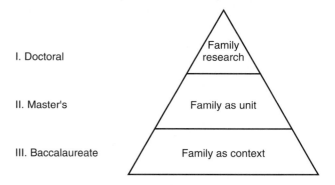

Figure 1–12 Levels of preparation for family nursing. (Adapted from Gilliss, C. L. [Ed.]. [1993]. *Readings in family nursing* [p. 36]. Philadelphia: JB Lippincott.)

and clinical supervision. At some schools of nursing, master's students (nurse practitioners and clinical nurse specialists) are required to take this kind of coursework. As in much of nursing education, master's preparation has a clinical specialty focus.

Finally, there is doctoral and postdoctoral education in nursing. The focus of doctoral study for those studying families (within or outside of nursing) is on family theory development and research. The National Institute of Nursing Research (NINR) is now funding institutional and individual National Research Service Awards (NRSA) to support graduate and postdoctoral students in family nursing research.

SUMMARY

This chapter provided an introduction to and broad overview of family health care nursing and why this information is important in today's family. The chapter explored definitions of "family," "family health," "family health care nursing," and "healthy families." It discussed theoretical concepts important to the nursing of families, as well as the history of families in the United States and the development of family nursing. Finally, implications for nursing theory, practice, research, and education were explicated. This chapter demonstrates that family health care nursing is ever changing and evolving due to the world and society that is around us all, and that family health care nursing is at the very center and heart of the nursing of families today.

References

American Medical Association. (2003). *International classification of diseases: Clinical modifications* (ICD-9-CM) (6th ed., 9th rev.). Chicago: American Medical Association.

American Nurses Association. (2003a). *Nursing's social policy statement* (2nd ed.). Washington, DC: American Nurses Association.

American Nurses Association. (2003b). *Nursing: Scope and standards of practice*. Washington, DC: American Nurses Association.

American Psychiatric Association. (2000). *Diagnostic and statistical manual of mental disorders* (DSM-IV-TRtm) (4th ed.). Washington, DC: American Psychiatric Association.

Anderson, K. H., & Tomlinson, P. S. (1992). The family health system as an emerging paradigmatic view for nursing. *Image: Journal of Nursing Scholarship, 24,* 57–63.

Beavers, W. R., & Hampson, R. B. (1993). Measuring family competence: The Beavers Systems Model. In F. Walsh (Ed.), *Normal family processes* (2nd ed.). New York: Guilford Press.

Becvar, D. S., & Becvar, R. J. (2000). *Family therapy: A systemic integration* (4th ed.). Boston: Allyn & Bacon.

Benner, P. (2001). *Novice to expert: Excellence and power in clinical nursing practice*. Menlo Park, CA: Prentice Hall.

Bomar, P. J. (Ed.). (2004). *Promoting health in families: Applying family research and theory to nursing practice* (3rd ed.). Philadelphia: Saunders/Elsevier.

Broderick, C. B. (1993). *Understanding family process: Basics of family systems theory*. Thousand Oaks, CA: Sage Publications.

Burgess, E. W., & Locke, H. J. (1953). *The family: From institution to companionship*. New York: American Book Company.

Curran, D. (1983). *Traits of a healthy family*. Minneapolis: Winston Press (Harper & Row).

Curran, D. (1985). *Stress and the healthy family*. Minneapolis: Winston Press (Harper & Row).

Doherty, W. J. (1985). Family intervention in health care. *Family Relations, 34,* 129–137.

Doherty, W. J. (2002). A family-focused approach to health care. In K. Bogenschneider (Ed.), *Family policy matters: How policy-making affects families and what professionals can do*. Mahway, NJ: Lawrence Erlbaum.

Doherty, W. J., & Campbell, T. L. (1988). *Families and health*. Newbury Park, CA: Sage.

Doherty, W. J., & McCubbin, H. I. (1985). Families and health care: An emerging arena of theory, research and clinical intervention. *Family Relations, 34,* 5–11.

Fields, J. (2001a, June). America's families and living arrangements: 2000. *Current population report* (pp. 20–537). Washington, DC: U.S. Census Bureau.

Fields, J. (2001b, April). Living arrangements of children: 1996. *Current population report* (pp. 70–74). Washington, DC: U.S. Census Bureau.

Fields, J. (2001c, April). 'The nuclear family' rebounds, Census Bureau reports [News release]. Washington, DC: U.S. Department of Commerce.

Ford, D. Y. (1994). An exploration of perceptions of alternative family structures among university students. *Family Relations, 43,* 68–73.

Friedemann, M. L. (1995). *The framework of systemic organization: A conceptual approach to families and nursing*. Thousand Oaks, CA: Sage.

Friedman, M. H., Bowden, V. R., & Jones, E. G. (2003). *Family nursing: Research, theory and practice* (5th ed.). Norwalk, CT: Appleton & Lange.

Gilliss, C. L., & Davis, L. L. (1993). Does family intervention make a difference? An integrative review and meta-analysis. In *The nursing of families: Theory, research, education, practice* (pp. 259–265). Newbury Park: Sage.

Gilliss, C. L., Roberts, B. M., Highley, B. L., & Martinson, I. M. (1989). What is family nursing? In C. L. Gilliss, B. L. Highley, B. M. Roberts, & I. M. Martinson (Eds.), *Toward a science of family nursing* (pp. 64–73). Menlo Park, CA: Addison-Wesley.

Gladding, S. T. (1998). *Family therapy: History, theory, and practice* (2nd ed.). Upper Saddle River, NJ: Merrill/Prentice Hall.

Greenstein, T. N. (2001). *Methods of family research*. Thousand Oaks: Sage Publications.

Ham, L. M., & Chamings, P. A. (1983). Family nursing: Historical perspectives. In I. Clements & F. B. Roberts (Eds.), *Family health care: A theoretical approach to nursing care* (Vol. 1, pp. 88–109). San Francisco: McGraw-Hill.

Hanson, S. M. H. (2001a). *Family health care nursing: Theory, practice, and research*. Philadelphia: FA Davis.

Hanson, S. M. H. (2001b). Family health care nursing: An introduction. In S. M. H. Hanson (Ed.), *Family health care nursing: Theory, practice, and research* (pp. 2–35). Philadelphia: FA Davis.

Hanson, S. M. H. (2001c). Family nursing assessment and intervention. In S. M. H. Hanson (Ed.), *Family health care nursing: Theory, practice, and research* (pp. 170–195). Philadelphia: FA Davis.

Hanson, S. M. H., & Heims, M. L. (1992). Family nursing curricula in U.S. schools of nursing. *Journal of Nursing Education, 31*(7), 305–308.

Kaakinen, J. R., & Hanson, S. M. H. (2004a). Family development and family nursing assessment. In M. Stanhope and J. Lancaster (Eds.), *Community & public health nursing* (6th ed., pp. 562–593). St. Louis: Mosby.

Kaakinen, J. R., & Hanson, S. M. H. (2004b). Theoretical foundations for family health nursing. In P. Bomar (Ed.), *Promoting health in families: Applying family research and theory to nursing practice* (pp. 93–116). Philadelphia: Saunders/Elsevier.

Kirschling, J. M., Gilliss, C. L., Krentz, L., Camburn, C. D., Clough, R. S., Duncan, M., et al. (1994). "Success" in family nursing: Experts describe phenomena. *Nursing and Health Care, 15*, 186–189.

Lamanna, M. A., & Riedmann, A. C. (2003). Issues for thought: Some facts about families in the United States today. In M. A. Lamanna & A. C. Riedmann (Eds.), *Marriages and families: Making choices in a diverse society* (8th ed., pp. 9–11). Belmont, CA: Thomson/Wadsworth.

Martin, K. S., & Scheet, N. J. (1992). *The Omaha System: Applications for community health nursing.* Philadelphia: WB Saunders.

Maslow, A. (1970). *Motivation and personality.* New York: Harper & Row.

McEwan, P. J. M. (1974). The social approach to family health studies. *Social Science and Medicine, 8*, 487–493.

NANDA. (1999). *Nursing diagnosis: Definitions and classification 1999–2000.* Philadelphia: North American Nursing Diagnosis Association.

National Center for Health Statistics. (2003). *Health, United States, 2000: Chartbook on trends in the health of Americans* (DHHS Publication No. 2003–1232). Washington, DC: U.S. Government Printing Office.

Neuman, B. (1995). *The Neuman systems model* (3rd ed.). Norwalk, CT: Appleton & Lange.

Nightingale, F. (1979). *Cassandra.* Westbury, NY: The Feminist Press.

Orem, D. (1995). *Nursing: Concepts of practice,* St. Louis: C.V. Mosby.

Otto, H. (1963). Criteria for assessing family strengths. *Family Process, 2*, 329–338.

Pender, N. (2001). *Health promotion in nursing practice* (4th ed.). Norwalk, CT: Appleton & Lange.

Pratt, L. (1976). *Family structure and effective health behavior: The energized family.* Boston: Houghton Mifflin.

Roy, C., & Andrews, H. A. (1999). *The Roy adaptation model* (2nd ed.). Englewood Cliffs, NJ: Prentice Hall.

Seccombe, K., & Warner, R. L. (2004). *Marriages and families: Relationships in social context.* Belmont, CA: Wadsworth/Thomson Learning.

Stinnett, N., Chesser, B., & DeFrain, J. (Eds.) (1979). *Building family strengths: Blueprints for action.* Lincoln, NE: University of Nebraska Press.

Stinnett, N., & DeFrain, J. (1985). *Secrets of strong families.* Boston: Little, Brown & Company.

Thornton, A., & Young-DeMarcho, L. (2001). Four decades of attitudes toward family issues in the United States: The 1960's through the 1990's. *Journal of Marriage and Family, 63*, 1009–1037.

U.S. Census Bureau. (2001, May). *Profiles of general demographic characteristics: 2000.* Retrieved from http://www.census.gov/prod/cen2000

Whall, A. L. (1993). The family as the unit of care in nursing: A historical review. In G. D. Wegner & R. J. Alexander (Eds.), *Readings in family nursing* (pp. 3–12). Philadelphia: JB Lippincott.

Wright, L. M., & Bell, J. M. (1989). A survey of family nursing education in Canadian universities. *Canadian Journal of Nursing Research, 21*(3), 59–74.

Wright, L. M., & Leahey, M. (1994). *Nurses and families: A guide to family assessment and intervention* (2nd ed.). Philadelphia: FA Davis.

Wright, L. M., & Leahey, M. (2000). *Nurses and families: A guide to family assessment and intervention.* Philadelphia: FA Davis.

Bibliography

Altergott, K. (Ed.). (1993). *One world, many families.* Minneapolis, MN: National Council on Family Relations.

Anderson, D. B., Ward, H., & Hatton, D. C. (2004). Family health risks. In M. Stanhope & J. Lancaster (Eds.), *Community & public health nursing* (6th ed., pp. 594–615). St. Louis: Mosby.

Bell, J. M., Watson, W. L., & Wright, L. M. (Eds.). (1990). *The cutting edge of family nursing.* Calgary, Alberta: University of Calgary.

Berkey, K. M., & Hanson, S. M. H. (1991). *Pocket guide to family assessment and intervention.* St. Louis: Mosby Year Book.

Bianchi, S. M. (1995). The changing demographic and socioeconomic characteristics of single-parent families. *Marriage and Family Review, 22*(1–4).

Boss, P. G., Doherty, W. J., LaRossa, R., Schrumm, W. R., & Steinmetz, S. K. (Eds.). (1993). *Source book of family theories and methods: A contextual approach.* New York: Plenum.

Broome, M. E., Knafl, I. K., Pridham, K., & Feetham, S. (Eds.). (1998). *Children and families in health and illness.* Thousand Oaks: Sage Publications.

Campbell, T. (1987). *Family's impact on health: A critical review and annotated bibliography* (DHHS Publication No. ADM861461). Washington, DC: U.S. Government Printing Office.

Candib, L. M. (1995). *Medicine and the family: A feminist perspective.* New York: Basic Books.

Craft-Rosenberg, M., & Denehy, J. (Eds.). (2001). *Nursing interventions for infants, children, and families.* Thousand Oaks, CA: Sage Publications.

Danielson, C. B., Hamel-Bissell, B., & Winstead-Fry, P. (Eds.). (1993). *Families, health and illness: Perspectives on coping and intervention.* St. Louis: Mosby.

Denham, S. (2003). *Family health: A framework for nursing.* Philadelphia: FA Davis.

Feetham, S. L. (1990). Conceptual and methodological issues in research of families. In J. M. Bell, W. L. Watson, & L. M. Wright (Eds.), *The cutting edge of family nursing.* Calgary, Alberta: University of Calgary.

Feetham, S. L., Meister, S. B., Bell, J. M., & Gilliss, C. L. (Eds.). (1993). *The nursing of families: Theory, research, education, practice.* Newbury Park, CA: Sage.

Feetham, S. L., & Meister, S. B. (1999). Nursing research of families: State of the science and correspondence with policy. In A. H. Hinshaw, S. L. Feetham, & J. L. F. Shaver (Eds.), *Handbook of clinical nursing research* (chap. 14). Thousand Oaks, CA: Sage Publications.

Gilliss, C. L. (1999). Family nursing research, theory and practice. In G. D. Wegner & R. J. Alexander (Eds.), *Readings in family nursing* (pp. 34–43). Philadelphia: JB Lippincott.

Gilliss, C. L., & Knafl, K. A. (1999). Nursing care of families in non-normative transitions: The state of science and practice. In A. H. Hinshaw, S. L. Feetham, & J. L. F. Shaver (Eds.), *Handbook of clinical nursing research* (chap. 13). Thousand Oaks, CA: Sage Publications.

Gordon, M. (1994). *Nursing diagnosis: Process and application* (2nd ed.). New York: McGraw Hill.

Hanson, S. M. H., Heims, M. L., Julian, D. J., & Sussman, M. B. (Eds.). (1995). *Single-parent families: Diversity, myths, and realities.* New York: Haworth.

Hanson, S. M. H., & Mischke, K. (1996). Family health assessment and intervention. In P. J. Bomar (Ed.), *Nurses and family health promotion: Concepts, assessment and interventions* (2nd ed., pp. 165–202). Philadelphia: WB Saunders.

Hinshaw, A. S., Feetham, S. L., & Shaver, J. L. F. (1999). *Handbook of clinical nursing research.* Thousand Oaks, CA: Sage Publications.

Levinson, D. (Ed.). (1996). *Encyclopedia of marriage and the family* (Vols. 1 & 2). New York: Macmillan.

Loveland-Cherry, C. J. (2004). Family health promotion and health protection. In P. J. Bomar (Ed.), *Nurses and family health promotion: Concepts, assessment and interventions* (pp. 61–92). Baltimore: Williams & Wilkins.

McCubbin, M. (1999). Normative family transitions and health outcomes. In A. H. Hinshaw, S. L. Feetham, & J. L. F. Shaver (Eds.), *Handbook of clinical nursing research* (chap. 12). Thousand Oaks, CA: Sage Publications.

McCubbin, M. A., & McCubbin, H. I. (1993). Families coping with illness: The resiliency model of family stress, adjustment, and adaptation. In C. B. Danielson, B. Hamel-Bissell, & P. Winstead-Fry (Eds.), *Families, health and illness: Perspectives on coping and intervention* (pp. 21–65). St. Louis: Mosby.

Moriarty, H. J. (1990). Key issues in the family research process: Strategies for nurse researchers. *Advances in Nursing Science, 12*(3), 1–14.

Olson, D. H., & Hanson, M. K. (Eds.). (1990). *2001: Preparing families for the future.* Minneapolis: National Council on Family Relations.

Price, S., & Elliott, B. (Eds.). (1993). *Vision 2010: Families and health care.* Minneapolis, MN: National Council on Family Relations.

Sawa, R. J. (Ed.). (1992). *Family health care.* Newbury Park, CA: Sage.

Stanhope, M., & Lancaster, J. (2004). *Community & public health nursing* (6th ed.). St. Louis: Mosby.

Vaughan-Cole, B., Johnson, M. A., Malone, J. A., & Walker, B. L. (Eds.). (1998). *Family nursing practice.* Philadelphia: WB Saunders.

Wegner, G. B., & Alexander, R. J. (Eds.). (1999). *Readings in family nursing* (2nd ed.). Philadelphia: JB Lippincott.

Wright, L. M., Watson, W. L., & Bell, J. M. (1997). *Beliefs: The heart of healing in families and illness.* New York: Basic Books.

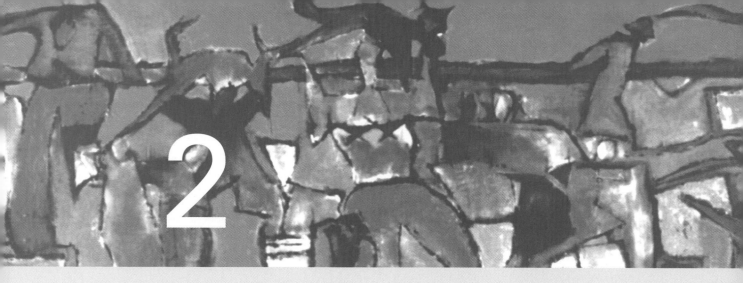

2

Family and Health Demographics

Lynne M. Casper, PhD • John G. Haaga, PhD

CRITICAL CONCEPTS

- Economic and cultural changes have increased family diversity. More families are maintained by single mothers, single fathers, cohabiting couples, and grandparents than in the past.

- Increases in women's labor force participation, especially among mothers, have reduced the amount of nonwork time that families have to attend to health care needs.

- Single-mother families are particularly vulnerable. They are more likely to be in poverty than are other families. These mothers are usually the sole wage earners and care providers in their families. Thus, these families are more likely than other families to be both monetarily poor and time-poor.

- Americans are more likely to live alone than they were a few decades ago. Thus, people are less likely to have family members living with them who can assist them when they become ill or injured.

- The aging of the population presents significant challenges for family nursing. Increasing proportions of the population will be older, increasing the need for nurses who specialize in caring for the elderly.

- More Americans are immigrants than was the case a couple of decades ago. More family nurses can expect to provide care for an ethnically, culturally, and linguistically diverse population.

INTRODUCTION

If there is one "mantra" about family life in the last half-century, it is that the family has undergone tremendous change. No other institution elicits as contentious debate as the American family. Many argue that the movement away from marriage and traditional gender roles has seriously degraded family life. Others view family life as amazingly diverse, resilient, and adaptive to new circumstances (Popenoe, 1993; Stacey, 1993).

Any assessment of the general "health" of family life in the United States and the health and well-being of family members, especially children, requires a look at what we know about demographic and socioeconomic trends that affect families. And a pragmatic approach to family nursing requires an understanding of the broader changes in family and health within the population to be treated. The latter half of the 20th century was characterized by tumultuous change in the economy, in civil rights, and in sexual freedom and by dramatic improvements in health and longevity. Marriage and family life felt the reverberations of these societal changes.

In the early 21st century, as we reassess where we have come from and where we are, one thing stands out. Our rhetoric about the dramatically changing family may be a step behind the reality. Recent trends suggest a quieting of changes in the family, or at least of the pace of change. There was little change in the proportion of two-parent or single-mother families during the 1990s. The living arrangements of children stabilized, as did the living arrangements of young adults and the elderly. The divorce rate had been in decline for more than two decades. The rapid growth in cohabitation among unmarried adults has also slowed (Casper & Bianchi, 2002).

Yet family life is still evolving. Age at first marriage rose as more young adults postponed marriage and children to complete college and settle into a labor market increasingly inhospitable to poorly educated workers. Accompanying this delay in marriage was the continued increase in births to unmarried women, though here, too, the pace of change slowed in the 1990s (Ventura et al., 1995).

Within marriage or marriage-like relationships, the appropriate roles for each partner are shifting as American society accepts and values more equal roles for men and women. The widening role of fathers has become a major agent of change in the family. There are an increasing number of father-only families, a shift toward shared custody of children by fathers and mothers after divorce, and increased father involvement with children in two-parent families.

Whether the slowing, and in some cases cessation, of change in family living arrangements is a temporary lull or part of a new, more sustained equilibrium will only be revealed in the first decades of the 21st century. New norms may be emerging about the desirability of marriage, the optimal timing of children, and the involvement of fathers in child rearing and mothers in breadwinning. Understanding the ever-evolving American family and the implications these changes have for family nursing requires taking the pulse of contemporary family life from time to time. This chapter describes the American family and changes in the health and health behaviors of adults, children, and adolescents so that we can understand what these changes portend for family health care nursing during the first half of this century. Many different family and health demographic statistics derived from various data sources are described in this chapter (see Box 2–1). To ensure that students understand the implications of these demographic patterns for practicing family nursing, the practice, research, education, and policy implications for nurses are discussed within each section of the chapter. This departs from the format of other chapters in this book that have a separate section on implications for nursing.

A CHANGING ECONOMY AND SOCIETY

Consider the life of a young woman reaching adulthood in the 1950s or early 1960s. Such a woman was likely to marry straight out of high school or to take a clerical or retail sales job until she married. She would have moved out of her parents' home only after she married, to form a new household with her husband. This young woman was likely to marry by age 20 and begin a family soon after. If she were working when she became pregnant, she would probably have quit her job and stayed home to care for her children and husband while her husband had a steady job that paid enough to support the entire family. Thus, there was usually someone at home with the time to care for the health needs of family members, to schedule routine checkups with doctors and dentists, and to take family members to these appointments.

Fast-forward to the beginning of the 21st century. A young woman reaching adulthood in the early 21st century is not likely to marry before her 25th birthday. She will probably attend college and is likely to live by herself, with a boyfriend, or with roommates before

Box 2–1 SOURCES OF INFORMATION ON DEMOGRAPHY AND PUBLIC HEALTH

Many of the statistics discussed in this chapter draw on information from the **Current Population Surveys** (CPS) collected by the U.S. Census Bureau. This is a continuous survey of about 60,000 households, selected at random to be representative of the national population. Each household is interviewed monthly, for two 4 month periods while it is included in the sample. The main purpose of the survey is to produce monthly estimates of the unemployment rate for the Bureau of Labor Statistics and official annual estimates of income and poverty for the Census Bureau. During February through April of each year, the CPS collects additional demographic and economic data, including data on health insurance coverage, from each household. This Annual Demographic Supplement (often called the "March CPS Supplement," as it used to be collected only for one month) is the most frequently used source of data on demographic and economic trends in the United States and is the data source for the majority of statistics presented in this chapter regarding changes in the family.

The CPS data can be used to estimate rates and trends for the whole nation or for very large groups (such as the population of California, or all households outside metropolitan areas, or all African-American families). It cannot be used for estimates for small areas or for small groups, because the sample size is insufficient for stable estimates. For more detailed comparisons, demographers often use data from the "long form" of the **Decennial Census,** which collects data from one-sixth of all households. The census collects a range of economic and demographic information, including incomes and occupations, housing, disability status, and grandparent responsibility for children. The census data can be used for estimates for fairly small areas, such as neighborhoods, or for small populations, but it cannot match the detail found in more specialized surveys. For example, there are only four short questions measuring disability for children; surveys designed for precise and complete estimates of disabilities will usually have dozens of such questions. Beginning in 2004, the **American Community Survey** replaced the sample data from the census and provides a more continuous flow of estimates for states, cities, counties, and even towns and rural areas, for which estimates used to come only once a decade.

The census also conducts the **Survey of Income and Program Participation**—a longitudinal survey that collects information in households every 4 months for 4 years. This is a nationally representative survey of about 50,000 households and collects detailed information on changes in people's work histories, income, and participation in public assistance programs. It also routinely collects information on change in family composition, education, assets, and disability status. Several supplements are collected on a rotating basis to provide information on such subjects as child care, child well-being, fertility, and health care utilization. This survey is the source of the majority of the detailed disability statistics presented in this chapter.

Several health-related surveys are conducted by the National Center for Health Statistics (NCHS). The **National Health Interview Survey** (NHIS) is a large, continuous survey of about 43,000 households per year, covering the civilian, noninstitutionalized population of the United States. The NHIS is the major source of information on health status and disability, health-related behaviors, and health care utilization for all age groups. The **National Health and Nutrition Examination Survey** (NHANES) includes physical examinations, mental health questionnaires, dietary data, analyses of urine and blood, and immunization status from a random sample of Americans (about 10,000 in each 2-year cycle). NHANES also collects some basic demographic and income data. It is the major source of information on trends in obesity, cholesterol status, and a host of other conditions in the national population, and in particular age groups, racial and ethnic groups, and so on. The **National Survey of Family Growth** (NSFG) is the primary source of information on marriage and divorce trends, pregnancy, contraceptive use and fertility behaviors, and the ways in which they vary among different groups and over time. The NSFG is fielded every few years. The most recent version, in 2002, collected data for the first time from men as well as from women.

Birth and death certificates, sent by hospitals and funeral homes to state offices of vital events registration, provide the raw material for calculating fertility and mortality rates and life expectancy. The data are collected from the states and analyzed by the National Center for Health Statistics.

(continued on page 42)

> BOX 2–1   **SOURCES OF INFORMATION ON DEMOGRAPHY AND PUBLIC HEALTH**
> *(Continued)*
>
> The national surveys previously listed draw new samples of households and individuals to interview each year. They are used mainly to track changes in rates *for the whole population* or to analyze differences in rates between groups. To study how individuals change over time—for example, how many children lose insurance coverage when their parents separate, or how many people retire early after a major illness—requires data from *panel surveys*, which reinterview the same people over a long period of time. Panel surveys often used by researchers interested in family demography, economics, and health include the **Survey of Income and Program Participation, Panel Survey of Income Dynamics,** and, for older people, the **Health and Retirement Study** and the **National Long-Term Care Survey.**
>
> Trends and recent data from all these sources can be found in the annual reports published by the Department of Health and Human Services (such as *Health 2003*), survey and birth/death registration reports published by the NCHS (www.nchs.gov), and annual reports on children and families published by the U.S. Census Bureau (www.census.gov), the Interagency Forum on Child and Family Statistics (www.childstats.gov), and the KIDS COUNT network (www.kidscount.org). The Websites and publications of the Population Reference Bureau (www.prb.org) and Child Trends (www.childtrends.org) contain a wide variety of health- and family-related data and analyses. Links to more detailed research on these topics are provided by the National Institute of Child Health and Human Development (www.nichd.nih.gov) and the National Institute on Aging (www.nia.nih.gov), which fund much of the research on families, demography, and health.

marrying. She may move in and out of her parents' house several times before she gets married. Like her counterpart reaching adulthood in the 1950s, she is likely to marry and have at least one child, but the sequence of those events may well be reversed. She probably will not drop out of the labor force after she has children, although she may curtail the number of hours she is employed to balance work and family. She is much more likely to divorce and possibly even to remarry, compared with a young woman in the 1950s or 1960s. Because she is more likely to be a single mother and to be working outside of the home, she is also not as likely to have the time necessary to devote to caring for the health of family members.

A dramatic change in women's participation in market work (work for pay) occurred after 1970, as mothers with young children began entering the labor force in greater numbers. Historically, unmarried mothers (either never married or formerly married) of young children had higher labor force participation rates than married mothers. These women often were the only earners in their families. One notable change has been the increase in the combination of paid work and mothering among married mothers. In 1960, only 19 percent of married mothers with children under the age of 6 were in the labor force. By 2001, the proportion increased to 63 percent (Casper & Bianchi, 2002; U.S. Census Bureau, 2003a). Another truly remarkable change has been the increase in the labor force participation of never-married mothers from 49 percent to 70 percent between 1990 and 2001. This change reflects, in part, never-married mothers' responses to new welfare reform rules requiring welfare recipients to work or look actively for jobs. What does this trend imply for family nursing? The majority of families with young children in the mid-20th century had mothers who were home full-time to care for the health needs of family members, whereas at the beginning of the 21st century such families were in the minority.

Changes in the Economy

Many of the timing changes of when women (and men) marry, have children, and enter the labor force reflect changed economic circumstances since the 1950s. After World War II, the United States enjoyed an economic boom characterized by rapid economic growth, full employment, rising productivity, higher wages, low inflation, and increasing earnings. A man with a high-school education in the 1950s and 1960s could secure a job that paid enough to allow him to purchase a house, support a family, and join the swelling ranks of the middle class.

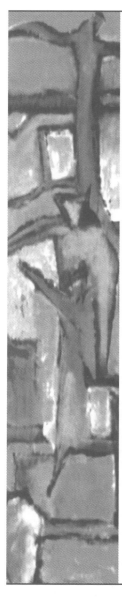

RESEARCH BRIEF

Sample and Setting

The data used in this study are from Wave 9 of the Survey of Income and Program Participation (SIPP), collected in fall 1995 by the U.S. Census Bureau. The sample consisted of 6189 children aged 5 to 13 years from across the United States.

Methodology

The Wave 9 SIPP interviewed 17,583 households in 1995, representing a total sample loss of 27 percent since the panel began in 1993. Data are collected either in person or over the phone by Census Field Representatives. Respondents identified as the designated parent—the mother, if she is in the household—responded to a variety of questions for the four youngest children under age 15 about the child care arrangements used during the designated parent's work and nonwork hours.

Findings

Sixteen percent of children aged 5 to 13 are primarily in self-care during the time they are not at school. Percentages range from 7 percent for children aged 5 to 7 to 25 percent for those aged 11 to 13. One of the most important factors associated with parents selecting self-care over some other primary supervised child care arrangement is full-time work. Parents who work more hours have to cover more hours with child care than do parents who work part-time or don't work, and this care can be expensive. Parents who work full-time may use self-care as a way to cut down on the high costs of child care. Children who are more responsible and mature and those who live in neighborhoods with safe places to play outside are more likely to care for themselves than those who are less responsible and mature or who live in unsafe neighborhoods.

Implications

Nurses dealing with families with grade-school-age children should be aware that some children care for themselves on a regular basis. Children in these situations do not have parental supervision all of the time. Thus, parents may not be home when a child gets hurt or when a sick child requires medication (Casper & Smith, 2004).

Casper, L. M., & Smith K. E. (2004). Self care: Why do parents leave their children unsupervised? *Demography, 41*(2), 285–301.

The economic realities of the 1970s and 1980s were quite different. The two decades following the oil crisis in 1973 were decades of economic change and uncertainty marked by a shift away from manufacturing and toward services, stagnating or declining wages (especially for less-educated workers), high inflation, and a slowdown in productivity growth. The 1990s were just as remarkable for the turnaround: sustained prosperity, low unemployment, and economic growth that seems to have reached many in the poorest segments of society (Farley, 1996; Levy, 1998).

When the economy is on such a roller coaster, family life often takes a similar ride. Marriage oc-curred early and was nearly universal in the decades after World War II; mothers remained in the home to rear children, and the baby-boom generation was born and nurtured. When baby boomers hit working age in the 1970s, the economy was not as hospitable as it had been for their parents. They postponed entry into marriage, delayed having children, and found it difficult to establish themselves in the labor market.

Many of the baby boomers' own children began reaching labor force age in the 1990s and 2000s, when individuals' economic fortunes were increasingly dependent on their educational attainment. Those who attended college were much more likely to become self-sufficient and to live independently from their parents. High-school graduates who did not go to college discovered that jobs with high pay and benefits were in relatively short supply. A high-school graduate lucky enough to land such a job earned about 25 percent less than a comparable job would have paid 20 years earlier (Farley, 1996). The increasing benefits of a college education probably encouraged more young men and women to delay marriage and attend college.

Due in part to changes in the economy, both men and women are remaining single longer and are more likely to leave home to pursue a college education, to live with a partner, and to launch a career before taking on the responsibility of a family of their own. The traditional gender-based organization of home life (in which mothers have primary responsibility for care of the home and children, and fathers provide financial support) has not disappeared, but young women today can expect to be employed while raising children, and young men are more likely to share in some child-rearing and household tasks. Thus, in the first decade of this century, men are more likely to play a role in looking after the health of family members than they were in previous decades.

Changing Family Norms

In 1950, there was one dominant and socially acceptable way for adults to live their lives. Those who deviated could expect to be censured and stigmatized. The idealized family was composed of a homemaker-wife, a breadwinner-father, and two or more children. Americans shared a common image of what a family should look like and how mothers, fathers, and children should behave. These shared values reinforced the importance of the family and the institution of marriage (McLanahan & Casper, 1995). This vision

of family life showed amazing staying power, even as its economic underpinnings were eroding.

For this 1950s-style family to exist, Americans had to support distinct gender roles and the economy had to be vibrant enough for a man to support a family on his own financially.

Government policies and business practices perpetuated this family type by reserving the best jobs for men and discriminating against working women when they married or had a baby. After 1960, with the civil rights movement and an energetic women's liberation movement, women and minorities gained legal protections in the workplace and discriminatory practices began to recede.

A transformation in attitudes toward family behaviors also took place. People became more accepting of divorce, cohabitation, and sex outside marriage; less sure about the universality and permanence of marriage; and more tolerant of blurred gender roles and of a mother's working outside the home (Bumpass & Sweet, 1989; Casper & Bianchi 2002; Cherlin, 1992; Thornton & Young-DeMarco, 2001). Society became more open-minded about a variety of living arrangements, family configurations, and lifestyles.

Although the transformation of many of these attitudes occurred throughout the 20th century, the pace of change accelerated in the 1960s and 1970s. These years brought many political, social, and medical developments, including the highly publicized, although unsuccessful, attempt to pass the Equal Rights Amendment (ERA); the development of new, effective contraception; the legalization of abortion; and the dawn of the sexual revolution and an era of "free love." A new ideology was emerging during these years that stressed personal freedom, self-fulfillment, and individual choice in living arrangements and family commitments. People began to expect more out of marriage and to leave bad marriages that failed to

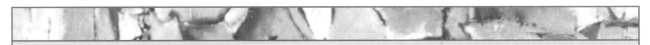

The ERA was first introduced in Congress in 1923. It stated that "equality or rights under the law shall not be denied or abridged by the United States or by any State on account of sex." After nearly a half-century, the amendment was passed by Congress in 1972. The first campaign to ratify the proposed 27th Amendment to the U.S. Constitution—the Federal Equal Rights Amendment—ended on June 30, 1982, three states shy of the 38 required for ratification.

National Women's Conference Committee, *National Plan of Action Update* (Washington, DC: 1986).

fulfill their expectations. These changes in norms and expectations about marriage may have followed rather than preceded increases in divorce and delays in marriage; however, such cultural changes have important feedback effects, leading to later marriage and more divorce.

An Aging Society

For Americans born in 1900, the average life expectancy was less than 50 years. But the early decades of the 20th century brought such tremendous advances in the control of communicable diseases of childhood that life expectancy at birth increased to 70 years by 1960. Rapid declines in mortality from heart disease—the leading cause of death—significantly lengthened life expectancy for those aged 65 or older after 1960 (Treas & Torrecilha, 1995). By 2001, life expectancy at birth was nearly 77 years. An American woman who reached age 65 in 2001 could expect to live an additional 19 years, on average, and a 65-year-old man would live another 16 years (National Center for Health Statistics, 2003a). Women continue to outlive men, though the gender gap is shrinking as women's and men's rates of cancer and heart disease converge (Casper & Bianchi, 2002). Nonetheless, the gap in life expectancy between men and women means that women tend to outlive their husbands, and they predominate in the older age groups. Nearly two-thirds of Americans aged 75 and over are women.

Partly because more Americans are surviving until older ages, and partly because of a long-term decline in fertility rates, the proportion of the population aged 65 or older has grown. In 1900, only 1 of every 25 Americans was aged 65 or older. By 2000, the proportion was one in eight. By 2011, the first of some 78 million baby boomers will reach their 65th birthday, and the rate of increase of the elderly population will accelerate. By 2030, it is expected that one in five Americans will be aged 65 or older.

People do not suddenly become old on their 65th birthday, of course. Along with improvements in life expectancy have come improvements in the disability rates at older ages, so that Americans are not only living longer than in the past but also enjoying healthy lives longer than in the past. At age 65, most people can look forward to many more years of life without chronic illness or disabilities. But 65 is a convenient marker for "old age" in health policy terms, because it is the age at which the great majority of Americans

become eligible for medical and hospital insurance provided through Medicare. By 65, as well, most workers (both men and women) have left full-time work, though many work part-time, or for part of the year, often at different jobs than those they pursued during most of their working lives.

The aging of the population is often considered a major cause of increasing demand for medical services and of the growth in medical expenditures. Population aging is one factor, but the increase in medical expenditures per older person is due more to changes in medical technology and in the usage and prices of pharmaceuticals than to the rate of growth of the elderly population (Reinhardt, 2003).

Increased life expectancy translates into extended years spent in family relationships. A couple who marry in their 20s could easily spend the next 50 years together, assuming they remain married. Couples in the past were much more likely to experience the death of one spouse earlier in their adult years. All family members today have more years together as adults now than they did during the early 1900s. Longer lives (along with lower birth rates) also mean that people spend a smaller portion of their lives parenting young children. More parents live long enough to be part of their grandchildren's and even great-grandchildren's lives. Many adults are faced with caring for extremely elderly parents about the time they reach retirement age and begin to experience health limitations of older age themselves.

Immigration and Ethnic Diversity

In 1965, Congress amended the Immigration and Naturalization Act to create a fundamental change in the nation's policy on immigration. Visas for legal immigrants were no longer to be based on quotas for each country of origin; instead, preference would be given to immigrants joining family members in the United States. The legislation removed limitations on immigration from Asia. The numbers of legal immigrants to the United States increased, to an average of 900,000 persons per year in the 1990s and first years of the new century. In 2001, 63 percent of legal immigrants were admitted because family members already living in the United States petitioned the government to grant them entry. Immigrant visas were granted for economic reasons, including employers petitioning the government for admission of persons considered to have special skills the employers need. Visas were also granted for political reasons, including asylum granted to refugees because of well-founded fear of persecution in their home countries. In addition to legal immigrants, an estimated 7 to 9 million illegal immigrants are in the country at any one time, either because they entered without detection or because they stayed longer than allowed by a temporary visa. In 2002, the Census Bureau estimated that there were 32.5 million U.S. residents born outside the country, 11.5 percent of the total population. Because immigrants tend to arrive in the United States early in their working careers, they are younger on average than the total U.S. population and account for a larger share of young families. In 2002, for example, 23 percent of all births in the United States were to women born outside the country. It is too early to tell the long-term effects on immigration of the terrorist attacks of September 11, 2001, or the economic recession that began the same year, but the preliminary estimates are that immigration has continued at the same high pace as in the late 1990s.

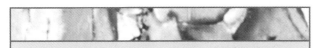

In recent decades, the majority of immigrants have come from Latin America (51 percent of immigrants during the 1990s) and Asia (30 percent of immigrants in the 1990s). Immigration has contributed to the rapid growth of the Latino and Asian-American populations in the United States.

Estimates based on the 2000 Census show that 47 million people over age 5 speak a language other than English at home, the most common being Spanish (28 million) and Chinese (2 million). About a quarter of the adult (age 25 to 44) Latino population of the United States—and one-third of Mexican-origin adults—reported that they could not speak English well (Saenz, 2004). Keep in mind, however, that the overwhelming majority of those who do not speak English well are recent immigrants. Over 97 percent of Latino adults born in the United States report that they can speak English well.

The majority of foreign-born U.S. residents live in states that are the traditional "gateways" to immigrant populations: California, New York, Florida, Texas, and Illinois. In recent decades, however, there have been significant increases in the immigrant populations of

most parts of the country, including the rural South and the Upper Midwest, that had seen few immigrants for most of the 20th century. This spreading of the immigrant population throughout the country, coupled with the increased number of immigrants, has meant that patient populations in many regions are more diverse than in the past. Nurses throughout the country work with families whose cultural backgrounds, perceptions of sickness, and expectations of healers may be very different from those with which they are familiar. Everyone providing health care may face both the challenges and the professional rewards of adapting to new ways of providing service. To take just one example, medical records technicians must get used to filing and retrieving records for patients whose family name comes before their given names or who use both maiden and husbands' surnames.

Implications for Family Nursing

The aging and the growing diversity of the American population, combined with shifts in the economy and changing norms, values, and laws, alter the context of family health care nursing.

As the population ages, the demand will increase for nurses who specialize in caring for the elderly. Improvements in health among those aged 60 to 70 reduce the need for care among this group. Yet rates of population growth are greatest for those aged 80 and over, implying an increased demand for care among the "oldest old" who are likely to suffer from poorer health and to require substantial care. Because women continue to outlive men, on average, nurses are more likely to be dealing with the health care needs of older women than of men. Extended lives and delayed child bearing have increased the chances that adults will experience the double whammy of having to provide care and financial support for their children and their parents. And families in these situations can face considerable time and money pressures.

At the same time that changing gender roles point to more men in families taking on caregiving duties, more women are in the labor force and unavailable to care for family members, and it is doubtful that the increase in men's time in caregiving will fully compensate for the decrease in women's time. Societal changes also influence individuals' life course trajectories. All these changes in individual lives and family relationships are transforming U.S. households and families and in turn changing the context in which health needs are defined and both formal and informal health care are provided.

> **"**The aging and growing diversity of the American population, combined with shifts in the economy and changing norms, values, and laws, alter the context of family health care nursing.**"**

LIVING ARRANGEMENTS

The term "family" carries rich social and cultural meanings, and it has deep personal significance for most people. But for statistical purposes, a family is defined as two or more people living together who are related by blood, marriage, or adoption (Casper & Bianchi, 2002). Most households—which are defined by the U.S. Census Bureau as one or more people who occupy a house, apartment, or other residential unit (but not "group quarters" such as dormitories)—are maintained by families. The social and economic transformation of the family in recent decades means that the family share of U.S. households has been declining. In 1960, 85 percent of households were family households; by 2003, just 68 percent were family households (authors' calculations from 2003 March Current Population Survey; U.S. Census Bureau, 2003b). Two-parent family households with children dropped from 44 percent to 23 percent of all households between 1960 and 2003 (authors' calculations from 2003 March Current Population Survey; U.S. Census Bureau, 2003b). At the same time, non-family households, which consist primarily of people who live alone or who share a residence with roommates or with a partner, have been on the rise. The fastest growth was among persons living alone. The proportion of households with just one person doubled from 13 percent to 26 percent between 1960 and 2003. Thus, as we move forward in the new millennium, fewer people will live with family members who can help care for them when they are ill or injured.

Elderly Americans

Improvements in the health and financial status of older Americans helped generate a revolution in lifestyles and living arrangements among the elderly. Older Americans now are more likely to spend their later years with their spouse or living alone than with adult children. The options and choices differ between elderly women and elderly men, however, in large part because women live longer than men yet have fewer financial resources and smaller pensions.

At the beginning of the 20th century, more than 70 percent of people aged 65 or older resided with kin (Ruggles, 1994). By 1980, only 23 percent of elderly people lived with relatives other than their spouses, and by 1998, the percentage had slipped to 20 percent (Casper & Bianchi, 2002). Meanwhile, living alone increased dramatically among the elderly in the latter half of the 20th century. Just 15 percent of widows aged 65 or older lived alone in 1900, for example, whereas 24 percent lived alone in 1950, and more than 70 percent lived alone in 1998 (Lugaila, 2000; McGarry & Schoeni, 2000; Ruggles, 1996).

The improvements in life expectancy among elderly Americans have meant more years in retirement and a greater likelihood of spending those years with a spouse. Accordingly, married couples without children under age 18 make up an increasing share of American households. Both men and women aged 65 and older were more likely to be living with a spouse in 2003 than in 1960.

A woman is likely to spend more years living alone after a spouse dies than will a man because life expectancy is about 3 years longer for an elderly woman than for an elderly man and because women usually marry men older than themselves. Men aged 65 or older were nearly twice as likely as were women to be living with their spouse in 2003 (70 percent versus 40 percent). In sharp contrast, women were more than twice as likely as were men to be living alone (40 percent versus 19 percent) and thus without anyone in the house to take care of them should they become ill or sustain an injury (authors' calculations from March Current Population Surveys).

Women were also almost twice as likely as were men to be living with nonrelatives (20 percent versus 11 percent), in part because they tend to live longer and reach advanced ages when they are most likely to need the physical care and the financial help others can provide. Men generally receive companionship and care from their wives in the latter stages of life, whereas women are more likely to live alone with assistance from grown children, to live with other family members, or to enter a nursing home (Kramarow, 1995; Silverstein, 1995; Weinick, 1995).

Elderly men and women have a variety of living options including living alone, living with family members or roommates, or living in a retirement community or nursing home, either with or without assisted care. To explain trends in living arrangements among the elderly, researchers have focused on a variety of constraints and preferences that shape people's living arrangement decisions. These constraints and preferences fall under three general categories: availability and accessibility of relatives, feasibility, and preferences (Goldscheider & Jones, 1989).

Availability and Access

The number and gender of children generally govern the availability and accessibility of relatives with whom an elderly person might live. The greater the number of children, the greater the chances there will be a son or daughter who can take care of an elderly parent. Daughters are more likely than are sons to provide housing and care for an elderly parent, presumably as an extension of the traditional female caretaker role. Geographical distance from children is also a key factor; having children who live nearby promotes coresidence when living independently is no longer feasible for the elderly person (Crimmins & Ingegneri, 1990; Spitze & Logan 1990).

Feasibility

The feasibility of living alone, with relatives, or in a nursing home is tied to economic resources and health status. Older Americans with higher income and better health are more likely to live independently (Crimmins & Ingegneri, 1990; Holden, 1988; Mutchler, 1992; Wolf & Soldo, 1988; Woroby & Angel, 1990). Growth in Social Security benefits accounts for half of the increase in independent living among the elderly since 1940 (McGarry & Schoeni, 2000; Ruggles & Goeken, 1992). By contrast, elderly Americans in financial need are more likely to live with relatives (Speare & Avery, 1993).

Preferences

Finally, social norms and personal preferences determine the choice of living arrangements for the elderly (Wister, 1984; Wister & Burch, 1987). Many elderly individuals are willing to pay a substantial part of their incomes to maintain their own residence, which suggests strong personal preferences for privacy and independence. Social norms involving family obligations and ties also have an effect on residence patterns and may be especially important when examining racial and ethnic differences in the living arrangements of the elderly.

Despite the trend toward independent living among older Americans, many of them are not able to live alone without assistance. It is important for family health care nurses to keep in mind that many families who have older kin in frail health provide extraordinary care. One study in New York City, for example, found that 40 percent of those who reported caring for an elderly relative devoted 20 or more hours per week to such informal care, and 80 percent of caregivers had been providing care for over a year (Navaie-Walsier et al., 2001). Despite the growth of home health services and adult day-care centers, most informal caregivers report that they have no assistance from formal care providers (Navaie-Walsier et al., 2001). Adult women, in particular, are likely to have primary responsibility for home care of the frail elderly, often including parents-in-law, and there is some evidence that female caregivers experience greater levels of stress than do male caregivers (Yee & Schulz, 2000).

Young Adults

The young-adult years (ages 18 to 30) have been referred to as "demographically dense" because these years involve many interrelated life-altering transitions (Rindfuss, 1991). Between these ages, young people usually finish their formal schooling, leave home, develop careers, marry, and begin families, but these events do not always occur in this order. Delayed marriage extends the period during which young adults can experiment with alternative living arrangements before they adopt family roles. Young adults may experience any number of independent living arrangements before they marry, as they change jobs, pursue education, and move into and out of intimate relationships. They may also return home for periods of time, if money becomes tight or if a relationship breaks up.

In 1890, one-half of American women had married by age 22 and one-half of American men had married by age 26 (U.S. Census Bureau, 2003c). The ages of entry into marriage dipped to an all-time low during the post–World War II baby-boom years, when median age at first marriage reached 20 years for women and 23 years for men in 1956. Age at first marriage then began to rise and reached 25 years for women and 27 years for men by 2002 (U.S. Census Bureau, 2003c). In 1960, it was unusual for a woman to reach age 25 without marrying; only 10 percent of women aged 25 to 29 had never married (Casper & Bianchi, 2002). In 2000, a woman in her late 20s who had never been married was more common because two-fifths of women aged 25 to 29 had not been married. Moreover, in 2000, 52 percent of men were still unmarried at that age.

This delay in marriage has shifted the family behaviors in young adulthood in three important ways. First, later marriage coincides with a greater diversity and fluidity in living arrangements in young adulthood. Second, delaying marriage has accompanied an increased likelihood of entering a cohabiting union before marriage. Third, the trend to later marriage affects childbearing in two important ways. It tends to delay entry into parenthood and, at the same time, increases the chances that a birth (sometimes planned but more often unintended) may happen before marriage (Bianchi & Casper, 2000).

Many demographic, social, and economic factors influence young adults' decisions about where and with whom to live (Casper & Bianchi, 2002). Family and work transitions are influenced greatly by fluctuations in the economy as well as by changing ideas about appropriate family life and roles for men and women. Since the 1980s, the transition to adulthood has been hampered by recurring recessions, tight job markets, slow wage growth, and soaring housing costs, in addition to the confusion over roles and behavior sparked by the gender revolution (Goldscheider & Goldscheider, 1994). Even though young adults today may prefer to live independently, they may not be able to afford to do so. Many entry-level jobs today offer low wages, yet housing costs have soared, putting independent living out of reach for many young adults. Higher education, increasingly necessary in today's labor market, is expensive, and living at home may be a way for families to curb college expenses. Even when young adults attend school away from home, they still frequently depend on their parents for financial help and may return home after graduation if they cannot find a suitable job.

66 Young adults may experience any number of independent living arrangements before they marry, as they change jobs, pursue education, and move into and out of intimate relationships. 99

Married living declined dramatically between 1970 and 2003, among both young men and young women. As a declining share of young adults chose married life, a greater share lived with parents or on their own. The percentage of young men living in their parents' homes was 55 percent in 2003, about the same as in 1970, whereas the percentage increased for young women from 39 percent to 46 percent (authors' calculations based on the March Current Population Surveys).

Americans were leaving their parents' homes at increasingly younger ages throughout most of the 20th century. In the 1980s, however, this trend reversed for both young men and young women. Not only are recent cohorts leaving home later, but also they are more likely to return home—a "backward" transition out of the adult role and back into the role of a dependent. By the 1980s, about 40 percent of young adults who left home eventually returned for a time, a marked increase from less than 25 percent of those reaching adulthood before World War II (Goldscheider & Goldscheider, 1994).

Young adults who leave home to attend school, join the military, or take a job have always had, and continue to have, high rates of returning to the nest. The "return rate" is nearly as high for those young adults who leave home to live with a partner or to form another type of nonmarital family. Those who leave home to get married have had the lowest likelihood of returning home, although returns to the nest have increased over time even in this group. Historically, moving away for independence was associated with very low rates of returning home—less than 20 percent prior to World War II. This pattern has changed over time so that currently about 40 percent of those who first leave for independence return to the nest.

American parents routinely take in their children after they return from the military or school or when they are between jobs. In the past, however, many American parents apparently were reluctant to take children in if they had left home simply to gain "independence." This is not true today. Demographers Frances Goldscheider and Calvin Goldscheider argue that in the past, leaving home for simple independence was probably the result of friction within the family, whereas today, leaving and returning home seems to be part of a successful transition to adulthood. In the past, a young adult may have been reluctant to move back in with parents because a return home implied failure; there is less stigma attached to returning home these days (Casper & Bianchi, 2002). Changes in the economy have also contributed to this trend. It may be more difficult to sustain an independent residence today than in the past.

Changing demographic behaviors among young adults have implications for family health care nursing. On the one hand, these trends mean that young adults today are less likely to be covered by health insurance and to be financially independent, reducing the likelihood that they will receive routine checkups or go to a doctor when the need arises. On the other hand, if more adult children are living with their parents, there are more adults potentially available among these families to help with caregiving responsibilities and to pay medical bills.

Unmarried Couples

One of the most significant household changes in the second half of the 20th century was the increase in men and women living together without marrying. The rise of cohabitation outside marriage appeared to counterbalance the delay of marriage among young adults and the overall increase in divorce. Unmarried-couple households made up less than 1 percent of U.S. households in 1960 and 1970 (Casper & Cohen, 2000). This share rose to 2.2 percent by 1980, to 3.6 percent in 1990, and to nearly 5 percent by 1998 (Bianchi & Casper, 2000). Unmarried-couple households also are increasingly likely to include children. In 1978, 29 percent of unmarried-couple households included children under age 18; by 1998, 43 percent included children (Casper & Bianchi, 2002).

The number of unmarried-couple households surged from 1.3 million in 1978 to 3.0 million in 1988 and to 4.9 million in 1998. These figures suggest that the growth in cohabitation from 1978 to 1998 could account for 38 percent of the decline in marriage over the period, assuming that all the cohabitants would have married (Casper & Cohen, 2000). Although a relatively small percentage of U.S. households consists of an unmarried couple—1 in 20 households in 1998—many Americans have lived with a partner outside marriage at some point, which means that cohabitation is a large and growing component of U.S. family life. The 1987/1988 National Survey of Families and Households found that 25 percent of all adults and 45 percent of adults in their early 30s had lived with a partner outside marriage. More than one-half of the couples who married in the mid-1990s had lived together before marriage, up slightly from 49 percent in 1985/1986 and a big jump from just 8 percent of first marriages in the late 1960s (Bumpass, 1990; Bumpass & Sweet, 1989; Bumpass & Lu, 2000).

Why has cohabitation increased so much since the 1970s? Researchers have offered several explanations, including increased uncertainty about the stability of marriage, the erosion of norms against cohabitation and sexual relations outside of marriage, the wider availability of reliable birth control, economic reasons, and increased individualism and secularization. Youth reaching adulthood in the past two decades are much more likely to have witnessed divorce than any generation before them. Some have argued that cohabitation allows a couple to experience the benefits of an intimate relationship without committing to marriage. If a cohabiting relationship isn't successful, one can simply move out; if a marriage isn't successful, one suffers through a sometimes lengthy and messy divorce.

Nevertheless, most adults in the United States eventually do marry. In 2000, 91 percent of women aged 45 to 54 had been married at least once. An estimated 88 percent of U.S. women born in the 1960s will eventually marry (Raley, 2000). However, the meaning and permanence of marriage may be changing. Marriage used to be the primary demographic event that marked the formation of new households, the beginning of sexual relations, and the birth of a child. Marriage also implied that an individual had one sexual partner, and it theoretically identified the two individuals who would parent any child born of the union. The increasing social acceptance of cohabitation outside marriage has meant that these linkages could no longer be assumed. Unmarried couples began to set up households that might include the couple's children as well as children from previous marriages or other relationships. Similarly, what it meant to be single was no longer always clear, as the personal lives of unmarried couples began to resemble those of their married counterparts.

The increase in unmarried-couple households is slowing from the frantic pace of the 1970s and 1980s. The number of households with unmarried couples increased 67 percent in the 5 years between 1978 and 1983 but just 23 percent in the 5 years between 1993 and 1998 (Casper & Bianchi, 2002). The pace of growth varied among the three largest racial and ethnic groups. In 1978, single non-Hispanic white women were least likely to cohabit outside marriage, whereas single Hispanic women were most likely to cohabit. By 1998, 10 percent of single non-Hispanic white women lived with a male partner, compared with 9 percent of single Hispanic women and 7 percent of single non-Hispanic black women (Casper & Bianchi, 2002).

Cohabiting households can pose unique challenges for family health care nurses. Because cohabiting relationships are not legally sanctioned in most states, partners do not generally have the right to make health care decisions on behalf of each other or of the other's children. Cohabiting couples are not as healthy as married couples and have lower incomes, on average (Waite & Gallagher, 2000). Thus, although they are more likely to need health care services, they are less likely to have the financial ability to secure them.

PARENTING

Even with the rise in divorce and cohabitation, postponement of marriage, and decline in childbearing, most Americans have children and most children live with two parents. In 2002, 72 percent of families with children were two-parent families (U.S. Census Bureau, 2003d). But the changes in marriage, cohabitation, and nonmarital childbearing over the past few decades have had a profound effect on American families with children and are changing our images of parenthood.

Cohabitation

Changes in marriage and cohabitation tend to blur the distinction between one-parent and two-parent families. The increasing acceptance of cohabitation as a substitute for marriage, for example, may reduce the chance that a premarital pregnancy will lead to marriage before the birth (Raley, 1999). A greater share of children today are born to a mother who is not currently married than in previous decades, but some of those children are born to cohabiting parents and begin life in a household that includes both their parents. The percentage of unmarried mothers who were cohabiting grew from 5 percent to 13 percent between 1978 and 1998 (Casper & Bianchi, 2002). Cohabitation increased for unmarried mothers in all race and ethnic groups but especially among whites. Cohabiting couples account for up to 16 percent of the white mothers classified as unmarried mothers in 1998, compared with 8 percent of black mothers and 10 percent of Hispanic mothers (Casper & Bianchi, 2002).

Demographers Larry Bumpass and R. Kelly Raley show that the increase in cohabitation among Americans may be reducing the time children spend in a single-parent household. They found that the number of years a mother spent as a single parent declined by one-fourth when they took into account the time she and her children shared a home with a partner (Bumpass & Raley, 1995). African-American women with children spent half as many years as a single parent after adjusting for the years they lived with an unmarried partner (Bumpass & Raley, 1995).

Many single-father families may also effectively be two-parent families because the father is living with his children and another woman. Demographers Steven Garasky and Daniel Meyer used census data from 1960 through 1990 to track the increase in the percentage of families that are father-only families.

When they ignored the increase in cohabitation, they estimated that father-only families rose from 1.5 percent to 5.0 percent of families with children between 1960 and 1990. When they removed fathers who are likely to be cohabiting, the 1990 figure fell to 3.2 percent of all families with children (Garasky & Meyer, 1996).

Unmarried fathers living with children are much more likely than unmarried mothers to be living with a partner: 33 percent of the 2.1 million "single" fathers lived with a partner in 1998, more than twice the percentage for single mothers. About 1.4 million American men were raising their children on their own, without a wife or partner, in 1998 (Bianchi & Casper, 2000).

Single Mothers

How many single mothers are there? This turns out to be a more difficult question to answer than it would first appear. Over time, it is easiest to calculate the number of single mothers who maintain their own residence. Between 1950 and 2002, the number of such single-mother families increased from 1.3 million to 8.0 million (U.S. Census Bureau, 2003d). These estimates do not include single mothers living in other persons' households but do include single mothers who are cohabitating with a male partner. The most dramatic increase was during the 1970s, when the number of single-mother families was increasing at 8 percent per year. The average annual rate of increase slowed considerably during the 1980s and was near zero after 1994 (Casper & Bianchi, 2002). By 2002, single mothers who maintained their own households accounted for 22 percent of all families with children, up from 6 percent in 1950 (U.S. Census Bureau, 2003d). Almost 2 million more single mothers live in someone else's household—1.6 million with relatives and 370,000 with nonrelatives (cohabitating or with roommates)—bringing the total number of single mothers to nearly 10 million (Casper & Bianchi, 2002).

Single mothers with children at home face a multitude of challenges. They usually are the primary breadwinners, disciplinarians, playmates, and caregivers for their children. They must manage the financial and practical aspects of a household and plan for the family's future. Most mothers cope remarkably well, and many benefit from financial support and help from relatives and from their children's fathers.

Most single mothers are not poor, but they do tend to be younger, earn lower incomes, and be less educated than married mothers (Casper & Bianchi, 2002). Women earn less than men, on average, and because single mothers are younger and less educated than other women, they are often at the lower end of the income curve. Never-married single mothers are particularly disadvantaged; they are younger, less well educated, and less often employed than are divorced single mothers and married mothers. Single mothers often must curtail their work hours to care for the health and well-being of their children.

Single Mothers in Poverty

Despite the fact that the majority of single mothers are not poor, they are much more likely to be poor than are other parents. Never-married single mothers are the poorest of all. The family income of children who reside with a never-married mother is less than one-fourth that of children in two-parent families (Bianchi & Casper, 2000). Almost three of every five children who live with a never-married mother are poor. Mothers who never married are much less likely to get child support from the father than are mothers who are divorced or separated. Whereas 60 percent of divorced mothers with custody of children under age 21 received some child support from the children's father, less than 20 percent of never-married mothers reported receiving regular support from their child's father (Bianchi & Casper, 2000).

Children who live with a divorced mother tend to be much better off financially than are children of never-married mothers. Although the family income of divorced mothers is less than one-half the income of two-parent families and rates of poverty are greater, divorced mothers are substantially better educated and more often employed than are mothers who are separated or who never married. Home ownership is also significantly higher among families of divorced mothers, although not as high as among two-parent families.

Single mothers with children in poverty are particularly affected by major welfare reform legislation, such as the Personal Responsibility and Work Opportunity Reconciliation Act (PRWORA), signed into law by President Clinton in August 1996 (see Box 2–2). President Clinton claimed that the law would "reform welfare as we know it," and the changes embodied in PRWORA—time limits on welfare eligibility and mandatory job-training requirements, for example—seemed far-reaching. Some argued that this legislation would end crucial support for poor mothers and their children; several high-level government

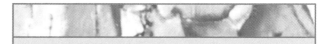

Why has welfare receipt become such a contentious issue? In part, it was because many people were alarmed by the dramatic increase in the second half of the 20th century in the numbers of single mothers. When legislation to protect poor women and children was enacted with the Social Security Act of 1935, most single mothers, poor as well as nonpoor, were widows. That changed dramatically in the 1960s and 1970s as the divorce rate soared. After 1980, the delay in marriage and the increase in the proportion of births to unmarried mothers meant that never-married mothers accounted for an increasingly significant component of the growth in single-parent families. Cash payments to single mothers under the Aid to Families with Dependent Children program were considered by some analysts and politicians to have encouraged or facilitated the increase in childbearing by never-married women.

officials resigned because of the law (Aber, 2000). Others heralded PRWORA as the first step toward helping poor women gain control of their lives and making fathers take responsibility for their children. Many states had already begun to experiment with similar reforms (Cherlin, 2000).

Single Motherhood Characterized

Why have mother-child families increased in number and as a percentage of American families? Explanations tend to focus on one of two trends. First is women's increased financial independence, either through their own wages as more women entered the labor force and women's incomes rose relative to those of men, or because of expanded welfare benefits for single mothers. Women today are less dependent on a man's income to support themselves and their children, and many can afford to live independently rather than stay in an unsatisfactory relationship. Second, the job market for men has tightened, especially for less-educated men. As the U.S. economy experienced a restructuring in the 1970s and 1980s, the demand for professionals, managers, and other white-collar workers expanded while the jobs available for semiskilled

Box 2–2 WELFARE REFORM

Federal and state programs to aid low-income families have been transformed during the past decade. The 1996 Personal Responsibility and Work Opportunity Reconciliation Act (PRWORA) was the legislative milestone at the federal level. PRWORA

- replaced the Aid to Families with Dependent Children program, an entitlement for poor families, with a program of block grants to the states called Temporary Assistance to Needy Families (TANF);
- required states to impose work requirements on at least 80 percent of TANF recipients;
- forbade payments to single mothers under age 18 unless they lived with an adult or in an adult-supervised situation;
- set limits of 60 months on TANF for any individual recipient (and 22 states have used their option to impose shorter lifetime limits);
- gave states more latitude to let TANF recipients earn money or get child support payments without reduction of benefits and to use block grants for child care.

Welfare-reform proponents often supported efforts to "make work pay" as well as to discourage long-term dependence on welfare. The Earned Income Tax Credit, for example, was expanded several times during the 1980s and 1990s and now provides twice as much money to low-income families, whether single- or two-parent families, as does TANF. Funding for child care was also expanded during the decade, though child care remains a problem for low-income working families in most places.

PRWORA accelerated a decline in welfare caseloads throughout the country. Because of a concern that former welfare recipients entering the workforce would lose insurance coverage through Medicaid for their children, the 1997 Balanced Budget Act set up the new State Child Health Insurance Program (SCHIP), providing federal money to states in proportion to their low-income population and recent success in reducing the proportion of uninsured children.

When it was enacted in 1996, welfare reform was supposed to be reauthorized after 5 years. Congress has been unable to agree on new provisions and has simply extended the 1996 law several times during 2001–2004. The major controversies concern proposals for more stringent work requirements and for increased funding for child care.

and unskilled workers declined. The wages for men in lower-skilled jobs have declined in real terms over the past two decades. Men still earn more than women, on average, but the income gap narrowed during the 1970s and 1980s as women's earnings increased and men's earnings remained flat or declined (Cotter et al., 2004, Fig. 14). Many men without a college degree cannot earn enough to support a family of four.

Ethnic Disparities in Single Parenthood

Rates of single parenthood have grown for each of the largest racial and ethnic groups—African-Americans, Hispanics, and whites—but there are large differences in the rates across groups (McLanahan & Casper, 1995; Ruggles, 1994; Spain & Bianchi, 1996). In 1980, 85 percent of white family households with children

under age 18, 76 percent of Hispanic households, and 50 percent of black households were maintained by married couples (U.S. Census Bureau, 2003e). By 2002, 77 percent of white, 70 percent of Hispanic, and 42 percent of black households were maintained by married couples. The percentage of mother-only family households remains much higher for African-Americans (51 percent) than for Hispanics (24 percent) and whites (18 percent). During the 1980s and 1990s, the percentage of single-father households nearly tripled for whites and Hispanics and doubled for African-Americans.

❝The remarkable increase in the number of single-mother households with women who have never married was driven by a dramatic shift to childbearing outside marriage.❞

Never-Married Single Mothers

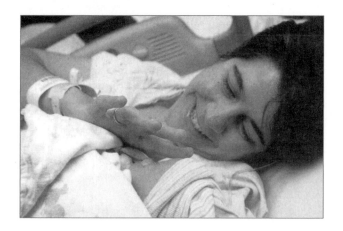

In the early years of the 20th century, higher mortality rates made it more common for children to live with only one parent (Uhlenberg, 1996). As falling death rates reduced the number of widowed single parents, there was a counterbalancing increase in single-parent families because of divorce. Still, at the time of the 1960 census, almost one-third of single mothers living with children under age 18 were widows (Bianchi, 1995). As divorce rates rose precipitously in the 1960s and 1970s, most single-parent families were created through divorce or separation. By the end of the 1970s, only 11 percent of single mothers were widowed and two-thirds were divorced or separated. During the past two decades, the path to single motherhood has increasingly bypassed marriage. In 1978, about one-fifth of single mothers had never married but had a child and were raising that child on their own. By 2000, two-fifths of single mothers had never married (Bianchi & Casper, 2000).

The remarkable increase in the number of single-mother households with women who have never married was driven by a dramatic shift to childbearing outside marriage. The number of births to unmarried women grew from less than 90,000 per year in 1940 to nearly 1.4 million per year in 2002 (National Center for Health Statistics, 2003b). Less than 4 percent of all births in 1940 were to unmarried mothers compared with 34 percent in 2002. The rate of nonmarital births—the number of births per 1000 unmarried women—increased from 7.1 in 1940 to 43.7 in 1999. The nonmarital birth rate peaked in 1994 at 46.2 and leveled out in the latter 1990s (Bianchi & Casper, 2000).

Trends in nonmarital fertility are connected to broad trends in marriage and fertility. The delay in marriage, for example, can lead to an increase in the number of births outside marriage even if the birth rate for unmarried women remains the same. When women remain single longer, they spend more years at risk of becoming pregnant and having a child outside marriage. At the same time, married women are having fewer children, which means that children born to unmarried women make up a greater share of all births. In the 1960s and 1970s, the delay in marriage and decline in fertility within marriage were the major factors contributing to the increase in the proportion of births outside marriage. During the past two decades, the increase in the birth rates of unmarried women has been a much more important factor and, indeed, has raised concerns about the move away from marriage and a breakdown of social sanctions against out-of-wedlock childbearing (Morgan, 1996).

The proportion of births that occur outside marriage is as high or higher in some European countries than in the United States. But unmarried parents in European countries are more likely than are unmarried parents in the United States to be living together, with their biological children (Council of Europe, 1999; Heuveline et al., 2003). In the United States, the tremendous variation in rates of unmarried childbearing among population groups suggests that there may be a constellation of factors that determine whether women have children when they are not married. More than two-thirds (68 percent) of the babies born to African-American mothers in 2001 were born to unmarried mothers, as were more than one-half (60 percent) of babies of Native American mothers (National Center for Health Statistics, 2003b). The percentage is relatively low for Cuban-Americans (30 percent) and for Asian-Americans and Pacific Islanders (15 percent). The rates are extremely low for Chinese-Americans (9 percent) and Japanese-Americans (10 percent).

Single-mother families present challenges for family health care nurses providing care for this vulnerable group. Single mothers today are younger and less educated than they were a few decades ago. This presents problems because these mothers have less experience with the health care system and are likely to have more difficulty reading directions, filling out forms, communicating effectively with doctors and nurses, and understanding their care instructions. These mothers are also more likely to be poor and uninsured, making it less likely they will seek care and more likely they will not be able to pay for it.

Consequently, when the need arises, these women are more likely to resort to emergency rooms for noncritical illnesses and injuries. Time is also in short supply for single mothers. With the advent of welfare reform, more of them are working, which conceivably takes away from the time they used in the past to care for themselves and their children. Moreover, although many of these mothers can rely on their families for help, they are apt to have tenuous ties with their children's fathers.

Fathering

A new view of fatherhood emerged out of the feminist movement of the late 1960s and early 1970s. The new ideal father was a coparent who was responsible for and involved in all aspects of his children's care. The ideal has been widely accepted throughout U.S. society; people today, as opposed to those in earlier times, believe that fathers should be highly involved in caregiving (Pleck & Pleck, 1997). Fathers do spend more time with their children and are doing more housework than in earlier decades. In 1998, married fathers in the United States reported spending an average of 4.0 hours per day with their children, compared with 2.7 hours in 1965 (Bianchi, 2000). Parallel findings emerge from data collected on children and the individuals with whom they spend time. Studies of fathers' time with their children in other industrialized countries, including Great Britain and Australia, also indicate that fathers are becoming more involved in parenting (Bittman, 1999; Fischer et al., 1999; Sandberg & Hofferth, 1999).

At the same time, other trends increasingly remove fathers from their children's lives. When the mother and father are not married, for example, ties between fathers and their children often falter. Family demographer Frank Furstenberg uses the label "good dads, bad dads" to describe the parallel trends of increased commitment to children and child rearing on the part of some fathers at the same time that there seems to be less connection to and responsibility for children on the part of other fathers (Furstenberg, 1998).

It is difficult to measure "father involvement" in the United States; until recently, there had been little scientific research that focused on men as parents. In 1880, 42 percent of men aged 18 to 75 lived with their own biological children or stepchildren (Goldscheider et al., 2001). This dropped to 33 percent in 1940 and to 28 percent in 1990—a decline that parallels declines in the birth rate. The major interruption to this long-term trend was the baby-boom years, captured in the 1950 through 1970 censuses. Almost one-half of adult men lived with an "own child" in these years, a higher percentage than in 1880 (Goldscheider et al., 2001).

How many years do men spend as parents? Demographer Rosalind King has estimated the number of years that men and women will spend as parents of biological children or stepchildren under age 18 if the parenting patterns of the late 1980s and early 1990s continue throughout their lives (King, 1999). Almost two-thirds of the adult years will be "child-free" years in which the individual does not have biological children under age 18 or responsibility for anyone else's children. Men will spend about 20 percent of their adulthood living with and raising their biological children, whereas women will spend more than 30 percent of their lives raising biological children. Whereas women, regardless of race, spend nearly all of their parenting years rearing their biological children, men are more likely to live with stepchildren or a combination of their own children and stepchildren. Among men, whites will spend about twice as much time living with their biological children as will African-Americans.

Single Fathers

One of the new aspects of the American family in the last 50 years has been an increase in the number of families maintained by the father without the mother present. Between 1950 and 2002, the number of households with children that were maintained by an unmarried father increased from 229,000 to 1.9 million (U.S. Census Bureau, 2002e). An additional 328,000 unmarried fathers lived with their children in someone else's household, bringing the total count of single fathers to about 2.2 million for 2002.

> ❝ One of the new aspects of the American family in the last 50 years has been an increase in the number of families maintained by the father without the mother present. ❞

Recent demographic trends in fathering have changed the context of family health care nursing. The growth in single fatherhood and joint custody, together with the increased tendency for fathers to perform household chores, means that family health care nurses are more likely today than in decades past to be interacting with the fathers of children.

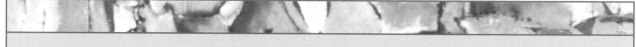

Although mothers generally get custody of children after divorce, shared physical custody—in which children alternate between their mother's and father's households—has become more common in recent years. Although divorced fathers rarely are granted sole custody of their children, shared custody promotes close involvement in all aspects of their children's lives (Cancian & Meyer, 1996).

In one of the few analyses of child custody trends, researchers Maria Cancian and Daniel Meyer examined the custody outcomes of divorce cases in Wisconsin between 1986 and 1994 (Cancian & Meyer, 1996). Their study found little change in the percentage of cases in which fathers were awarded sole custody of children; fathers got sole custody in about 10 percent of divorce cases throughout the period. The percentage of cases in which mothers were awarded sole custody declined, however, from 80 percent to 74 percent, and the percentage of cases with shared physical custody between the mother and father rose from 7 percent to 14 percent over the period. If trends in other states are similar to Wisconsin's, fathers are becoming more involved in the lives of their children after divorce, not as sole custodians but as increased participants in legal decisions (joint legal custody) and in shared physical custody arrangements.

Grandparents

One moderating factor in children's well-being in single-parent families can be the presence of grandparents in the home. Although the image of single-parent families is usually that of a mother living on her own, trying to meet the needs of her young child or children, many single mothers live with their parents. In 1998, about 17 percent of unmarried mothers with children lived in the homes of their parents, compared with 10 percent of single fathers (Casper & Bianchi, 2002). However, this is a snapshot at one point in time; a much higher percentage of single mothers (36

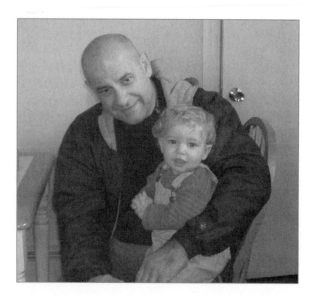

percent) live in their parents' home *at some point* before their children are grown. Black single mothers with children at home are more likely than are others to live with a parent at some time.

The involvement of grandparents in the lives of their children who become single parents is receiving increased attention. Court cases are ruling on grandparents' visitation rights. The 2000 census included a new set of questions, mandated as part of welfare reform, on grandparents' support of grandchildren.

Children whose parents for one reason or another cannot take care of them also live with their grandparents. In 1970, 2.2 million or 3.2 percent of all American children lived in their grandparents' household. By 2002, this number had risen to 3.7 million, or 5.1 percent (U.S. Census Bureau, 2003f). Substantial increases occurred among all types of households maintained by grandparents, regardless of the presence or absence of the grandchildren's parents, but increases were greatest among children with only one parent in the household.

Emerging research shows that grandparents play an important role in multigenerational households, which is at odds with the traditional image of grandparents as family members who require financial and personal support. Although early studies assumed that financial support flowed from adult children to their parents, more recent research suggests that the more common pattern is for parents to give financial support to their adult children (Eggebeen & Hogan, 1990; Mancini & Blieszner, 1989; Rossi & Rossi, 1990).

In most multigenerational households, the grandparents bring their children and grandchildren into a household that the grandparents own or rent. In 1997, three-fourths of multigenerational households were of this type. In nearly one-third of the grandparent-maintained families, grandparents lived with their grandchildren without the children's parents (Bryson & Casper, 1999). Grandparents who own or rent homes that include grandchildren and adult children are younger, healthier, and more likely to be in the labor force than are grandparents who live in a residence owned or rented by their adult children. Grandparents who maintain multigenerational households are also better educated (more likely to have at least a high-school education) than are grandparents who live in their children's homes (Bryson & Casper, 1999; Bianchi & Casper, 2000; Casper & Bianchi, 2002).

Parents who maintain a home that includes both dependent children and dependent parents have been referred to as the "sandwich" generation, because they provide economic and emotional support for both the older and younger generations. Although grandparents in parent-maintained households tend to be older, in poorer health, and not as likely to be employed, many are in good health and are, in fact, working (Bryson & Casper, 1999; Bianchi & Casper, 2000; Casper & Bianchi, 2002). These findings suggest that the burden of maintaining a "sandwich family" household may be somewhat overstated in the popular press. Many of the grandparents who are living in the houses of their adult children are capable of contributing to the family income and helping with supervision of children.

The type of family structure among families with coresident grandparents also makes a difference for the financial well-being of family members. Grandmothers living in households with their grandchildren are about twice as likely to be poor as are grandfathers (21 percent compared with 12 percent) (Casper & Bianchi, 2002). Families in which parents are absent and single grandmothers provide homes for their grandchildren have the highest poverty rates—57 percent of such families live below the poverty line.

Many grandparents step in to assist their children in times of crisis. Some provide financial assistance or child care, whereas others are the primary caregivers for their grandchildren. The recent increase in the numbers of grandparents raising their grandchildren is particularly salient to family health care nurses because both grandparents and grandchildren in this situation often suffer significant health problems (Casper & Bianchi, 2002). Researchers have documented high rates of asthma, weakened immune systems, poor eating and sleeping patterns, physical disabilities, and hyperactivity among grandchildren being raised by their grandparents (Dowdell, 1995; Minkler & Roe, 1996; Shore & Hayslip, 1994). Grandparents raising grandchildren are in poorer health than are their counterparts. They have higher rates of depression, poorer self-rated health, and more multiple chronic health problems (Dowdell, 1995; Minkler & Roe, 1993). These families are also more likely to face economic hardship, having disproportionately high poverty rates (Bryson & Casper, 1999; Chalfie, 1994; Fuller-Thomson et al., 1997; Rutrough & Ofstedal, 1997).

It is important to keep in mind that although many of the grandparents who live in their adult children's homes are in good health, some of these grandparents require significant care. Nursing students should also be aware that there are also adults who provide care for their parents who are not living with them, a situation that was not discussed in this section. Adults who provide care for both generations are likely to face both time and money concerns.

HEALTH DEMOGRAPHICS

So far this chapter has highlighted profound changes in families and households, and the ethnic diversity and age composition of the American population, all setting the social context in which health care is provided and demands are made on providers. The next section reviews no less profound changes in demographic measures of health status and its more direct determinants.

Adults: Mortality, Morbidity, and Disability

The health status of the American population has improved greatly during the last half-century. This improvement can be measured most precisely by looking at mortality indicators. Since the mid-1950s, age-standardized mortality rates have improved nearly every year, at an average rate of around 1 percent a year (Fuchs & Garber, 2003). Disability is a less precisely definable outcome of ill health. There are different definitions and measures of different aspects of physical health and functioning (see Box 2–3). But despite the difficulties of comparing over time and across data sources, the disability trends confirm the picture of improving health. Among Americans aged 65 and over, age-standardized disability rates have also

Box 2–3 **DEFINITIONS OF DISABILITY STATUS, SEVERE DISABILITY, FUNCTIONAL LIMITATIONS, ACTIVITIES OF DAILY LIVING (ADLS), AND INSTRUMENTAL ACTIVITIES OF DAILY LIVING (IADLS)**

Demographers and epidemiologists use various ways to measure disability within the population. In recent U.S. Census Bureau studies using data from the Survey of Income and Program Participation, individuals 15 years old and over are typically identified as having a disability if they meet any of the following criteria (McNeil, 2001):

1. Use a wheelchair, a cane, crutches, or a walker
2. Have difficulty performing one or more **functional activities** (seeing, hearing, speaking, lifting/carrying, using stairs, walking, or grasping small objects)
3. Have difficulty with one or more **activities of daily living** (the **ADLs** include getting around inside the home, getting into or out of bed or a chair, bathing, dressing, eating, and toileting)
4. Have difficulty with one or more **instrumental activities of daily living** (the **IADLs** include going outside the home, keeping track of money and bills, preparing meals, doing light housework, taking prescription medicines in the right amount at the right time, and using the telephone)
5. Have one or more specified conditions (a learning disability, mental retardation or another developmental disability, Alzheimer's disease, or some other type of mental or emotional condition)
6. Have any other mental or emotional condition that seriously interferes with everyday activities (frequently depressed or anxious, trouble getting along with others, trouble concentrating, or trouble coping with day-to-day stress)
7. Have a condition that limits the ability to work around the house
8. If age 16 to 67, have a condition that makes it difficult to work at a job or business
9. Receive federal benefits based on an inability to work

Individuals are considered to have a **severe disability** if they meet criteria 1, 6, or 9; if they have Alzheimer's disease, mental retardation, or another developmental disability; or if they are unable to perform or need help to perform one or more of the activities in criteria 2, 3, 4, 7, or 8.

been declining during the same decades at a rate of about 1 percent a year, with some variation among different data sources (Freedman et al., 2002).

Demographers and epidemiologists usually adjust for differences in the proportions of a population in different age groups when they compare mortality rates at different times or across different countries. This is because the risk of mortality for any individual is closely associated with age, rising from the lowest point at about age 10. Among persons aged 15 to 24 years in the United States in 2000, there were 80 deaths per 100,000 people. Among those over age 65, there were close to 5200 deaths per 100,000 people.

The general picture of progress in adult health holds true for segments of the U.S. population defined by race and ethnicity, by levels of income and education, or by geography. But disturbing inequalities in health outcomes persist, posing a challenge for the health care system and society at large. African-

American males have a life expectancy at birth more than 6 years lower than white American males (68.2 years compared with 74.8), and African-American women have a life expectancy at birth about 5 years lower than white American women (74.9 years compared with 80.0).

Latinos and Asian-Americans, by contrast, have lower age-adjusted mortality rates than do non-Hispanic whites in the United States (National Center for Health Statistics, 2003a, Table 28). In large part, this advantage is associated with "immigrant selectivity." Leaving one's native country to move to a new one has always required a certain degree of good health and optimism. There is also evidence that many immigrant families maintain healthy diets, social and family connections, and other behaviors that promote health and well-being. These advantages appear to dissipate as subsequent generations assimilate to the larger culture and patterns of behavior (Hernandez, 1999).

The Americans with Disabilities Act of 1990 (ADA) defines "disability" as a substantial limitation in a major life activity. In 1997, 52.6 million people (19.7 percent of the population) had some level of disability and 33.0 million (12.3 percent of the population) had a severe disability, according to a recent Census Bureau report (McNeil, 2001). African-Americans are the most likely to be disabled. For all ages, the prevalence of severe disability was 9 percent for Asians and Pacific Islanders, 10 percent for Hispanics (not statistically different from the rate for Asians and Pacific Islanders), 12 percent for non-Hispanic whites, and 16 percent for African-Americans. Some of the overall differences among the different race/ethnic groups reflect differences in the age distributions of the populations. For the population 25 to 64 years old, 8 percent of Asians and Pacific Islanders were severely disabled compared with 11 percent of non-Hispanic whites, 12 percent of Hispanics (not statistically different from non-Hispanic whites), and 19 percent of African-Americans. For individuals 65 years old and over, non-Hispanic whites fared considerably better— 35 percent of non-Hispanic whites were severely disabled compared with 49 percent of Asians and Pacific Islanders, 47 percent of Hispanics, and 52 percent of African-Americans.

About 10.1 million individuals (3.8 percent of the population) needed personal assistance with one or more activities of daily living (ADLs include getting around inside the home, getting into or out of bed or a chair, bathing, dressing, eating, and toileting) or instrumental activities of daily living (IADLs include going outside the home, keeping track of money and bills, preparing meals, doing light housework, taking prescription medicines in the right amount at the right time, and using the telephone) (McNeil, 2001). Among the population 15 years old and over, 2.2 million used a wheelchair (1 percent of the population). Another 3 percent or 6.4 million used some other ambulatory aid such as a cane, crutches, or a walker. About 7.7 million individuals 15 years old and over had difficulty seeing the words and letters in ordinary newspaper print; of them, 1.8 million were unable to see.

The ability to work is one of the major activities affected by the chronic conditions of the disabled. In 1997, 18.5 million individuals 16 to 64 years old were identified as having a work disability (McNeil, 2001). Individuals with a severe disability had an employment rate of 31.4 percent and median earnings of $13,272, compared with 82.0 percent and $20,457 for those with a nonsevere disability and 84.4 percent and $23,654 for those with no disability. Needless to say,

many people with disabilities live in poverty. The poverty rate among the population 25 to 64 years old with no disability was 8.3 percent; it was 27.9 percent for those with a severe disability.

Obesity

One of the most disturbing trends in health over the past decade has been the increase in the proportion of the population that is obese or overweight. Epidemiological studies have shown that increased body weight is associated with an increased risk of mortality. Overweight and obese people are more likely than are those of normal weight to suffer from heart disease, diabetes, and some types of cancer. Hypertension, musculoskeletal problems, and arthritis tend to be more severe in obese and overweight people. Obesity increased little in the population between the early 1960s and 1980. Since 1980, however, obesity has increased dramatically. Thirteen percent of adults were obese in the early 1960s. This figure rose slightly to 15 percent by the mid-to-late 1970s but skyrocketed to 31 percent by 1999/2000 (the most recent results available from the National Health and Nutrition Examination Survey, National Center for Health Statistics, 2003a, Table 68). The proportions of overweight individuals also increased dramatically over this period, from 47 percent in the mid-1970s to 64 percent by 1999/2000. Women are more likely than are men to be obese or overweight.

Adults: Behavioral Risk Factors

In 1990, at the urging of the surgeon general of the United States, the federal government published a national agenda for health promotion, entitled *Healthy People 2000*, which identified 319 objectives for health promotion and set measurable goals for achieving them. (See National Center for Health Statistics, 2001, for a complete list of objectives and an assessment of progress toward their achievement.) Many of the objectives for the decade dealt with behavior, including physical activity and exercise; tobacco, alcohol, and drug use; violent and abusive behaviors; safe sexual practices; and behaviors designed to prevent or mitigate injuries. The effort was never meant to be the responsibility of the health care, or even the public health, sector alone. Rather, these were set as national objectives to be realized through a combination of public- and private-sector, community, and individual efforts. The results were mixed, with considerable success in some areas, including increases in moderate physical activity; moderate improvements in some others, including decreases in binge drinking and increases in safe sexual practices; and little progress or worsening in some other behavioral objectives, including marijuana use and tobacco use during pregnancy (National Center for Health Statistics, 2001). A new set of objectives and measurable goals, *Healthy People 2010*, was adopted for the first decade of this century. The relevant *Healthy People* goals provide a good way to assess changes in behaviors that affect susceptibility to illness and injury. Numerous tables in the statistical yearbooks published by the National Center for Health Statistics form a "scorecard" for this national effort. Among the behaviors with the greatest impact on public health are tobacco use, use of alcohol and other drugs, lack of physical activity, and unsafe sexual practices.

Smoking

Smoking has declined steadily among adults in the United States. In 1965, more than half of adult men smoked, as did a third of adult women. The prevalence has declined more rapidly for men than for women, and the gap has narrowed. By 2001, just over 25 percent of adult men, and just under 21 percent of adult women, were current smokers (National Center for Health Statistics, 2003a, Table 59, unadjusted rates). African-Americans are somewhat more likely to smoke than are white men, whereas African-American women are less likely to smoke than are white women (National Center for Health Statistics, 2003a, Table 59, unadjusted rates).

Alcohol and Drug Use

Use of alcohol is a risk factor for a wide range of poor physical and mental health outcomes. Alcohol use is legal for adults, though drunk driving and, to a lesser extent, public drunkenness are banned. Alcohol use is illegal for minors, though widely tolerated. In 2001, 69 percent of adult men and 57 percent of adult women reported that they currently drank alcohol. Of the current drinkers, 43 percent of men and 21 percent of women reported "binge drinking" (defined as five or more drinks on one occasion) during the preceding year (National Center for Health Statistics, 2003a, Table 65, unadjusted). Non-Hispanic whites were more likely than were either African-Americans or Latinos to be current drinkers or binge drinkers.

The prevalence of drug use, the particular drugs used, and the methods in which they are taken vary considerably over time, among racial and ethnic groups, across social and economic classes, and among regions of the country or even neighborhoods. In 2000, nearly 6 percent of Americans aged 18 who were interviewed in confidential household surveys reported that they had used one or more illicit drugs during the preceding 30 days.

In popular discussions, and sometimes among professionals, health-related behaviors are treated as resulting solely from conscious choice by individuals, who are to blame if their risky behavior leads to poor health outcomes. Many health activists, by contrast, seek to place blame on commercial interests that profit from these behaviors or on government policies that protect them. Research on the causes of risky behaviors is much less developed than is research on their consequences, but even so, it is clear that behaviors are the results of multiple causes and can be influenced by health policy in multiple ways (Singer & Ryff, 2001; Berkman & Mullen, 1997). Obesity, for example, has a genetic component, as well as dietary, environmental, and economic correlates. Health promotion is concerned with generating improvements through whatever works. This orientation leads to combined approaches of research, public education, changes in the physical and social environment, regulation or even banning of disease-promoting activities, and improved access to high-quality health care.

Nursing Implications of Adult Disability and Risk Factors

What implications do these health demographics have for family nursing? Lower mortality means that more people will need care at older ages. But declines in disability mean that seniors are probably less likely than they used to be to require intensive, round-the-clock care, at least in their 60s and 70s. Fewer adults smoke, so the incidence of diseases stemming from tobacco use such as lung cancer and emphysema may decline. However, obesity is on the rise, increasing the need for counseling on diet, nutrition, and exercise.

Children

In many ways, the physical health of American children has never been better. When parents are asked to assess the overall health of their children, the vast majority (83 percent in 2001) rate their children's physical health as very good or excellent (Federal Interagency Forum on Child and Family Statistics, 2003). But fewer poor parents (71 percent) than nonpoor parents (86 percent) rate their children's overall health this well. Fewer African-American (74 percent) and Hispanic (77 percent) children are reported to be in very good or excellent health when compared with white children (87 percent). Younger children are generally reported to be in better health than are older children. The overall health of children was reported to be better in 2001 than in 1990 for children in each age, race/ethnic, and economic group.

Another indicator of the general health of American children is activity limitations that result from chronic conditions. Very few children who suffer from chronic health conditions have activity limitations requiring help from other people with personal-care needs, such as eating, bathing, dressing, getting around inside the home, or walking. In 2001, only 8 percent of children aged 5 to 17 had limitation of activities associated with physical, mental, or psychological chronic conditions (Federal Interagency Forum on Child and Family Statistics, 2003). Almost twice as many boys as girls are reported to have limitations in their activities. This difference exists mainly because more boys experience limitations associated with the need for special education. White and African-American children are more likely to have activity limitations than are Hispanic children. Poor children are more likely than are nonpoor children to experience limitations.

Although the U.S. infant mortality rate remains higher than in many other industrialized countries, both infant and child mortality rates have dropped significantly since 1960 (National Center for Health Statistics, 2003a, Table 22). Many serious illnesses, such as diphtheria and polio, have been greatly reduced through widespread inoculation campaigns. Most children may not enter school unless they have been vaccinated against several major childhood diseases. A significant increase in the likelihood that children receive all immunizations occurred in the latter part of the 1990s, although minority children are still less likely than are white children to receive these vaccines (Figure 2–1). Poor children (74 percent) are less likely to be immunized than are higher-income children (82 percent) (Federal Interagency Forum on Child and Family Statistics, 2003).

Infant mortality continues to decline while the percent of low birth weights has been stable or slightly rising (Table 2–1). These two trends may be intertwined, as more premature babies are kept alive by improvements in technology than in the past. The most striking finding is that the proportion of African-American infants that are low birth weight is about twice as high as that for white, Hispanic, Asian/Pacific-Islander, and Native-American/Alaska-Native infants. The infant mortality rate among African-American births is similarly more than twice as high as the white, Hispanic, and Asian/Pacific-Islander rates and substantially higher than the Native-American/Alaska-Native rate. The source of this difference is poorly understood. One might speculate that the difference exists because the African-American population, on average, is more likely to be poor and less educated than is the white population. However, if poverty and low education were the root cause, one would expect that the mortality rates of Hispanics and Native Americans would be higher as well, as they are also more likely to be in poverty and have low educations. In addition, African-American infant mortality rates are higher than white rates within each socioeconomic group. One reason for the increase in low-birth-weight infants is that the number of multiple births has also been rising, and multiple births such as twins, triplets, and so forth are much more likely to be of low birth weight (Federal Interagency Forum on Child and Family Statistics, 2003).

Adolescents

Once children survive the first year of life, their risk of death decreases dramatically. However, it rises again in the teen years as youths, especially males and minority youth, are subject to heightened risk of fatal motor vehicle accidents and homicides. Black males are extremely likely to be the victim of a homicide in their teenage years (Federal Interagency Forum on Child and Family Statistics, 2003). Boys' mortality rates are usually at least twice as high as girls' mortality rates for all of the most common causes of death. Hispanic teenage girls have the lowest mortality rates, and black teenage boys have the highest rates. Car accidents account for more deaths among white adolescents than among minority adolescents for both boys and girls.

As is the case with the older population, the percentage of teenagers who are overweight has been increasing dramatically. In the mid-1980s only 5 percent of children were overweight (Federal Interagency Forum on Child and Family Statistics, 2003). By 2000, the percentage had tripled and 15 percent of teenagers were overweight. Boys and girls are about equally likely to be overweight. Minority teenagers are more likely to be overweight than are whites. In 2000, slightly more than 1 in 10 white

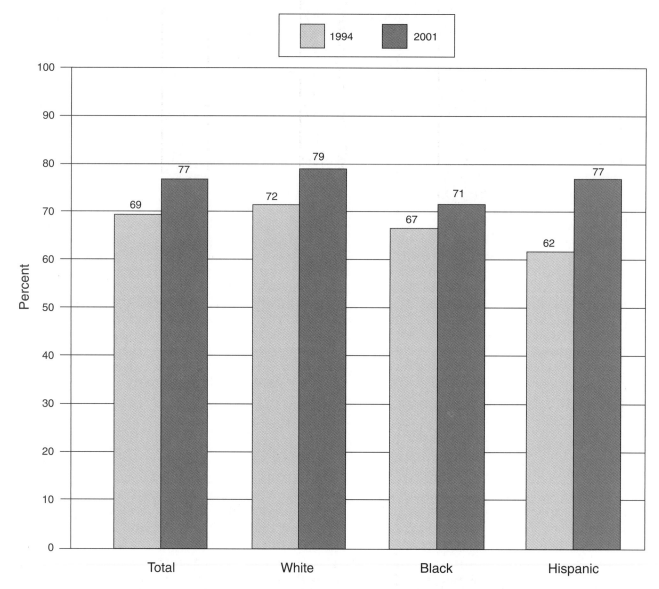

Figure 2–1   Percent of children 19–35 months with complete immunization[a]/vaccination: 1994 and 2001.
[a]Complete immunizations include four doses of diptheria, tetanus toxoids, pertussis vaccine (DPT), three doses of polio vaccine, measles containing vaccine (MCV), and three doses of Haemophilus influenzae-type b vaccine (Hib).
Note: Race/ethnicity categories are White, non-Hispanic; Black, non-Hispanic; and Hispanic.
Source: Federal Interagency Forum on Child and Family Statistics, 2003.

teenagers were overweight compared with about one in four of African-American and Mexican-American teenagers.

The teen years become the time of heightened experimentation with behaviors that engender health consequences. From 1991 to 2001, adolescent smoking and alcohol consumption remained relatively stable over the period, and the use of illicit drugs increased substantially (Table 2–2). However, there was a worrisome increase in regular cigarette use among high-school seniors from 19 percent in 1990 to 25 percent in 1997, but this rate declined to 17 percent by 2001 (Federal Interagency Forum on Child and Family Statistics, 2003). Interestingly, the risky

Table 2–1   LOW BIRTH WEIGHT (<2500 G) AND INFANT MORTALITY BY RACE, 1980 TO 2000

	1980	1990	2000
Percent Low Birth Weight			
Total	6.8	7.0	7.7
White	5.7	5.6	6.8
Black	12.7	13.3	13.1
Hispanic	6.1	6.1	6.5
Asian/Pacific Islander	6.7	6.5	7.3
American Indian/Alaska Native	6.4	6.1	6.8
Infant Mortality Rate (per 1000)[a]			
Total	10.9	8.9	6.9
White	9.2	7.2	5.7
Black	19.1	16.9	13.6
Hispanic	9.5	7.5	5.6
Asian/Pacific Islander	8.3	6.6	4.9
American Indian/Alaska Native	15.2	13.1	8.3

[a]Infant mortality rates are for 1983 rather than 1980, and 1997 rather than 1998.
Note: Unless otherwise noted, race/ethnicity categories are White, non-Hispanic; Black, non-Hispanic; Hispanic; Asian/Pacific Islander and American Indian/Alaska Native.
Source: Federal Interagency Forum on Child and Family Statistics, 2003.

behaviors of smoking, alcohol use, and drug use are all much more likely among whites than among minority youth (Casper & Bianchi, 2002). African-Americans were the least likely to report engaging in any of these behaviors. Research with new large data sets, such as the National Study of Adolescent Health, are just beginning to untangle the effects of peer influences, family factors, school climate, and neighborhood contexts on youth risk-taking behavior (Duncan et al., 2001; Harris et al. 2002).

❝ The teen years become the time of heightened experimentation with behaviors that engender health consequences. ❞

Children's Material Hardship

Living conditions for children have improved in many ways—especially in the poorest households (Mayer & Jencks, 1989). Poor children are increasingly better housed over time. The percentage of low-income chil-

dren living in homes without a complete bathroom or with leaky roofs, holes in the floor, no central heat, no electric outlets, or no sewer or septic system has declined substantially.

Poor children today are also more likely to receive medical attention than in the past. The percentage of children who had not visited a doctor in the previous year declined, especially during the 1970s. Poor children are more likely to be immunized than in the past. Children at the bottom of the income distribution became more likely to live in families that owned an air conditioner and had telephone service. In sum, children's general health has been improving, more children are receiving the inoculations, and mortality rates have improved, as have many of the health indicators for poor children. By contrast, obesity and illicit drug use are on the rise among teenagers. Family nursing students should be aware of these negative trends, but more important, they should note that poor and minority children are likely to fare worse on nearly all of these measures.

Table 2–2   SELECTED RISKY BEHAVIORS OF ADOLESCENTS

		1991	2001
Adolescent Birth Rate (per 1000)			
Age	15–17	38.7	24.7
	18–19	94.4	76.1
Percent Smoking Daily in Past 30 Days			
8th grade		7.2	5.5
10th grade		12.6	12.2
12th grade		18.5	19
Percent Consuming 5+ Drinks in a Row in Past 2 Weeks			
8th grade		12.9	13.2
10th grade		22.9	24.9
12th grade		29.8	28.6
Percent Using Illicit Drugs in Past 30 Days			
8th grade		5.7	11.7
10th grade		11.6	22.7
12th grade		16.4	25.7

Source: Federal Interagency Forum on Child and Family Statistics, 2000 and 2003.

SUMMARY

Families change in response to economic conditions, cultural change, and shifting demographics such as the aging of the population and immigration. The United States has gone through a particularly tumultuous period in the last few decades, resulting in rapid change in family behaviors. Families have emerged more diverse: there are more single-mother and single-father families and more families with all parents in the labor force than was true in the past. This translates into less time for parents to take care of the health needs of the family. Single mothers may find it particularly challenging to meet the health care needs of their families because they tend to have the least time and money to do so. More fathers are taking responsibility for caring for their children and will be increasingly likely to be the parent with whom the nurse interacts. More grandparents are raising their grandchildren, and children who are being raised by grandparents tend to suffer from more health problems than do other children. Many families maintained by grandparents are in poverty, and many of the grandparents in these families suffer from poor health

themselves. Family nurses may be increasingly likely to provide care to grandparent families, and they should be aware of the unique health and financial challenges these families face.

As mortality rates at the older ages continue to improve and baby boomers move into their retirement years, increasing proportions of the population will be elderly. This demographic shift will increase the need for nurses who specialize in caring for the elderly. With the aging of the population, more adults will have children and parents whom they must care for. Family nurses should be aware that meeting the needs of both groups will be challenging for working families, in terms of both time and money.

Today, more Americans come from other countries than was true in the past. Many of these Americans speak a language other than English. Because immigrants are more evenly spread out across the country than they used to be, many more family nurses will be providing care for a more ethnically and culturally diverse population.

Demographic health data indicate that mortality rates, disability, and smoking have been declining in the adult population. However, obesity is on the rise, increasing the need for nurses who specialize in diet, nutrition, and exercise. The general health of children has improved over the past decade, but racial and economic disparities still exist, with minority and poor children faring the worst. Increasing proportions of teenagers are overweight, and more of them are using illicit drugs.

Economics and family relationships remain intertwined. Issues growing in importance include balancing paid work with child rearing, gender income inequality, fathers' parenting roles, and relationship changes due to the increase in life expectancy. Families have been amazingly adaptive and resilient in the past; one would expect them to be so in the future.

The findings and opinions expressed are attributable to the authors and do not necessarily reflect those of the National Institute on Aging or the National Institute of Child Health and Human Development.

STUDY QUESTIONS

1. List two ways in which single-parent families are formed.

2. Name a demographic health trend for adults that has been worsening over the past decade.

3. Name a demographic health trend for teenagers that has been worsening over the past decade.

4. Discuss additional implications for nurses of the following demographic trends:
   a. Increases in single-mother families
   b. Increases in single-father families
   c. Increases in cohabiting-couple families
   d. Increases in grandparent-maintained families
   e. Declines in married-couple families with children
   f. Changes in living arrangements among young adults and the elderly
   g. Increases in the immigrant population
   h. The aging of the population

5. Identify two national statistical agencies and describe the types of data provided by each and the major sources of the data.

6. Describe why it is important to standardize health and family statistics by age.

7. Discuss why it is important to take into account race/ethnicity and socioeconomic status in caring for patients.

References

Aber, J. L. (2000). Welfare reform at three—Is a new consensus emerging? *News and Issues, 10*(1), 1. National Center for Children in Poverty.

Berkman, L. F., & Mullen, J. M. (1997). How health behaviors and social environment contribute to health differences between black and white older Americans. In L. G. Martin & B. J. Soldo (Eds.), *Racial and ethnic differences in the health of older Americans* (pp. 163–182). Washington, DC: National Academy Press.

Bianchi, S. M. (1995). The changing demographic and socioeconomic characteristics of single-parent families. *Marriage and Family Review, 20,* 71–97.

Bianchi, S. M. (2000). Maternal employment and time with children: Dramatic change or surprising continuity? *Demography, 37*(4), 401–414.

Bianchi, S. M., & Casper, L. M. (2000). American families. *Population Bulletin, 55*(4), 1–44.

Bittman, M. (1999). *Recent changes in unpaid work.* Occasional paper. Sydney: Social Policy Research Centre, University of New South Wales.

Bryson, K., & Casper, L. M. (1999). Coresident grandparents and grandchildren. *Current Population Reports* (P23–198). Washington, DC: U.S. Census Bureau.

Bumpass, L. L. (1990). What's happening to the family? Interactions between demographic and institutional change. *Demography, 27*(4), 483–493.

Bumpass, L. L., & Lu, H. (2000). Trends in cohabitation and implications for children's family contexts in the United States. *Population Studies, 54*(1), 29–41.

Bumpass, L. L., & Raley, R. K. (1995). Redefining single-parent families: Cohabitation and changing family reality. *Demography, 32*(1), 97–109.

Bumpass, L. L., & Sweet, J. A. (1989). National estimates of cohabitation. *Demography, 26*(4), 615–625.

Cancian, M., & Meyer, D. R. (1998). Who gets custody? *Demography, 35*(2), 147–158.

Casper, L. M., & Bianchi, S. M. (2002). *Continuity and change in the American family.* Thousand Oaks, CA: Sage.

Casper, L. M., & Cohen, P. (2000). How does POSSLQ measure up? Historical estimates of cohabitation. *Demography, 37*(2), 237–245.

Chalfie, D. (1994). *Going it alone: A closer look at grandparents rearing grandchildren.* Washington, DC: American Association of Retired Persons.

Cherlin, A. J. (1992). *Marriage, divorce, remarriage.* Cambridge, MA: Harvard University Press.

Cherlin, A. J. (2000). How is the 1996 welfare reform law affecting poor families? In A. J. Cherlin (Ed.), *Public and private families: A reader* (2nd ed.). New York: McGraw-Hill.

Cotter, D. A., Hermsen, J. M., & Vannemena, R. (2004, forthcoming). *Gender inequality at work.* Washington, DC: Population Reference Bureau and Russell Sage Foundation.

Council of Europe. (1999). *Recent demographic developments in Europe 1999.* Brussels: Council of Europe Publishing.

Crimmins, E. M., & Ingegneri, D. G. (1990). Interaction and living arrangements of older parents and their children. *Research on Aging, 12*(1), 3–35.

Dowdell, E. B. (1995). Caregiver burden: Grandparents raising their high-risk children. *Journal of Psychosocial Nursing, 33*(3), 27–30.

Duncan, G. J., Harris, K. M., & Boisjoly, J. (2001). Sibling, peer, neighbor and schoolmate correlations as indicators of the importance of context for adolescent development. *Demography, 38*(3), 437–447.

Eggebeen, D. J., & Hogan, D. P. (1990). Giving between generations in American families. *Human Nature, 1*(3), 211–232.

Farley, R. (1996). *The new American reality: Who we are, how we got here, where we are going.* New York: Russell Sage Foundation.

Federal Interagency Forum on Child and Family Statistics. (2003). *America's children: Key national indicators of well-being, 2003.* Washington, DC: U.S. Government Printing Office.

Fischer, K., McCulloch, A., & Gershuny, J. (1999). *British fathers and children.* Working paper. Essex, U.K.: Institute for Social and Economic Research, University of Essex.

Freedman, V., Martin, L., & Schoeni, R. (2002). Recent trends in disability and functioning among older adults in the United States: A systematic review. *Journal of the American Medical Association, 288*(24), 3137–3146.

Fuchs, V. R., & Garber, A. M. (2003). Health and medical care. In H. J. Aaron, J. M. Lindsay, & P. S. Nivola (Eds.), *Agenda for the nation* (pp. 145–182). Washington, DC: Brookings Institution Press.

Fuller-Thomson, E., Minkler, M., & Driver, D. (1997). A profile of grandparents raising grandchildren in the United States. *Gerontologist, 37*, 406–411.

Furstenberg, F., Jr. (1998). Good dads–bad dads: Two faces of fatherhood. In A. J. Cherlin (Ed.), *The changing American family and public policy* (pp. 193–218). Washington, DC: The Urban Institute.

Garasky, S., & Meyer, D. R. (1996). Reconsidering the increase in father-only families. *Demography, 33*(3), 385–393.

Goldscheider, C., & Goldscheider, F. K. (1994). Leaving and returning home in 20th century America. *Population Bulletin, 48*(4). Washington, DC: Population Reference Bureau.

Goldscheider, C., & Jones, M. B. (1989). Living arrangements among the older population. In F. K. Goldscheider & C. Goldscheider (Eds.), *Ethnicity and the new family economy* (pp. 75–91). Boulder, CO: Westview Press.

Goldscheider, F., Hogan, D., & Bures, R. (2001). A century (plus) of parenthood: Changes in living with children, 1880–1990. *History of the Family, 6*, 477–494.

Harris, K. M., Duncan, G. J., & Boisjoly, J. (2002). Evaluating the role of 'nothing to lose' attitudes on risky behavior in adolescence. *Social Forces, 80*(3), 1005–1039.

Hernandez, D. J. (Ed.). (1999). *Children of immigrants: Health, adjustment, and public assistance.* Washington, DC: National Academy Press.

Heuveline, P., et al. (2003). Shifting child rearing to single mothers: Results from 17 Western nations. *Population and Development Review, 29*(1), 47–71.

Holden, K. C. (1988). Poverty and living arrangements among older women: Are changes in economic well-being underestimated? *Journal of Gerontology: Social Sciences, 43*(1), S22–S27.

King, R. B. (1999). Time spent in parenthood status among adults in the United States. *Demography, 36*(3), 377–385.

Kramarow, E. (1995). Living alone among the elderly in the United States: Historical perspectives on household change. *Demography, 32*(2), 335–352.

Levy, F. (1998). *The new dollars and dreams.* New York: Russell Sage Foundation.

Lugaila, T. (2000). Marital status and living arrangements: March 1998 (update). *Current Population Reports, P20–514: Detailed Tables.* U.S. Census Bureau. Retrieved October 18, 2000, from http://www.census.gov/prod/99pubs/p20-514u.pdf

Mancini, J., & Blieszner, R. (1989). Aging parents and adult children: Research themes in intergenerational relations. *Journal of Marriage and the Family, 51*, 275–290.

Mayer, S. E., & Jencks, C. (1989, March). Growing up in poor neighborhoods: How much does it matter? *Science, 243*, 1441–1446.

McGarry, K., & Schoeni, R. F. (2000). Social security, economic growth, and the rise in elderly widows' independence in the twentieth century. *Demography, 37*(2), 221–236.

McLanahan, S., & Casper, L. (1995). Growing diversity and inequality in the American family. In R. Farley (Ed.), *State of the union: America in the 1990s* (Vol. 2, pp. 1–46). New York: Russell Sage Foundation.

McNeil, J. (2001). Americans with disabilities, 1997. *Current Population Reports,* P70–P73.

Minkler, M., & Roe, K. M. (1993). *Grandmothers as caregivers: Raising children of the crack cocaine epidemic.* Newbury Park, CA: Sage.

Minkler, M., & Roe, K. M. (1996). Grandparents as surrogate parents. *Generations, 20,* 34–38.

Morgan, S. P. (1996). Characteristic features of modern American fertility. In J. B. Casterline, R. D. Lee, & K. A. Foote (Eds.), *Fertility in the United States: New patterns, new theories* (pp. 19–66). New York: The Population Council.

Mutchler, J. (1992). Living arrangements and household transitions among the unmarried in later life. *Social Science Quarterly, 73,* 565–580.

National Center for Health Statistics. (1999, December). United States life table, 1997. *National Vital Statistics Reports, 47*(28).

National Center for Health Statistics. (2000, July). Deaths: Final data for 1998. *National Vital Statistics Reports, 48*(11).

National Center for Health Statistics. (2001). *Healthy People 2000 final review.* Hyattsville, MD: Public Health Service.

National Center for Health Statistics. (2003a). *Health, United States 2003, with chartbook on trends in the health of Americans.* Hyattsville, MD: Public Health Service.

National Center for Health Statistics. (2003b, December). Births: Final data for 2002. *National Vital Statistics Reports, 52*(10).

National Women's Conference Committee. (1986). *National plan of action update.* Washington, DC: Author.

Navaie-Walsier, M., et al. (2001). The experiences and challenges of informal caregivers: Common themes and differences among whites, blacks, and Hispanics. *Gerontologist, 41*(6), 733–741.

Pleck, E. H., & Pleck, J. H. (1997). Fatherhood ideals in the United States: Historical dimensions. In M. E. Lamb (Ed.), *The role of the father in child development* (3rd ed., pp. 33–48). New York: John Wiley & Sons.

Popenoe, D. (1993). American family decline, 1960–1990: A review and appraisal. *Journal of Marriage and the Family, 55*(3), 527–555.

Raley, R. K. (1999). *Then comes marriage? Recent changes in women's response to a non-marital pregnancy.* Presented at the annual meeting of the Population Association of America, New York.

Raley, R. K. (2000). Recent trends and differentials in marriage and cohabitation. In L. Waite (Ed.), *Ties that bind: Perspectives on marriage and cohabitation* (pp. 19–39). New York: Aldine de Gruyter.

Reinhardt, U. E. (2003). Does the aging of the population really drive the demand for health care? *Health Affairs, 22*(6), 27–39.

Rindfuss, R. R. (1991). The young adult years: Diversity, structural change, and fertility. *Demography, 28*(4), 493–512.

Rossi, A. S., & Rossi, P. H. (1990). *Of human bonding: Parent-child relations across the life course.* New York: Aldine de Gruyter.

Ruggles, S. (1994). The transformation of American family structure. *American Historical Review, 99*(1), 103–127.

Ruggles, S. (1996). Living arrangements of the elderly in America: 1880–1990. In T. Harevan (Ed.), *Aging and generational relations: Historical and cross-cultural perspectives* (pp. 254–263). New York: Aldine de Gruyter.

Ruggles, S., & Goeken, R. (1992). Race and multigenerational family structure in the United States, 1900–1980. In S. South & S. Tolnay (Eds.), *The American family: Patterns and prospects* (pp. 15–42). Boulder, CO: West Wind Production.

Rutrough, T. S., & Ofstedal, M. B. (1997, March). *Grandparents living with grandchildren: A metropolitan-nonmetropolitan comparison.* Presented at annual meeting of the Population Association of America, Washington, DC.

Saenz, R. (2004, forthcoming). *Latinos and the changing face of America*. Washington, DC: Population Reference Bureau.

Sandberg, J. F., & Hofferth, S. L. (1999). *Changes in parental time with children, U.S. 1981–1997*. Paper presented at the annual meeting of the International Association of Time Use Research, University of Essex, Colchester, England, October 6–8, 1999.

Shore, R. J., & Hayslip, B., Jr. (1994). Custodial grandparenting: Implications for children's development. In A. E. Gottfried & A. W. Gottfried (Eds.), *Redefining families: Implications for children's development* (pp. 171–218). New York: Plenum.

Silverstein, M. (1995). Stability and change in temporal distance between the elderly and their children. *Demography, 32*(1), 29–46.

Singer, B. H., & Ryff, C. D. (Eds.). (2001). *New horizons in health: An integrative approach/ Committee on Future Directions for Behavioral and Social Sciences Research at the National Institutes of Health, Institute of Medicine*. Washington, DC: National Academy Press.

Spain, D., & Bianchi, S. M. (1996). *Balancing act: Motherhood, marriage and employment among American women*. New York: Russell Sage Foundation.

Speare, A., Jr., & Avery, R. (1993). Who helps whom in older parent-child families? *Journal of Gerontology: Social Sciences, 48*(2), S64–S73.

Spitze, G., & Logan, J. R. (1990). Sons, daughters, and intergenerational social support. *Journal of Marriage and the Family, 52*(2), 420–430.

Stacey, J. (1993). Good riddance to 'the family': A response to David Popenoe. *Journal of Marriage and the Family, 55*(3), 545–547.

Thornton, A., & Young-DeMarco, L. (2001). Four decades of trends in attitudes toward family issues in the United States: The 1960s through the 1990s. *Journal of Marriage and the Family, 63*(4), 1009–1037.

Treas, J., & Torrecilha, R. (1995). The older population. In R. Farley (Ed.), *State of the union: America in the 1990s* (Vol. 2, pp. 47–92). New York: Russell Sage Foundation.

Uhlenberg, P. (1996). Mortality decline in the twentieth century and supply of kin over the lifecourse. *Gerontologist, 36*, 681–685.

U.S. Census Bureau. (2003a). *Statistical abstract of the United States 2003*. Washington, DC: U.S. Government Printing Office.

U.S. Census Bureau. (2003b). Households, by type: 1940 to present. Table HH-1 retrieved March 24, 2004, from *http://www.census.gov/population/www/socdemo/hh-fam.html*

U.S. Census Bureau (2003c). Estimated median age at first marriage, by sex: 1890 to the present. Table MS-2 retrieved March 24, 2004, from *http://www.census.gov/population/www/ socdemo/hh-fam.html*

U.S. Census Bureau. (2003d). Families by presence of own children under 18: 1950 to present. Table FM-1 retrieved March 24, 2004, from *http://www.census.gov/population/www/schdemo/ hh-fam.html*

U.S. Census Bureau. (2003e). All parent/child situations, by type, race, and Hispanic origin of householder or reference person: 1970 to present. Table FM-2 retrieved March 24, 2004, from *http://www.census.gov/population/www/socdemo/ hh-fam.html*

U.S. Census Bureau. (2003f). Grandchildren living in the home of their grandparents: 1970 to present. Table CH-7 retrieved March 24, 2004, from *http://www.census.gov/population/www/ socdemo/hh-fam.html*

Ventura, S. J., et al. (1995). The demography of out-of-wedlock childbearing. In National Center for Health Statistics (Ed.), *Report to Congress on out-of-wedlock childbearing* (pp. 1–133). Washington, DC: U.S. Department of Health and Human Services.

Waite, L. J., & Gallagher, M. (2000). *The case for marriage: Why married people are happier, healthier and better off financially*. Garden City, NY: Doubleday.

Weinick, R. M. (1995). Sharing a home: The experiences of American women and their parents over the twentieth century. *Demography, 32*(2), 281–297.

Wister, A. V. (1984). Living arrangement choices of the elderly: A decision-making approach. Ph.D. thesis, University of Western Ontario.

Wister, A. V., & Burch, T. K. (1987). Values, perceptions, and choice in living arrangements of the elderly. In E. F. Borgatte & R. J. V. Montgomery (Eds.), *Critical issues in aging policy* (pp. 180–198). Newbury Park, CA: Sage Publications.

Wolf, D. A., & Soldo, B. J. (1988). Household composition choices of older unmarried women. *Demography, 25*(3), 387–403.

Woroby, J. L., & Angel, R. J. (1990). Functional capacity and living arrangements of unmarried elderly persons. *Journal of Gerontology: Social Sciences, 45*(3), S95–S101.

Yee, J. L., & Schulz, R. (2000). Gender differences in psychiatric morbidity among family caregivers: A review and analysis. *Gerontologist, 40*(2), 147–164.

Bibliography

Bianchi, S. M. (2000). Maternal employment and time with children: Dramatic change or surprising continuity? *Demography, 37*(4), 401–414.

Bianchi, S. M., & Casper, L. M. (2000). American families. *Population Bulletin, 55*(4), 1–44. Washington, DC: Population Reference Bureau.

Bumpass, L. L. (1990). What's happening to the family? Interactions between demographic and institutional change. *Demography, 27*(4), 483–493.

Casper, L. M., & Bianchi, S. M. (2002). *Continuity and change in the American family*. Thousand Oaks, CA: Sage.

Casterline, J. B., Lee, R. D., & Foote, K. A. (Eds.). (1996). *Fertility in the United States: New patterns, new theories*. New York: The Population Council.

Cherlin, A. J. (1992). *Marriage, divorce, remarriage*. Cambridge, MA: Harvard University Press.

Decade in review: Understanding families into the new millennium. (2000). *Journal of Marriage and the Family* (Special Issue). Minneapolis: National Council on Family Relations.

Farley, R. (1996). *The new American reality: Who we are, how we got here, where we are going*. New York: Russell Sage Foundation.

Federal Interagency Forum on Child and Family Statistics. (2003). *America's children key national indicators of well-being, 2003*. Washington, DC: U.S. Government Printing Office.

Fields, J., & Casper, L. M. (2001). America's families and living arrangements, 2000. *Current Population Reports* (Series P20–537). Washington, DC: U.S. Census Bureau.

Levy, F. (1998). *The new dollars and dreams*. New York: Russell Sage Foundation.

Mayer, S. E. (1997). *What money can't buy: Family income and children's life chances*. Cambridge, MA: Harvard University Press.

McGarry, K., & Schoeni, R. F. (2000). Social security, economic growth, and the rise in elderly widows' independence in the twentieth century. *Demography, 37*(2), 221–236.

McLanahan, S., & Casper, L. (1995). Growing diversity and inequality in the American family. In R. Farley (Ed.), *State of the union: America in the 1990s* (Vol. 2, pp. 1–46). New York: Russell Sage Foundation.

McLanahan, S., & Sandefur, G. (1994). *Growing up with a single parent: What helps, what hurts?* Cambridge, MA: Harvard University Press.

McNeil, J. (2001). Americans with disabilities 1997. *Current Population Reports* (Series P70–73). Washington, DC: U.S. Census Bureau.

National Center for Health Statistics. (2001). *Healthy People 2000 final review*. Hyattsville, MD: Public Health Service.

National Center for Health Statistics. (2003). *Health, United States 2003, with chartbook on trends in the health of Americans.* Hyattsville, MD: Public Health Service.

Nock, S. L. (1998). *Marriage in men's lives.* New York: Oxford University Press.

Peters, H. E., Peterson, G. W., Steinmetz, S. K., & Day, R. D. (Eds.). (2000). *Fatherhood: Research interventions and policies.* New York: Haworth Press.

Ruggles, S. (1994). The transformation of American family structure. *American Historical Review, 99*(1), 103–127.

Spain, D., & Bianchi, S. M. (1996). *Balancing act: Motherhood, marriage, and employment among American women.* New York: Russell Sage Foundation.

Waite, L. J., Bachrach, C. A., Hinden, M., Thomson, E., & Thornton, A. T. (2000). *The ties that bind: Perspectives on marriage and cohabitation.* New York: Aldine de Gruyter.

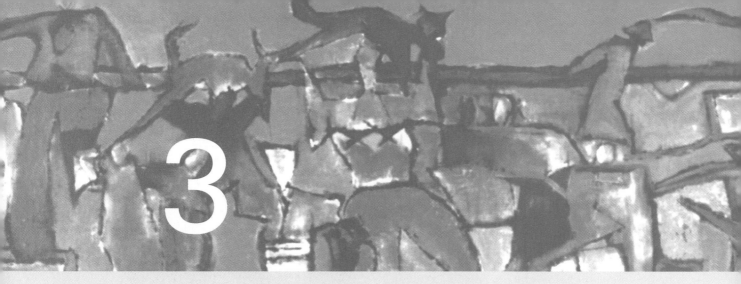

3

Theoretical Foundations for Nursing of Families

Shirley May Harmon Hanson, RN, PMHNP, PhD, FAAN, CFLE, LMFT
• Joanna Rowe Kaakinen, RN, PhD

CRITICAL CONCEPTS

- Using knowledge of nursing theory, practice, and research, nurses can consider options and interventions to support families. By understanding theories and models, the nurse is prepared to think creatively and critically about how the illness event is affecting the family client. Theories and models provide different ways of understanding issues that may be affecting families. As a result, theories offer choices for action.

- No single theory or conceptual framework adequately describes the complex relationships of family structure, function, and process.

- The major function of theory in family nursing is to provide knowledge and understanding that improves nursing care of families.

- The theoretical/conceptual frameworks and approaches that provide the foundations for nursing of families have evolved from three major traditions and disciplines: family social science, family therapy, and nursing.

- Nurses who use one theoretical approach to working with families limit the possibilities for families. By integrating several theories, nurses acquire different ways to conceptualize problems, thus enhancing thinking about interventions. Nurses who use an integrated theoretical approach build on the strengths of families in creative ways.

INTRODUCTION

Students often struggle to understand how theory relates to nursing practice. It is not uncommon for students to negate the importance of theory in practice. The saying "Theory and research inform family nursing practice, while this practice informs further family nursing theory development and research" appears not to be a concept readily understood by students. Basically the reciprocal relationship between theory, practice, and research is that each aspect informs the other, thereby expanding knowledge and nursing interventions to support families. By understanding theories and models, the nurse is better prepared to think creatively and critically about how the illness event is affecting the family client. Theories and models open doors to different ways of understanding issues that may be affecting families, and thereby offer options for action.

Vaughan-Cole, Johnson, Malone, and Walker (1998) presented numerous case studies of nurses working with families across the continuum of health care. Each family story was viewed from three different theoretical approaches: family systems theory, ecological framework for family nursing, and the resiliency model of family stress. In each case, the authors describe excellent family nursing. Significantly the authors discovered that by using different lenses to view the family health care problems, different solutions, options for care, and interventions surfaced. No one theoretical perspective stood out as yielding the "best" family nursing care. However, nurses who understand multiple theories and models are able to offer multiple solutions for families to consider in their adaptation to the health issue of the family. Nurses who draw from multiple theoretical lenses will integrate a variety of approaches into their care, thereby providing more holistic, family-centered nursing.

This chapter starts out with a review of components of a theory and how theories are analyzed and how they contribute to the nursing of families. Next the chapter will explore theories that serve as the foundation for the nursing of families: family social science, family therapy, and nursing. The chapter concludes with a discussion of integrated models for nursing care of families that are explained in more detail in Chapter 8.

WHAT IS THEORY?

Science is fundamentally concerned with ideas, data, and the relationships between them. *Theory* exists in

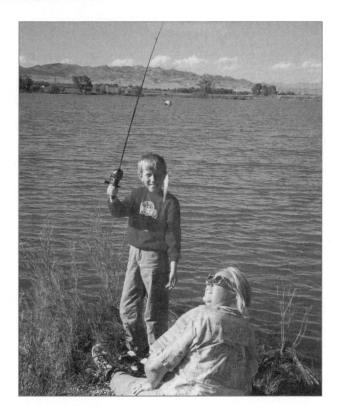

the realm of ideas (White and Klein, 2002, p. 3). *Theories* are abstract, general ideas that are subject to rules of organization. All theories are composed of concepts and the relationships between concepts. Theories are designed to make sense of the world—to show how one thing is related to another and how together they make a pattern that can predict the consequences of certain clusters of characteristics or events. All theories serve the function of describing, explaining, or making predictions about phenomena (LoBiondo-Wood & Haber, 2002). Nursing theories ideally represent logical and intelligible patterns that make sense of the observations a nurse makes in practice and enable the nurse to predict what is likely to happen to clients (Fawcett, 1999). The major function of theory in family nursing is to provide knowledge and understanding that improve nursing services to families.

> ❝The major function of theory in family nursing is to provide knowledge and understanding that improve nursing services to families.❞

Concepts, which are the building blocks of theory, are words that are mental images or abstract representations of phenomena. Concepts, or the major ideas expressed by a theory, may exist on a continuum from empirical (concrete) to abstract (Powers & Knapp, 1995). For example, family and health are highly abstract concepts; the routines and rituals of the family dinner are more concrete. The more abstract the concept, the greater the range of its definitions. For example, there are many ways in which to define and thus measure the concept of *family*, and there are even more definitions and ways to assess the concept of *health*.

Propositions are statements about the relationship between two or more concepts (Powers & Knapp, 1995). A proposition might be a statement, such as "The family as a unit interacts with the health of the individual members of the family." The word *interact* links the two concepts of family and health. A *hypothesis* is a way of stating an expected relationship between concepts. For example, using the concepts of family and health, one could hypothesize that there is an interactive relationship between how a family is coping and the health of family members. In other words, the family's ability to cope with stress affects the health of individual family members, and, in turn, the health of these individual members has an impact on the family's ability to cope. This hypothesis may be tested by a research study that measures family coping strategies and family members' health over time and uses statistical procedures to look at the relationships between the two concepts.

A *conceptual model* is a set of general propositions that integrates concepts into a meaningful configuration or pattern (Fawcett, 2000). Conceptual models in nursing are based on the observations, insights, and deductions that combine ideas from several fields of inquiry. Conceptual models provide a frame of reference and a coherent way of thinking about nursing phenomena. A conceptual model is more abstract and more comprehensive than a theory. Like a conceptual model, a conceptual framework is a way of integrating concepts into a meaningful pattern, but conceptual frameworks are often less definitive than models. They provide useful conceptual approaches or ways in which to look at a problem or situation rather than a definite set of propositions.

In this chapter, the terms *conceptual model* and *framework* are often used interchangeably, as are the terms *theory* and *theoretical framework*. In part, this is because there is no single, firm theoretical basis for the nursing of families. Rather, nurses draw from many theoretical conceptual foundations using a more pluralistic and eclectic approach. The interchangeable use of these various terms reflects the fact that there is considerable overlap between ideas in the various theoretical perspectives and conceptual models/frameworks and that there are many "streams of influence" that are important for family nurses to incorporate into practice.

As might be expected, there has been a substantial amount of cross-fertilization between disciplines, such as social science and nursing, and concepts originating in one theory or discipline have been translated into similar concepts for use in another discipline. At present, no single theory or conceptual framework adequately describes the complex relationships between family structure, function, and process, nor does one theoretical perspective give nurses a sufficiently broad base of knowledge and understanding to guide assessment and interventions with families. Box 3–1 lists the criteria for evaluating family theories that are useful for nursing of families.

In sum, theories help nurses accumulate and organize research findings into coherent patterns and to develop and test hypotheses or predictions of what the world will look like. Theories are systematic sets of ideas that make it possible to articulate ideas more clearly and specifically than in everyday language. Theories demonstrate how ideas are connected to each other. Most importantly theories explain what is happening; they provide answers to *how* and *why* questions, help to interpret and make sense of phenomena, and predict or point to what could happen in the future.

In nursing, the relationship of theory to practice constitutes a dynamic feedback loop rather than a static linear progression. That is, theory grows out of observations made in practice and is tested by research. Tested theory informs practice, and practice, in turn, facilitates the further refinement and development of theory. Figure 3–1 depicts the dynamic relationship between theory, practice, and research. Thus, theory, practice, and research related to the nursing of families are mutually dependent on each other.

THEORETICAL AND CONCEPTUAL FOUNDATIONS FOR THE NURSING OF FAMILIES

The theoretical/conceptual frameworks and approaches that provide the foundation for the nursing of families evolved from three major traditions and disciplines: family social science, family therapy,

Box 3–1 **CRITERIA FOR EVALUATING FAMILY THEORIES**

Internal consistency: A theory that does not contain logically contradictory assertions.

Clarity or explicitness: The ideas in a theory are expressed in such a way that they are unambiguous. They are defined and explicated where necessary.

Explanatory power: A theory explains well what it is intended to explain.

Coherence: They key ideas are integrated or interconnected and loose ends are avoided.

Understanding: A theory provides a comprehensible sense of the whole phenomenon being examined.

Empirical fit: A large portion of the tests of a theory have been confirmatory or, at least, have not been interpreted as not disconfirming.

Testability: The theory can be empirically supported or refuted.

Heuristic value: A theory has generated or can generate considerable research and intellectual curiosity (including a large number of empirical studies, as well as much debate or controversy).

Groundedness: A theory has been built from detailed information about events and processes observable in the world.

Contextualization: A theory gives serious consideration to the social and historical contexts affecting or affected by its key ideas.

Interpretive sensitivity: A theory reflects the experiences practiced and felt by the social units to which it is applied.

Predictive power: A theory can successfully predict phenomena that have occurred since the theory was formulated.

Practical utility: A theory can be readily applied to social problems, policies, and programs of action (i.e., it is useful for teaching, clinical work, political action, or some combination of these).

Source: Adapted from White, J. M., & Klein, D. M. (2002). *Family theories* (2nd ed.). Thousand Oaks, CA: Sage Publications.

and nursing. Figure 3–2 shows the theoretical frameworks that influence the nursing of families. Box 3–2 lists theoretical foundations used in family nursing practice. Of these sources of theory, family social science theories are best developed and informative

about family phenomena, such as family function, the environment-family interchange, interactions and dynamics within the family, changes in the family over time, and the family's reaction to health and illness. However, it is somewhat difficult to use family social

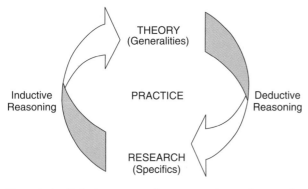

Figure 3–1 Relation among theory, practice, and research. Adapted from Ingoldsby, B., Smith, S., & Miller, J. (2004). *Exploring family theories*. Los Angeles: Roxbury.

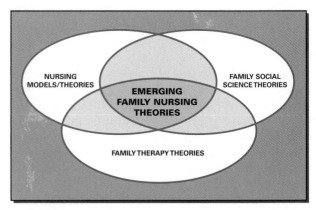

Figure 3–2 Theoretical frameworks that influence the nursing of families.

Table 3–1 DIFFERENCES AMONG FAMILY SOCIAL THEORIES, FAMILY THERAPY THEORIES, AND NURSING MODELS AND THEORIES

CRITERIA	FAMILY SOCIAL SCIENCE THEORIES	FAMILY THERAPY THEORIES	NURSING THEORIES
Purpose of theory	Descriptive and explanatory (academic models); to explain family functioning and dynamics	Descriptive and prescriptive (practice models); to explain family dysfunction and guide therapeutic actions	Descriptive and prescriptive (practice models); to guide nursing assessment and intervention efforts
Discipline focus	Interdisciplinary (although primarily sociological)	Marriage and family therapy; family mental health; new approaches focus on family strengths	Nursing focus
Target population	Primarily "normal" families (normality-oriented)	Primarily "troubled" families (pathology-oriented)	Primarily families with health and illness problems

Adapted from Jones, S.L., & Dimond, S.L. (1982). Family theory and family therapy models: Comparative review with implications for nursing practice. *Journal of Psychiatric Nursing and Mental Health Services, 20(10), 12-19.*

science theories as a basis for nursing assessment and intervention because of the abstract nature of these theories. In recent years, nursing scholars have made strides in extrapolating and developing these theories for application in nursing practice (Berkey & Hanson, 1991; Bomar, 2004; Danielson, Hamel-Bissell, & Winstead-Fry, 1993; Friedemann, 1995; Friedman, Bowden, & Jones, 2003; Hanson, 2001; Kaakinen & Hanson, 2004; Vaughn-Cole, Johnson, Malone, & Walker, 1998; Wright & Leahey, 2000). Table 3–1 shows the differences between family social science theories, family therapy theories, and nursing models.

Family therapy theories are newer and less well-developed than family social science theories, but they are more relevant to the nursing of families because they emanate from a practice discipline rather than an academic discipline. Thus, today family nursing theory, practice, research, and education draw heavily from family therapy theories. Family nurses are urged to reformulate existing family therapy theories to fit the nursing paradigm.

Finally, of the three types of theories, nursing conceptual frameworks are the least developed. During the 1960s and 1970s, nurses placed great emphasis on the development of nursing models. However, many of these models originated from an individualized medical paradigm and few have evolved to be useful for the nursing practice or interventions with families.

Family Social Science Theories

Family social science theories were developed from various social science disciplines, primarily sociology. These ideas emerged during the first half of the 20th century, and by the early 1950s, scholars were beginning to organize the accumulated conceptual knowledge on the family. Historically, structural-functional theory, symbolic interaction theory, and developmental theory have been described as family social science theory. However, much can be learned about working with families from other theories, such as systems theory, stress theory, and change theory. All of these theories are reviewed in the next sections. Table 3–2 is a summary of the key social science theories addressed in this chapter.

Family social science theories were originally developed with little thought for practical use by clinicians. Over the last several decades, however, three major works explored the development of family social science with emphasis on its usefulness for practice. Boss, Doherty, Schumm, and Steinmetz (1993) traced

Box 3–2 THEORETICAL FOUNDATIONS USED IN FAMILY NURSING PRACTICE

Family Social Science Theories

- Structural-functional theory
- Systems theory
- Family developmental theory
- Family interactional theory
- Family stress theory
- Change theory
- Others
    - Chaos theory
    - Social exchange theory
    - Conflict theory
    - Ecological theory
    - Anthropological/multicultural theory
    - Phenomenological theory

Family Therapy Theories

- Structural family therapy theory
- Family systems therapy theory
- Interactional family therapy theory
- Others
    - Psychodynamic therapy theory
    - Experiential therapy theory
    - Humanistic therapy theory
    - Strategic therapy theory
    - Behavioral/cognitive therapy theory

- Narrative therapy theory
- Solution-oriented therapy theory

Nursing Models and Theories

- Systems theory
    - King
    - Roy
    - Neuman
    - Orem
    - Rogers
    - Friedemann
    - Parse
    - Denham
- Others
    - Leininger
    - Watson
    - Peplau
    - Barnard
    - Newman

Integrated

- Hanson & Mischke
- Friedman
- Wright & Leahey
- McCubbin & McCubbin

the development of family theory from its origins in religion and philosophy through the construction of theory and methodology in the mid-20th century to the latest emerging models. Their book emphasizes the interaction between theories and methods. White and Klein (2002) reviewed the major theoretical frameworks from the social sciences perspective that are used to understand families further. In addition to symbolic interaction framework, family life course development framework, and the systems framework, they discuss social exchange and choice frameworks, conflict frameworks, feminist frameworks, and ecological frameworks. Winton (1995) summarized frameworks used by scholars and researchers in analyzing families. Sources such as these that synthesize the literature serve to make the knowledge base of the family social sciences more accessible for practice disciplines. The next section summarizes the major theories from the family social sciences that have been useful to the understanding of families and the practice of family nursing. (See Table 3–2.)

Structural-Functional Theory

In *structural-functional theory*, the family is considered a small group that has features common to all small groups. The family is viewed as a social system. This theory assumes that social systems carry out functions that serve individuals and society. The individuals in the family act in accordance with a set of internalized norms and values, which are learned primarily through socialization.

Family analysis involves examining the arrangement of members within the family, relationships between the members, and relationships of the members to the whole (Artinian, 1994; Hanson & Kaakinen, 2001; Friedman, Bowden, Jones, 2003). The family is viewed in terms of its relationships with other major social

Table 3–2 **SUMMARY OF SOCIAL SCIENCE THEORIES**

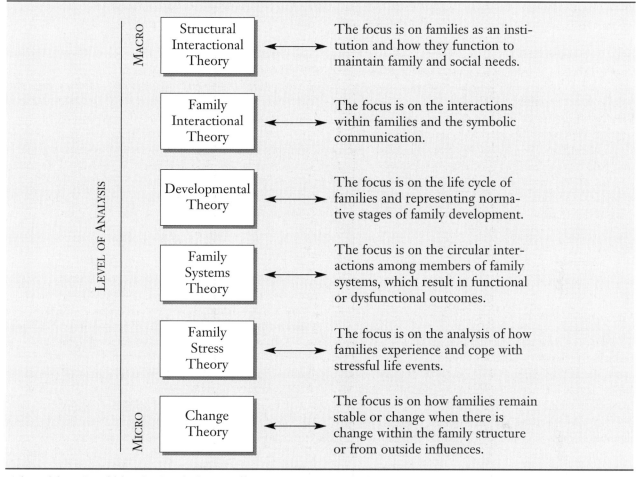

Adapted from Ingoldsby, G., Smith, S., & Miller, J. (2004). *Exploring family theories.*
Los Angeles: Roxbury.

institutions, such as health care, religion, education, government, and the economy. The primary aim of this theoretical perspective is to consider the family in the overall structure of society and see how family patterns interact with other institutions. From this perspective, the basic functions of families are considered to be economic, reproductive, protective, cultural, social, status conferring, relationship developing, and health maintaining (Hanson, 2001; Kaakinen, Hanson, & Birenbaum, 2004). A central issue is how well the family structure allows the family to perform its functions. Family theorists who use this approach want to understand the social or family system and its relationship to the overall social system (Nye & Berardo, 1981).

Family is characterized as open to outside influences while maintaining its boundaries. The family, however, is seen as a passive adapting institution rather than an agent of change. This approach tends to take a static view of the societal structure and to neglect change as a structural dynamic. The illness of a family member inevitably brings alterations in the family structure and function. For example, if a single mother is ill, she cannot carry out her usual and various roles, so grandparents or siblings may have to assume child care responsibilities. Clearly the illness of the single mother changes the power structure and communication patterns of the family. Assessment includes determining whether the changes caused by the mother's illness will affect the family's ability to carry out its functions. The terminal or chronic illness of a family member also affects family structure and functioning. Using the structural-functional perspective, assessment questions during the chronic illness of a family member might include these: What family roles were altered by the onset of the chronic illness? How did the illness alter the family structure? Intervention becomes necessary when changes in family structure alter the family's ability to function. Interventions might include assisting families to use existing support structures and community resources and assisting families to modify their organization so that role responsibilities can be redistributed.

The major strength of the structural-functional approach to family nursing practice is that it is comprehensive and views families within the context of the broader community. The major weakness of this approach is that it is static and tends to view families at one moment in time rather than as a social system that changes over time.

Interactional Theory

The *family interactional theory* is derived from a major theory in social psychology and sociology called symbolic interaction theory (Hill & Hansen, 1960; Rose, 1962; Turner, 1970). In the interactional approach, the family is viewed as a unit made up of interacting personalities. It examines internal family dynamics, including communication processes, roles, decision making and problem solving, and socialization patterns (Rose, 1962).

The interactional approach places major emphasis on family roles. That is, each member of the family is considered to occupy formal and informal positions. Family members expect to perform their roles in certain ways, depending on their perceptions of role demands by the family as a whole and by other individuals in the family. Family members judge their own behavior by obtaining feedback from others in the family. The responses of these other family members serve to challenge or reinforce the way that an individual family member carries out its roles (Nye, 1976). That is why the theory is called *interactional*.

Understanding families via the interactional approach is particularly useful in family nursing because its focus is on internal processes of social interaction within families rather than on the outcomes of these interactions. The major problem with this interaction focus is that the family is seen as existing in a vacuum, with no consideration of the environment or the family's history, culture, or socioeconomic status. In the interactional approach, families are considered to be comparatively closed units, and the external world is thought to have little effect on what occurs within the family. This view ignores the influence of the external world on the family and interactions within the family.

Working from an interactional perspective, the family health care nurse assesses interaction and communication between family members, family roles and power distribution, family coping, and family socialization patterns, as well as relationships between marital partners, siblings, and parent/children. The nurse intervenes on the basis of the family's needs for health promotion, health maintenance, or health restoration in these areas.

Developmental Theory

Developmental theory lies at the core of nursing. Developmental stages have been elaborated by Erikson, Piaget, and others, and every nursing student learns these stages for individuals. According to developmental theory, human beings have specific tasks at specific periods in their life span, and successful achievement of the tasks at one stage of life leads to happiness and success with later tasks. Failure to achieve tasks leads to unhappiness, disapproval, and difficulty in achieving later tasks. Table 3–3 outlines the traditional family life-cycle stages and tasks.

Duvall (1977) and Duvall & Miller (1985) applied the principles of individual development to the family as a unit. Duvall identified overall family tasks that need to be accomplished for each stage of family development, beginning with a couple's marriage and ending with death. Development implies movement to a higher level of functioning or unidirectional progression. Disequilibrium occurs during the transitional periods from one stage to the other. The family has a predictable natural history; the first stage involves the simple husband-wife pair and the group becomes more complex over time with the addition of new positions or members. When the younger generation leaves home to take jobs or marry, the family group becomes less complex again.

Even though there are family developmental needs and tasks that must be performed at each family life-cycle stage, developmental tasks are general goals rather than specific jobs that are completed at once. Achievement of family developmental tasks enables individuals in the family to achieve their own individual tasks.

Table 3–3 TRADITIONAL FAMILY LIFE-CYCLE STAGES AND DEVELOPMENTAL TASKS

STAGES OF FAMILY LIFE CYCLE	FAMILY DEVELOPMENTAL TASKS
Married couple	• Establishing relationship as a married couple • Blending of individual needs, developing conflict and resolution approaches and communication and intimacy patterns
Childbearing families with infants	• Adjusting to pregnancy and then infant • Adjusting to new roles: mother and father. • Maintaining couple bond and intimacy
Families with preschool children	• Understanding normal growth and development • If more than one child in family, adjusting to different temperaments and styles of children • Coping with energy depletion • Maintaining couple bond and intimacy
Families with school-age children	• Working out authority and socialization roles with school • Supporting child in outside interests and needs • Determining disciplinary actions and family rules and roles
Families with adolescents	• Allowing adolescent to establish own identity but still be part of family • Thinking about the future, education, jobs, working • Increasing role of adolescent in family, cooking, repairs, and power base
Families with young adults—launching	• After member moves out, reallocating roles, space, power, and communication • Maintaining supportive home base • Maintaining parental couple intimacy and relationship
Middle-aged parents	• Refocusing on marriage relationship • Ensuring security after retirement • Maintaining kinship ties
Aging families	• Adjusting to retirement, grandparent roles, death of spouse, and living alone

Source: Adapted from Duvall, E. M., & Miller, B. (1985). *Marriage and family development* (6th ed.). New York: Harper & Row.

According to this developmental theory, every family is unique in its composition and in the complexity of its expectations of members at different ages and in different roles. Families, like individuals, are influenced by their history and traditions and by the social context in which they live. Furthermore, families change and develop in different ways because their internal and external demands and stimulations differ. Families may also arrive at similar developmental levels through different processes. However, despite their differences, families have enough in common to make it possible to chart family development over the life span in a way that applies to most, if not all, families.

By looking at the movement of families over time, developmental theory goes beyond the large-scale view of the family in the structural-functional framework and the small-scale analysis used in the interactional framework discussed previously. It attempts to integrate small- and large-scale analyses while viewing the family as an open system in relation to other configurations and systems in society (Hanson & Kaakinen, 2001). Developmental theory explains what changes occur (and how they occur), more or less uniformly, to all human organisms or family groups over time.

A major strength of the developmental approach is that it provides a framework for predicting what a family will experience at any period in the family life cycle. Family nurses can assess a family's stage of development, the extent to which the family has achieved the tasks associated with that stage of family development, and problems that exist. Clinical problems can be more easily anticipated. Family strengths

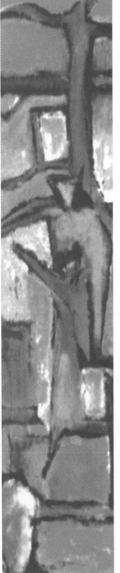

RESEARCH BRIEF

Purpose of Study

The purpose of this study was to understand coping in dual-career families. Do coping strategies differ by stage in the family life cycle? Are there differences in how dual-career women and men cope with stressful life circumstances?

Methodology

Data were collected from a purposive sample of dual-career couples. Subjects (329 couples) were recruited through professional organizations and word of mouth. The Dual-Employed Coping Scales (DECS) and an investigator-constructed questionnaire were completed by subjects. MANOVA and factor analysis with varimax rotation were used for statistical analysis.

Results

Coping strategy use differs significantly by gender and life-cycle stage. Women utilize the coping strategies of cognitive restructuring, delegating, limiting avocational activities, and using social support significantly more often than do men. Coping strategy use differ by life-cycle stage as well as by gender. Dual-career men and women without children at home use compartmentalizing significantly less frequently than those with children. When children are not a factor at home, both genders are more involved in their careers and experience less pressure.

Implications

Findings have potential implications for both male and female nurses. A number of different coping strategies are used according to gender and stage in the family life cycle. This information can be made available to nurses and their employers. Couples can be made aware of cognitive restructuring whereby focusing on the positive aspects of dual-career lifestyle can help reduce emotional responses such as guilt, anxiety, and frustration. Employers can implement career track models that offer greater flexibility in professional advancement for men and women wherever they are in the family life cycle. Further research needs to be done on the linkages between work and family in order to best optimize nursing resources and prevent burnout.

Source: Schnittger, M. H., & Bird, G. W. (1990). Coping among dual-career men and women across the family life cycle. *Family Relations, 31,* 199–205.

and available resources are easier to identify as they are based on assisting families to achieve developmental milestones and handling problems. Thus, this conceptualization provides a neat framework, both for assessing families and for intervening when necessary. A major weakness of the developmental framework is that it originated when the "traditional nuclear family" was considered the norm. Today, families vary widely in their makeup and in their roles. The traditional view that a family moves in a linear fashion from getting married, raising children, and then tracking these children through the children's adulthood to old age and death is no longer applicable. Families may not involve a marriage, a couple may go through divorce or adopt children, or they may become families with two sets of stepchildren through multiple divorces. Also, families may be made up of single parents and their children or same-sex parents. There are many types of families and many trajectories of families that do not fit within the traditional developmental framework.

Today the developmental framework remains useful as long as it is viewed as a general model for families, despite all the variations of families. In using the developmental model to conduct an assessment of families, there are several questions that can be asked: Where does this family lie on the continuum of family life-cycle stages? What are the developmental tasks that are and are not being accomplished? Depending on the assessment, nursing intervention strategies using this perspective might include helping families to understand individual and family growth and developmental stages and helping families recognize the transitions that must occur in moving from one developmental stage to the next (e.g., in moving from the tasks of the school-aged family to the tasks of an adolescent family). Interventions might also include helping the family understand the normalcy of disequilibrium in these transitional periods. Family nurses must recognize that in every family, both individual and family developmental tasks must be accomplished for every stage of the individual and family life cycle. Therefore, it is important for the nurse to keep in mind the needs and requirements of both the family as a whole and the individuals making up the family.

Systems Theory

Systems theory has been the most influential of all the family social science frameworks. This approach to understanding families was derived from physics and biology (von Bertalanffy, 1950, 1968). A system is composed of a set of interacting elements; each system is identifiable as distinct from the environment in which it exists. An open system exchanges energy and matter with the environment, while a closed system is isolated from its environment. Systems depend on both positive and negative feedback to maintain a steady state (homeostasis). Figure 3–3 shows how families maintain homeostasis from positive and negative feedback. The systems perspective assumes that family systems are greater than and different from the sum of their parts. The family system is an organized whole, and individuals in the family are interdependent and interactive. There are boundaries, however, in the system, which can be open, closed, or random. Further, there are hierarchies within the family system (mother-child) and logical relationships between subsystems (family-community). Every family system has features designed to maintain stability or homeostasis, although these features may be adaptive or maladaptive. At the same time, the family changes constantly in response to stresses and strains from the external environment, as well as from the internal family environment. Cause and effect are modified by feedback loops. Figure 3–4 depicts the feedback loop in systems theory. The patterns of family systems are circular rather than linear. The family system increases in complexity over time, and as a system the family increases its ability to adapt and to change.

The family system perspective encourages nurses to see individual clients as participating members of a family system. Figure 3–5 is a mobile that shows a family system in balance. For example, nurses who are using this perspective assess the effects of illness or injury on the entire family and the effects of family functioning on the individual with the illness or injury. Emphasis is on the whole rather than on individuals. Assessment questions that might be asked from this

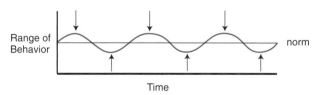

Figure 3–3 Family homeostatic response to positive and negative feedback from the environment. Adapted from Goldberg, I., & Goldberg, H. (2004). *Family therapy: An overview* (3rd ed.). Upper Saddle River, NJ: Merrill/ Prentice Hall.

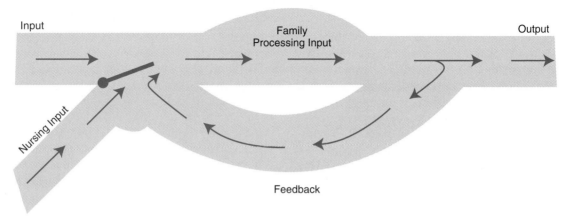

Figure 3–4   Family systems feedback loop. Adapted from Goldberg, I., & Goldberg, H. (2004). *Family therapy: An overview* (3rd ed.). Upper Saddle River, NJ: Merrill/ Prentice Hall.

perspective include the following: Who is in the family system? How has a family member's critical illness affected the family and its members? Interventions by family nurses must address individuals, subsystems within the family, and the whole family relative to process and function.

The strengths of the general systems framework is that this theory covers a large array of phenomena and views the family and its subsystems within the context of its suprasystems (the larger community in which it is embedded). Moreover, this is an interactional and holistic theory that looks at processes within the family rather than at the content and relationships between the members. The family is viewed as a whole, not as merely a sum of its parts. Unfortunately the strengths of the theory are also its limitations. Because this theoretical orientation is broad and general, it is difficult to apply to nursing practice.

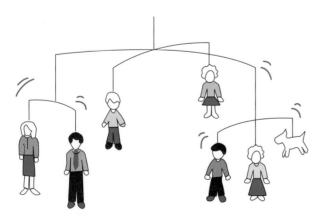

Figure 3–5   Mobile depicting family system.

Specific concepts and practice guidelines have to be developed outside the theory.

Family Stress Theory

The foundation for *family stress theory* comes from Hill's (1949) classic research on war-induced separations and reunions in families during World War II (McKenry & Price, 2000). Hill found that the experiences of families facing separations and reunions sometimes resembled a roller coaster. The stress of separation often led to crisis, and crisis led to a decline in family functioning or even disorganization in the family. The downward spiral, however, would be followed by an upward recovery curve resulting in a new higher level of family organization and functioning. Hill (1965) formulated his ABC-X theory of family crisis, which may be stated as follows:

A (the provoking or stressor event) is influenced by B (the family's resources or strengths), which is influenced by C (the definition or meaning attached to the event by the family), which results in X (stress or crisis). Furthermore, A is the event or stressor that, with its associated hardships, leads to changes in the family system. B refers to the strengths or resources of the family that enable it to deal with stressors. These resources include religious faith, financial resources, social support, physical health, family flexibility, and family coping mechanisms. C refers to the family's appraisal of the seriousness of stressor events or the subjective meaning that the family attaches to that event.

It is essential for the family nurse to understand that the family's definition of an event determines how they will deal with it and how stressful it will be for them. Nurses who view the family problem from the nurse's own perspective are at risk for not accurately understanding the way a family reacts to a specific event. A family will react to its own appraisal or definition rather than to the reality of the event. A, B, and C all influence the family's ability to prevent crisis as a result of stressor events. Changes created by stressors may lead to a crisis, which is X, or the amount of disruption of the family system caused by the stressful event. Families are more susceptible to crisis if they lack family resources and if they tend to appraise or define stressors or hardships as crisis-producing. See Figure 3–6, which shows the ABC-X model of family stress/crisis.

According to the family stress model, unexpected or unplanned events are usually perceived as stressful and have the potential to be disruptive to families. However, stressful events within families, such as serious illness, can be more disruptive than stressors that occur outside the family, such as floods, economic depression, or war. Ambiguous events, which the family has difficulty deciphering, are even more stressful than events that can be easily interpreted. If a family has not had previous experience with stressor events, the family is more likely to see events as stressful.

A dichotomous classification often used by family stress scholars is normal or predictable events versus nonnormative, unpredictable or situational events. Normal events are part of everyday life representing transitions inherent in the family life cycle such as birth, death, and retirement. Normative stressors are of short duration although they disturb system equilibrium. These events can lead to crisis if the family does not cope with the changes brought about by these events. Nonnormative events occur in a unique situation that was not predicted and is not likely to be repeated. Examples include natural disasters, loss of a job, or an automobile accident. Unexpected events that are not disastrous, such as winning the lottery, may also be stressful for families. The clustering of normative and/or nonnormative causes a "stress pileup," which could result in a major crisis.

McCubbin and Patterson (1983) expanded on Hill's ABC-X model by adding postcrisis/poststress factors to explain how families achieve a satisfactory adaptation to stress or crisis. Their model consisted of an ABC-X model followed by their "Double ABC-X" configuration. The *Double A* factor refers to the stressor pileup in the family system coming from unresolved aspects of the initial stressor, the changes and events that occur regardless of the initial stressor, and the consequences of the family's effort to cope with the hardships of the situation. The family's resources, the *Double B* factor, come from two courses: resources that are already available to the family that minimize the impact of the initial stressor, and personal, family, and social coping resources that are strengthened or developed in response to the stress. *Double C* refers to the perception of the initial stressor event, and the perception of the stress or crisis. *Double X* includes the original family crisis/stress response and subsequent adaptation. Figure 3–7 depicts the Double ABC-X Model of Family Stress/Crisis.

More recently, family scholars assessed family stress outcomes from a family strengths perspective (McCubbin & McCubbin, 1993; McKenry & Price, 2000). McCubbin and McCubbin (1993) developed the *Resiliency Model of Family Stress, Adjustment, and Adaptation.* See Figure 3–8, which shows the resiliency Model. According to the resiliency model, families are more likely to adapt successfully to an illness if

- They have fewer other family stressors or demands occurring at the same time.
- They have family types or patterns of functioning that are more adaptive (e.g., there is more emotional closeness between family members and they are more flexible and able to change roles, boundaries, and rules when necessary).

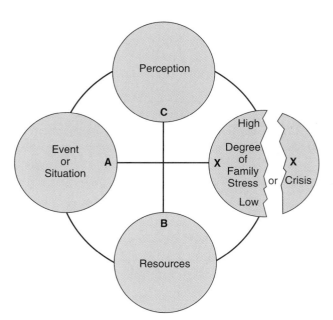

Figure 3–6 ABC-X model of family stress/crisis. Adapted from Hill, R. (1958), Social Stresses on the family: General features of families under stress. *Social Casework*, February, 139–150.

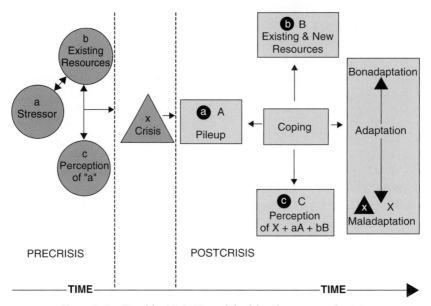

Figure 3–7 Double ABC-X model of family stress and crisis.

- They define the situation positively and view it as something they can master and have control over.
- They have good coping and communication skills.

Factors that influence how families respond to a member's illness include family stressors, family types, family resources, family appraisal, and family problem-solving, communication, and coping.

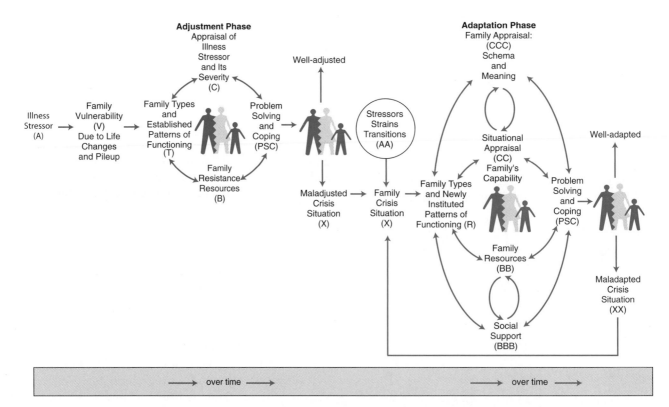

Figure 3–8 Resiliency Model of Family Stress, Adjustment, and Adaptation.

Family Stressors

"A stressor is a demand placed on the family that produces, or has the potential of producing, changes in the family system" (McCubbin & McCubbin, 1993, p. 28). Families are more vulnerable if they experience an accumulation or pileup of demands at the time that a member becomes ill. Demands on the family unit may include financial problems; work stresses; conflicts among family members, with the extended family or with former spouses; childbearing or child care strains; transitions of members in and out of the family; other illness or family care strains, such as care of an aging parent; recent losses of close relatives or friends; or legal violations (e.g., family member being arrested, sent to jail, or running away from home). Families rarely have to deal only with one member's illness. They also need to manage other normal expected transitions, as well as work and family demands. Existing strains in the family, such as spousal conflicts or parent-child tensions, may be exacerbated by illness. In addition, the illness itself brings new demands and changes. Negotiation with the health care system and decisions about treatment can go smoothly or become agonizingly difficult. There may be uncertainty about the diagnosis, the treatment options, and the prognosis. Complex conditions may require many types of providers, who may offer conflicting opinions about what the patient and family should do.

Family Resources

Family resources are those attributes and supports that are available for use by the family. McCubbin and McCubbin (1993) identified three different sources and levels of resources: the individual, the family unit, and the community. Resources from individual family members may include intelligence, personality traits, knowledge, skills, physical health, and psychological health. Family resources may include cohesion, adaptability, decision-making skills, organization, and conflict-resolution abilities. Resources from the community include personal support and institutional support (e.g., support from health care providers and other professionals). To date, social support is the community resource that has received the most attention in the study of family adaptation to illness.

Family Appraisal

The family appraisal of the illness, or the way the family sees the illness, is a critical factor in family adaptation. How do family members define the illness, and what does the illness mean to them? Do they see the illness as having an impact on them? Do they believe they have the resources and capabilities to handle what is happening? Are the family's goals, priorities, and expectations changed by the illness? Are these changes viewed as temporary or more permanent?

Family members will appraise the situation differently depending on their age, gender, role in the family, and experience. Coming to a shared understanding of the situation is difficult and demanding, and it is achieved only through perseverance, patience, negotiation, understanding, and shared commitment (McCubbin & McCubbin, 1993).

Family Problem Solving, Communication, and Coping

Family problem-solving communication influences family adaptation to illness. Two types of family communication have been found to predict family adaptation after the diagnosis of a child's congenital heart condition (McCubbin & McCubbin, 1993). Incendiary communication is characterized by bringing up old unresolved issues, failing to calmly talk things through to reach a solution, yelling and screaming at other family members, and walking away from conflicts without much resolution. This type of communication increases the stress. Affirming communication, as the name implies, is more supportive. It is characterized by being careful not to hurt other members emotionally or physically, taking time to hear what others have to say, conveying respect for others' feelings, and ending conflicts on a positive note. Families with more affirming communication and less incendiary communication are better able to adapt to the demands created by a member's illness.

Process of Family Adaptation to Illness

Families make trial-and-error efforts to sort out all the information they receive and decide on strategies to manage the illness situation. All families rely on previously established ways of functioning and coping to manage the initial crisis of a family member's illness. This period is the *family adjustment* phase in the resiliency model. Initially the family may totally reorganize around the member's illness, focusing only on the illness and neglecting other family needs. For short-term acute conditions, where recovery is predictable and complete, this adjustment on the part of the family system can work. In chronic illnesses and acute illnesses with prolonged recovery times, what seems to work at first may be detrimental to meeting the needs of family members and the family unit as a whole over the long haul. This is called the *family adaptation* phase in the model (Figure 3–8). For example, a mother may take time off from work to spend most of her time at the hospital bedside with an ill child, while the father tries to manage his work and the other children at home. This approach may work at first, but if the child's illness is prolonged, the workplace may not continue to tolerate the mother's absence, problems of reduced income and potential job loss may surface, and the other children may begin to feel neglected. Further, both parents can become exhausted with this arrangement. The family system is then in a state of *crisis*.

This does not mean the family is sick and needs fixing. It indicates that change is needed and new patterns of functioning should be tried. For instance, the mother may return to work part-time; the father may spend more time at the hospital; both parents may try to spend time with the siblings left at home; additional help from relatives may be sought to ease the burden on the parents; and if financial resources permit, outside help with household tasks and chores may be obtained. The family thus tries to achieve adaptation. In the resiliency model, this adaptation represents a fit at two levels of functioning: a fit of the individual and the family system (ensuring the care and well-being of family members and the family unit) and the fit of the family system with the community (including satisfactory relationships in the workplace and hospital).

Change Theory

Change theory is also relevant for family nurses. According to Bateson (1979), systems of relationships have a tendency toward progressive change. The proverb "the more something changes, the more it remains the same" (Wright & Leahey, 2000) underscores the paradoxical relationship between persistence (stability) and change. According to Maturana (1978; Maturana & Varela, 1992), changes in the family's structure occur as compensation for outside influences (perturbations) on the family system and paradoxically have the purpose of maintaining stability within the family. Watzlawick, Weakland, and Fisch (1974) considered that family changes are either first- or second-order changes. In first-order change, the system itself remains unchanged, although one or several of its parts undergo some type of change. For example, when parents learn a new behavioral strategy to discipline a child, the family remains the same, but with the new approach, the child, a part of the family, changes. Second-order change occurs, for instance, in the system itself. In second-order change, there are actual changes in the rules governing the system, and, therefore, the system is transformed structurally or in its communications. Second-order change occurs when parents begin to treat their teenager as a growing adult instead of as a young child. Because the teenager is no longer viewed as a child, the whole family system is now different.

Families do not change smoothly or in a linear fashion; rather, changes occur in leaps, creating patterns that did not exist before. Bateson (1979) stated that we are unaware of most changes and that we become accustomed to a new way of being before our senses advise us. Wright and Watson (1988) noted that "the most profound and sustaining changes [within a family] will be those that occur within the family's belief system (cognition)" (p. 425).

Wright and Leahey (2000) pointed out that change is dependent on the perception of the problem. Therefore, family nurses must recognize that there are as many truths or realities as there are members of a given family. The nurse must accept all these perceptions and offer the family another, more comprehensive view of their problem(s). Change is dependent on context so that efforts to promote change in the family system must take into account the family's larger context and the connections between the family and the larger community.

A family nurse working from the perspective of change theory must realize that helping families change depends on the family goals. These goals must be mutually developed between nurses and families with a realistic time frame for accomplishing them. Without family input, nurses are likely to set unrealistic or the wrong goals for families. One of the primary goals in family nursing is to assist families to see a problem differently so that it can develop new behavioral, cognitive, and affective responses to the problem.

Understanding that a problem exists is not enough to bring about change in a family: Change occurs when the family believes or sees that there are alternatives to a current state. Change does not occur equally in all family members. Some family members change more dramatically and quickly than others, in part because change is the result of many different factors and because it is often difficult to tell what exactly leads to change in one person or in a whole family.

Families who get stuck in the search for *why* will not move or change, but spiral in a circular fashion around the same problem. It is more productive to assist the family to focus on *what* can be done to solve the problem. Nurses cannot make families change: Nurses create the context that makes change more possible. The disadvantage to this model is that it takes considerable time to work with families to bring about change.

Family Therapy Theories

Although family therapy is a relatively new field, developed over the past 40 years, it has made great strides. Unlike family social science theories, family therapy models are all influenced by general system theory and are practice oriented. They have been developed to work with troubled families, and, therefore, most focus primarily on family pathology (Box 3–2; Table 3–1). Nevertheless, these conceptual models describe family dynamics and patterns that are found, to some extent, in all families. Because these models are concerned with what can be done to facilitate change in "dysfunctional" families, they are both descriptive and prescriptive. That is, they not only describe and explain observations made in practice; they also suggest treatment or intervention strategies.

Family therapy models have been influenced by theories in psychology and sociology. Just as there is no single approach to family nursing, there is no single approach to family therapy that can be put forth as the "right" or "wrong" approach. Different models offer alternative explanations of family phenomena and suggest alternative approaches to family assessment, diagnosis, and treatment.

Three prominent family therapy models are summarized in the following sections: (1) structural family therapy, (2) family systems therapy, and (3) family interactional and communications therapy (Goldenberg & Goldenberg, 2004).

Structural Family Therapy Theory

Structural family therapy was developed by Minuchin and his associates (Minuchin, 1974; Minuchin & Fishman, 1981; Minuchin, Rosman, & Baker, 1978; Nichols, 2004). This systems-oriented approach uses spatial and organizational metaphors to describe problems and develop solutions (Goldenberg & Goldenberg, 2004). From this perspective, the family is viewed as an open sociocultural system that is continually faced with demands for change, both from within and from outside the family. Within the context of the family, individuals must learn to adapt to these demands and the resulting stresses. The family's underlying organizational structure (i.e., its enduring transactional patterns and flexibility in responding to demands for change) helps determine how well the family functions.

In structural family therapy, transactional patterns, or the ways in which family members generally interact, are viewed as laws that govern the conduct of family members. Transactional patterns help the family to be stable or homeostatic. The family structure comprises a covert set of functional demands that organize family interactions. The ability to mobilize these alternative transactional patterns to meet external and internal demands for change determines the adaptability of the family. Dysfunctional transactional patterns lead to poor adaptation and to family dysfunction.

The family system differentiates and carries out its affective and socialization functions through subsystems. These subsystems may be individual members of the family or interpersonal subsystems, such as the marital subsystem or the parent/child and sibling subsystems. Family subsystems are differentiated by boundaries. The clarity of these boundaries is an indicator of how well the family functions. The two pathological extremes in boundaries are the disengaged family and the enmeshed family. In the disengaged family, boundaries are so rigid that there is little cohesiveness between family members. In the enmeshed family, the boundaries are so diffuse or porous that subsystems do not function autonomously or independently. As Minuchin (1974) explained, in the enmeshed family, when one person sneezes, everyone runs for the Kleenex.

The goal of structural family therapy is to facilitate restructuring of the family. This approach is present centered, action oriented, and problem focused. Clarifying boundaries and power hierarchies helps the family to understand its structure and then with the help of the therapist, family members can restructure to make the family more functional.

The family nurse who is working from this theoretical perspective assesses families by asking questions, observing family transactions, and asking family members to interact with each other about a particular situation. It is important to evaluate the whole family system, its subsystems, boundaries, and coalitions, as well as family transactional patterns and covert rules. It is also important to show respect for the current family structure. Nurses who intervene to

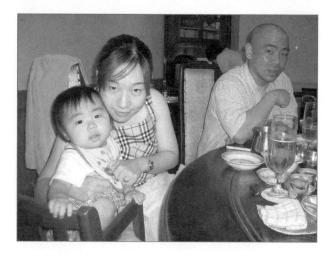

help the family should encourage and reinforce family successes through praise and support.

Structural family therapy is a clear, well-integrated, and well-tested approach. However, the approach calls for a very directive, active, and even confrontational role on the part of the family therapist or family nurse. Some practitioners or families may feel uncomfortable with this approach.

Interactional Family Therapy

The *interactional family therapy model* was originally developed at the Mental Research Institute (MRI) in Palo Alto, California, by Don Jackson, John Weakland, Paul Watzlawick, and Virginia Satir (Becvar & Becvar, 2000; Goldenberg & Goldenberg, 2004). This approach views the family as a system of interactive or interlocking behaviors or communication processing. Emphasis is on the here and now rather than on the past. The key question is "what is being processed?" not "why?". This approach is based on the fundamental rules of communication developed by Watzlawick, Beavin, and Jackson (1967). The first rule is that human beings cannot *not* behave, and therefore, they cannot *not* communicate. All behavior is communication at some level, and to be fully understood, all behavior must be examined in its context. Furthermore, all systems, such as the family system, are characterized by rules that maintain homeostatic balance and preserve the system.

Interactional family therapy is based on the dynamics of interchanges between individuals, and that is why it is called *interactional*. The approach assumes that emotional problems result from the way people interact with each other in the context of the family. In the normal or functional family, rules are clear and communication is clear; this kind of family can maintain its basic integrity even during stressful periods and accommodate change when it is needed. A breakdown in family functioning occurs when dysfunctional communication is predominant and the rules of communication are ambiguous. Dysfunctional families are said to be "stuck." Individual symptoms reflect family system dysfunction and these symptoms persist only if they are maintained by that family system (Goldenberg & Goldenberg, 2004). The individual symptoms maintain the family's current equilibrium, and the family avoids change even when change is needed.

Virginia Satir (1982), a well-known interactional family therapist, said that the natural movement of all individuals is toward positive growth and development and that symptoms indicate an impasse in the growth process. Satir assumed that all individuals possess the resources necessary for growth and development. Each person is in charge of their own growth. Therapy provides a supportive context for such change and development, and the role of the therapist is to facilitate the process. Primary goals of family therapy include understanding the communication rules and processes that troubled families use and teaching the family to use more functional communication.

Key interventions using this theoretical orientation focus on establishing clear, congruent communication, and clarifying and changing family rules (Jackson, 1965; Satir, 1982). This approach is very useful for family nurses because it stresses the interactions between family members. The weakness of the interactional approach is that it looks only at internal family behavior and not how the family is affected by the larger environment.

Family Systems Therapy Theory

Family systems therapy theory was first developed by Murray Bowen (1978). Bowen was a pioneer in the field of family therapy and he is still recognized as the founder of family systems therapy theory. Since his death in 1990, his work has been continued by David Freeman (1992) and Michael Kerr (Kerr and Bowen, 1988). Murray Bowen's particular version of family systems theory begins with the assumption that anxiety is an inevitable, omnipresent part of life (Gladding, 2001; Goldenberg & Goldenberg, 2004). Chronic anxiety is the basic cause of dysfunction in individuals and in families. The only antidote for chronic anxiety is "resolution through differentiation" (Goldenberg & Goldenberg, 2004, p. 186). Box 3–3 lists the eight

Box 3–3	**BOWEN'S FAMILY SYSTEMS THEORY: EIGHT INTERLOCKING CONCEPTS**

- Differentiation of self
- Nuclear family emotional system
- Multigenerational transmission process
- Family projection process
- Triangles
- Sibling position
- Emotional cutoff
- Societal regression

interlocking concepts of Bowen's family systems theory.

In Bowen's view, the key to healthy function is *differentiation of self*, or the ability of persons to distinguish themselves from their family of origin, both emotionally and intellectually. According to Bowen, there are two counterbalancing life forces, togetherness and individuality, which exist at two ends of a continuum. On one end of this continuum is autonomy, which is an ability to see oneself separately from others, think through a situation without confusing self with others, and separate feelings from rational thought. At the other end of the continuum is undifferentiated egomass, which implies emotional dependence on the family of origin, even if one is living away from the family. People can be ranked on a scale of differentiation of self. The more differentiated the individual, the more that individual is able to use logical reasoning and adapt to stress and change in the surroundings. Thus, a well-differentiated person is less apt to experience emotional difficulties. Figure 3–9 shows the Bowen continuum of self differentiation.

The nuclear family is viewed as a *family emotional system*. In this system, the coping strategies and patterns that are used tend to be passed on from generation to generation, a phenomenon that Bowen called the *multigenerational transmission process*. Thus, families who are dysfunctional have usually carried the problematic behaviors over several generations. Further, families tend to perpetuate their level of differentiation. That is, people tend to marry partners at their own level of differentiation and couples tend to produce offspring at the same level of differentiation as themselves.

Parents who are anxious and have poor differentiation of self tend to transfer their anxiety and low level of differentiation to a susceptible child. Therefore, a susceptible child is seen as the problem in the family. This phenomenon is called the *family projection process*.

According to Bowen, *triangulation* is a way that families use to deal with anxiety. In a triangle, which Bowen says is a basic building block of any emotional system, the tension between two persons is projected onto another object or person in the family. In certain stressful situations, anxiety may spread from a triangle within the family to triangles that include persons outside the family.

Sibling position is another important concept in family systems therapy. From this perspective, people are seen as developing fixed personality characteristics based on their birth order in their family of origin (Toman, 1961). A person is likely to carry out their sibling position from their family of origin in their family of procreation. For example, if a youngest child marries an oldest child, the marriage is more likely to be a functional one. If an oldest child marries an oldest child, the couple is more likely to compete for power and leadership.

Emotional cutoff occurs when children have unresolved attachments to parents. Children who are

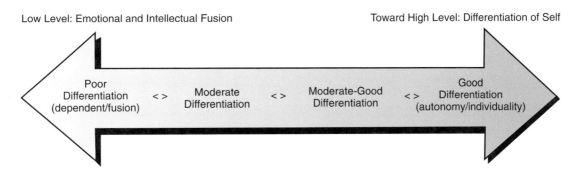

Figure 3–9 Bowen's continuum of self-differentiation. Adapted from Gladding, S.T. *Family therapy. History, theory, and practice* (3rd ed.). Upper Saddle River, NJ: Merrill/Prentice Hall.

emotionally fused to their parents and family of origin may live near or far from them. They may try to withdraw from parents and stay emotionally distanced from the family, but they are fused regardless of their physical proximity.

Societal regression is where the emotional process in society influences the emotional process in families—like a background influence affecting all families. The concept of social emotional process describes how a prolonged increase in social anxiety can result in a lowering of the functional level of differentiation in families. For example, feminists believe that sexism is a societal emotional process that affects families in a negative way. When a society is under too much stress, societal regression occurs because of toxic forces countering the achievement of differentiation.

Bowen's family systems therapy focuses on promoting differentiation of self from family and promoting differentiation of intellect from emotion (Becvar & Becvar, 2000). Family members are encouraged to examine the processes described above to gain insight and understanding into their past and present. Presumably they are then free to choose how they will behave in the future.

Using Bowen's approach, a family nurse or therapist would have individuals or couples investigate their family tree. The nurse would serve as coach and teacher, asking questions about people's history while helping the clients to construct a family tree, called a multigenerational genogram. In this approach, families are encouraged to ask questions of their own family members to gain an understanding of the past and the ways they currently interact. The goal is to help family members reduce triangulation, develop relationships with individual family members, and end emotional withdrawal. Because this approach to the family is objective and neutral, it takes the blame out of what problems people bring to the family therapist. However, this type of therapy emphasizes understanding the past to help deal with problems in the present. This kind of therapy requires a long commitment. Many people are not inclined to stay with such therapy to completion, and today many health plans are not inclined to pay for it.

Nursing Models and Theories

Formal nursing theories are not very evident in the nursing of families (Whall & Fawcett, 1991). Other than the Neuman Systems Model (Neuman, 1983), which was based on several family social science theories, the majority of the classic nursing theorists from the 1970s were originally focused on the individual patient and not the family. King (1987) and Roy (Roy & Roberts, 1981) revisited their original works and ultimately incorporated family into their theories. Other nursing theories have also been adapted to the nursing of families. For example, Rogers has been expanded by Casey (1996) and Orem was revised by Gray (1996). More recently Freidemann (1995) and Denham (2003) have developed conceptual nursing frameworks specifically for working with families.

The nursing models, in large part, represent a deductive approach to the development of nursing science (i.e., they move from the general to the specific). Although they embody an important part of our nursing heritage, these nursing conceptual frameworks and their deductive approach are being viewed more critically today. More inductive approaches to nursing theory development (i.e., approaches that move from the specific to the general) are now being advocated. That is, there is more focus today on making empirical observations, whether quantitative or qualitative, and generalizing from those observations to develop concepts and propositions to formulate new theory. In addition, nursing intervention studies need to be conducted to test and provide evidence that these approaches to working with families are best practice. It is imperative that family nurses build a body of knowledge that stems from theory and is based in research. It is important to establish that the family-as-client is fully accepted in nursing (Whall & Fawcett, 1991; ANA, 2003). Family nursing is clearly a component of the nursing discipline, even though "there remains virtually no evidence of formal middle-range family theory that is unique or distinctive to nursing" (Whall & Fawcett, 1991, p. 15). Gilliss (1991) aptly cautioned that it is not appropriate to simply substitute the word *family* for the word *individual* in nursing theories because doing so ignores the complexity of family systems. Whall and Fawcett (1991) restated the three central propositions in nursing theory from the perspective of family nursing.

1. Family nursing is concerned with the principles and laws that govern family process, family well-being, and optimal function of families in various states of illness and wellness.
2. Family nursing is concerned with the patterning of family behavior in interaction with the environment in normal life events and critical life situations.

3. Family nursing is concerned with the processes by which positive changes in family health status may be effected (pp. 3–4).

According to Whall and Fawcett (1991), the family nurse must consider environmental influences on family health and the effect of actions taken by nurses on behalf of or in conjunction with the family. In addition, the practitioner must work from a comprehensive biopsychosocial or holistic perspective on health and focus on family well-being rather than on family pathology (Whall & Fawcett, 1991, p. 4).

Although nursing theories are the least influential type of theory used in the nursing of families, it is important to be familiar with the ways nursing theories guide nurses in practice with families. In this section, several specific nursing theories or models that address the nursing of families are summarized.

Florence Nightingale

From a historical and chronological perspective, the first nurse theorist to incorporate family in nursing was *Florence Nightingale*. Nightingale described the family as having both positive and negative influences on the outcome of clients (Nightingale, 1859; Nightingale, 1979). In 1852, she wrote, "The family uses people not for what they are, not for what they are intended to be, but for what it wants them for—for its own uses" (Nightingale, 1859, p. 37). At the same time, Nightingale noted that the family was a supportive institution throughout the lifespan for its individual family members. She firmly believed in home health nursing and maintaining ill persons in the home environment.

Imogene King

Imogene King's *theory of goal attainment* (1981, 1987) is derived from systems theory. Early in her work, the family was seen as having an influence on individual development. The individual's role in the family contributes to the socialization and development of each member. She defined family as a small group of individuals bound together for the socialization of the members. The family was the vehicle for transmitting values and norms of behavior across the life span (King, 1983; Whall, 1986; Frey & Sieloff, 1995), which includes the role of a sick family member and transmitting the health care function of the family.

Later, King came to view the family as both an interpersonal and a social system. She focused on the integration of the personal system, interpersonal systems, and social systems (George, 2001; Parker, 2001). Many components of King's theory are relevant for working with families, such as the concepts of interaction, communication, transaction, role, self, growth and development, time, perception, and personal space. The role of the nurse in King's model capitalizes on the importance of the interaction between the nurse and the family-as-client.

Sister Callista Roy

Sister Callista Roy (1976; Roy & Roberts, 1981) viewed the individual as an adaptive system that responds to environmental stimuli in four response modes: physiological, self-concept, role function, and interdependence. *Roy's adaptation model* was derived primarily from von Bertalanffy's (1968) general systems theory and adaptation theory. The family was originally incorporated in this model from a family-as-context perspective, which means that the family influenced the individual's development across the lifespan and adaptation in times of change. In 1981, Roy and Roberts expanded this individualistic view to describe the "family as an adaptive system that, like the individual, has inputs, internal control and feedback processes and output" (Whall & Fawcett, 1991, p. 23).

Roy's theory of adaptation holds promise for describing and explaining how adaptation occurs in family and offers insight into ways to assist families to adapt to health issues. Moreover, Roy's theory stresses health promotion and the importance of assisting clients in coping with their environment, which are important elements of family nursing.

Betty Neuman

The *Neuman Systems Model*, developed by Betty Neuman (1983, 1995), is based on several family social science theories, including systems and stress theories. Neuman defined the family as "a group of two or more persons who create and maintain a common culture; its most central goal is one of continuance" (1983, p. 241). She viewed the family as a system composed of family member subsystems. The relationships between individual family members or subsystems are the central focus of her model.

The family's primary goal is to maintain its stability by preserving the integrity of its structure (Whall & Fawcett, 1991). The family system becomes threatened when it is exposed to stressors that affect its stability (equilibrium) and influence its state of wellness. The family has the ability to open or close its boundaries to protect its members and preserve the integrity of the family as a whole. Families vary in how well they balance and interact with the various subsystems that affect the well-being of their members.

One of the strengths of this model is that it addresses family health promotion, family reaction when a stressor affects the family and restoration of the family via family functions to achieve balance or equilibrium. It is a fluid model that depicts the family in motion and not a static view of family from one perspective. Further delineation of this theoretical model is contained in Chapter 8.

Dorothea Orem

Dorothea Orem's *self-care deficit theory* (1985) depicts the family as the basic conditioning unit, in which the individual learns culture, roles, and responsibilities. Specifically, family members learn how to act when one is ill. Orem's specific focus is on the role of family in helping its individual family members achieve self-care. Thus, the family is portrayed primarily as supportive of the individual from a family-in-context perspective, not as a client or recipient of care. Nevertheless, Orem (1985) suggested that people receive health care not only as individuals but also as members of a multiperson unit, the family.

Gray (1996) further expanded Orem's work to include families. Specifically, Gray (1996, p. 88) identified the following ways families addresses self-care for their members.

1. Self-care of families can be evaluated in a variety of situations. For example, the self-care potential of families can be assessed as it relates to health promotion and health protection. Each individual family member is a self-care agent who makes continual contributions to his or her own health.
2. Self-care reflects the personal values and health beliefs of the family. The family's self-care behavior evolves through a combination of social and cognitive experiences that have been learned through interpersonal relationships, communication, and culture, which are unique to each family.
3. Self-care can be administered to families by individual self-care agents. Thus, family members, either individually or collectively, can initiate and perform self-care, based on their

views of health and their ability to perform self-care behaviors.

4. The concept of self-care can be used to promote health in families and to recognize and evaluate areas where diminished health may exist.

Martha Rogers

Martha Rogers' (1970, 1986, 1990) *theory of unitary human beings* is an abstract theory based on general systems theory and draws on many fields of study, including anthropology, sociology, astronomy, religion, philosophy, history, and mythology (George, 2001; Parker, 2001).

Rogers viewed the human being as a unitary multidimensional energy field that is engaged in a continuous mutual process with the environment. The individual was the primary focus in her writings. Fawcett (2000) elucidated Rogers' theory by explaining that the family is a constant open-system energy field that is ever-changing in its interactions with the environment. Casey (1996) explained the application of Rogers' theory to family nursing as follows (pp. 56–57):

1. The family unit is a whole; it is composed of subsystems that are interdependent and that together form a unity that is different from the sum of the family subsystems.
2. The family is an open system in constant interaction with the environment through exchange of matter and energy.
3. Families are continuously influenced by information in the environment and, depending on the degree of permeability of their boundaries, they are constantly responding to this input.
4. The family system is subject to change along a space-time axis. The family moves through stages of development in a sequential, unidirectional manner.
5. The family has the capacity for feeling, knowing, and comprehending and for using these processes to determine patterns, make choices, and recognize its environment.

Marie-Louise Friedemann

Marie-Louise Friedemann's (1995) *framework of systemic organization* is built on the view of the family-as-client. The family is described as a social system that has the expressed goal of transmitting culture to its members. Consistent with general systems theory, her framework is based on the following assumptions:

1. The family, which is embedded in the civil or social system, transmits culture (i.e., the total of human patterns and values).
2. The family and the civil system and environment at large share responsibility for providing physical necessities and safety, teaching social skills to its members, fostering personal growth and development, allowing emotional bonding of family members, and promoting a purpose for life and meaning through spirituality.
3. The family satisfies its members' needs for control over their environment and helps them find their place in the network of systems through spirituality.
4. All family processes include collectively accepted and coordinated behaviors or strategies that aim to regulate space, time, energy, and matter in pursuing family stability, growth, control, and spirituality.
5. Family processes fall into four dimensions: system maintenance, system change, coherence, and individualization. These dimensions are interdependent but also exist independently in that no single dimension is emphasized at the expense of another in healthy families (pp. 16–17).

The elements that are central to Friedemann's theory are family stability, family growth, family control, and family spirituality. The family offers safety to its members as they learn group values, norms, and acceptable behaviors. As its members grow, the family grows and interacts with other systems, such as schools, church, and work. Family growth is facilitated by communication among its members. By selectively opening or closing its boundaries, the family can serve as a buffer between its members and the demands of society. Family control is maintained through the structure of the family. Family spirituality connects family members emotionally and encourages self-growth of the individual members (Friedemann, 1995).

Rose Marie Parse

Rose Marie Parse developed the *human becoming theory* in 1992. According to Parse (1992, 1998) the family makeup includes individuals that family members consider to be "part of the family." The concept of family and who makes up the family is continually

becoming and evolving. The role of the nurses is to use therapeutic communication to invite each member of the family to uncover his or her understanding of the meaning of the experience, learn what the meaning of the experience is for each other, and discuss the meaning of the experience for the family, as a whole. Nurses remain nonjudgmental and do not provide advice or direction, but work with the family to discover a course of action. Nurses ask questions such as the following: What has this situation been like for you and your family? What are you most concerned about? How is what you are most concerned about similar or different from how others in your family see the problem? What would you like to know more about? How would you like to change your situation? (Alligood & Tomey, 2002; Marriner-Tomey, 1998; Tomey & Alligood, 2002) The role of the nurse is to support the family members while they work through the difficult process of change (Alligood & Tomey, 2002; Marriner-Tomey, 1998; Tomey & Alligood, 2002),

Sharon Denham

The *family health model* by Sharon Denham (2003) draws from a broad base of literature and existing research about individual and family health but is primarily based on the ecological model from qualitative research with Appalachian families. Family health is viewed as a process over time of family member interactions and health-related behaviors. The model assumes that family health involves all members who reside within a household and includes their interactions with one another and their environments. Family health is described in relationship to contextual, functional, and structural domains, which address unique member traits, family characteristics, geographic location, household factors, broad environmental aspects, time, and societal and political influences.

Individual family members act independently but also cooperatively through dyadic and triadic relationships, which potentiates, mediates, or negates family health. Seven core functional processes—caregiving, cathexis, celebration, change, communication, connectedness, and coordination—are used to explain effects on individual and family health. These core functions largely characterize how the family views itself and have implications for family-focused care.

Family health routines are dynamic behavioral patterns, germane to individual and family health outcomes. These routines tend to be dynamic, have unique qualities, and often involve multiple family members. The six categories of family health routines identified in the model are self-care, safety and prevention, mental health behaviors, family care, illness care, and family caregiving.

Integrated Approaches to the Nursing of Families

Integrated families are complex small groups in which multiple processes and dynamics occur simultaneously. Families do not function in one way alone. No single theory or conceptual framework from family social science, family therapy, or nursing fully describes the dynamics of family life. Thus, nurses who use only one theoretical approach to working with families are, in essence, limiting the possibilities for families. Integrating theories allows nurses to view the family from a variety of perspectives, which increases the probability that the interventions selected will be implemented by the family, because they "fit" the structure, processes, and style of functioning for that family. By integrating several theories, nurses acquire different ways in which to conceptualize problems, and this enhances their thinking about interventions. Instead of fragmented knowledge and piecemeal interventions, nursing practice is based on an organized, realistic conceptualization of families. Nurses who use an integrated theoretical approach build on the strengths of families in creative ways.

Several nursing scholars have taken integrated approaches to working with families. General systems theory was merged with the Neuman Systems Model (Neuman, 1995) to develop the *Family Assessment Intervention Model* and *Family Systems Stressor Strength Inventory* (FS³I) (Berkey & Hanson, 1991; Hanson, 2001). Similarly Friedman combined general systems theory, developmental theory, and structural-functional theory into an assessment instrument (*Friedman Family Assessment Model* [long and short form]) that provides a macroscopic view of families (Friedman, Bowden, & Jones, 2003). The *Calgary Family Model* (Wright & Leahey, 2000; Wright, Watson, & Bell, 1997) integrates general systems theory, communication theory, change theory, and cybernetics in a unique approach to working with families. The model draws on sociological theories and other theories, such as Maturana and Varela's (1992) theory of the biology of knowing, Bateson's (1979) theory of the mind, and constructivist and narrative approaches (Wright, Watson, & Bell, 1997). All three of these integrated family assessment models are described in detail in Chapter 8.

Using one theoretical perspective does not give nurses a sufficiently broad base of knowledge on which to assess and intervene with families. Nurses must draw on multiple theories to be effective in tailoring interventions for specific families with unique needs. The number of possibilities for interventions is increased when nurses use multiple ways of conceptualizing families.

SUMMARY

- No single theory or conceptual framework adequately describes the complex relationships of family structure, function, and process.
- The major function of theory in family nursing is to provide knowledge and understanding that improves nursing care of families.
- The theoretical/conceptual frameworks and approaches that provide the foundations for nursing of families have evolved from three major traditions and disciplines: family social science, family therapy, and nursing.
- Family social science theories are the most well developed and informative with respect to the functioning of families, the environment and family interchange, interactions within the family, family changes over time, and the family's reaction to health and illness.
- Since family therapy is also a practice discipline and not only an academic discipline, these theories are more easily applied in family nursing practice.
- The importance of the nursing models for family nursing lies in the rich understanding they provide of human responses and the relationships between individuals, health, the environment, and nursing.
- Nurses who use one theoretical approach to working with families limit the possibilities for families.
- By integrating several theories, nurses acquire different ways to conceptualize problems, thus enhancing the possibilities of successful interventions.

STUDY QUESTIONS

1. The conceptual and theoretical frameworks that provide the foundation for family nursing

have evolved from the following three major traditions and disciplines: _____, _____, and _____.

2. Discuss why it is important for nurses to integrate conceptual and theoretical frameworks when working with families.

3. Select a research article that investigates a question or describes family function. Review it to determine the conceptual framework or theoretical approach(es) used to support the study and the findings. Was the article approached from any of the three disciplines and traditions discussed in the chapter? Did the researchers use an integrated approach to make sense out of the concept studied? How did the theoretical concepts they studied contribute or limit the findings about families? How will this knowledge assist nurses in caring for families?

References

Alligood, M. R., & Tomey, A. M. (2002). *Nursing theory: Utilization and application* (2nd ed.). St. Louis: Mosby, Inc.

American Nurses Association. (2003). *Nursing's social policy statement 2003*. Washington, DC: American Nurses Association.

Artinian, N. T. (1994). Selecting model to guide family assessment. *Dimensions of Critical Care Nursing, 14*(1), 4–16.

Bateson, G. (1979). *Mind and nature*. New York: E. P. Dutton.

Becvar, D. S., & Becvar, R. J. (2000). *Family therapy: A systemic integration*. Boston: Allyn and Bacon.

Berkey, K. M., & Hanson, S. M. H. (1991). *Pocket guide to family assessment and intervention*. St. Louis: C. V. Mosby.

Bomar, P. J. (2004). *Promoting health in families: Applying family research and theory to nursing practice*. (3rd ed.). St. Louis: Mosby/WB Saunders/Elsevier.

Boss, P. G., Doherty, W. J., Schumm, W. R., & Steinmetz, S. K. (Eds.) (1993). *Sourcebook of family theories and methods: A contextual approach*. New York: Plenum Publishing Corporation.

Bowen, M. (1978). *Family therapy in clinical practice*. New York: Jason Aronson.

Casey, B. (1996). The family as a system. In C. Bomar (Ed.), *Nurses and family health promotion: Concepts, assessment, and interventions* (2nd ed.) (pp. 49–59). Philadelphia: Saunders.

Danielson, C. B., Hamel-Bissell, B., Winstead-Fry, P. (1993). *Families, health and illness: Perspectives on coping and intervention.* St. Louis: CV Mosby.

Denham, S. (2003). *Family health: A framework for nursing.* Philadelphia: FA Davis.

Duvall, E. M. (1977). *Marriage and family development* (5th ed.). Philadelphia: Lippincott.

Duvall, E. M., & Miller, B. (1985). *Marriage and family development* (6th ed.). New York: Harper & Row.

Fawcett, J. (1999). *The relationship of theory and research* (3rd ed.). Philadelphia: FA Davis.

Fawcett, J. (2000). *Analysis and evaluation of contemporary nursing knowledge: Nursing models and theories*. Philadelphia: FA Davis.

Freeman, D. S. (1992). *Multigenerational family therapy*. New York: The Haworth Press.

Frey, M., & Sieloff, C. (Eds.). (1995). *Advancing King's systems framework and theory of nursing*. London: Sage.

Friedman, M. M., Bowden, V. R., & Jones, E. G. (2003). *Family nursing: Research, theory, and practice* (5th ed.). Upper Saddle River, NJ: Prentice Hall.

Friedemann, M-L. (1995). *The framework of systemic organization: A conceptual approach to families and nursing.* Thousand Oaks, CA: Sage Publications.

George, J. B. (2001). *Nursing theories: The base for professional nursing practice* (5th ed.). Upper River Saddle, NJ: Prentice Hall.

Gilliss, C. (1991). Family nursing research. *Image, 23*(1), 19–22.

Gladding, S. T. (2001). *Family therapy: History, theory, and practice* (3rd ed.). Upper Saddle River, NJ: Merrill/Prentice Hall.

Goldenberg, I., & Goldenberg, H. (2004). *Family therapy: An overview* (6th ed.). Pacific Grove, CA: Brooks/Cole – Thomas Learning.

Gray, V. (1996). Family self-care. In C. Bomar (Ed.), *Nurses and family health promotion: Concepts, assessment, and interventions* (2nd ed., pp. 83–93). Philadelphia: Saunders.

Hanson, S. M. H., & Kaakinen, J. R. (2001). Theoretical foundations for family nursing. In S. M. H. Hanson (Ed.), *Family health care nursing: Theory, practice and research* (2nd ed., pp. 36–59). Philadelphia: FA Davis.

Hill, R. (1949). *Families under stress*. New York: Harper and Brothers.

Hill, R. (1965). *Challenges and resources for family development: Family mobility in our dynamic society*. Ames, IA: Iowa State University.

Hill, R., & Hansen, D. (1960). The identification of conceptual frameworks utilized in family study. *Marriage and Family Living, 22*(4), 299–311.

Jackson, D. D. (1965). Family rules: Marital quid quo. *Archives of General Psychiatry, 12*, 589–594.

Jones, S. L., & Dimond, S. L. (1982). Family theory and family therapy models: Comparative review with implications for nursing practice. *Journal of Psychiatric Nursing and Mental Health Services, 20*(10), 12–19.

Kaakinen, J. R., & Hanson, S. M. H. (2004). Theoretical foundations for family health nursing practice. In P. Bomar (Ed.), *Promoting health in families* (3rd ed., pp. 93–116). St. Louis: WB Saunders/Mosby/Harcourt.

Kaakinen, J. R., Hanson, S. M. H., & Birenbaum, L. K. (2004). Family development and family nursing assessment. In M. Stanhope & J. Lancaster (Eds.), *Community and public health nursing* (6th ed., pp. 562–593). St. Louis: Mosby, Inc./Elsevier.

Kerr, M., & Bowen, M (1988). *Family evaluation: An approach based on Bowen's theory*. New York: Norton.

King, I. (1981). *Family therapy: A comparison of approaches*. Bowie, MD: Brady.

King, I. (1983). King's theory of nursing. In I. W. Clements & J. B. Roberts (Eds.), *Family health: A theoretical approach to nursing* (pp. 177–187). New York: John Wiley & Sons.

King, I. (1987, May). *King's theory*. Paper presented at Nursing Theories Conference, Pittsburgh, PA. (Cassette recording.)

LoBiondo-Wood, G., & Haber, J. (2002). *Nursing research: Methods, critical appraisal, and utilization* (5th ed.). St. Louis: CV Mosby.

Marriner-Tomey, A. (Ed.) (1998). *Nursing theorists and their work* (4th ed.). St. Louis: C. V. Mosby.

Maturana, H. (1978). Biology of language: The epistemology of reality. In G. Millar & E. Lenneberg (Eds.), *Psychology and biology of language and thought* (pp. 27–63). New York: Academic Press.

Maturana, H. R., & Varela, F. J. (1992). *The tree of knowledge: The biological roots of human understanding*. Boston: Shambhala (Random House).

McCubbin, H. I., & Patterson, M. (1983). The family stress process: The double ABCX model of adjustment and adaptation [Special issue]. *Marriage and Family Review, 6*, 7–27.

McCubbin, M. A., & McCubbin, H. I. (1993). Family coping with illness: The resiliency model of family stress, adjustment, and adaptation. In C. Danielson, B. Hamel-Bissell, & P. Winstead-

Fry (Eds.), *Families, health and illness* (pp. 21–64). St. Louis, MO: C. V. Mosby.

McKenry, P. C., & Price, S. J. (Eds.) (2000). *Families & change: Coping with stressful events and transitions*. Thousand Oaks, CA: Sage Publications.

Minuchin, S. (1974). *Families and family therapy*. Cambridge, MA: Harvard University Press.

Minuchin, S., & Fishman, H. G. (1981). *Family therapy techniques*. Cambridge, MA: Harvard University Press.

Minuchin, S., Rosman, B. L., & Baker, L. (1978). *Psychosomatic families. Anorexia nervosa in context*. Cambridge, MA: Harvard University Press.

Neuman, B. (1983). Family intervention using the Betty Neuman health care systems model. In I. W. Clements & F. B. Roberts (Eds.), *Family health: A theoretical approach to nursing care*. New York: John Wiley & Sons.

Neuman, B. (1995). *The Neuman systems model* (3rd ed.). Stanford, CT: Appleton & Lange.

Nichols, M. P. (2004). *Family therapy: Concepts and methods* (6th ed.). Boston: Pearson/Allyn & Bacon.

Nightingale, F. (1859). *Notes on nursing: What it is, and what it is not*. London: Harrison. Reprinted 1980. Edinburgh: Churchill Livingstone.

Nightingale, F. (1979). *Cassandra*. Westbury, NY: The Feminist Press.

Nye, F. I. (1976). *Role structure and analysis of the family* (Vol. 24). Beverly Hills, CA: Sage.

Nye, F. I., & Berardo, F. (Eds.) (1981). *Emerging conceptual frameworks in family analysis*. New York: Praeger.

Orem, D. (1983a). The family coping with a medical illness: Analysis and application of Orem's theory. In I. Clements & F. Roberts (Eds.), *Family health: A theoretical approach to nursing care* (pp. 385–386). New York: John Wiley & Sons.

Orem, D. (1983b). The family experiencing emotional crisis: Analysis and application of Orem's self-care deficit theory. In I. Clements & F. Roberts (Eds.), *Family health: A theoretical approach to nursing care* (pp. 367–368). New York: John Wiley & Sons.

Orem, D. (1985). *Nursing: Concepts of practice* (3rd ed.). New York: McGraw-Hill.

Parker, M. E. (2001). *Nursing theories and nursing practice*. Philadelphia: FA Davis.

Parse, R. R. (1992). Human becoming: Parse's theory of nursing. *Nursing Science Quarterly, 5*, 35–42.

Parse, R. R. (1998). *The human becoming school of thought: A perspective for nurses and other health professionals*. Thousand Oaks, CA: Sage.

Powers, B., & Knapp, T. (1995). *A dictionary of nursing theory and research* (2nd ed.). Newbury Park, CA: Sage.

Rogers, M. (1970). *Introduction to the theoretical basis of nursing*. Philadelphia: FA Davis.

Rogers, M. (1986). Science of unitary human beings. In V. Malinski (Ed.), *Explorations on Martha Rogers' science of unitary human beings* (pp. 3–8). Norwalk, CT: Appleton-Century-Crofts.

Rogers, M. (1990). Nursing: Science of unitary, irreducible, human being: Update, 1990. In E. Barret, *Visions of Rogers' science-based nursing* (pp. 5–11). New York: National League for Nursing.

Rose, A. M. (1962). *Human behavior and social processes*. Boston: Houghton Mifflin.

Roy, C. (1976). *Introduction to nursing: An adaptation model*. Englewood Cliffs, NJ: Prentice-Hall.

Roy, C., & Roberts, S. (1981). *Theory construction in nursing: An adaptation model*. Englewood Cliffs, NJ: Prentice-Hall.

Satir, V. (1982). The therapist and family therapy: Process model. In A. M. Horne & M. M. Ohlsen (Eds.), *Family counseling and therapy* (pp. 12–42). Itasca, IL: F. E. Peacock.

Schnittger, M. H., & Bird, G. W. (1990). Coping among dual-career men and women across the family life cycle. *Family Relations, 31*, 199–205.

Toman, W. (1961). *Family constellation: Its effects on personality and science behavior*. New York: Springer.

Tomey, A. M., & Alligood, M. R. (2002) *Nursing theorist and their work* (5th ed.). St Louis: Mosby, Inc.

Turner, R. H. (1970). *Family interaction*. New York: John Wiley & Sons.

Vaughan-Cole, B., Johnson, M. A., Malone, J. A., & Walker, B. L. (1998). *Family nursing practice*. Philadelphia: Saunders.

von Bertalanffy, L. V. (1950). The theory of open systems in physics and biology. *Science, 111*, 23–29.

von Bertalanffy, L. W. (1968) *General systems theory: Foundations, development, and applications*. New York: George Braziller.

Watzlawick, P., Beavin, J., & Jackson, D. (1967). *Pragmatics of human communication*. New York: W. W. Norton.

Watzlawick, P., Weakland, J., & Fisch, R. (1974). *Change: Principles of problem formulation and problem resolution*. New York: W. W. Norton.

Whall, A. L. (1986) *Family therapy theory for nursing*. East Norwalk, CT: Appleton & Lange.

Whall, A., & Fawcett, J. (Eds.). (1991). *Family theory development in nursing: State of the science and art*. Philadelphia: FA Davis.

White, J. M., & Klein, D. M. (2002). *Family theories* (2nd ed.). Thousand Oaks, CA: Sage Publications.

Winton, C. A. (1995). *Frameworks for studying families*. Guilford, CT: Dushkin.

Wright, L. M., & Leahey, M. (2000). *Nurses and families: A guide to family assessment and intervention* (3rd ed.). Philadelphia: FA Davis.

Wright, L. M., & Watson, W. L. (1988). Systemic family therapy and family development. In C. J. Falicox (Ed.), *Family transitions: Continuity and change over the life cycle* (pp. 407–430). New York: Guilford Press.

Wright, L. M., Watson, W. L., & Bell, J. M. (1997). *Beliefs: The heart of healing in families and illness*. New York: Basic Books.

Bibliography

Barth, R. P. (1990). Theories guiding home-based intensive family preservation services. In L. M. Tracy, & C. Booth (Eds.). *Reaching high risk families: Intensive family preservations in human services*. New York: Aldine deGruyter.

Broderick, C. B. (1993). *Understanding family process*. Newbury Park, CA: Sage Publications.

Broome, M. E., Knaftl, K., Pridham, K., & Feetham, S. (1998). *Children and families in health and illness*. Thousand Oaks, CA: Sage.

Carlson, J., & Lewis, J. (1991). *Family counseling: Strategies and issues*. Denver: Love.

Casper, L. M., & Bianchi, S. M. (2002) *Continuity & change in the American family*. Thousand Oaks, CA: Sage Publications.

Clements, I. W., & Buchanan, D. M. (1982). *Family therapy: A nursing perspective*. New York: John Wiley & Sons.

Day, R. D. (2003). *Introductions to family processes* (4th ed.). Mahwah, NJ: Lawrence Erlbaum Associates, Publishers

Day, R. D., Gilbert, K. R., Settles, B., & Burr, W. R. (1995). *Research and theory in family science*. Pacific Grove, CA: Brooks Cole.

Donaldson, S. K., & Crowley, D. M. (1978). The discipline of nursing. *Nursing Outlook, 26*, 103–120.

Edelman, C. L., & Mandle, C. L. (2002). *Health promotion through-out the lifespan* (5th ed.). St. Louis: Mosby.

Feetham, S. L., & Meister, S. B. (1999). Nursing research of families: State of the science and correspondence with policy. In A. S. Hinshaw, S. L. Feetham, & J. L. Shaver. *Handbook of clinical nursing research* (pp. 251–272). Thousand Oaks, CA: Sage Publications.

Gilliss, C. L., & Knafl, K. A. (1999). Nursing care of families in non-normative transitions: The state of science and practice. In

A. S. Hinshaw, S. L. Feetham, & J. L. Shaver, *Handbook of clinical nursing research* (pp. 231–250). Thousand Oaks, CA: Sage Publications.

Gilliss, C. L., Highley, B. L., Roberts, B. M., & Martinson, I. M. (Eds.). (1989). *Toward a science of family nursing.* Menlo Park, CA: Addison-Wesley.

Greenstein, T. N. (2001). *Methods of family research.* Thousand Oaks, CA: Sage Publications.

Hanson, S. M. H., & Kaakinen, J. (2000). Nursing of families in the community. In M. Stanhope & J. Lancasters (Eds.), *Community health nursing: Promoting health of aggregates, families, and individuals* (5th ed.). St. Louis: C. V. Mosby.

Hanson, S. M. H., Kaakinen, J., & Friedman, M. M. (1998). Theoretical approaches to family nursing. In M. M. Friedman, *Family nursing: Research, theory and practice* (4th ed., pp. 75–98). Norwalk: Appleton & Lange.

Hill, R., Katz, A. M., & Simpson, R. L. (1957). An inventory of research marriage and family behavior: A statement of objectives and progress. *Marriage and Family Living, 19,* 89–92.

Hinshaw, A. S., Feetham, S. L., & Shaver, J. L. (1999). *Handbook of clinical nursing research.* Thousand Oaks, CA: Sage Publications.

Ingoldsby, G., Smith, S., & Miller, J. (2004). *Exploring family theories.* Los Angeles: Roxbury Publishing Company.

Lamanna, M. A., & Riedmann, A. (2003). Marriages and families: Making choices in a diverse society. Belmont, CA: Wadsworth/ Thomson Learning.

McCubbin, M. (1999). Normative family transitions and health outcomes. In A. S. Hinshaw, S. L. Feetham, & J. L. Shaver, *Handbook of clinical nursing research* (pp. 201–230). Thousand Oaks, CA: Sage Publications.

McCubbin, M., & McCubbin, H. (1996). Resiliency in families: A conceptual model of family adjustment and adaptation in response to stress and crisis. In H. McCubbin, A. Thompson, & M. McCubbin (Eds.), *Family assessment: Resilience, coping and adaptation—Inventories for research and practice* (pp. 1–64). Madison: University of Wisconsin System.

Meleis, A. I. (1992). Directions for nursing theory development in the 21st century. *Nursing Science Quarterly, 5*(3), 112–117.

Meleis, A. I. (1996). Theory development: A blueprint for the 21st century. In P. Walker & B. Neuman (Eds.), *Blueprint for the use of nursing models.* New York: NLN Press.

Meleis, A. I. (1997). *Theoretical nursing: Development and progress* (3rd ed.). Philadelphia: Lippincott.

Minuchin S., & Nichols, M. P. (1998). Structural family therapy. In F. M. Dattilio (Ed.), *Case studies in couple and family therapy: Systematic and cognitive perspectives.* New York: Guilford Press.

Nicoll, L. H. (Ed.). (1997). *Perspective on nursing theory.* Philadelphia: Lippincott.

Nightingale, F. (1949). Sick nursing and health nursing. In I. Hampton, et al., *Nursing of the sick: 1893.* New York: McGraw-Hill.

Olsen, D. H., & DeFrain, D. (2000). *Marriages and families: Intimacy, diversity, and strengths* (4th ed.). Boston: McGraw-Hill.

Price, S. J., McKenry, P. C., & Murphy, M. J. (Eds.) (2000). *Families across time: A life course perspective.* Los Angeles: Roxbury Publishing Company.

Seccombe, K., & Warner, R. L. (2004). *Marriages and families: Relationships in social context.* Belmont, CA: Wadsworth/Thomson Learning.

Selye, H. (1950). *The physiology and pathology of exposure to stress.* Montreal, Quebec: ACTA. Out of print.

Stanhope, M. (1996). Family theories and development. In M. Stanhope & J. Lancaster (Eds.), *Community health nursing: Process and practice for promoting health* (pp. 562–593). St. Louis: C. V. Mosby.

Strong, B., DeVault, C., Sayad, B. W., & Cohen, T. F. (2001). *The marriage and family experience* (8th ed.). Belmont, CA: Wadsworth/Thomson Learning.

Thomas, M. B. (1992). *An introduction to marital and family therapy: Counseling toward healthier family systems across the lifespan.* New York: Merrill/Macmillan Publishing Company.

Timpson, J. (1996). Nursing theory: Everything the artist spits is art. *Journal of Advanced Nursing, 23,* 1030–1036.

Wegner, G. D., & Alexander, R. J. (Eds.) (1999). *Readings in Family Nursing.* Philadelphia: Williams & Wilkins.

White, M., & Epston, D. (1990). *Narrative means to therapeutic ends.* New York: W. W. Norton.

Wicks, M. (1995). Family health as derived from King's framework. In M. Frey & C. Sieloff (Eds.), *Advancing King's systems framework and theory of nursing.* London: Sage.

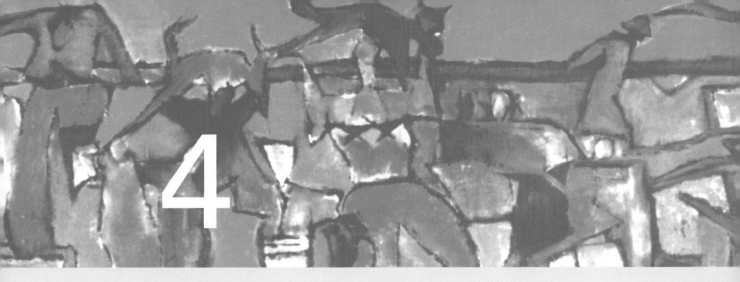

4

Research in Families and Family Nursing

Gail M. Houck, RN, PMHNP, PhD • *Sheila Kodadek, RN, PhD* • *Catherine Samson, RN, BSN, MPH*

CRITICAL CONCEPTS

- The relationships between the various ways we develop knowledge for nursing care, especially the relationship between nursing theories and research-based knowledge, are important ones.

- Many of the family nursing studies have not explicated their assumptions or theoretical frameworks. Studies that did often relied on concepts and methods from other disciplines.

- Although nursing has much to learn from the social sciences and family therapy, these disciplines cannot guide nursing practice.

- One reason for the lack of theory in family nursing is the apparent dissonance between considering the family as the client and fully appreciating the freedom and uniqueness of each family member.

- Family nurses need research methods and theories that facilitate their ability to see the complexities of the whole family unit as well as to yield the important potential contributions of each family member.

- The most practical question that faces a family researcher is who to include in the study.

- What is important is whether the researcher obtains information from an individual about the family or from the family as a whole at one time, and it is important because of the application of findings to practice. If family interventions are to be successful, they cannot rest on family-related research alone.

- The choice of who should be the source of data collection, or the unit of analysis, should make sense in terms of the purpose of the study, the theoretical orientation and research question, and whether the researcher wants to generalize about the family as a whole or focus on the individual's perceptions about the family.

- A variety of methods are used to describe characteristics of families, including surveys, structured interviews, and intensive observations in the laboratory, the clinical setting, or in the family home.

- A primary concern with sampling is whether the families who participate in a study are representative of the populations or groups to whom findings and conclusions can be generalized.

- What is important in the conduct of family research is to determine potentially relevant variables and then to identify respondents that illustrate this range of variables.
- Criteria for including and excluding families from the sample must be clear to ensure that the sample represents the group of interest.
- Family research and theory cannot be assumed to have cross-cultural applicability.
- Generally speaking, family research is *multivariate* in nature; multiple concepts and, therefore, multiple variables are of interest in our efforts to understand families. Thus, family research typically involves multivariate statistics.
- Most of the significant family nursing interventions are applied in a natural environment where very few of the processes and conditions other than the intervention can be controlled.
- Nursing practice is caring for the patient and family—not managing the disease—and therefore research should reflect the complexity of the lives for which it is providing evidence to alter clinical practice.

HISTORICAL PERSPECTIVE

Nursing's interest in families is not new. Throughout its history, the profession of nursing has been concerned with family influences in the health and well-being of individual members. Perhaps the most enduring example of this is the focus on families, which has characterized community health nursing practice for generations. However, in the 1970s, nurses became significantly more appreciative of the influence families exert on the health-related beliefs, attitudes, and behaviors of their individual patients. They systematically began to ask questions about relationships between families, health, and illness.

Consequently, nurse researchers interested in family issues began moving away from individually focused studies, choosing instead to focus on families. Discussions about what constituted family research were frequent and lively and continue today.

Classic review articles provide a glimpse of the remarkable upsurge in family nursing research that occurred during the 1970s and early 1980s and can give the reader an appreciation of the creativity and clinical grounding of the researchers involved. In 1983, Gilliss' paper, "The Family as a Unit of Analysis: Strategies for the Nurse Researcher," was published in *Advances in Nursing Science* (Gilliss, 1983). In this paper, Gilliss examined the nature of the family as a research phenomenon, reviewed and critiqued approaches that had been used to study the family, and identified strategies appropriate to the nature of nursing research (pp. 50–51). Gilliss concluded that family research remained flawed, despite creative strategies, and suggested attention to "the logical consistencies among what is measured, about whom, from whom, and for what purpose" (p. 58).

In 1984, Feetham's paper "Family Research: Issues and Directions for Nursing" was published in the *Annual Review of Nursing Research*. In this landmark paper, Feetham reviewed research in nursing to date, using the categories of family characteristics, family as environment of the individual, external environment and the family, nursing interventions with families, and family-related research. She suggested that a single definition of family by nurses is not essential, but what is essential is that each investigator define family within the context of the research. She recommended that researchers focus on "how families help each other, how they cope, and how they grow" (Feetham, 1984, p. 20).

Despite an upsurge in family nursing research, Gilliss (1991) and, separately, Hayes (1995) later identified a dearth of research with nontraditional families and families from nondominant cultures. Hayes also found little research on families of the elderly and healthy, and well-functioning families. Whall and Loveland-Cherry (1993) reviewed family unit-focused research published from 1984 to 1991, finding that family as the unit of analysis still was not defined consistently or even often. The majority of studies continued to be descriptive or exploratory in nature.

(continued on page 99)

Gilliss and Knafl (1999) found in their subsequent review of family nursing research publications that they were unable to make definitive statements about what had been learned about family response to chronic illness. However, in their most recent synthesis of research literature on family functioning in the context of chronic illness (Knafl & Gilliss, 2002), the conclusions were more heartening. Consistent with recent trends toward interdisciplinary research and knowledge development, these authors focused on the current state of knowledge and not the disciplinary source of the knowledge. They additionally focused on research that addressed how the family system responded to a member's chronic illness rather than research that might be more focused on individual family roles. Their analysis of research articles published over the past decade (1990–1998) revealed that although two-thirds of the studies could be characterized as descriptive and focused on describing or conceptualizing how families responded to or experienced the impact of illness, one-third of the studies were more explanatory in nature.

The criteria for research of families proposed by Feetham in 1984 were subsequently applied as guidelines for the development and review of research with families, thereby serving science policy. These criteria have since been revised and reformulated for family researchers with a notable, additional standard that directs the scientist to "provide guidance to institutions and agencies" (Feetham & Meister, 1999, p. 266). Feetham and Meister (1999) urged the inclusion of policy recommendations in addition to traditional clinical implications in publications of research findings. Most recently, this urging was extended to research with vulnerable families. Among many important issues identified in their discussion, Feetham and Deatrick (2002) made two particularly salient points. First they recognized the mandate that vulnerable populations must be studied in the context of the family, their culture, and their community in order to be understood. They asserted, then, that to do such relevant research requires interdisciplinary research training and experience and credibility with vulnerable populations.

COMMON THEORETICAL PERSPECTIVE

The relationship between the various ways we develop knowledge for nursing care, especially the relationship between nursing theories and research-based knowledge, is an important one. This relationship is complicated by the ongoing debate regarding the state of theory distinctive to nursing. Baumann (2000, 2002) most recently bemoaned the dearth of quality theory drawn from nursing research and argued instead for a perspective of human sciences. Baumann (2002) drew from the work of Dilthey, a philosopher, in defining the human science perspective in nursing and other health care research. Accordingly human science is described as uncovering universal lived experience, in which commonalities and differences are open to being inspected and interpreted (Baumann, 2002). Although this sounds phenomenological, he made the distinction that, because human science engages a reflective reader in the dialectic between experiences and interpretations, it is not phenomenological.

Baumann (2000) concluded that although there has been considerable growth in the number of nurses conducting family research over the past two decades, it remains unclear what family nursing and family nursing theory are. He argued that many of the family nursing studies have not explicated their assumptions or theoretical frameworks and that studies have often relied on concepts and methods from other disciplines that are suspect in their ability to guide nursing practice. Although Baumann (2000) acknowledged the value of the interdisciplinary understanding of families as vital, he called for greater clarity about what family nursing theory has to offer. By contrast, the work of other family scientists in nursing holds interdisciplinary work as salient to the understanding of family phenomena (Knafl & Gilliss, 2002; Feetham & Dietrick, 2002).

Nonetheless, Baumann's point is well-taken and echoed by Hanson and Kaakinen (2001) in their review of the theoretical foundations of family nursing. In essence, they concluded that family nursing today draws on three types of theory: family social science theories, family therapy theories, and nursing models and theories. Family social science theories remain abstract and have not been extended to clinical intervention, whereas family therapy theories are not readily applicable to healthy families or families with health problems that are physiological (Hanson & Kaakinen,

2001). Nursing models and theories have originated largely with an individual focus, and they remain the least developed. Contrary to Baumann, however, Hanson and Kaakinen concluded that the nursing profession has come to recognize that family nursing has roots in all three genres of theory (Hanson, 2001).

It is this perspective of the profession that guided the development of this chapter on research in families and family nursing. It is worth reiterating, therefore, the definition for family adopted by this textbook (p. xxx): "Family refers to two or more individuals who depend on one another for emotional, physical, and economic support. The members of the family are self-defined." It is additionally critical to reiterate the definition of family health adopted by this textbook (p. xxx): "Family health is a dynamic, changing, relative state of well-being that includes the biological, psychological, spiritual, sociological, and cultural factors of the family system."

As Hanson noted (2001), this approach refers to individual members as well as to the whole family unit. In addition, the biopsychosocial perspective for individuals and families embedded in cultural context is inherently the nursing perspective. This common theoretical perspective is evident in the emerging research on vulnerable families conducted by nurse scientists (e.g., Horowitz, Ladden, & Moriarty, 2002; Shepard, Orsi, Mahon, & Carroll, 2002). This research provides direction to the discipline's efforts to understand vulnerable populations in the context of the family, culture, and the community (Feetham & Deatrick, 2002).

Finally the standards for family scientists revised by Feetham and Meister (1999) are worth noting: (1) Be conceptually and methodologically rigorous; (2) focus on circumstances in which families are likely to need help; (3) contribute to the development and testing of interventions and assessment of strategies; (4) be conducted in the broadest context of relevance to the individual and family, such as the community, health system, environment, and social and health policy; and (5) provide guidance to institutions and agencies (Feetham & Meister, 1999, p. 265). The standards are consistent with the theoretical perspective reflected in the work of family nurse researchers and certainly set the parameters of what must be considered in the review of family research.

DEFINING RESEARCH SUBJECTS

Before delving into research questions, designs, and methods, it is important first to define the research subjects. The nursing discipline has a long-standing tradition of concern for the well-being of families and their individual members. Beginning in the early 1970s, nursing's research interest in families and family nursing became a significant focus for the profession (Ganong, 1995), with the goal of strengthening its knowledge base in family practice. As the discipline's interest in and conduct of research on families have grown, so has the need to specify and define what constitutes the family. This is probably the most practical question that faces a family researcher: who to include in the study. In family research, it is a complex issue.

In the first chapter, Hanson described four approaches to family nursing: the family as the context for individual development, the family as a client, the family as a system, and the family as a component of society. To build the science for these approaches, researchers must be certain that the subjects of the study and the information collected are consistent with how the findings will be used. For instance, research findings about how family members support a chronically ill child's psychosocial development, when the emphasis is on the family as context, may provide information about family caring activities. However, the findings from such a study will not necessarily be able to answer questions about how the family as a whole adapts to a child's chronic illness.

Families as a Research Subject

However we define families, it is clear that they are a special form of small group, with unique dimensions that challenge researchers (Ganong, 1995). Ganong summarized the characteristics that make families difficult to study as follows:

- An ethic of privacy governs nearly every aspect of family life.
- Family systems are value-laden.
- Families, similar to other small groups, have unique attributes, such as organization around gender and generation.
- Families are structurally, ethnically, and culturally diverse.
- Families are "ongoing" and exist multigenerationally over time.
- Families are influenced by the sociocultural context.

All of these characteristics contribute to the complexity of research on families. At the same time, these characteristics speak to the necessity for systematically derived knowledge about families to guide the practitioner of family nursing about nursing interventions with families. In this regard, the unit of analysis is twofold: *outcomes* of family nursing interventions (whether targeted for an individual member, a dyad, or the family system) and the *process* of the intervention (Bell, 1995a). Both are needed, because the *how* one intervenes can significantly influence the efficacy of the outcome. From a definitional standpoint, it seems crucial also to distinguish between mere treatment provision and the more sensitive alternative of caring interventions, because, according to Frank's (1995) personal accounts, their respective, consequent family experiences differ considerably. Ultimately, it is in the lives of families that family researchers and family nurses strive to make a difference.

Distinctions and Unit of Analysis

Two sets of distinctions have characterized discussions about research with families. The first set concerns those distinctions between family-related research and family research (Feetham, 1990), and the second set concerns distinctions between individual persons and families in research (Robinson, 1995). These distinctions bear on the issue of the exact subject or "unit of analysis" in family research. Research that focuses on relationships between selected family members, using

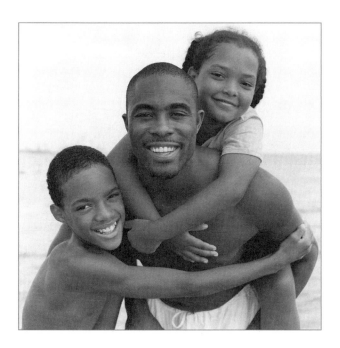

data reported from individuals, often is referred to as *family-related research*. A classic example of family-related research is research on parent-child relationships. In contrast, research that focuses on the family unit as a whole is referred to as *family research* (Feetham, 1990). Studies of the family experience of chronic illness often are true family studies. What is important is whether the researcher obtains information from an individual about the family or from the family as a whole at one time, and it is important because of the application of findings to practice. If family interventions are to be successful, they cannot rest on family-related research alone.

Family-Related versus Family Research

Data from an individual family member about the family represent the individual's perspective. The assumption underlying this approach is that the individual's perspective is a valuable source of information about the family (Uphold & Strickland, 1989). In particular, the individual family member is the appropriate unit of analysis when the family is viewed as the context for individual growth, development, well-being, and adaptation. In such cases, the individual's perceptions of the family's influence on his or her development, health, illness, or treatment are the focus of study. From a pragmatic standpoint, this approach to researching families is less expensive and has fewer statistical analysis problems than does collecting data from more than one family member. The principal disadvantage is that one person's view of the family cannot be extrapolated to a family view. His or her perceptions of the family may or may not correspond to the family's view as a whole.

Family-level information usually is derived through an interview with the whole family, an observational method, or a method of data analysis, such as combining the responses or test scores of several family members. Family-level data are obtained from multiple family members as informants. Although one may obtain greater insight into families through study of the family as the unit of analysis, several problems may occur (Uphold & Strickland, 1989). First, there may be a bias if not all members of a given family are willing to participate. Recruitment, retention, and coordination of whole families can be difficult or even impossible from a practical standpoint. Second, there are scoring problems when data from multiple family members are used because most instruments are designed for one person. However, several approaches to scoring, which will be discussed later in this chapter, address this problem. The important point is that the choice of who should be the source of data collection, or the unit of analysis, should make sense in terms of the purpose of the study, the theoretical orientation and research question, and whether the researcher wants to generalize about the family as a whole or focus on the individual's perceptions about the family.

Research of Individuals versus Research of Families

The second distinction is between research of individuals and research of families. Robinson (1995) argued against this separation, which takes an either/or approach. Instead, she proposed a schema in which both the individual and the family are considered, with each serving as background for the other. Accordingly there should be four units of analysis or interest in nursing research:

- Individual family member
- Individual family subgroup (marital dyad, parents, parent-child, siblings)
- Family group
- Individual family system (Robinson, 1995)

How do research questions vary according to the unit of analysis? Fisher, Terry, and Ransom (1990) concluded a decade ago that family researchers can focus selectively on family subsystems or identifiable parts of the family. They asserted that a family focus is not violated when certain elements within the family are identified and assessed while other elements are not. Again, this focus is apparent in the four approaches to family nursing described in the first chapter. With these notions in mind, it is useful to consider Robinson's distinctions about family as background or foreground as a way of categorizing research questions.

RESEARCH QUESTIONS ABOUT FAMILIES AND FAMILY NURSING

The ability to ask the right research question for a study can be thought of as both an art and a science. The following is a discussion of some of the challenges of asking questions in family research.

Individual Family Member

Nursing research on the *individual family member* strives to eliminate the separation between individual and family member. According to this focus, the family is background, and the person as individual, as family member, or as both individual and family member is foreground (Robinson, 1995). The unit of analysis may be as follows:

- Individual—physiological measurements or self-reporting
- Relational—data from two or more "related" persons about the individual or family
- Transactional—data from family members in interaction.

See Berkey and Hanson (1991) or Robinson (1995) for more detailed discussion of these levels of analysis.

Research questions that illustrate a focus on the individual family member include those pertaining to battered women. In this body of research, for instance, family violence is the background and the battered woman, mother, wife, or partner is the foreground. Research questions that pertain to transition to parenthood also reflect this emphasis. For example, family relationships and social support may be the background, but the parenting experience of the mother or father is in the foreground. Overall, research on the individual family member involves family phenomena as the context for the individual, and informs us not only about the individual but about the family as well.

SAMPLE RESEARCH QUESTIONS

Individual Family Member

How do mothers learn to care for a child who has been diagnosed with diabetes?

Individual Family Subgroup

What is the impact of a child's diabetes on the parental relationship?

(continued on page 103)

Family System or Family Group

How do families manage vacations when a child has diabetes?

Individual and Family System

How does family management style impact siblings of a child with diabetes?

Individual Family Subgroup

When the *individual family subgroup* is the focus of interest, it is possible to focus on persons as individuals and as family members, as well as on their relationship to the family (Robinson, 1995). The focus is on the relationship as a subgroup of the family, from the perspective of persons individually and in interaction. Research questions may concern the marital relationship as perceived by the individual partners or as observed by researchers, and it may concern individual characteristics that attend the relationship. Research questions about parent-child relationships also reflect this focus, with attention paid both to the assessment of individual characteristics that may contribute to the relationship and to the assessment of the relationship itself. Other examples of this focus are research on individual adjustment or development (child or adult) and marital and parental adjustment to life events (Benson & Deal, 1995).

Family System or Family Group

In research on the *family system or group*, the individual family members and their relationships become background and the family is foreground (Robinson, 1995). In this focus, the family is the unit of analysis and is distinct from individuals and family members. This emphasis does not represent the "whole" family or a "holistic" perspective because it does not include the parts of the family or the individual's and subgroup's perspectives (Fisher, Terry, & Ransom, 1990; Robinson, 1995). This focus characterizes much of the family sociological research before the 1970s (Benson & Deal, 1995). Individual and relational levels of data can be used to inform us or to make statements about the family. For measures of the family per se, transactional data would be collected to reflect a characteristic or property of the family without accounting for the contribution of particular family members or relationship patterns between members. Research questions that typify this focus pertain to family functioning during crisis or transition, family adaptation to chronic illness, and family experiences with specific events.

Individual and Family System

Research on the *individual and family system* involves consideration of the influence of family on individuals and individuals on family (Robinson, 1995). This focus of research, a trend beginning in the 1970s, includes both the individual family member and the family as foreground. The essential idea is that an integrated focus on the person as individual and family member, as well as on the family, allows the researcher to question how the individual as a separate, autonomous person contributes to the family system variables and vice versa (Benson & Deal, 1995). Research questions typical of this focus address spousal caregivers of persons with Alzheimer's disease or other chronic illnesses and conditions, parental caregivers of children with chronic conditions, and children in families in which the mother has breast cancer. The key is consideration of individual characteristics, including those embedded in the family member role, and assessment of the family as a family system. Data from individual, relational, and transactional levels are relevant. This approach to research holds much promise in addressing the complexities inherent to family life and, therefore, in family nursing practice.

OVERVIEW OF DESIGNS FOR FAMILY RESEARCH

A study is designed to fit the research questions asked about specific phenomena. The research design includes the plan, structure, and procedures for collecting and analyzing the data to answer the research questions. Two issues are central: (1) Does the design fit the research question(s)? and (2) Is the design both practical and economical? There are several ways of classifying research designs, none of which is universally accepted. This overview addresses exploratory, descriptive, correlational, experimental, and longitudinal designs.

Exploratory

Exploratory studies are conducted when little is known about a phenomenon of interest. The purpose of exploratory research is to generate ideas, insights, or understandings about family phenomena that are not well understood. In other words, exploratory studies are conducted to find out what the important issues and variables are. Both quantitative and qualitative methods are appropriate for this design, which relies on subjective insights. Although such research may be less structured and more flexible in approach, this does not mean that it proceeds without a plan or systematic procedure. A well-executed exploratory study can develop and refine ideas about family phenomena and can build family theory. For example, Oxley and Weekes (1997) used an exploratory design "to explore and describe the meaning African American adolescents give to the experience of being pregnant and strategies they used to manage the pregnancy experience" (p. 168).

Descriptive

Descriptive research is distinguished from exploratory research by its specification of variables about families that it seeks to describe or assess in a population. It is not flexible in the way exploratory research can be and does not rely on subjective insight in the same way (Miller, 1986). A variety of methods are used to describe characteristics of families, including surveys, structured interviews, and intensive observations in the laboratory, the clinical setting, or in the family home. The aim of a descriptive study is the complete and accurate description, characterization, and/or enumeration of selected variables within a given group of people or families. An example of a descriptive study question is "How do families with young children choose health care providers?"

Correlational

Correlational family studies assess the relationships between characteristics of families, family relations, and individual family members. The purpose of this research design is to examine specific relationships between two or more variables of interest. Correlational designs typically examine variables that are not under the control of the researcher or cannot be experimentally manipulated. Observations, questionnaires, and interviews are among the methods that can be used to collect data.

Correlational designs are common to family research because they tend to fit the research questions that interest investigators (Miller, 1986). Olsen and associates (1999) used a descriptive correlational design, for example, to examine how support and communication are related to hardiness in families who have young children with disabilities. They found that perceived family support was a predictor of family hardiness for both parents. Incendiary communication was negatively related to family hardiness for mothers, and income was positively associated with assessments of family hardiness by fathers (p. 275).

Experimental

Experimental designs allow the researcher to control or manipulate causal or independent variables and to assign families randomly to treatment and control groups. Experiments are designed to allow the inference of a functional or causal relationship between causal factors (independent variables or treatments) and individual or family outcomes (dependent variable). *Family intervention research* typically involves an experimental design by which one group of families receives or participates in an intervention and another group does not participate or receives a different intervention. In some designs, families who are not selected for the experimental intervention may be placed on a waiting list and, after comparisons on the outcomes, will subsequently receive the effective intervention. Other designs provide the "usual" intervention or program to one group of families and the experimental or demonstration intervention to another group and compare the outcomes. An experimental design compares interventions and their respective outcomes so that researchers can determine causes and effects.

One example of an experimental design is the use of a randomized clinical trial to evaluate the effectiveness of nursing and education support services in improving family functioning after cardiac surgery (Gilliss et al., 1993). The services were offered in the hospital and by telephone to 67 pairs of patients and caregivers after cardiac surgery. Although the study did not identify differences for the main effect of the intervention group, the main effect of time was significant, suggesting a pattern of response during recovery.

Longitudinal

Many family research questions are concerned with continuity, naturally occurring change, and predictability over time; *longitudinal designs*, in which the same families are studied over time, address such questions (Copeland & White, 1991). Individual development within the family can also be addressed readily through longitudinal design. The defining feature of longitudinal designs, which essentially are descriptive studies, is that the same families or family members are assessed at two or more points in time. For example, the question of how families adapt to a mother's diagnosis of breast cancer was studied by making a specified number of data collection visits to the same families—and studying the same family members—at specified intervals (e.g., Woods, Lewis, & Ellison, 1989; Lewis, 1993; Lewis, Hammond, & Woods, 1993; Lewis, Zahlis, Shands, Sinsheimer, & Hammond, 1996). Research that addresses parent-child interaction and child developmental outcomes at specified ages in infants, toddlers, and preschoolers is another example of longitudinal design (e.g., Houck, Booth, & Barnard, 1991; Houck & LeCuyer-Maus, 2002; Houck & LeCuyer-Maus, 2004; LeCuyer-Maus & Houck, 2002).

Several potential problems require attention with this design. First, if children are involved, the study must change to use measures that are appropriate for each developmental age. As the nature of the measures change according to age, however, there is concern for how comparable the measures actually are. Second, a question always arises in discovering a family change. Did the change come about because of the factors being studied or did it come about due to developmental, evolutionary, or other environmental factors? Finally attrition is a problem common to longitudinal research studies (Ryan & Hayman, 1996; Motzer, Moseley, & Lewis, 1997). Many subjects who initially participate will drop out of the study because they move or their circumstances change. Especially problematic for family researchers are changes in family constellations: Family members graduate, move away, or refuse to participate, and new members are added through birth or marriage. Not surprisingly longitudinal designs are as rare as they are informative.

QUANTITATIVE METHODS IN FAMILY RESEARCH

Once the study design is identified, the family researcher is faced with the challenge of how to get the information needed to answer the research question. There are significant methodological issues in family research. How these issues are addressed is central to the quality of family research and to the nurse who is evaluating family research for use in practice. This section will provide an overview of sampling, data collection, measurement, and analysis. While all four topics are of concern in both quantitative and qualitative family research, there also are significant differences in how they are addressed in each approach. Following the discussion of these four topics is an overview of qualitative methods in family research.

Sampling

The term sampling pertains to who or what is selected to be studied. More specifically, the term *sample* refers to a subset or part of a whole and sampling refers to how the sample or subgroup is chosen. *Quantitative approaches* to family nursing research typically sample populations of children, parents, and/or families. *Qualitative approaches* sample phenomena and the data are texts or transcripts of interview discourse.

A primary concern with sampling is whether the families who participate in a study are representative of the populations or groups to whom findings and conclusions can be generalized. For example, if one wishes to study families who are caring for a member with dementia, knowing the population characteristics of all families in similar situations will help determine what the sample should be.

Socioeconomic stratification is one way of characterizing a sample. Economic resources, social prestige, power, information, and lifestyle affect many family variables; the variables most frequently used to indicate socioeconomic level are occupation, income, and formal education (Smith & Graham, 1995). What is important in the conduct of family research is to determine potentially relevant variables and then to identify respondents that illustrate this range of variables. In the end, the key issue is whether the sample of participating families is representative; does it include a reasonable range? Researchers may also be interested in certain groups within a sample and linking certain kinds of interventions accordingly; for example, low education, low income, and "social risk." The ways in which these categories are defined by sampling criteria or demographic data are important.

Another sampling consideration involves restricting the families to those with a specific health condition, diagnosis, or circumstance. For example, researchers may want to investigate family responses to pregnancy in midlife, management strategies for cardiac disease, coping with parental death, or parenting a preschooler. Criteria for including and excluding families from the sample must be clear to ensure that the sample represents the group of interest.

One issue with sampling concerns cross-cultural family research. Family research and theory cannot be assumed to have cross-cultural applicability (Moriarty, Cotroneo, DeFeudis, & Natale, 1995). Cross-cultural research often requires collaboration across disciplines and among researchers of the ethnic groups under study. Challenges to the investigators include access to the population of interest and cultural competence in collecting and analyzing data. From the standpoint of research evaluation, at issue is whether there is cultural or ethnic representation within the study and how investigators account for cultural differences while conducting the study. Although many researchers have argued for cross-cultural comparisons, such findings often contribute to broad generalizations. Instead, investigators increasingly are urged to explore variation within cultural or ethnic groups rather than to compare cultural groups directly (Kelly, Power, & Wimbush, 1992).

Another sampling issue occurs in longitudinal research, which, as mentioned previously, has the problem of attrition. The loss of sample members over time occurs because families move, cannot be located, or refuse to continue their participation. With older families or families with ill members, some participants die and others may no longer be able to participate as a result of illness or disability. Thus, there is a potential threat of attrition bias. This bias exists when there are significant differences in the sample between the initial and subsequent data collections (Miller & Wright, 1995). It is important that reports of longitudinal research address the issue of attrition, including attrition bias, any measures taken to correct the bias, and any caveats applied in the interpretation of the findings.

Modes of Data Collection

Mode of data collection refers, in part, to whether the nature of the data is individual, relational, or transac-

tional (Berkey & Hanson, 1991; Feetham, 1990; Fisher et al., 1990). *Mode of data collection* also refers to the way researchers actually collect the information—through questionnaires, interviews, observations, etc. Individual data are collected from a single family member and reflect individual perceptions about the phenomenon of interest; there is no reference to the perceptions of other family members. Relational data are either (1) collected from individual family members and combined in some way (e.g., using means, sums, and difference scores) to address relationship dimensions; or (2) are obtained through the observation of or interview with a dyad. Family level or transactional data typically are obtained from naturalistic observation of family interaction, as well as by aggregating data from all individual family members. Keep in mind that responses will differ when the same questions are asked of family members individually and when they are in the presence of a partner, parent, or the entire family.

Self Reports

Self-reports are useful for obtaining information about subjective events and conditions (Copeland & White, 1991). Also called *survey method*, data collection by self-report consists of asking people questions directly through questionnaires, face-to-face interviews, or telephone interviews (Miller, 1986).

Questionnaires are surveys that can be mailed to respondents or administered in a group or family setting; the respondents mark the answers themselves with complete anonymity. Questionnaire data are cost-effective, but it is difficult or impractical to follow up on missing or incomplete data, so data quality may not be optimal. *Face-to-face interviews* entail an interviewer asking a respondent questions and recording the answers. These interviews can be more flexible, allowing the interviewer to probe for more information, clarify responses, or elicit elaboration. Interviews can yield more complete and accurate data, especially home interviews where family members are in their natural environments (Astedt-Kurki, Paavilainen, & Lehti, 2001). However, these advantages must be considered in light of the costs for training and evaluation of the interviewers and travel expenses for home interviews. Telephone interviews require significantly less staff time than do face-to-face interviews; for one thing, they eliminate travel time and costs. Thus, they are relatively inexpensive and have the advantage of being rather quick yet yielding high-quality data (Miller, 1986).

When self-report methods are used in research, thought goes into *how the questions are asked*. The questions should be clear and unambiguous and should use vocabulary that fits the education and experience of the participants. Attention must be paid to developing the right language and context (Shepard & Mahon, 2002). The questions should focus on a single idea, provide a clear frame of reference so that the responses are relevant, and ask only for information the respondent has, not speculation about how others think or feel. Closed-ended, fixed-response (multiple choice or true-or-false) formats are useful in large studies and can be objectively scored, but the responses may not reflect the issues the researcher intended to assess. Open-ended formats, especially useful for interviews, provide opportunities for clarification and elaboration but are also subject to interviewer bias and require interrater reliability to be established (Copeland & White, 1991).

66 The questions should focus on a single idea, provide a clear frame of reference so that the responses are relevant, and ask only for information the respondent has, not speculation about how others think or feel. 99

Observational Methods

Observational methods are systematic procedures for observing behavior and recording what happens. Direct observation of families and relationship interactions can provide objective information about the behavior of family members. Observational researchers assume that although the presence of an observer or camera may alter family members' behavior in some respects, people cannot change their behavior in any profound way by simply trying to do so. To further guard against "impression management," observational coding systems usually are designed to tap behaviors, dynamics, or characteristics that operate below the level of conscious control. For example, observation might include not only what a father says to a child, but also how his body is positioned, where his eyes are focused, and his facial expression. The family is also asked to engage in a task that is interesting in order to minimize the artificial nature of the situation and enhance the realism of its behavior. Of course the task must elicit the behavior or dynamics that represent the construct of interest.

Coding systems are developed to capture what is going on in the family as it is observed. Coding systems can assess: (1) interpersonal process, or *how* family members interact with each other, regardless of what they say; (2) verbal content, or *what* is said by whom; and (3) affective display, or the nonverbal expression of emotional tone. Within these categories, the researcher can code the interaction at a very specific level or can rate the interaction at a more global level. An observational checklist may require the observer to note whether or not many specific behaviors occur within a task or given time frame. Global ratings, on the other hand, involve entire interactions or larger segments of interaction. A rating or judgment is assigned on a carefully defined scale that assesses a dimension (e.g., control or power, communication, reciprocity, enmeshment, and adaptability) of a family or dyadic interaction over the period of observation. Observational coders require extensive training in order to use the coding systems effectively. Over time, investigators must establish intercoder or interrater reliability.

Secondary Data Sources

Secondary data sources include data sets from completed projects on related topics, family and social archives, large-scale surveys, and public records. *Secondary analysis* involves using previously collected data or secondary data sources to answer questions not asked by the original investigator or to ask similar questions in new ways (Moriarty et al., 1999). The secondary data sets may have been designed for other purposes or may have been collected for both current and future unspecified purposes. Interviews, written narratives, questionnaires, videotaped observation sequences, and demographic surveys all can be viewed from a new perspective and may even benefit from secondary analysis. Raw data may be available for coding in a new way, which is especially true of interviews, narratives, and observation sequences. For example, an interview of family caregivers may be coded first for caregiving tasks and their perceived difficulty and then later be recoded for clues to relationship qualities between the caregiver and receiver. In other cases, access to existing data may be available, such as demographic data, scores on questionnaires or tests, and observational codes. These data may be used to address new questions or relationships between different variables or to examine follow-up data or replication. Another source of data is the ongoing records of society that are collected for legal, medical, or political reasons. Examples of societal records include actuarial records, judicial records, census data, and governmental reports. Large national databases may be chosen for family research as well. In all cases of secondary analysis, there must be consistency among the theory, variables, and available data in the database, and the reliability and validity of the data need to be ascertained in the context of the theory (Shepard et al., 2002).

Measurement

Measurement is the process of linking theoretical ideas or concepts to empirical indicators or variables (Miller, 1986). The explicit procedures or instructions for linking abstract concepts to measures are found in operational definitions. These definitions describe the "operations" necessary to produce scores (Berkey & Hanson, 1991; Miller, 1986). Articulation of the logical linkages between conceptualization, operational definition, and measurement requires both precision and creativity. This has been a challenge to family researchers (see Feetham, 1990) and perhaps stems from the difficulty of finding a way to "measure" systematically (with numbers, observational classifications, or ratings) the dynamic interactions of family life.

Levels of Measurement

To read and evaluate family research, one must be mindful of the levels of measurement. *Nominal measurement* simply means naming, categorizing, or classifying. If a number is assigned to a category or classification, it is for the purpose of grouping data and does not reflect a numeric value. Gender, ethnicity, and marital status are typical nominal measurements.

> **"**Measurement is the process of linking theoretical ideas or concepts to empirical indicators or variables. (Miller, 1986)**"**

Ordinal-level measurement means that it is possible to rank subjects on the basis of the variable being assessed. Ordinal rankings do not reflect a quantity but rather a general amount or more or less of a characteristic (e.g., controllingness, sensitivity, rigidity). Ordinal measures have meaning only when compared with other ordinal measures. In contrast, interval-level measurement does reflect quantity, with equal distance between the points of measurement. *Ratio level measurement*, in addition to reflecting equal distance between measurement points, includes an

absolute zero, which represents that none of the characteristics being assessed is present. The important issue is for the researcher and the practitioner to be clear about the meaning of the measurement used in a given study, especially because many of the measures and observations in family research are also used as clinical assessments (Berkey & Hanson, 1991).

Reliability

Reliability of measurement is crucial to obtaining meaningful data about families. Reliability essentially refers to the dependability and consistency of a measure. Stability or consistency over time is one aspect of reliability; greater stability is expected for traits or consistent characteristics. Of course, development and growth also affect stability, and the challenge is to parse out what is real change. For example, if one is interested in family communication over time, one would expect the content of communication to change as children mature. One would not necessarily expect the patterns of communication to change, unless something happened to impact those patterns. Internal consistency is another aspect of reliability and reflects how well all parts of the measure are in correspondence or agreement. In other words, if a questionnaire purports to measure family cohesion, the question of internal consistency is whether all questions in the questionnaire measure the concept of family cohesion or some measure something else. Finally, as discussed with observational methods, interrater or intercoder reliability is concerned with the dependability of coders and how consistently two observers agree in their coding of observed family phenomena.

Validity

Validity is also central to the meaningfulness of research findings. *Validity* refers to the appropriateness of the specific use of a given measure; it answers the question, "Did the instrument actually measure what it was meant to measure?"

The issue of validity also raises the question of exactly what to measure. Fisher, Terry, and Ransom (1990) have advocated strongly for multiple measures: selecting from several family constructs, dimensions, or domains expected to be related to health, and sampling each one with multiple indicators to describe the domain thoroughly. Through broader family assessments with multiple indices, investigators can obtain more complete descriptions and better predictions of outcomes. These authors argued for *triangulation*, the use of two or more research methods in a single study. An example of triangulation would be the use of self-report, historical, interview, and observational methods both to obtain the unique perspectives of the family and integrate cross-method data in analyses to further our understanding of the complexities of the family unit

While multiple measures are clearly an answer, they can be difficult to administer because of time, expense, and burden. In addition, the results are not always clear, particularly when they result in conflicting data (Polit, Beck, & Hungler, 2001). The question of validity is always essential and rarely easy to address.

Data Analysis

The crux of data analysis in family and family nursing research is embodied in Feetham's (1990) caveat: Selection of a data analysis technique should not be arbitrary, but rather should be linked conceptually to the study and be appropriate to the data. Generally speaking, family research is *multivariate* in nature; multiple concepts and, therefore, multiple variables are of interest in our efforts to understand families. Thus, family research typically involves multivariate statistics. As a reader of family and family nursing research, it is important to be mindful that larger samples are needed to support such analyses, unless researchers perform certain *data reduction techniques*. Recognizing the inherent need for multivariate analyses in the face of the challenges in recruiting and retaining target families for research, Fisher, Terry, and Ransom (1990) explicated several effective strategies for managing large variable sets with relatively small samples.

Approaches to Data Analysis

Multivariate analysis aside, there are three broad approaches to data analysis:

- Descriptive analysis
- Assessment of relationships
- Determination of differences

Descriptive analysis basically describes the sample and the characteristics assessed. For example, families may be described in terms of parental marital status, family income level, education level of the partners or spouses, and number of children. Families may then be described in terms of the number and proportion who experience various types of conflict, presented

perhaps as classifications or as a score. The distribution of types or the average scores on a scale may be described in relation to national norms. The goal of such analysis is to describe selected family characteristics in a sample of individuals or families.

If the research questions were concerned with the relationships between family characteristics, the data analysis assesses the relationships between variables. Both correlational and regression analysis may be used. There are several types of correlation (e.g., Pearson's and canonical) and regression (e.g., linear, multiple, and logistic) analyses, but all generally require interval, ratio, or dichotomous (1/0) scores. Measures of association also may be used to assess the relationships between nominal variables and ordinal-level data (using nonparametric statistics).

When research questions are concerned with differences between families, data analysis assesses for group differences. The sample—individuals, married couples, parents, or families—are grouped on the basis of a classification or nominal characteristic to assess differences between those groups on a measure. The scores are usually at the interval or ratio level of measurement. At the most general level, t-tests determine differences between two groups; an analysis of variance techniques is applied to more than two groups. In both cases, one dependent measure is assessed for differences. When there is more than one dependent or outcome measure, multivariate analyses are used. If measures are applied over time, on repeated occasions, one should expect to see a repeated measures analysis.

These are some broad generalizations about what to expect in the data analysis of family research. However, analysis of such a complex social unit is becoming equally complex, and there are many exceptions to these generalities, many variations within these approaches, and new strategies and techniques for analyzing large data sets. The issue of concern in assessing a study is whether there is a logical consistency between the data analysis and the research questions, the central concepts or domains of concern, the design and measurement, and the conclusions.

QUALITATIVE METHODS AND FAMILY RESEARCH

Qualitative methods are a common approach to family research, and family nursing researchers are recognized both within and outside of the discipline for their knowledge and skill in qualitative research. Qualitative methods often are chosen for exploratory investigations (Miller, 1986) and are most valuable when researchers seek in-depth information about how and why people behave, think, and act as they do (Ambert, Adler, Adler, & Detzner, 1995). Qualitative research allows for the discovery or uncovering of perceptions, meanings, understandings, multiple realities, and psychosocial context in families. Although a qualitative approach to family research usually relies on the interview method, content analysis of written materials and participant observation of the family also may be used.

Within the qualitative approach, there are distinct methods. Each method emphasizes selected aspects of the phenomenon in question, with focus on specific aims and evidence. Sampling plans and data analysis differ markedly from quantitative methods, with effort generally focused on identifying research participants who have experience with the phenomenon under study. Regardless of the specific qualitative method, rigor in qualitative research is assessed in terms of the following:

- Credibility—faithfulness to the descriptions and interpretations of experience
- Applicability—fittingness to other contexts
- Consistency—the ability to audit or to follow the researcher's "decision trail"
- Confirmability (Sandelowski, 1986)

&&Qualitative research allows for the discovery or uncovering of perceptions, meanings, understandings, multiple realities, and psychosocial context in families.,,

Grounded Theory

Discovering theory about family or individual experiences in families is the aim of the *grounded theory* method in family research. Grounded theory methodology was developed and named in the mid-1960s by Glaser and Strauss (1967). Grounded theory researchers generate or construct theory from data provided by families; thus, the specific theory is connected closely with the data and is said to be "grounded" in data. This approach explicitly acknowledges the family and its members as experts in their own experience and allows nurses to explore areas of nursing experience that have not been adequately addressed by existing theories. Symbolic interaction theory underlies this method, a theory that helps to explain how a group of people—in this case, a family—defines reality through social interaction.

Wilson and Morse (1991) used grounded theory methods to examine the experience of husbands living with wives undergoing chemotherapy. Their analysis of the data resulted in a three-stage model of husbands' perceptions of their experience: Husbands moved from identifying the threat, to engaging in the fight, and finally, to becoming a veteran (p. 227). Recurrence of the cancer initiated the cycle once again.

Phenomenology

Hermeneutic phenomenology is an approach to the study of shared family meanings and family concerns (Chesla, 1995). Careful attention to context is essential to this approach; family and cultural history are important to the understandings derived from this research. Hermeneutic study emphasizes the everyday experience of families and focuses on their central concerns in living with life situations (Chesla, 1995).

The perspective of *interpretive phenomenology* embraces both the shared, everyday "lived experiences" of the family and the multiple realities of family members. It recognizes each family member's unique experience of the family and perception of reality. Thus, the researcher seeks to understand the lived experience of the different family members and their multiple realities (Hartrick & Lindsey, 1995). The focus is not on the facts of a situation but, instead, on the meaning of those facts to the various family members. Hartrick and Lindsey consider the "phenomenological attitude" as central to this method, as a way of coming to question human experience in an effort to uncover deeper meaning. An example of phenomenological research in family nursing is Chesla's use of hermeneutic phenomenology to guide her study of the caring practices of parents with their adult schizophrenic children (1994). The richness of this method can be seen in her interpretation of the meaning of those practices.

Narrative Inquiry

Narrative inquiry is another qualitative method by which the researcher seeks to understand the meanings of experiences from families and their individual members. As families and family members relate their experiences, they are telling their stories. This form of inquiry analyzes the narratives or created structures of the stories on the assumption that family members, as narrators telling their stories, select, order, and prioritize events based on their meaning for the individuals involved (Knafl, Ayres, Gallo, Zoeller, & Breitmayer,

1995). Narrative inquiry identifies the "plot" or the organizing framework of the story according to the temporal unfolding of the story (Poirier & Ayres, 1997), which reveals the context and meaning of the events and experiences for the narrator (Knafl, Ayres, Gallo Zoeller, & Breitmayer, 1995). The researcher notes inconsistencies, repetitions, and omissions to identify "secrets," or those issues that are to be avoided or that bring discomfort to the narrator (Poirier & Ayres, 1997). Ultimately the researcher is able to arrive at interpretations of story "types" through careful analysis and comparison of unique story features and similarities across stories. An example of this approach is the application of narrative analysis techniques to parents' stories of the events preceding their child's diagnosis of a serious chronic illness (Knafl, Ayres, Gallo, Zoeller, & Breitmayer, 1995). The analysis uncovered five major pathways to diagnosis (direct, delay, detour, quest, and ordeal) and information about what those pathways meant for parents (p. 411).

Ethnography

Leininger (1985) described *ethnography* as the systematic process of observing, detailing, describing, documenting, and analyzing patterns of a culture to understand the patterns of people in their familiar environment (p. 35). Ethnography generally is associated with anthropology but has been used in family research to understand patterns of behavior or lifestyles of families who share experiences. Recent examples of ethnographic research in family nursing include three ethnographic studies on family health of Appalachian families. One study examined the definition and practice of family health, the second examined family health during and after death of a family member, and the third examined family health in an economically disadvantaged population (Denham, 1999a, 1999b, 1999c).

CRITERIA FOR EVALUATING RESEARCH

The long-standing gap between family nursing research and practice has limited the extent to which research has enhanced practice. Dialogue between researchers and practitioners of nursing is even more crucial in the era of health care reform. After all, families are now carrying out many of the tasks that used to be hospital-based and taken care of by professional nurses. With limited resources, the family itself as a "resource" becomes crucial to the individual patient's well-being and, therefore, this function must be optimized. Furthermore, the "high users" of health care resources are complex, multiproblem cases that require professional nursing intervention with both individuals and their families. Toward this end, family and family nurse researchers must perform studies in the context of practice, present findings in clinical journals, and discuss how to apply findings. But until researchers become adept at doing so, it rests with the practitioners of nursing to evaluate family and family nursing research and to integrate relevant research into their practice. The following evaluation criteria should assist in this effort.

The first issue to be evaluated in family and family nursing research is whether an *explicit family conceptual or theoretical framework* is used. The basic assumptions the investigator holds about individuals and families in the conduct of the research must be clear. Family itself is likely to be the "lens" with which the problem under research is viewed, although the family as a whole may be considered or the family may be the context or environment for an individual's health and illness.

> **❝**It rests with the practitioners of nursing to evaluate family and family nursing research and to integrate relevant research into their practice.**❞**

Thus, another criterion for evaluation is a *concept of the family*, and this conceptualization must be consistent with the theoretical framework.. The family may be viewed as a system interacting with its environment (health care system, community), as an environment for the individual members, as a mediator or moderator for individual members, or as the cause of health or illness (Feetham, 1990). The researcher should be explicit about this, and the conceptualization should be clear to the reader.

It follows, therefore, that there must be a *definition of the family*. This involves a clear statement about who was included in the data-collection process. In other words, the definition of the family should be linked to the participants in the study. Here we are not only talking about a theoretical definition but how the definition of family is operationalized. Look for congruence between the theoretical framework, the concept of the family, the definition of family, and the persons who participate in the study.

There must be a *logical consistency* in the methods of family research. As this chapter has described, the research design, the modes of data collection, the measures, and the data analysis must be consistent with the foregoing criteria; all relate back to the unit of analysis. Throughout the methods section, actual or potential *ethical considerations* should be addressed. Finally, the findings must add to the *knowledge base* about families and should have *relevance* to nursing practice.

Critical evaluation of family research is too important to leave to researchers alone. Practicing family nurses have a responsibility to read and weigh the merits of family studies. Whatever they may lack in understanding of a particular design, method, or analytical technique, they bring to the evaluation a wealth of clinical knowledge with which to assess the clinical significance of the study.

EVIDENCE-BASED FAMILY NURSING

Hallberg (2003) provided a thought-provoking, overall perspective on the status of research in family nursing and potential pitfalls that lay on the horizon. She addressed not only the definition of "evidence-based" nursing and its implications for nursing research but also raised concern about the potential for losing the "humanistic" side of nursing if the definition of evidence-based care were to be strictly based on the medical model. In her editorial, Hallberg identified four fundamental questions facing family nursing research.

- What do we mean by evidence-based nursing?
- How are empirically developed knowledge and theoretically developed knowledge in nursing related to each other?
- Do we have the knowledge base needed to assert that we apply evidence-based nursing?
- How do we apply evidence-based knowledge in nursing practice, or rather what part of it are we going to apply?

What Do We Mean by Evidence-Based Nursing?

As Hallberg pointed out, the term *evidence-based nursing* is not currently a MeSH term in MEDLINE, in contrast to *evidence-based medicine*, defined as a MeSH term for a clinical learning strategy. (MeSH is the National Library of Medicine's vocabulary used for indexing articles for MELINE/PubMed. It provides a way to retrieve information that may use varying terminology for a concept.) In medicine, a clinical

learning strategy involves four steps: formulating a clear clinical question from a patient's problem; searching the literature for relevant articles; critically evaluating the evidence for its validity and usefulness; and implementing useful findings in clinical practice (Rosenberg & Donald, 1995). This is a rather strict interpretation of the application of research-based findings to clinical practice. By contrast, in the Cumulative Index of Nursing and Allied Health Literature (CINAHL), one finds a more inclusive definition of evidence-based medicine that features clinical expertise and patient choices.

Many of the emerging definitions of evidence-based practice in nursing draw on the definitions from medicine but stress the use of research findings as well as other sources of credible information (versus tradition) to guide practice. Stetler (2001) differentiated between external and internal evidence. External evidence refers to research findings and consensus reports of national experts. Internal evidence refers to

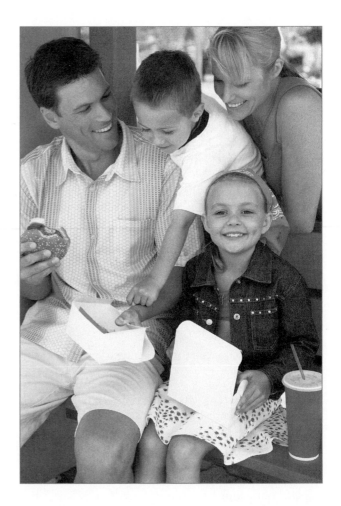

the other sources of credible information or data, including quality-improvement, operational, and evaluation data. Emerging definitions of evidence-based nursing practice recognize the centrality of individual clinical expertise, defined as the proficiency and judgment acquired by individual clinicians through clinical experience (Messecar & Tanner, 2003). Thus, external clinical evidence informs but does not replace clinical expertise. Instead, clinical expertise is necessary to decide whether given external evidence applies to the patient or family at all and how it should be integrated into a clinical decision (Messecar & Tanner, 2003). Accordingly evidence-based nursing practice may be understood as a process of clinical reasoning that uses external and internal evidence to inform a knowledge base in the context of factors that affect patient/family responses. This definition recognizes the value of clinical expertise in a model of patient/family-centered care (Messecar & Tanner, 2003).

How Are Empirically Developed Knowledge and Theoretically Developed Knowledge in Nursing Related to Each Other?

Implied in this question is another about whether family nursing research needs to base itself on its own unique theories and models or if it is acceptable for the research to employ frameworks and theories from other disciplines. In fact, can family nursing research assert itself as a unique discipline if it does not have a specific research theory base from which to grow? If we use theories based on concepts from other disciplines, is family nursing research able to adapt theory to the nursing perspective?

Hallberg (2003) encouraged those active in family nursing to reflect on how researchers develop knowledge for nursing practice. She urged the examination and comparison of theory development based on analytic and philosophical processes versus theory development based on empirical research. According to Hallberg, researchers need to grapple with how such variously derived knowledge is to be used when it comes to evidence-based nursing.

Fundamentally family nursing is about serving families. This means that we are willing to integrate evidence from a variety of disciplines into our knowledge base. The nursing perspective dictates what is included. In essence, knowledge and theory that address biopsychosocial domains, in cultural context, are relevant to family nursing.

Do We Have the Knowledge Base Needed to Assert That We Apply Evidence-Based Nursing?

Several important questions can be derived from this overriding question. When one looks at research, it is generally considered that longitudinal, prospective, and randomized-controlled clinical trials are stronger in providing "evidence" than cross-sectional and retrospective studies. Nursing research relies, to some extent, on qualitative studies that have limited generalizability and are more likely to suggest further research questions. However, when investigating diseases and processes within the context of the patient, confounding factors arise. At some point, these specific questions need to be more broadly addressed through further research. Hallberg suggested synthesizing all qualitative studies to build upon them further—which raises methodological questions. Nonetheless, it is important to evaluate interventions and be creative with them in order not to miss the larger context in which patients and families exist. Very few arenas in the nursing care of families lend themselves to the conditions of true experimental designs. Most of the significant family nursing interventions are applied in a natural environment where very few of the processes and conditions other than the intervention can be controlled.

In examining the knowledge base found in research, it is fundamental for researchers to have a dialogue with each other about where evidence and research overlap (Hallberg, 2003). As Hallberg reminds us, nursing practice is caring for the patient and family—not managing the disease—and therefore research should reflect the complexity of the lives for which it is providing evidence to alter clinical practice. Collaborative nursing research is needed to address the intrinsic difficulties of conducting research in the field and to address such issues as heterogeneity of age, socioeconomic conditions, disease and treatment, and other aspects (Hallberg, 2003). Only then can we build systematic knowledge within a given area of family nursing.

How Do We Apply Evidence-Based Knowledge in Nursing Practice, or Rather What Part of It Are We Going to Apply?

In addressing this question, Hallberg raised two fundamental concerns: (1) a fear of losing the humanistic values of nursing care when applying evidence-based nursing; and (2) the importance of examining and bearing in mind the difference between science and practice:

> *Science tries to simplify things, whereas practice is complex. Science means explanation, whereas practice means doing what can be done. Science claims general validity, whereas practice is specific to a particular situation. Science claims to be intersubjective, whereas practice is subjective and context bound. Last, science is collective, belonging to the international research community, whereas practice is individual from the perspective of both the patient and the caregiver.* (Hallberg, 2003, p. 19)

The definition and model of evidence-based practice offered by Messecar and Tanner (2003) should serve to alleviate these concerns, with their emphasis on clinical expertise as requisite for the evaluation and integration of evidence into patient-centered care. Accordingly, contextual factors and knowing the particulars of the patient/family are central and thereby contribute to the complexity of the research required for evidence.

NURSING IMPLICATIONS

There are a number of implications for nursing practice but among the ones most important to consider are privacy, informed consent, and the concept of research versus treatment.

Privacy and Informed Consent

A major consideration in the conduct of family research is disclosure of personal information. Often such information has not been revealed before this research process. Therefore, researchers must consider the balance between the risks to the participants by intrusive or threatening data collection procedures and the benefits to family science and society (Bussell, 1994).

Informed consent, as with any research, is essential. What is particular to family research, however, is the involvement of young children and adolescents. An important strategy is to include a child *assent* form that describes the purpose of the research and requests the child's or adolescent's agreement to participate. This consenting procedure is used with children who are able to read. Then researchers should obtain actual consent from the parents.

Another facet of informed consent pertains to the use of videotaped observations; the faces and voices are recorded and names are usually used in the obser-

vation period. Participants must be fully informed about how the videotaped data will be managed and stored, and who will see it. They must be informed when the videotapes will be destroyed and how they will have access to view the recordings or obtain a copy. One valuable strategy is to provide participants with a copy of the recording, if doing so does not violate the integrity of the research procedures.

The research setting presents other considerations. When data collection takes place in the home, several issues emerge. One is the issue of privacy if individual interviews take place or questionnaires are administered. It is critical to maintain the privacy and confidentiality of the individual member or couple and to avoid any undue influence by other family members. This caution is especially necessary for children, care receivers, and those who are vulnerable to other family members in terms of a power differential. Another consideration in the home setting concerns the visibility of the family's private living space. Researchers must be most careful not to draw unwarranted conclusions or assumptions about families based on their living environment.

Research and Treatment

If clinical information will be derived from certain measures (e.g., depression level), the consent form can state that subjects will be informed if they have scores that are in a clinical range on a given measure. In this way, participants are aware that they will receive clinically relevant feedback. At the same time, the consent forms typically state, quite clearly, that the investigators' work with the family is for scientific purposes and that researchers will not be expected to provide treatment. Investigators can avoid conflicts by establishing guidelines, before data collection begins, for when and how to intervene on a subject's behalf (Bussell, 1994).

This blurring of boundaries between research and treatment occurs in a similar way even with self-report data. The process of completing questionnaires about family issues is likely to trigger consideration of ideas and feelings that may not have been addressed previously. Although this self-reflection may serve as a benefit of the research process, alternatively, it can serve as a risk for unpleasant feelings (e.g., anxiety, anger, and regret) or adverse responses that require professional assistance. It is not uncommon, therefore, for a research team to be prepared to make referrals for crisis intervention or provide a list of relevant mental health or diagnosis-specific resources.

Future

Much work has been done in family nursing research. Family nursing researchers have given the discipline and family science knowledge about interactions between families and health and illness across the life span, including family health promotion, family management of acute and chronic illness, and family care giving. Research on aging families and healthy families is increasing steadily. Family nursing can be justifiably proud of this heritage.

However, there is much work to be done. Some of the gaps in family nursing research have narrowed during the last 30 years, while others have widened.

The following are areas for future work in family nursing research:

- Family intervention studies, using the wealth of exploratory, descriptive, and correlational studies in the literature
- Studies of families representing diversity in structure, ethnicity, and living situation
- Research to advance our understanding of vulnerable families
- Attention to mixed methods as research strategies to enhance the depth and breadth of our knowledge base in family nursing, especially regarding vulnerable families
- Studies that focus on relationships between families and other social systems
- Increased and consistent attention to the unit of analysis in family studies
- Attention to informing social and health policy with findings from family research
- Attention to theory development and theoretical consistency within and across studies
- Attention to biosocial research opportunities in family nursing, including the implications for families of the ever-increasing information on genetics (Feetham & Meister, 1999)

SUMMARY

- The relationships between the various ways we develop knowledge for nursing care, especially the relationship between nursing theories and research-based knowledge, are important ones.
- Many family nursing studies have not explicated their assumptions or theoretical frameworks. Studies that did often relied on concepts and methods from other disciplines.
- Although nursing has much to learn from the social sciences and family therapy, these disciplines cannot guide nursing practice.
- Another reason for the lack of theory in family nursing is the apparent dissonance between considering the family as the client and fully appreciating the freedom and uniqueness of each family member.
- The most practical question that faces a family researcher is who to include in the study.
- What is important is whether the researcher obtains information from an individual about the family or from the family as a whole at one time, and it is important because of the application of findings to practice. If family interventions are to be successful, they cannot rest on family-related research alone.
- The choice of who should be the source of data collection, or the unit of analysis, should make sense in terms of the purpose of the study, the theoretical orientation and research question, and whether the researcher wants to generalize about the family as a whole or focus on the individual's perceptions about the family.
- A variety of methods are used to describe characteristics of families, including surveys, structured interviews, and intensive observations in the laboratory, the clinical setting, or in the family home.
- A primary concern with sampling is whether the families who participate in a study are representative of the populations or groups to whom findings and conclusions can be generalized.
- Family research and theory cannot be assumed to have cross-cultural applicability.
- The researcher and the practitioner must be clear about the meaning of the measurement used in a given study, especially since many of the measures and observations in family research are also used as clinical assessments.
- Generally speaking, family research is *multivariate* in nature; multiple concepts and, therefore, multiple variables are of interest in our efforts to understand families.
- Grounded theory explicitly acknowledges the family and its members as experts in their own experience and allows nurses to explore areas of nursing experience that have not been adequately addressed by existing theories.
- Nursing practice is caring for the patient and family—not managing the disease—and therefore research should reflect the complexity of

the lives for which it is providing evidence to alter clinical practice. Collaborative nursing research is needed to address the intrinsic difficulties of conducting research in the field and to address such issues as heterogeneity of age, socioeconomic conditions, disease and treatment, and other aspects.

SQ STUDY QUESTIONS

1. How does the unit of analysis in family nursing research influence the nature of the research? How does it influence the type of research questions addressed? How does it influence the data received? Give an example of each.

2. Why is it important for family nurse researchers to define *family* explicitly in a study?

3. Choose one of the research designs used in family research and give an example of a family research question that would be appropriate for that design.

4. Briefly discuss two challenges associated with sampling in family research.

5. How questions are asked can make a significant difference in the quality of data when self-report methods are used in family research. Describe three strategies to improve the quality of the data collected.

6. Distinguish between reliability and validity of measurement in family research.

7. Why is quantitative family research *multivariate* in nature?

8. Give two reasons why a family nurse researcher might choose qualitative methods to answer a research question.

9. Briefly discuss three ethical considerations in family nursing research.

10. List six issues that should be evaluated in family and family nursing research.

11. The authors list seven areas for future work in family nursing research. Which area do you believe should be addressed first if the goal is improvement of family nursing practice? Why?

References

Ambert, A., Adler, P. A., Adler, P., & Detzner, D. F. (1995). Understanding and evaluating qualitative research. *Journal of Marriage and the Family, 57*, 879–893.

Astedt-Kurki, P., Paavilainen, E., & Lehti, K. (2001). Methodological issues in interviewing families in family nursing research. *Journal of Advanced Nursing, 35*, 288–293.

Baumann, S. L. (2000). Research issues. Family nursing: theory-anemic, nursing theory-deprived. *Nursing Science Quarterly, 13*, 285–290.

Baumann, S. L. (2002). Toward a global perspective of the human sciences. *Nursing Science Quarterly, 15*, 81–84.

Bell, J. M. (1995a). Wanted: Family nursing interventions. *Journal of Family Nursing, 1*, 355–358.

Bell, J. M. (1995b). What is "family"? Perturbations and possibilities. *Journal of Family Nursing, 1*, 131–133.

Benson, M. J., & Deal, J. E. (1995). Bridging the individual and the family. *Journal of Marriage and the Family, 57*, 561–566.

Berkey, K. M., & Hanson, S. M. H. (1991). Family nursing assessment/measurement instrumentation. In *Pocket guide to family assessment and intervention* (pp. 226–277). St. Louis: Mosby Year Book.

Bussell, D. A. (1994). Ethical issues in observational family research. *Family Process, 33*, 361–376.

Chesla, C. A. (1994). Parents' caring practices with schizophrenic offspring. In P. Benner (Ed.), *Interpretive phenomenology: Embodiment, caring, and ethics in health and illness* (pp. 167–184). Thousand Oaks, CA: Sage.

Chesla, C. A. (1995). Hermeneutic phenomenology: An approach to understanding families. *Journal of Family Nursing, 1*, 63–78.

Copeland, A. P., & White, K. M. (1991). *Applied social research methods series: Vol. 27. Studying families.* Newbury Park, CA: Sage.

Denham, S. A. (1999a). Part 1: The definition and practice of family health. *Journal of Family Nursing, 5*, 133–159.

Denham, S. A. (1999b). Part 2: Family health during and after death of a family member. *Journal of Family Nursing, 5*, 160–183.

Denham, S. A. (1999c). Part 3: Family health in an economically disadvantaged population. *Journal of Family Nursing, 5*, 184–213.

Feetham, S. L. (1984). Family research: Issues and directions for nursing. In H. H. Werley & J. J. Fitzpatrick (Eds.), *Annual review of nursing research* (pp. 3–26). New York: Springer.

Feetham, S. L. (1990). Conceptual and methodological issues in research of families. In J. M. Bell et al. (Eds.), *The cutting edge of family nursing* (pp. 35–49). Calgary, AB: Family Nursing Unit Publications.

Feetham, S. L., & Deatrick, J. (2002). Expanding science policy regarding research with vulnerable families. *Journal of Family Nursing, 8*, 371–382.

Feetham, S. L., & Meister, S. B. (1999). Nursing research of families: State of the science and correspondence with policy. In A. S. Hinshaw, S. L. Feetham, & J. L. Shaver (Eds.), *Handbook of clinical nursing research* (pp. 251–271). Thousand Oaks, CA: Sage.

Fisher, L., Terry, H. E., & Ransom, D. C. (1990). Advancing a family perspective in health research: Models & methods. *Family Process, 29*, 177–189.

Frank, A. W. (1995). Further reflections on illness (Review essay). *Journal of Family Nursing, 1*, 420–426.

Ganong, L. H. (1995). Current trends and issues in family nursing research. *Journal of Family Nursing, 1*, 171–206.

Gilliss, C. (1983). The nurse as a unit of analysis: Strategies for the nurse researcher. *Advances in Nursing Science, 5,* 50–59.

Gilliss, C. (1991). Family nursing research: Theory and practice. *Image: Journal of Nursing Scholarship, 23,* 19–22.

Gilliss, C., & Knafl, K. A. (1999). Nursing care of families in non-normative transitions. In A. S. Hinshaw, S. L. Feetham, & J. L. Shaver (Eds.), *Handbook of clinical nursing research* (pp. 231–249). Thousand Oaks, CA: Sage.

Gilliss, C., Gortner, S., Hauck, W., Shinn, J., Sparacino, P., & Tompkins, C. (1993). A randomized trial of nursing care for recovery from cardiac surgery. *Heart and Lung, 22,* 125–133.

Glaser, B., & Strauss, A. (1967). *The discovery of grounded theory.* Chicago: Aldine.

Hallberg, I. (2003). Evidence-based nursing, interventions, and family nursing: Methodological obstacles and possibilities. *Journal of Family Nursing, 9,* 3–22.

Hanson, S. M. H. (2001). Family health care nursing: An introduction. In S. M. H. Hanson (Ed.), *Family health care nursing: Theory, practice and research* (pp. 3–35). Philadelphia: Davis.

Hanson, S. M. H., & Kaakinen, J. R. (2001). Theoretical foundations for family nursing. In S. M. H. Hanson (Ed.), *Family health care nursing: Theory, practice and research* (pp. 36–59). Philadelphia: Davis.

Hartrick, G. A., & Lindsey, A. E. (1995). Part 2: The lived experience of family: A contextual approach to family nursing practice. *Journal of Family Nursing, 1,* 148–170.

Hayes, V. E. (1995). Response to L. H. Ganong: "Current trends and issues in family nursing research." *Journal of Family Nursing, 1,* 207–212.

Horowitz, J. A., Ladden, M. D., & Moriarty, H. J. (2002). Methodological challenges in research with vulnerable families. *Journal of Family Nursing, 8,* 315–333.

Houck, G. M., & LeCuyer-Maus, E. A. (2002). Maternal limit-setting patterns and toddler development of self-concept and social competence. *Issues in Comprehensive Pediatric Nursing, 25,* 21–41.

Houck, G. M., & LeCuyer-Maus, E. A. (2004). Maternal limit-setting during toddlerhood, delay of gratification, and behavior problems at age five. *Infant Mental Health Journal, 25,* 28–46.

Houck, G. M., Booth, C. L., & Barnard, K. E. (1991). Maternal depression and locus of control orientation as predictors of dyadic play behavior. *Infant Mental Health Journal, 12,* 347–360.

Kelly, M. L., Power, T. G., & Wimbush, D. D. (1992). Determinants of disciplinary practices in low-income black mothers. *Child Development, 63,* 573–582.

Knafl, K. A., & Gilliss, C. L. (2002). Families and chronic illness: A synthesis of current research. *Journal of Family Nursing, 8,* 178–198.

Knafl, K. A., Ayres, L., Gallo, A. M., Zoeller, L. H., & Breitmayer, B. J. (1995). Learning from stories: Parents' accounts of the pathway to diagnosis. *Pediatric Nursing, 21,* 411–415.

LeCuyer-Maus, E. A., & Houck, G. M. (2002). Mother-toddler interaction and the development of self-regulation in a limit-setting context. *Journal of Pediatric Nursing, 17,* 184–200.

Leininger, M. M. (1985). Ethnography and ethnonursing: Models and modes of qualitative data analysis. In M. M. Leininger (Ed.), *Qualitative research methods in nursing* (pp. 33–71). Orlando, FL: Grune & Stratton.

Lewis, F. M. (1993). Psychosocial transitions and the family's work in adjusting to cancer. Seminars in *Oncology Nursing, 9,* 127–129.

Lewis, F. M., Hammond, M. A., & Woods, N. F. (1993). The family's functioning with newly diagnosed breast cancer in the mother: The development of an explanatory model. *Journal of Behavioral Medicine, 16,* 351–370.

Lewis, F. M., Zahlis, E. H., Shands, M. E., Sinsheimer, J. A., & Hammond, M. A. (1996). The functioning of single women

with breast cancer and their school-aged children. *Cancer Practice, 4,* 15–24.

Messecar, D., & Tanner, C. A. (2003). Evidence-based practice. In L. A. Joel (Ed.), *Advanced practice nursing: Essentials for role development* (pp. 257–279). Philadelphia: Davis.

Miller, B. C. (1986). *Family studies text series: Vol. 4. Family research methods.* Beverly Hills, CA: Sage.

Miller, R. B., & Wright, D. W. (1995). Detecting and correcting attrition bias in longitudinal family research. *Journal of Marriage and the Family, 57,* 921–929.

Moriarty, H. J., Cotroneo, M., DeFeudis, R., & Natale, S. (1995). Key issues in cross-cultural family research. *Journal of Family Nursing, 1,* 359–381.

Moriarty, H. J., Deatrick, J. A., Mahon, M. M., Feetham, S. L., Carroll, R. M., Shepard, M. P., & Orsi, A. J. (1999). Issues to consider when choosing and using large national data bases for research of families. *Western Journal of Nursing Research, 21,* 143–153.

Motzer, S. A., Moseley, J. R., & Lewis, F. M. (1997). Recruitment and retention of families in clinical trials with longitudinal designs. *Western Journal of Nursing Research, 19,* 314–333.

Olsen, S. F., et al. (1999). Support, communication, and hardiness in families with children with disabilities. *Journal of Family Nursing, 5,* 275–291.

Oxley, G. M., & Weekes, D. P. (1997). Experiences of pregnant African American adolescents: Meanings, perception, appraisal, and coping. *Journal of Family Nursing, 3,* 167–188.

Poirier, S., & Ayres, L. (1997). Endings, secrets, and silences: Overreading in narrative inquiry. *Research in Nursing & Health, 20,* 551–557.

Polit, D. F., Beck, C. T., & Hungler, B. P. (2001). *Essentials of nursing research: Methods, appraisal, and utilization* (5th ed.). Philadelphia: Lippincott.

Robinson, C. A. (1995). Unifying distinctions for nursing research with persons and families. *Journal of Family Nursing, 1,* 8–29.

Rosenberg, R., & Donald, A. (1995). Evidence-based medicine: An approach to clinical problem solving. *British Medical Journal, 310*(6987), 1122–1126.

Ryan, E. A., & Hayman, L. L. (1996). The role of the family coordinator in longitudinal research: Strategies to recruit and retain families. *Journal of Family Nursing, 2,* 325–335.

Sandelowski, M. (1986). The problem of rigor in qualitative research. *Advances in Nursing Science, 8*(3), 27–37.

Shepard, M., & Mahon, M. (2002). Vulnerable families: Research findings and methodological challenges. *Journal of Family Nursing, 8,* 309–314.

Shepard, M., Orsi, A. J., Mahon, M. M., & Carroll, R. M. (2002). Mixed-method research with vulnerable families. *Journal of Family Nursing, 8,* 334–352.

Smith, T. E., & Graham, P. B. (1995). Socioeconomic stratification in family research. *Journal of Marriage and the Family, 57,* 930–940.

Stetler, C. B. (2001). Updating the Stetler model of research utilization to facilitate evidence-based practice. *Nursing Outlook, 49,* 272–279.

Uphold C. R., & Strickland, O. L. (1989). Issues related to the unit of analysis in family nursing research. *Western Journal of Nursing Research, 11,* 405–417.

Whall, A. L., & Loveland-Cherry, C. J. (1993). Family unit-focused research: 1984–1991. In H. H. Werley & J. J. Fitzpatrick (Eds.), *Annual review of research in nursing* (pp. 227–247). New York: Springer.

Wilson, S., & Morse, J. M. (1991). Living with a wife undergoing chemotherapy. *Image: Journal of Nursing Scholarship, 23,* 78–84.

Woods, N. F., Lewis, F. M., & Ellison, E. S. (1989). Living with cancer: Family experiences. *Cancer Nursing, 12,* 28–33.

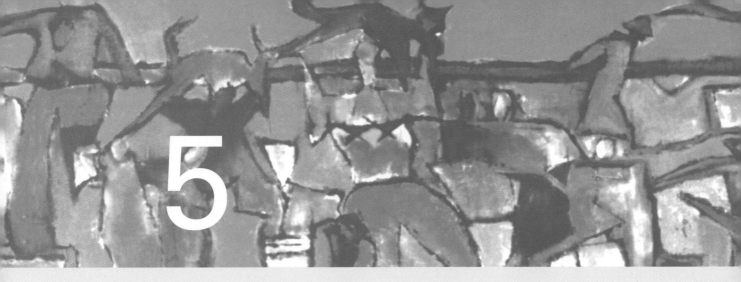

5

Family Structure, Function, and Process

Sharon A. Denham, RN, DSN

CRITICAL CONCEPTS

- The major factors for family analysis are family structure, function, and process.

- Family structure can be described in terms of family types, membership, and context.

- Traditional views of American families regarded them mainly as nuclear units, but today's families are just as apt to be stepparent, single-parent, blended, cohabitating, gay, or lesbian.

- Family is the socializing unit for most individuals and affects all aspects of members' lives including the ways they experience health and illness.

- Families have affective, reproductive, economic, and health functions that greatly impact the lives of individual family members.

- Family processes such as roles, communication, power, decision making, coping strategies, and marital satisfaction are the interactions through which members accomplish instrumental and expressive tasks.

- Family structure, function, and process greatly impact the ways in which individual members and families experience health and illness and define family health.

- Nurses have great potential to practice in ways that impact families' structure, functions, and processes and intervene in ways that promote health and wellness, as well as prevent illness risks, treat disease conditions, and manage rehabilitative care needs.

INTRODUCTION

Nurses often focus on individuals as the primary unit of health care and view family as the context for the individual. However, when family is considered the unit of care, nurses have much broader perspectives for approaching individual health care needs. The structure, functions, and processes of the family unit influence and are influenced by individuals' health status and the health of the family unit. For example, the health of a family and its members is influenced not only by heredity or genetics but also by access to health care, environmental conditions in the area of residence, economics, availability of employment, and even the ways the members respond to stress and conflict over time. Nurses need broad-based knowledge about families to provide optimum health care for individuals encountered in diverse health care settings. Understanding about families enables nurses to assess the family's health status, ascertain effects of the family on individuals' health status, predict the impact of alterations in health status on the family system, and work with members as they plan and implement action plans targeting health or illness outcomes. Knowledge about family structure, function, and process equips the nurse to provide care tailored to the uniqueness of family systems and suggests ways to optimize clinical practice. Learning about family structure, function, and process provides ways to evaluate standards for nursing actions with individual clients and families.

The reciprocal and interactive relationships that exist among family structure, function, and process should not be ignored. Nurses need knowledge about these concepts when completing assessments, developing care plans, identifying alternative interventions, and evaluating outcomes. Knowledge about family structure, function, and processes are essential keys for understanding the complex member interactions that impact health, illness, and well-being. Family concepts suggest a framework to discern ways the nurse can identify effective interventions. Many internal and external family variables affect individual members and the family as a whole. Variables influencing the family are related to internal factors (e.g., unique individual characteristics, communication, interactions) and external factors (e.g., location of family household, social policy, economic trends). Family members generally have complicated responses to these factors. Although some external factors may not be easily modifiable, nurses can assist family members to manage change, conflict, and care needs. For instance, a sudden downturn in the economy could result in the family breadwinner becoming unemployed. Although the nurse is unable to alter the situation directly, understanding the implications of the family situation provides a basis for planning more effective interventions. Nurses can assist members with things like coping skills, communication patterns, location of needed resources, effective use of information, or creation of family rituals or routines. Even a novice family nurse may assist family members in family interactions and responses to their environment.

Nurses who understand the concepts of family structure, function, and process can use these ideas to educate, counsel, and implement changes that enable individuals to cope with illness, family crisis, chronic health conditions, mental illness, or disabilities. Individual health alterations affect the entire family membership, and nurses prepared to work with families can assist them with needed life transitions. For example, when a member experiences a chronic condition such as diabetes, family roles, routines, and power hierarchies may be challenged. Nurses need to be prepared to address the complex and holistic family problems resulting from the illness, as well as to care for the individual's medical needs. This chapter provides explanations about family structure, function, and process and suggests relationships with health and illness needs.

FAMILY STRUCTURE

Family *structure* is the ordered set of relationships among family parts and between the family and other social systems. The most clear-cut change in the American family during the past few decades has been in its structure. In determining the family structure, the nurse needs to identify the following:

- The individuals that compose the family
- The relationships between them
- The interactions between the family members
- The interactions with other social systems

Family patterns of organization tend to be relatively stable over time; however, they are modified gradually throughout the family life cycle and often change radically when divorce, separation, or death occurs. Norms that control family relationships, although influenced by the culture, are not clearly prescribed by the culture. Family customs, practices, and traditions have evolved as the family interacts with various social institutions over time. The traditional view of family structure was the nuclear family with a mother, father, and often two to three children as members. Today's family structures differ widely. The structural family types are numerous, but some examples include the following:

- Single-parent never-married families with children fathered by a single male
- Single-parent never-married families with children fathered by more than one male
- Single-parent divorced families with shared custody of the children
- Partnering male and female relationships with children but no marriage
- Gay and lesbian families with children born to one of the partners
- Gay and lesbian families with adopted or in vitro–conceived children
- Grandparent families caring for grandchildren belonging to one of their own children

66 Knowledge about family structure, function, and process equips the nurse to provide care tailored to the uniqueness of family systems and suggests ways to optimize clinical practice. 99

In today's information age and global society, several ideas about the rightness of various types of family structure coexist simultaneously. Different family types have their strengths and limitations, which can directly or indirectly affect individual and family health. *Family health* has been described as a complex phenomenon that includes interactions of multiple systems, dynamics, relationships, and processes that have the potential to enhance individual and family well-being (Denham, 2003a). Many families still adhere to more customary forms and patterns, but many of today's families fall into categories more clearly labeled "nontraditional." Transitions from traditional to nontraditional families continue to evolve. Nurses are likely to confront families structured differently from their own family of origin and encounter family types that conflict with personal value systems. For nurses to work effectively with families, they must maintain open and inquiring minds.

Understanding family structure can enable nurses to assist families to identify effective coping strategies for daily life disturbances, health care crises, wellness promotion, and disease prevention. Additionally, nurses are in a position to help advocate and develop social policies relevant to family health care needs. For example, taking political action to increase the availability of appropriate care for children could reduce the financial and emotional burden of many working and single-parent families when faced with the problem of how to provide care for a sick child. Similarly, caregiving responsibilities and health care costs for acutely and chronically ill family members place increasing demands on family members. Nurses who are well-informed about family structure can better identify specific needs of unique families, provide appropriate clinical care to enhance family resilience, and act as change agents to enact social policies that reduce family burdens.

66 Many families still adhere to more customary forms and patterns, but many of today's families fall into categories more clearly labeled "nontraditional." 99

Diversity in the American Family

The family can be conceptualized as a social institution, a social system, and a social group (Eshleman, 1997). In our society, family aspects have been constantly evolving for decades. The family is a societal institution that undergoes dynamic changes over time in order to meet the needs of the larger society. Nurses need to understand the family as a social institution, in the context of other societal institutions. Consequently, understanding the ways family is impacted by society as well as ways it influences society requires knowledge about the historical, social, cultural, economic, political, psychological, and spiritual context in which families evolve.

Discussions of family structure often begin with a focus on the decline of the nuclear family and the emergence of diverse family types in American society during the late 20th century. *Contemporary families* may take one of several different forms, including single-parent (biological, adoptive, step), intact nuclear (biological, adoptive), intergenerational, extended without parent, same-sex, cohabiting or domestic partnerships, and institutions (foster care, group homes, residential or treatment centers). However, the traditional nuclear family remains the standard by which many still evaluate family forms (Ganong, Coleman, & Mapes, 1990; Spanier, 1989). A *nuclear family* can be defined as one with parents and children only. Extended family is the nuclear family plus other blood-related kin or relationships formed by a marriage tie. Multiple family types coexist, each type with its own strengths and weaknesses. A dichotomy often exists between abstract notions of the ideal family as nuclear and what actually exists within society. Following World War II, the number of nuclear families consisting of parents and children but no other immediate or distant family members started to grow. This meant, in much of the nation, that grandparents lived alone, siblings dispersed to remote geographic sites, and the extended family became less enmeshed.

The nuclear family is becoming a demographic oddity as Americans redefine ideas. Although it is not uncommon to hear people say that today's family is unstable and its future uncertain, evidence suggests that much of what has been viewed as truth about families is merely myth (Coontz, 1988, 1992, 1997). Many of the perceptions about families ignore the diversity that has always existed (Allen, Fine, & Demo, 2000). Much interest has focused on an alleged breakdown of the traditional family, but the 2000 census data indicates that throughout much of the United States, the majority of children under 18 years of age still live in households headed by a married couple.

The proportion of U.S. families with children under age 18 headed by married couples reached an all-time low in the mid-1990s, about 72.9 percent in 1996, and has since stabilized at 73 percent in 2000 (Blankenhorn, 2002). The proportion of all U.S. children living in two-parent homes reached a low of 68 percent in the mid-1990s but rose to 69.1 percent in 2000. Findings from the 2000 census indicate that race and ethnicity are important factors for characterizing households. For example, although 84 percent of Asian children and 79 percent of non-Hispanic whites lived with two parents, only 38 percent of black children did. Thus, it is important to consider demographic characteristics prior to making broad assumptions about families.

> ❝Contemporary families may take one of several different forms, including single-parent (biological, adoptive, step), intact nuclear (biological, adoptive), intergenerational, extended without parent, same-sex, cohabitating or domestic partnerships, and institutions (foster care, group homes, residential or treatment centers).❞

Family Types

American perspectives on family membership, like those of many other Westernized nations, continue to shift from traditional views to acceptance of more nonconventional forms. Although some nations continue to adhere fervently to family structures and traditions honored for centuries, others, influenced by societal changes, look more like those found in the United States. See Box 5–1 for a comparison of American and traditional family structures.

Although nearly everyone marries, nearly half of recent first marriages ended in divorce (Kreider & Fields, 2001). The last-reported U.S. divorce rate for a calendar year (2001) is 0.40 percent per 1000 persons, the provisional estimate for the year ("Births, Marriages, Divorces and Deaths," 2002). Numbers about divorce are somewhat confusing and sometimes difficult to interpret. First, because every divorce involves two people, the percentage might be somewhat more meaningful if it is doubled. Second, four

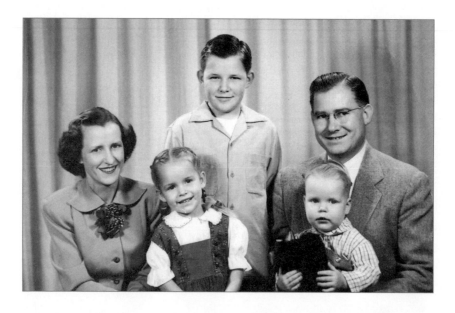

Box 5–1

In the United States, views of traditional family structure are often epitomized by stereotypical views that suggest ways a "normal" or "average" family is characterized. Americans are diverse and have pluralistic cultural values and traditional influences that impact their unique structures. In America, if a married couple gets divorced, decisions about custody are affected by multiple factors. Sometimes decisions about custody are based on friendly agreements between parents, a child may be old enough to decide, or a court may mandate what will occur. Mothers, in earlier times, would be granted custody of the children without question because a father was not viewed as a capable caregiver. Now, fathers are considered when custody is awarded, and parents frequently obtain joint custody. Other factors influencing custody may include parental economics, employment responsibilities, social supports, parenting abilities, or location of residence.

By contrast, a family from another culture may have a family structure that is influenced by a different set of cultural values and traditions. For example, many Asian families living in their native lands have very different practices when a divorce occurs. Although arranged marriages are less common, they still occur and infidelity in these marriages may not be uncommon. Women who ask for a divorce may be told to leave with only their clothes or other personal items and are expected to leave their children behind. Women experiencing physical abuse from their spouse may stay in the relationship because they fear that leaving would mean deprivation and loss of ties to their children. It is not unusual to find mothers in China, Japan, or other Asian nations who have been stripped of their children if they choose to divorce.

states (i.e., California, Colorado, Indiana, and Louisiana) do not report divorce rates. Marriages are most susceptible to divorce during the first 5 years, with about 10 percent ending in divorce, and another 10 percent divorced by the 10th year (Kreider & Fields, 2001). In the 1996 data, 40 percent of married white non-Hispanic and Hispanic women and 48 percent of black women were divorced from their first marriage, but only 24 percent of married Asian and Pacific Islanders were divorced from their first marriage (Kreider & Fields, 2001).

Between 1960 and 1990, the percentage of children living apart from their biological fathers more than doubled, from 17 percent to 36 percent (Popenoe, 1999). Some statistical data reflect that more people are paying child support to children who are part of another household. In 1997, 7.2 million people paid a median of $2940 a year in financial assistance. In 2002, although the median payment to custodial parents should have been $5044 each, the median amount received was $3160, or a national shortfall of $13 billion (U.S. Census Bureau, 2002a). In 2002, about five of every six custodial parents were mothers (84.4 percent) and one in six were fathers (15.6 percent), proportions statistically unchanged since 1994 (U.S. Census Bureau, 2003a).

Despite the growing numbers of nontraditional families in American society, far less is known about them than nuclear families. Nontraditional families have both similarities to and differences from traditional nuclear families. A *traditional family* is what is perceived to be the norm or mainstream, usually two parents with consanguineously related children where roles and power are related to gender. For example, today many families could be classified as remarried, blended, or reconstituted, a family with a male and a female where at least one has been married before and where children may or may not be living in the household. The number of households without children is rising because of the increased length of the post-parental stage of the family life cycle. Reconstituted families, stepfamilies, adoptive families, blended families, and gay and lesbian families are increasingly common. A more comprehensive knowledge base about families could be achieved in the future through research that is more focused on nontraditional families (Allen & Demo, 1995).

Single-Parent Family

The *single-parent family* is one in which the head of the household has never been or is not currently married. Although these families are more visible today, they have always existed, with the death of one parent being a common cause prior to the 20th century. The changing status of women, unintended pregnancy, and marital dissolution are common reasons for today's single-parent families (see Box 5–2). Greater

Box 5–2

According to the 2000 U.S. census, while 26 million two-parent families exist in the nation, another 11 million families are headed by single mothers, another 2 million by single fathers, and 2.2 million by cohabiting partners. Those statistics also demonstrate that 34 percent of the single mothers and 16 percent of the single fathers were living at or below the poverty level. The National Fatherhood Initiative (2002) reported that 1.35 million or 33 percent of births in 2000 occurred out of wedlock. Due to things like the high divorce rate and increased births to adolescents, 24 million or 34 percent of children live in households absent their biological father and nearly 20 million or 27 percent of children live in single-parent homes (National Fatherhood Initiative, 2002). High rates of fatherless homes mean that 40 percent of these children have not seen their father during the past year. About 26 percent of fathers and children live in different states, and 50 percent of children from single-parent homes may never set foot in their father's home. About 12 percent of children living with single mothers and those living apart from both parents were most likely to be in households receiving public assistance (U.S. Census Bureau, 2002b).

employment opportunities for women and somewhat better wages have made it easier for single parents to bear and raise children outside of marriage (Spain & Bianchi, 1996). Single-parenthood has become one of the more debated issues of our time with many social scientists researching its issues. Much is being learned about relevant issues, such as parental and child adjustment, economic impact, and child behavioral, education, and health outcomes. Study of diverse single-parent variables, however, produces different findings (Amato, 2000).

Studies have found that the success of single-parent families varies not only by race and ethnicity but also by variables such as parental gender and age, level of education, employment status, type of living arrangement, and societal factors. Based on the 2000 census data, the number of homes with single fathers has grown from 393,000 in 1970 to 2 million. According to McKinnon (2003), in 2002, there were 8.8 million African-American families in the United States. About 48 percent of all African-American families were married-couple families; another 43 percent of black families were maintained by women without a spouse present, and about 9 percent were families with black men as head of household. Whereas 25 percent of Caucasians had never been married, 43 percent of black individuals had never married.

Few differences have been found between children raised in single-parent families headed by mothers and children raised in single-parent families headed by fathers (Downey, Ainsworth-Parnell, & Dufur, 1998). However, the single-parent structure alters the relationship between men and women (Guttentag & Secord, 1983) and between parents and children

(Aquilino, 1994; Cooksey & Fondell, 1996; Hanson, McLanahan, & Thomson, 1996; MacDonald & DeMaris, 1995). In addition, single-parent families have high rates of poverty, a factor with ominous implications both for children and for society. The number of single mothers (9.8 million) has remained constant over the past 3 years, but the number of single fathers has grown from 1.7 million in 1995 to 2.1 million in 1998; men now compose one-sixth of the nation's 11.9 million single parents (U.S. Census Bureau, 1998).

Cohabitating Couples

Cohabitating couples are heterosexual couples who choose to live together outside of the marriage covenant, a phenomenon that has become increasingly more common over the last two decades. Cohabitation provides an alternative lifestyle for sexual partners who do not wish to marry or who, because of legal proscription, cannot marry. Reasons for cohabitation might relate to mistrust of the sense that traditional dating patterns can provide the certainty needed for marriage and a belief that cohabitation provides a means to test the worth of the relationship. Other reasons such as personal finances, sexual freedom, and marriage risks may also determine the choice for cohabitation over marriage. Persons in cohabitating relationships may be more likely to be nonmonogamous than married persons (Rutter & Schwartz, 2000). Some choose cohabitation as a trial that sometimes leads to marriage, but others view cohabitation as a statement of a monogamous relationship. Although children are often the reason marriage occurs, more

Box 5–3 COHABITATION

Cohabitation now may be viewed as one step in a continuum that sometimes leads to marriage (Ross, 1995):

- No partner
- Partner outside the household
- Living with partner in the household
- Living with married partner in the household

and more cohabitating couples are choosing to raise children outside the boundaries of matrimony.

> "Reasons such as personal finances, sexual freedom, and marriage risks may determine the choice for cohabitation over marriage."

Measurement of cohabitation has been somewhat problematic because of the fact that most surveys rarely include questions about nonmarital cohabitating relationships. Although measurement problems continue, it is assumed that the number of unmarried heterosexual couples that live together has increased markedly since 1970 (Cherlin, 1992). By 1986, 6 percent of all unmarried adults in the United States were cohabitating (Glick, 1988). Although cohabitation has not resulted in a decrease in the marriage rate, it has altered the timing of marriage, with many young adults postponing marriage until later in their lives. More and more, cohabitation seems to be a part of the courtship process, not an alternative to marriage (see Box 5–3). The Persons of the Opposite Sex Sharing Living Quarters (POSSLQ) measure has commonly been used to determine numbers of cohabitants even though it has problematic assumptions. An Adjusted POSSLQ households measure has been suggested to include cohabitating adults "living together" alone, with any combination of other relatives, or with other unrelated adults (Casper, Cohen, & Simmons, 1999). Use of the Adjusted POSSLQ suggests that earlier estimates may have been undercounted. Thus, estimates in 1977 to 1997 reflect that opposite-sex cohabitation has increased from 13 percent of the population to about 18 percent (Box 5–4).

It is thought that about 25 percent of cohabitating families marry within a year, 50 percent marry within 5 years, and 60 percent of stepparent families created by cohabitation are still intact after 5 years (Bumpass, Raley, & Sweet, 1994). Cohabitation prior to marriage has been associated with a higher divorce rate, and divorced people are more likely to cohabit after their divorces (Brown & Booth, 1996). It is reported that 31.1 percent of children in cohabitating households

Box 5–4 IDENTIFICATION OF OPPOSITE-SEX COHABITANTS

A variety of key household composition scenarios are possible, making identification of cohabitating partners especially difficult. The Adjusted Persons of the Opposite Sex Sharing Living Quarters (POSSLQ) measure includes the following:

- *Man* or *woman* with opposite-sex partner and no other adults present
- *Man* or *woman* with opposite-sex partner, children under 15, and no other adults present
- *Man* or *woman* with opposite-sex partner, children 15+, and no other adults present
- *Man* or *woman* with opposite-sex partner and other unrelated adults
- *Man* or *woman* with opposite-sex non-partner, children under 15, and no other adults present
- *Man* or *woman* with opposite-sex non-partner, children 15+, and no other adults present

Casper, L. M., Cohen, P. N., & Simmons, T. (1999). How does POSSLQ measure up? *Historical estimates of cohabitation.* Population Division, U.S. Bureau of the Census. Retrieved January 30, 2004, from http://www.census.gov/population/www/documentation/twps0036/twps0036.html

were poor in 1989 compared with 9.1 percent of children living with married couples and 45.2 percent of children living with a single mother (Manning & Lichter, 1996). Some facts about cohabiting families seem especially alarming. For example, white and Hispanic teens living with a mother and her boyfriend are more likely to have emotional and behavioral problems and to be suspended or expelled from school than are teens living with a single mother alone (Nelson, Clark, & Acs, 2001).

Gay and Lesbian Families

The assignment of gender at birth is accompanied by societal expectations about social relationships, gender roles, and reproductive patterns. American males, for example, are generally socialized to assume the provider role, be independent, and display masculine virility. Biological sex assignment results in assumptions that sexual expression is innate and that preparation of male-female role orientations is natural. Pop-psychology books such as *Men Are from Mars, Women Are from Venus* (Gray, 1992) emphasize societal notions of gender differences. Although heterosexual relationships provide gendered scripts of male and female expectations about intimate interactions, few people ever fully live up to these expectations. Individuals with same-sex attractions, rather than heterosexual ones, have nevertheless been socialized with the same societal pressures related to gender roles and values related to the importance of bonding with another person. Persons with different sexual orientations also desire the intimacy of sharing life with another person. This type of intimacy develops into another type of family increasingly more common in our society, the same-sex family. *Same-sex families* include male or gay partners or female or lesbian partners who cohabitate. These families may or may not include children.

Before getting involved in an intimate relationship, homosexual persons usually go through processes of self-recognition, acknowledgement of their failure to meet societal expectations related to gendered norms, and "coming out" to family, friends, and others. For many years, gay, lesbian, bisexual, and transgendered family types were ignored or viewed as deviant by mainstream society, researchers, and clinicians. The American Psychological Association viewed homosexuality as a psychiatric disorder until 1973 when a vote by 58 percent of the membership influenced the Board of Trustees to delete homosexuality from the diagnostic manual. Debate continues about whether homosexuality is a finite or genetically based trait or one that is related to choice. Although some researchers have identified homosexuality as innate and related to some genetic factors, religious arguments have largely supported the idea that sexual orientation is a choice. Today, most scientists agree that sexual orientation is shaped at an early age and most likely linked to the complex interaction of environmental, cognitive, and biological factors.

Same-sex families should not be stereotyped any more than their heterosexual counterparts should. The 2000 census identified nearly a million gays and lesbians as members of same-sex couples, the first authoritative record of homosexuals in America. According to the last census figures, same-sex households make up just over one-half of 1 percent of the 105.5 million U.S. homes. Census officials and gay rights activists believe that this number is likely an underestimation, as the census did not count partnered relationships when the two did not share the same household. Nor did it consider the prejudice and discrimination that still keeps many gays and lesbians from divulging their sexuality (Smith & Gates, 2001). Nevertheless, the census confirmed that same-sex couples were found in every part of the nation or 99.3 percent of U.S. counties, not just in San Francisco and New York City. In fact, 15 percent of gay and lesbian families are living in rural settings.

Although much more is now understood about same-sex families than in years past, much is still to be learned (Demo & Allen, 1996). In discussing gay and lesbian families, the literature has tended to focus more on families where parents are heterosexual but children are gay, lesbian, or bisexual (Savin-Williams & Esterberg, 2000). Our society currently lacks models of healthy same-sex unions, and it has been acknowledged only recently that such relationships are possible. Things such as communication, honesty, trust, mutual respect, adequate personal space, and support are fundamental to relationships, whether they are heterosexual or same-sex. Dr. John Gottman and his colleagues conducted a 12-year study of same-sex couples and found the following:

- Gay and lesbian couples are more upbeat in the face of conflict.
- Gay/lesbian couples use fewer controlling, hostile emotional tactics.
- In a fight, gay and lesbian couples take it less personally.
- Unhappy gay and lesbian couples tend to show low levels of "physiological arousal."
- In a fight, lesbians show more anger, humor, excitement, and interest than conflicting gay men.

- Gay men need to be especially careful to avoid negativity in conflict (Gottman Institute, 2001).

Still, little is yet known about the ways gay and lesbian couples make transitions to parenthood, the unique problems families encounter, and the levels of support available from families of origin, extended family, and other communities. Television programs such as *Queer as Folk*, *Queer Eye for the Straight Guy*, and the recently syndicated groundbreaking program titled *The L Word* hold promise to challenge some stereotypical views. In a classic study of same-sex and heterosexual couples on the ways they handle money, work, and sexuality, a high commitment to equality was found among lesbian couples (Blumstein & Schwartz, 1983). Same-sex couples tend to share more leisure activities than heterosexual ones do, which often results in higher rates of relationship satisfaction. Kurdek (1995) has used longitudinal data to study the stability and quality, social support, and division of labor in cohabitating and heterosexual relationships. His findings indicate that gay and lesbian couples were more likely to divide household tasks equitably, to share responsibilities, and to be less focused on gender roles than heterosexual couples were. However, same-sex relationships have needs for committed relationships, levels and types of conflict, and satisfaction similar to those of heterosexual couples.

> **"** Just as heterosexual families vary widely, same-sex families are also not monolithic and should not be stereotyped any more than should their heterosexual counterparts. **"**

The cohabitation patterns of homosexual couples have been less visible than those of other couples. Since 1950, data on unmarried and unrelated adults of the same sex 25 years and older who share a household have been included in the census. The data are limited, however, because these householders may or may not be sexual partners. Although the urge to bond with another person is often present for same-sex pairs, there has been little societal support for a federally sanctioned legal commitment (Box 5–5). Same-sex couples are denied certain benefits offered to other American citizens because of the inability to marry. Such benefits include clarity about rights for children being raised, economic arrangements that affect property, and taxes perquisites (Chambers, 1996). Issues such as child custody, visitation rights, adoption, and

---

Box 5–5 INCREASED SUPPORT FOR SAME-SEX COUPLES PARENTING CHILDREN

Children who are born to or adopted by one member of a same-sex couple deserve the security of two legally recognized parents. The American Academy of Pediatrics supports legislative and legal efforts to provide the possibility of adoption of the child by the second parent or coparent in these families. The American Academy of Pediatrics recognizes that a considerable body of professional literature provides evidence that children with parents who are homosexual can have similar advantages and expectations for health, adjustment, and development as children whose parents are heterosexual. Children need the permanence and security provided by two fully sanctioned and legally defined parents. The Academy supports the legal adoption of children by coparents or second parents[a].

Numerous studies over the last three decades consistently demonstrate that children raised by gay or lesbian parents exhibit the same level of emotional, cognitive, social, and sexual functioning as children raised by heterosexual parents. This research indicates that optimal development for children is based not on the sexual orientation of the parents but on stable attachments to committed and nurturing adults. The research also shows that children who have two parents, regardless of the parents' sexual orientations, do better than children with only one parent.

The American Psychiatric Association supports initiatives that allow same-sex couples to adopt and coparent children and supports all the associated legal rights, benefits, and responsibilities that arise from such initiatives[b].

[a]Committee on Psychosocial Aspects of Child and Family Health. (2002). Co-parent or second-parent adoption by same-sex parent. *Pediatrics, 109*(2), 339–340.
[b]The American Psychiatric Association. (2002). Adoption and co-parenting of children by same-sex couples: Position statement. Approved by the Board of Trustees and by the Assembly.

Box 5–6 DEFENSE OF MARRIAGE ACT

Introduced to Congress on May 7, 1996, the Defense of Marriage Act (DOMA) does two things. First, it provides that no state shall be required to give effect to a law of any other state with respect to a same-sex "marriage." Second, it defines the words "marriage" and "spouse" for purposes of federal law. The first substantive section of the bill is an exercise of Congress's power to allow each state (or other political jurisdiction) to decide for itself whether it wants to grant legal status to same-sex marriage. The second substantive section of the bill amends the U.S. Code to make explicit what has been understood under federal law for over 200 years: that a marriage is the legal union of a man and a woman as husband and wife, and a spouse is a husband or wife of the opposite sex. Senators voted 85–14 for the Defense of Marriage Act, the House overwhelmingly passed the bill, and President Clinton signed it into action. Although much discussion continues across the nation, the majority of states have now passed legislation favoring this amendment.

legal rights regarding children of same-sex relationships continue to be areas of concern for these families. Currently, marriage is not a legal alternative for homosexual couples in most states, and many same-sex pairs still face various forms of discrimination (Box 5–6). Although many same-sex families are becoming more visible and part of the mainstream in some American communities, a large number of such families remain insular.

Family Households

According to the 2000 U.S. census, a *household* consists of all the people who occupy a housing unit, which could be a house, an apartment, or some other group of rooms. A single room is regarded as a housing unit when it is occupied or intended for occupancy as separate living quarters, when the occupants do not live and eat with any other persons in the structure, and when there is direct access from the outside or through a common hall. A household includes the related family members and all the unrelated people, such as lodgers or foster children, who share the housing unit. Households do not include group quarters. *Family households* are ones maintained by a family householder and include any unrelated people who may reside there. *Non-family households* consist of a householder living alone or a household shared by people who are not related (Tables 5–1 and 5–2).

Although marriage was viewed as an institution for organizing family households in the early 20th century, the last 50 years have seen conflicting views about its importance. Other factors affecting household composition include increasing widowhood at older ages, women bearing fewer children at later ages, and increasing numbers of women in the workforce. Every family type experiences some strains when dealing with both daily hassles and crises. Households headed by married couples usually have more resources to draw on in dealing with day-to-day strains. Single-parent families, especially those headed by women, tend to have fewer resources in terms of time, energy, and money and are particularly vulnerable to stress and strains. Cohabitating families, both heterosexual and homosexual, have additional stressors such as social censure and legal restraints. These varied relationships have created diverse ways to view families.

> ❝Although marriage was viewed as an institution for organizing family households in the early 20th century, the last 50 years have seen conflicting views about its importance.❞

Additionally, the size of households has decreased during the past few decades. Declines in birth rates have reduced the number of large families, and reduced mortality rates have increased the proportion of post-parental families. More individuals are choosing to live alone. In 1998, approximately 28 million households were composed of one person (U.S. Census Bureau, 1998). The only trend that seems to offset this decline in household size is the tendency for adult children to return temporarily to their parents' home. In 1998, 59 percent of men and 48 percent of women between 18 and 24 years of age lived at home, compared with 52 percent of men and 35 percent of women in 1960 (U.S. Census Bureau, 1999). During the same time frame, 15 percent of men and 8 percent of women aged 25 to 34 years lived at home compared with 11 percent of men and 7 percent of women in 1960 (U.S. Census Bureau, 1999).

Table 5–1 SOCIAL FAMILIES' LIVING ARRANGEMENTS, 1997–1999

	TOTAL U.S.		
	1997 (%)	1999 (%)	DIFFERENCE
Single-mother families	27.0	26.7	−0.4
Lives independently	16.9	15.1	−1.8*
Lives with parents	3.1	3.0	−0.1
Cohabits[a]	4.1	5.6	+1.5*
Lives with other adults[b]	2.1	2.1	+0.0
Lives in complex/multigenerational setting[c]	0.9	1.0	+0.1
Married-couple families	66.8	67.5	+0.7
Traditional married couple[d]	61.8	62.2	+0.4
Extended married couple[e]	5.1	5.3	+0.3
Other types of families[f]	6.1	5.8	−0.3

Source: Urban Institute calculations from the 1997 and 1999 NSAF.
*Statistically significant difference at the 90 percent confidence level.
Note: A broad definition of "family" consists of children, their guardians or parents, other adult relatives, partners of all the adults, and any relatives of the partners who live in the same household.
[a] Single mothers cohabitating with parent(s) are classified as living with parents if under 30 years of age.
[b] Single mothers who live with their parents and with other adults who are neither their parents nor their partners are classified as living with their parents; those who cohabit and live with other adults are considered to be cohabitating.
[c] Complex/multigenerational single-mother families include arrangements such as two sisters who are both single mothers living together, or a single mother whose daughter is also a single mother.
[d] Traditional married-couple families are families in which no other adult resides.
[e] Married couples caring for grandchildren are classified as extended married-couple families.
[f] "Other types of families" represents those not elsewhere classified, such as single-father families or child-grandparent families.

Current Trends Altering Family Patterns

Variations on the traditional family are attributable to many societal trends, some of which will be discussed in the following sections.

Divorce Rates

A change that has had great impact on family structure is the high divorce rate. The divorce rate rose from the middle of the 19th century through the 1980s, and by 1974, more marriages ended in divorce than in death (Cherlin, 1992). In the 1980s, the divorce rate began to decline slightly but remained higher than in the 1960s. From 1960 to 1980, the rise in the divorce rate was greater than would have been predicted by the trend line. What accounted for this? Divorces tend to increase after wars and decrease in times of economic difficulty. Therefore, the Vietnam War, the burgeoning economy, and a high level of individualism probably contributed to the high divorce rate from 1960 to 1980. In addition, options available for women outside of marriage improved. In 1996, about 40 percent of men and women between the ages of 45 and 55 years had divorced from their first marriage (Kreider & Fields, 2001).

The social and economic consequences of the divorce rate for women and children have been well-documented (Weitzman, 1985). At the current divorce rate, almost half of all marriages end in separation or divorce. The majority of children will live in a single-parent household headed by their mother for at least 5 years before their mother remarries or they reach 18 years of age. The long-term impact of high rates of

Table 5–2 CHILDREN'S LIVING ARRANGEMENTS, 1997–1999

	TOTAL U.S.		
	1997 (%)	1999 (%)	DIFFERENCE
Married biological/adoptive parents	59.8	60.2	10.4
Married blended parents[a]	8.3	8.3	+0.0
Single mother	21.3	19.2	–2.1*
Single father	2.9	2.7	–0.2
Cohabitating parents with common children[b]	2.0	2.8	+0.8*
Cohabitating partners with no children in common[c]	2.6	3.2	+0.6*
No parents (foster, kinship, or nonrelative parents)	3.1	3.5	+0.5*
Other	0.1	0.1	+0.0

Source: Urban Institute calculations from the 1997 and 1999 NSAF.
*Statistically significant difference at the 90 percent confidence level.
[a] The category "married blended parents" refers to children living with a biological parent
   who is married to either a stepparent or an adoptive parent.
[b] Children living with cohabitating parents with common children are living with both of
   their biological parents, who are unmarried.
[c] Children living with cohabitating partners with no children in common are living with one
   biological parent and that parent's boyfriend or girlfriend.

marital dissolution on adult children and on society is just beginning to become apparent (Amato & Booth, 1996; Aquilino, 1994; Cherlin, 1999; Spitze, Logan, Deane, & Zerger, 1994).

Social Network Affecting Family Structure

People outside of the home who engage in activities of an affective or material nature with the members of the household constitute the family's social network. The presence of a strong social network often improves family member health status and life satisfaction. For individuals, one of the best single predictors of the size and richness of the social network is education. That is, better-educated individuals are more likely to have more substantial social networks than are families with less-educated members. Familial social networks are altered with changes in marital status, the family's developmental level, and their geographical location. An individual's social network generally changes markedly after divorce or separation. Remarried or blended families might have larger social networks than married couples have, however, due to continued contact with ex-spouses and their extended families.

The family's social network provides both instrumental and expressive support. This is particularly true of the extended family, which, contrary to popular myth, remains a major source of social support for many American families. However, families of different racial, ethnic, and cultural traditions and geographical locations may differ in their networks. For example, Appalachian families are likely to live near extended family and have close kin and friendship networks, which means they have less need to become entangled with others (Denham, 1996). Intergenerational interaction is the norm, not the exception (Stull & Borgatta, 1987). Familial support offered by extended family members is especially important for the frail elderly, single parents, and families caring for children with disabilities or chronic illness. However, the quality of intergenerational relationships is altered by many variables and may change over time (Umberson & Slaten, 2000).

Many elderly people who need either material or affective support depend on family members to provide it. Elderly persons often live within a short traveling time of at least one child and usually maintain contact with other adult children and their families. However, the availability of support may diminish as the elder parent and adult children age. As many as one-third of Caucasian, urban elderly individuals in their 80s and 90s have no family members who can respond when needed (Johnson & Troll, 1996).

Families seem to go out of their way to help single parents; this is particularly true when it comes to helping African-American mothers (Spitze, Logan, Deane, & Zerger, 1994). Black communities often form an extensive system of kin networks. Nonetheless, despite the presence of the extensive kin network, only a quarter of never-married mothers receive financial assistance from their kin and fewer than a fifth receive child care help (Jayakody, Chatters, & Taylor, 1993). In contrast to single-parent families, married families have the advantage of seeking and obtaining support from both families of origin. In order to determine accurately the viability of a family's social network, evaluate the following:

- The type of support provided
- Proximity of the network
- Interaction within the network
- Affinity of the kin

Nurses, as citizens and as health professionals, need to play an active role in enacting social policies to reduce strain on all families. For example, more available child care could significantly reduce the burden on many families. Families are continually being asked to assume more responsibilities for health care. They are expected to care for acutely and chronically ill family members, who were once cared for by health professionals. This warns of disaster for families already strained to the limit. Until social policies are enacted that reduce the burden on families, nurses, through counseling and education, need to help families develop more adaptive interaction patterns and more effective coping strategies.

Cultural Diversity and Family Structure

Many American students have little understanding about international perspectives and little knowledge about families in other parts of the world. Frequently, nurses come in contact with individuals and families who are from other nations and who have different values, traditions, and practices. Knowledge about global conditions, world trends, population growth, diseases in other nations, and political and social problems can be especially helpful to nurses employed in geographic regions and institutions where persons from diverse cultures may reside. Cultural issues such as religious beliefs, customs, traditions, celebrations, and rituals influence the family structure and have far-reaching implications for family functions and processes. Americans are becoming increasingly diverse, and this likely will continue over the next decades. It is essential that nurses be well prepared to address family issues related to cultural diversity and have an awareness and understanding about people from dissimilar backgrounds (Box 5–7).

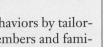

Box 5–7 **TIPS FOR PROVIDING CULTURALLY COMPETENT CARE TO FAMILIES**

Cultural competence is the ability to provide care to those with diverse values, beliefs, and behaviors by tailoring care delivery to meet the unique social, cultural, and linguistic needs of diverse family members and families as a whole. To ensure that individuals and families receive culturally competent health care, heed the following tips:

- Be sensitive to your personal bias and prejudice and find ways not to project these upon others.
- Promote attitudes, behaviors, knowledge, and skills that are affirming and open and that enable you to work respectfully and effectively with culturally diverse persons and families.
- Create culturally welcoming environments including methods for outreach, office spaces, intake forms, confidentiality policies, staff training, and client interviews.
- Listen to what clients and families are saying and do not assume that you know what is best.
- Utilize culturally and linguistically appropriate services, policies, and procedures in care delivery.
- Access education and training that prepares you to be culturally and linguistically competent in diverse work environments.
- Ensure that clients with limited English proficiency have access to bilingual or interpretation services.
- Develop health information that is written at the appropriate literacy levels and is targeted to the language and cultural norms of specific family populations.

FAMILY FUNCTION

A functional perspective has to do with the ways a family serves its members. One way to describe the *functional aspect of family* is to see the unit as made up of intimate, interactive, and interdependent persons who share some values, goals, resources, responsibilities, decisions, and commitment over time (Steinmetz, Clavan, & Stein, 1990). *Family functioning* has been described as "the individual and cooperative processes used by developing persons as to dynamically engage one another and their diverse environments over the life course" (Denham, 2003a, p. 277). Specific functional aspects include the ways a family reproduces offspring, interacts to socialize its young, cooperates to meet economic needs, and relates to the larger society. When concerned with functional aspects of the family, one might ask the question, "In what ways do specific characteristics factor into achieving family and/or societal goals?"

Several theoretical ideas strongly influence the ways in which functional perspectives of family are viewed. Parsons and Bales (1955) suggested that the nuclear family was necessary for the urban industrial society and that gender-based divisions of labor were necessities for appropriate sex-role development. Feminist theory challenges these views about the nuclear family and legitimizes the values of diverse family forms as effective ways to socialize children. Symbolic interactionist theory relies more on ideas about the ways in which one member's behavior influences that of another. Individuals are viewed as having great latitude in behaviors that can result in meaningful responses. Both feminist and interactionist theories rely less on stereotypical masculine-feminine roles by allowing for greater flexibility in role expectations and acceptance of gendered social roles.

Family function has to do with the purposes that the family serves in relation to the individual, the family, other social systems, and society. Family function is very difficult to describe, however, as one can quickly get caught in circular reasoning. Although family function is a consequence of family structure, the structure exists to fulfill one or more functions. Thus, in everyday life, the function of the family is usually questioned only when a social need is not being met. For example, several social trends, such as increases in societal violence, substance abuse, and problems of teenage pregnancies, have been attributed to the family's ineffectiveness in transmitting values. However, this is a simplistic explanation for complex problems that ignores things such as personal choice, peer influ-

ences, media messages, economics, and other community or social influences. The complexity of these multiple relationships or diverse variables makes describing family function difficult. Most families can benefit from health teaching or counseling that provides meaningful information to promote individual and family health.

Families' functional processes such as socialization, reproduction, economics, and health care provision are areas that nurses can readily address during health care encounters. Nurses' actions can enhance the family's protective health function when teaching and counseling are tailored to explicit learning needs. Families' cultural context and individuals' health literacy needs are closely related to functional needs of families. Nurses become therapeutic agents as they assist families to identify social supports and locate community resources during times of family transitions and health crisis. However, having conceptual understandings about families' functional aspects and establishing a theoretical basis for appreciation for families provides a substantial framework for practice.

> ❝Families' functional processes such as socialization, reproduction, economics, and health care provision are areas that nurses can readily address during health care encounters.❞

Family Boundaries

Family systems have boundaries that include some people as members but exclude others. Boundaries, although relatively stable, are not necessarily stationary and may be redrawn. Some family types allow for greater boundary ambiguity, which leaves the guidelines about the members who compose the family and how they should interact vaguer. One theory that relates to family boundaries involves scripting (Simon & Gagnon, 1986). This theory suggests that societal scripts, personal scripts, scenes, and mutual scripts can explain the interactions that occur with family members and guide the way members interact with those outside the family. Scripting helps families define whom they allow into and whom they block out of their family circle. It is also useful in describing the things families do, the places they go, and the ways they choose to interact with others in their neighborhood, workplace, and community. These family scripts often are translated into action and set the tone for the ways in which families form boundaries.

As social systems, families operate on a continuum from a closed to an open system in their interaction with the outside world (Kantor & Lehr, 1975). A *closed family system*, functioning in isolation from other social systems and social institutions, is impossible to sustain. Families who operate as a closed system maintain only essential contact with the outside world; their primary interaction with the outside world is through work. Closed families may send their children to school but fail to become involved in school activities. They may have no visitors and only nodding acquaintances with neighbors. They may choose not to become involved in community activities such as church and other social groups. An extremely closed family may be deeply enmeshed, mistrust outsiders, and be unlikely to seek help or resources outside the kin network. Under ordinary circumstances, the closed family may be able to maintain its homeostasis, but they may be poorly equipped to deal with change, illness risks, or stressors.

At the opposite extreme, an *open family system* encourages interchange with the outside world. An open system tends toward multiple activity involvement inside and outside the family. Visitors are welcome and encouraged. Family members may be involved in multiple social outlets, both individually and as a family. Although trust and loyalty may be important for members of an open family system, they may accept the merit of external voices without closely scrutinizing their long-term value to the family's well-being. The open family system's boundaries may become blurred because of multiple external social influences, leaving members vulnerable to distractions that might threaten the family structure. Neither open nor closed families are inherently good or bad. Families are not likely to be at either extreme but may have some tendencies in one direction or another. A healthy family generally has some clearly defined boundaries but enough flexibility to be able to accommodate stressors and capitalize on contacts with the outside world.

Family as a Socializing Agent

In order for the family to meet society's needs, the family unit has to maintain its integrity as a social system, in other words, as a group of persons viewed as a whole as they interact with the larger society. Survival as a social system entails meeting certain functional prerequisites, such as adaptation, goal attainment, integration, pattern maintenance, and tension management (Parsons, 1951). These inner workings of the family are essential elements for meeting the family's daily material or instrumental needs, providing a caring milieu that promotes members' physical growth and emotional development, and socializing children to fit into the larger societal context. Member socialization may operate differently over time.

Adaptation

Adaptation refers to the necessity of the family to accommodate its external and internal environments. The external environment includes the physical environment, other social systems with which the family interacts, and the predominant culture. The internal environment is composed of the family members as biological organisms and as personalities. In order to adapt, the family must carry out a range of tasks (Bell & Vogel, 1960). Therefore, the family must obtain the resources, the skills, and the motivation to perform the tasks. For example, one of the basic human needs of the family members is to obtain nourishment. One or more family members have to assume the responsibility for making the money to buy or to grow the food, someone has to purchase and cook food that is compatible with the family members' biological needs and their cultural prescriptions, the family members have to be motivated to eat the food, and someone has to clean up afterward. Failure to perform these tasks puts the individual family members in physical jeopardy and can lead to the breakdown of the family as a social system.

Goal Attainment

The family defines what is important or valuable to them, but individual members may not always be in agreement. Although not always a conscious act, family values are sometimes used to describe goals and identify the means for attainment. Family values are those ideals and principles that serve as guiding influences for the ways the family identifies itself and interacts with others. Sometimes, goals are inferred from the actions of the family members. At other times, the actions of the family members seem incongruous with identified goals. For example, parents may state that spending quality time with their children is a top priority. However, when caught in the bind between job demands and family, they may attend to their jobs first. As goals are identified and attained, the family member with the most influence in the decision-making process may vary from situation to situation. However, over time, the leadership structure of the family is fairly stable, and parental units tend to promote the family's goal attainment. Successful outcomes rely on the commitment and motivation of all family members.

Integration

Integration, unlike adaptation and goal attainment, refers strictly to activities within the family system. Integration is the means by which a family acquires cohesion, solidarity, and identity—important aspects that enable family members to maintain close relationships over time. The overt and covert expression of affection promotes family cohesion, as do family routines, rituals, traditions, and celebrations. Symbols of family solidarity and integration include photograph albums, heirlooms, family stories, and favorite jokes. Family ties operate to preserve the family system and motivate members to abide by the family's norms.

Pattern Maintenance and Tension Management

Like integration, pattern maintenance and tension management are functional prerequisites that deal primarily with the family's internal state. As members interact with one another, they develop expectations about personal and group behaviors. Family survival depends to some extent on the values that regulate family activities and interactions within and external to the family system. Families allowing for some flexibility permit some deviation from expected norms and may experience less stress and greater resilience than inflexible ones. For example, a family that expects everyone to be present for a 6 P.M. dinner needs to make allowances when a family member is delayed by a traffic jam. Furthermore, resilient families modify their value systems and behavioral expectations as the family develops over time. For instance, early constraints placed on a child's travel outside the home are reduced as the child ages.

Specific Functions of Family

Family units have four functional prerequisites that influence their stability or intactness during chaotic times and their resilience or ability to cope with internal and external stresses. These prerequisites are related to adaptation, goal attainment, integration, and pattern maintenance or tension management and greatly impact functional capacities of the family. When the family is ineffective in meeting these prerequisites, the family's functional status becomes less effective. Families unable to accomplish functional prerequisites are more prone to dissolution and may fail to serve the needs of the larger society. They may also fail to accomplish specific family functions such as reproduction, socialization of children, and stabilization of adult personalities. These primary family functions play major roles in family members' health outcomes.

Reproductive Functions of the Family

The survival of a society is linked to patterns of reproduction. Sexuality serves the purposes of pleasure and reproduction, but associated values differ from one society to another. Traditionally, the family has been organized around the biological function of reproduction. Reproduction was viewed as a major concern for thousands of years when populating the earth was continually threatened by famine, disease, war, and other life uncertainties. In America today, the fertility rate or the actual number of births is well below the fecundity or potential rate. Norms about sexual intercourse affect the fertility rate. Birth control has always had a place (Freed & Freed, 1993), and things such as religious rules about sexuality and norms concerning sexual relationships during breast-feeding and menstruation have always been used to control birth rates. Global concerns about overpopulation and environmental threats, as well as personal views of morality and financial well-being, have been reasons for limiting numbers of family births.

During the past two decades, the reproductive function has become increasingly separated from the family (Robertson, 1991). Individuals tend to organize themselves into families based on cultural prescriptions and basic human needs. As cultural prescriptions change, families change. In the past, the primary function of the family in society was the regulation of reproduction, but today's families have less control over these behaviors (Robertson, 1991). Abstinence, various forms of contraception, tubal ligation, vasectomy, family planning, and abortion have various degrees of social acceptance as means to control reproduction. For centuries, the state, religion, and family have fought over rights to control reproduction. In 1973, in the *Roe v. Wade* decision, based on the privacy rights, the U.S. Supreme Court ruled that during the first trimester of pregnancy states could not interfere with decisions about terminating pregnancy. The abortion issue continues to be debated with strong "pro-choice" and "pro-life" positions taken by some, with others giving assent to abortion in some situations but not others.

The ethical dilemmas mirrored in the abortion controversy seem compounded by technological advances affecting reproduction and problems of infertility. Reproductive technologies are guided by few legal, ethical, or moral guidelines. Artificial insemination by husband or donor, in vitro fertilization, surrogate mothers, and artificial embryonation, in which a woman other than the wife donates an egg for fertilization, create financial and moral dilemmas when pregnancy cannot occur through usual reproductive processes. Although assistive reproductive technologies can provide a biological link to the child, some families are choosing to adopt children. Many are wrangling over the issues implicit in cross-racial and cross-cultural adoptions. Reproductive technologies and adoption are being considered by all family types to add children to the family unit. Religious, legal, moral, economic, and technological challenges will continue to cause debates in the years ahead about family control over reproduction (Box 5–8).

The national teen pregnancy rate, between 1995 and 1996, fell 4 percent from 101.1 to 97.3 pregnancies per 1000 women aged 15 to 19 (Henshaw, 1999). This is a 17 percent decline since the pregnancy rate peaked in 1990. Eighty percent of this decline is a result of improved contraceptive use among sexually active teenagers, but 20 percent is attributable to increased abstinence (Saul, 1999). According to the *National Vital Statistics Report* ("Teen Pregnancy Rates," 2003), the pregnancy rate for young teenagers 15 to 17 years was 56 per 1000 in 1999. Pregnancy rates declined steadily for teenagers, by 25 percent overall; the rate fell from its peak in 1990, 116.3 per 1000 aged 15 to 19 years, to 86.7 in 1999. The 1999 rate for teenagers was the lowest ever reported since this series of pregnancy estimates began in 1976. The teen birth rate fell to 43 births per 1000 females aged 15 to 19 in 2002, a record low. These new figures represent a 5 percent decline from 2001 and a 28 percent decline from 1990 (Hamilton, Martin, & Sutton, 2003).

Pregnancy rates differ depending on the age of the teenager and her partners. Teenage girls with older

---

Box 5–8 FAMILY ISSUES AND REPRODUCTIVE TECHNOLOGIES

Today, individuals and families are faced with choices resulting from growing knowledge and successes with reproductive technologies that have never been encountered before. Artificial insemination, in vitro fertilization, donor eggs for women in their 40s and 50s, genetically enhanced embryos, rejuvenation of older women's eggs, cryobanks of anonymous sperm, and possibilities of cloning are just some of the options facing women who encounter infertility. High financial costs are often associated with uncertain outcomes related to the technologies, and potential parents have to cope with possibilities of success and failure when they seek procedures.

Many issues of concern are related to reproductive technologies. Some associated problems include the lack of standards and regulation in reproductive medicine, multiple births that may present financial and social risks to families, ownership of frozen embryos when divorce occurs, and determination of the best interest of the child. Across the nation are many for-profit fertility clinics whose main purpose is to make money. Nurses working with families need to be well-informed about reproductive issues and explicit needs for support and counseling.

Want to learn more about reproductive technologies? See information about the public television *Frontline* program entitled "Making Babies" at http://www.pbs.org/wgbh/pages/frontline/shows/fertility/.

Additional information can be obtained from these organizations:

- American Association for Reproductive Medicine, http://www.asrm.org/
- American Infertility Organization, http://www.americaninfertility.org/
- California Cryobank, http://www.cryobank.com
- Infertility Resources, http://www.ihr.com/infertility/
- RESOLVE: The National Infertility Association, http://www.resolve.org/main/national/index. jsp?name= home

partners are more likely to become pregnant. For example, teenage girls aged 15 to 17 with partners 6 or more years older were 6.7 percent more likely to become pregnant than those with partners no more than 2 years older (Darroch, Landry, & Oslak, 1999). Teen mothers have a 50 percent higher infant mortality rate than mothers older than 20, and nearly 75 percent of teen mothers eventually seek welfare services within 5 years after giving birth (Annie E. Casey Foundation, 1998).

According to Hamilton, Martin, and Sutton (2003), the birth rate for women aged 20 to 24 years declined by 3 percent to 103.5 per 1000 in 2002 compared with 2001, whereas the rate for women aged 25 to 29 years was essentially unchanged (113.6). The birth rate for women aged 30 to 34 years decreased slightly from 91.9 per 1000 in 2001 to 91.6 in 2002. Birth rates for women aged 35 to 39 years and 40 to 44 years continued to rise, increasing 2 percent for both. Childbearing among women over 45 years of age has remained unchanged. However, birth rates for unmarried women between ages 15 and 44 were down slightly in 2002 to 43.6 births per 1000. In 2002, the number of births to unmarried women increased by 1 percent, but births to unmarried teenagers declined by 4 percent.

Socialization of Children

This is another functional task that falls into the hands of families. Families have great variability in the ways they address physical, emotional, and economic needs of children, and these patterns are influenced by the larger society and the historical point in time (Coontz, 2000). Children are born into families without knowledge of the values, language, norms, or roles of the society in which they will become members. A major function of the family is to socialize the child about family and societal identity. Although the family is not the only institution that participates in children's socialization, it is generally viewed as having primary responsibility. When children fail to meet societal standards, it is not unusual to blame family deficits and parental inadequacies.

Although Americans have traditionally viewed the nuclear family as the optimum type, other societies have spread the responsibility of child rearing among several adults. For example, division of labor was different in hunting-gathering societies with task assignment by age and gender. Thus, men might do the hunting and women the foraging, but all had responsibility for caring for the children. An African saying, "It takes a village to raise a child," suggests that socialization can be a community as well as a parental responsibility. Children have been viewed differently in other historical periods, and age expectations have changed dramatically. The closeness and value placed on children today replaces century-old viewpoints of children as miniature adults. Today, patterns of socialization require appropriate developmental care that fosters dependence and leads to independence.

An important function of the family in American society is the socialization of children. Socialization is the primary way in which children acquire the social and psychological skills needed to take their place in the adult world. Parents combine social support and social control as they equip children to meet future life tasks (Peterson & Rollins, 1985). Parental figures interact in multiple roles such as friends, lovers, child care providers, housekeepers, recreation specialists, and counselors. Children growing up within families learn the values and norms of their parents and extended families.

The hierarchy of the nuclear family with its formal authority structure seems to be effective in preparing children for adult roles (Nock, 1988). In 1998, nuclear families with children under 18 years of age constituted 36 percent of all family households (U.S. Census Bureau, 1998). Census data (2000) show that in most areas of the United States, the majority of children under 18 live in households headed by a married couple, but these households may or may not include both of the child's parents. The proportion of all U.S. children living in two-parent homes reached an all-time low in the mid-1990s, but it has stabilized. In fact, the proportion of children in two-parent homes increased slightly from 68 percent in 1999 to 69.1 percent in 2000, and about 25 percent lived with a single parent (Blankenhorn, 2002). Children raised in two-parent homes seem to have fewer health and behavioral problems than children reared in some other family types have (Aquilino, 1994; Dawson, 1991). Attitudes and values learned within families are internalized. Consequently, the child reared in a family setting with clear lines of authority and power, for example, may be more effective and successful in hierarchical environments such as school or work.

Remarried or blended families seem to experience more problems with child rearing. The role of a stepparent has been less clearly defined, and in the past, some negative connotations have been associated with it. Some literature suggests that stepparents show less warmth, communicate less well with stepchildren, and participate in fewer child-related activities (Thomson, McLanahan, & Curtin, 1992). Although lack of parental engagement with children has potential to contribute to behavioral problems, this may also occur in traditional families. Fathers in two-parent families are unlikely to spend as much time with children as mothers do (Barnett & Shen, 1997). Close relationships between children and fathers have been viewed as very important to a child's healthy development, although some have found that this presence makes little difference in child outcomes (Snarey, 1993; Williams & Radin, 1999). It appears that American children do best when close relationships with both parents exist, regardless of whether this occurs within a traditional family structure or a diverse family structure.

Some have thought that parents use differential treatment with boys and girls as they socialize their children into what are viewed as appropriate masculine and feminine roles. Consistent differences in child-rearing practices have been found in several areas: (1) boys tend to be punished more frequently, (2) boys receive more praise, (3) infant boys receive more physical stimulation and encouragement, and (4) gender-type behavior is encouraged whereas cross-gender behavior is discouraged (Macoby & Jacklin, 1974). These early studies have been criticized over the years. A meta-analysis found few patterns of differences in warmth and responsiveness, encouragement, interaction patterns, discipline, communication, or use of reasoning (Lytton & Romney, 1991). The encouragement of sex-type activities and more frequent use of punishment with boys were the main areas where gender socialization seemed to differ. Information about gender-type differential treatment and roles continues to be studied.

Another role of families in the socialization process is to guide children through various rites of passage. Rites of passage are ceremonies that announce a change in status in the ways members are viewed. Examples include events such as baptism, communion, circumcision, puberty rituals, graduation, weddings, and funerals. These occasions signal to others that role relationships are changed and new expectations are present. Understandings about families' unique rites of passage can assist nurses working with diverse health care needs.

Stabilization of Adult Personalities

Stabilization of adult personalities has been viewed as a function of the American family. Family is an institution where adult members engage in roles involving mutual nurturance, emotional exchanges, and socialization. Adults seek opportunities to interact in reciprocal relationships through alternative family structures. Although the dynamics of marriage have changed remarkably over the last few decades, resulting in fewer formal or social controls governing the ways interactions occur, adults still seek intimate relationships as a means to finding happiness and adding value to life.

Adults, whether heterosexual or same-sex, married or cohabiting, tend to form intimate relationships because of needs of trust, reciprocity, and the ability to share resources. Although marriage often provides stability and protection for individuals, it also presents risks. In the past, marriage contracts decreed expectations about division of labor and assigned property ownership. Formerly couples reached agreements about religious beliefs, roles, and life tasks prior to marriage, but today most discussion and negotiation take place after marriage or cohabitation occurs. What effect does individual happiness have on the relationship between marriage and health? A decrease in marital satisfaction may offset the buffering effect of marriage on health status. Traditionally, personal happiness has been positively correlated with marriage. However, in the past two decades, the difference in happiness between married and never-married persons has decreased (Lee, Seccombe, & Shehan, 1991). Among the never married, both men and women demonstrate an increase in personal happiness. Among the married, women, particularly young women, report a decrease in personal happiness. This change is most pronounced among employed mothers, who are trying to balance multiple demanding roles. However, married people still tend to be happier than unmarried people. The increased economic, psychological, and social support available to married people serves to stabilize their personalities and, consequently, enhance their health.

> **❝**Today many families could be classified as remarried, blended, or reconstituted, a family with a male and a female where at least one has been married before and where children may or may not be living in the household.**❞**

Changes in today's marital status bring questions about the ways in which close family relationships stabilize, threaten, and introduce stress for adult personalities. Given the high rates of divorce, separation, remarriage, and changes in cohabiting partners, we must monitor changes over time in families and households in order to come to meaningful conclusions about long-term effects on adult and child members. Health histories that include information about previous marriages, cohabiting partnerships, and length of relationships could be important variables needed to understand the effects of family type on adult personalities. Questions in this area abound. For example, are married adults healthier than cohabiting or single adults? Does the psychological stress from the loss of a marriage increase one's susceptibility to illness? Are same-sex partners more or less likely than heterosexual partners to develop healthy lifestyle patterns?

Affective Functions of the Family

Affective function has to do with the ways in which family members relate to one another and those outside the immediate family boundaries. The family provides a sense of belonging and identity to its members. This identity often proves to be vitally important throughout the entire life cycle. Within the confines of family, members learn dependent roles that later serve to launch them into independent ones. Family serves as a place to learn about intimate relationships and establishes the foundation for future personal interactions. The family provides the initial experience of self-awareness, which includes a sense of knowing one's own gender, ethnicity, race, religion, and personal characteristics. Family helps members become acquainted with who they are and experience themselves in relationships with others. Family provides the substance for self-identity as well as a foundation for other-identity. Within the confines of family, individuals learn about love, care, nurture, dependence, and support. Although one hopes for early family-of-origin experiences to produce resilient members, it does not always occur. Resilience implies an ability to rebound from stress and crisis, the capacity to be optimistic, solve problems, be resourceful, and develop caring support systems. Although unique traits alter potentials for emotional and psychological health, individuals exposed to resilient family environments tend to have greater potential to achieve normative developmental patterns and positive sibling and parental relationships.

Research on parent-child interactions needs to consider the quantity and quality of time spent together, the kinds of activities engaged in, and patterns of interaction in order to better understand member feelings toward each other. More needs to be known

about relationships with nonresidential parents. Variables such as the quality of the couple's relationship, the ways in which family conflict is handled, whether abuse or violence has previously occurred in the household or in members' lives, frequency of children's contact with nonresidential parents, shared custody arrangements, and emotional relationships between parents and children seem important predictors of family affective functions. Affective functions can best be understood by gathering information from the various members involved within a household rather than merely responses from one or two individuals.

Economic Functions of the Family

During the 20th century, the most obvious change in family function is related to economics. In the early stages of American history, the household was the major source of commodity production (Coontz, 1988). In the past, families worked under the leadership of a household head, usually a man, and family economics reflected these familial relationships. However, it has always been true that some women, because of the death of their husbands or fathers, assumed positions as family head and exerted more power. With the emergence of capitalism in the early 19th century, the household and its patriarchal system served as a source of workers. The household head, who received the wage for the family, contributed family members as workers for the fledgling industries. Later in the 20th century, young and unmarried women constituted an important part of the labor pool in World War I. With the rise of capitalism in the late 19th and early 20th centuries, the division between work and home, or what was viewed as men's and women's work, increased. During World War II, many women moved back into the labor force.

After the war, the majority of women returned home, but many elected to remain in the labor force. In 1950, 29.6 percent of women were in the nation's workforce, but by 2002 the number had risen to 43.3 percent (Women's Bureau, 2003). Over the years since then, the shift from an industrial to a service economy has meant an increased number of women in the labor force. Wage differences and familial desires for broader services have been reasons why dual-wage earners have become more common. In 56 percent of married couples, both the husband and wife are in the labor force, and 68 percent of women with children less than 18 years of age in the home work outside the home (U.S. Census Bureau, 1998). Comparing mothers with children under 6 years of age in the labor force from 1955 (18.2 percent) to 2001 (64.3 percent) provides evidence that the economic well-being of today's families is supported by women working (Bureau of Labor Statistics, 2003a). According to the Bureau of Labor Statistics (2003a), the unemployment rate for mothers of children under 1 year of age increased from 7.7 percent in 2001 to 9.4 percent in 2002, but the rate for unmarried mothers of children less than 1 year of age grew from 16.7 percent to 19.6 percent. Of the nation's 74.2 million families, 82.4 percent had at least one employed member in 2002, down by 0.4 percent from 2001 (Bureau of Labor Statistics, 2003b). Unemployment was higher for black families (13.1 percent) than for either white families (7.0 percent) or Hispanic families (11.2 percent). Young men, in particular, are experiencing a worsening of their economic position, and older men are leaving the labor force in record numbers.

The family plays an important function in keeping the nation's economy viable. Married men and married women earn more money than those who are unmarried, but although this remains true for men at all ages, it is only true for women at younger ages. Women who never married tend to be higher wage earners by the time they turn 35 years of age (Cohen & Bianchi, 1999). Although employment plays an important role in determining family financial status, it is not the only determining factor related to economic well-being.

Family income provides a substantial part of family economics, but an equally important aspect has to do with economic interactions and consumerism related to household consumption and finance. For example, despite the fact that family size has decreased from 3.1 people per household in 1970 to 2.6 people per household in 2002, the size of new single-family homes increased from 1500 square feet to over 2200 square feet between 1970 and 2000 (U.S. Census Bureau, 2003c). Money management, housing decisions, consumer spending, insurance choices, retirement planning, and savings are just some of the issues affecting family capacity to care for the economic needs of its members. Financial vulnerability and bankruptcy have increased even for middle-class families as they have assumed greater debt, opted to use more credit cards, paid higher interest rates, and made increasingly larger credit payments. The ability of the family to earn sufficient income and to manage their finances wisely is a critical factor related to economic well-being.

Health Care Functions of the Family

Family members often serve as the primary health care providers to their families. Individuals regularly seek services from a variety of health care professionals, but it is within the family that health instructions are followed or ignored. Family members tend to be the primary caregivers and support persons for individuals. They influence well-being, prevention, illness care, maintenance care associated with chronic illness, and rehabilitative care. Family members care for one another's health conditions from the cradle to the grave. Although nurses continually interact with individuals around health and illness issues, far less is known about the ways family interactions occur within the household. Much of the information provided and interactions that occur tend to focus around biophysical problems rather than on the functions and processes of families. Families have feelings, questions, and stressors associated with health care that go far beyond medical interventions; these are areas where nurses can intervene. Families can become particularly vulnerable when they encounter health threats, and family-focused nurses are in positions where they can provide education and counseling and assist with locating resources. Family-focused care implies that when a single individual is the target of care, the entire family is still viewed as the unit of care (Denham, 2003a). Health literacy is an area where nurses can address vocabulary, sentence structure, organization of ideas, and design elements so that information provided is free of unnecessary barriers.

To ascertain the effect of the family on the individual's and the family's health status, the function of the American family must be analyzed at two levels. At the micro-level, the consequences of health care functions of an individual family greatly affect the growth and development of its members. On the macro-level, the effect of the family, as a social institution, is examined. For example, living in a safe and decent neighborhood promotes well-being whereas residence in high-risk neighborhoods threatens members emotionally, psychologically, physically, and socially (Edin & Lein, 1997; Yinger, 1995). Poor housing options, especially those for minorities, not only restrict available life options but also create a context of hardship within a larger message of abundance.

Health care functions of the family include many aspects of family life. Family members have different ideas about health and illness, and often these ideas are not discussed within families until problems arise.

Availability of health care insurance is a concern for many families, but many families lack clarity about what is and is not covered until they encounter a problem. Lifestyle behaviors, such as healthy diet, regular exercise, and alcohol and tobacco use, are areas that family members may not associate with health and illness outcomes. Risk reduction, health maintenance, rehabilitation, and caregiving are areas where families often need information and assistance. Family members spend far more time taking care of health issues than professionals do and are much more engaged in the daily functions affecting health outcomes. Nurses have multiple possibilities to intervene in ways that can affect individual and family health.

Health care functions of a family are greatly affected by the availability of basic resources such as food, clothing, shelter, transportation, and insurance. Poverty and the unavailability of health care insurance have been repeatedly identified as factors affecting family well-being and health of the individual members. Connections between these factors and ill health may extend beyond the years of childhood and continue to affect outcomes throughout the life cycle. The stresses of living in poverty often result in additional frustrations and exhaustion for families despite the family structure. The duration and extent of poverty are variables that need to be considered in relation to levels of happiness, anxiety, and health outcomes (McLeod & Shanahan, 1993; Sherman, 1994). Mothers play important roles in the health of their children as they (1) teach health information and provide health care, (2) serve as gatekeepers for access to health care providers, (3) assume responsibility for dispersion of family resources, and (4) address health risks (Denham, 2003a).

A large body of literature has suggested that married men and women have better physical and mental health than never-married, separated, divorced, or widowed persons do (Barnett, Marshall, & Pleck, 1992; Gove, 1973; Hahn, 1993; Verbrugge, 1979). Older persons who have never married may have a higher rate of mental disorders than married individuals of similar age do. In one study, widows were found to be five times more likely to be institutionalized in long-term care facilities than married persons were, and separated or divorced persons were 10 times more likely (Stull & Borgatta, 1987). Married persons have much lower age-standardized death rates. Unmarried persons have death rates above average from cirrhosis of the liver, pneumonia, motor vehicle accidents, suicide, and homicide. However, the cause of the inverse relationship between marriage and poor health for both men and women is unclear.

Marriage certainly seems to have a buffering effect on the health status of both men and women, but the effect seems stronger for men. The marital role, both as spouse and as father, may be more central to men's physical and mental health (Barnett, Marshall, & Pleck, 1992). In a satisfactory marriage, both men and women receive psychological support from each other, which may improve their immunological response. Married men and women are more likely to engage in health-enhancing activities (Hahn, 1993). This is particularly true of married men, who tend to rely on their wives in many health-enhancing activities such as the provision of a balanced diet. Socioeconomic status is positively related to health status and may be a confounding variable in the relationship between marriage and health (Rogers, 1995). Married women have a higher family income, are more likely to own a home, and are more likely to have health insurance than single women are. However, more needs to be known about health outcomes in specialized populations of families such as institutionalized or group populations, ethnic and racial minorities, gays and lesbians, and adoptive and foster families.

FAMILY PROCESSES

Family process is the ongoing interaction between family members through which they accomplish their instrumental and expressive tasks. In part, this is what makes families unique. Families with a similar structure and function may interact very differently. Family process, at least in the short term, seems to have a greater effect on the family's health status than family structure and function do and, in turn, seems to be more affected by alterations in health status. Family process certainly seems to have the greatest implications for nursing actions. For example, for the chronically ill, an important determinant for successful rehabilitation is the ability to assume one's familial roles. In order for rehabilitation to occur, family members have to communicate effectively, make decisions about atypical situations, and use a variety of coping strategies. The usual familial power structure may be threatened or may need to change to address unique individual needs. Ultimately, the success or failure of the adaptation processes will affect individual and family well-being.

Alterations in family processes are most likely to occur when the family faces a transition brought about by things such as developmental change, an illness, or other crises. The family's current modes of operation may be ineffective, and members are confronted with needs to learn new ways to cope with change. For example, when coping with the stress of a chronic illness, the family experiences alterations in role performance and in power. When individuals are unable to perform usual roles, other members are expected to assume them. A shift in family roles may result in the loss of individual power. During times of change, the family nurse can help family members communicate, make decisions, identify ways to cope with multiple stressors, reduce role strain, and locate needed resources.

Family communication patterns, member interactions, and interaction with social networks are a few areas in which nurses may want to complete assessments related to family processes. Nursing interventions that promote resilient family processes vary with the degree of strain faced by the family. Families have complex needs related to adaptation, goal attainment, integration, pattern, and tension management. When family processes are ineffective or disrupted, the family and its members may be at risk for problems pertinent to health outcomes and could be in danger of disintegrating. Family therapy by a nurse in advanced practice or another health professional is often needed to assist the family with deeply integrated and unresolved problems connected with family processes (Bulechek & McCloskey, 1992).

Coping with Multiple Stressors over Time

Families each have their own repertoire of coping strategies, which may or may not be adequate in times of stress. Coping consists of "constantly changing cognitive and behavioral efforts to manage specific external and/or internal demands that are appraised as taxing or exceeding the resources of the person" (Lazarus & Folkman, 1984, p. 141). Coping strategies are numerous and may be classified into three broad categories: (1) responses that change the stressful event, (2) responses that control the meaning of the stressful event, and (3) responses that control the stress itself (Pearlin & Schooler, 1982). Family coping is influenced by the family's structure, function, and process. The family's resources such as time, energy, money, knowledge, skills, and past experiences also influence the ways members solve problems and cope with stress and crisis. For example, many middle-class families have children involved in multiple after-school activities. Although these activities may be important aspects for enriching children's lives, they

also bring with them stress. Families often pay a price for these activities in terms of time, money, division of resources, and ability to address health-related practices. Meeting tight time schedules often means forfeiting healthy meals and spending more money eating at fast-food restaurants.

Even families that function at optimal levels may experience difficulties when stressful events pile up. Ineffective coping does not necessarily reduce or control stress (Measley, Richardson, & Dimico, 1989). The outcomes of coping are difficult to evaluate in the short term. The long-term impact of various coping strategies and styles is best understood over time. For example, an individual's grieving may appear adaptive during the first few weeks after the death of a family member. Others may even comment that the mourner is "taking it well." Years later, however, another lesser loss may evoke a disproportionate grief response. Many have viewed the grieving process as one having various stages or responses. Rando (1993) suggested that there are three phases: avoidance, confrontation, and accommodation. Complicated grief generally reflects the fact that the mourner did not effectively grieve in the earlier situation. Among those who have provided us with theories about grief are Sigmund Freud, Erich Lindemann, John Bowlby, Colin Murray Parkes, William Worden, Alan Wolfelt, and Therese Rando (Box 5–9 and Box 5–10).

Today's families encounter many challenges that leave them vulnerable to a myriad of stressors. Vulnerability comes in the forms of things like poverty, illness, abuse and violence, and even the location of the family residence. Coping capacities are enhanced whenever families demonstrate resilience or the capacity to survive in the midst of struggle, adversity, and long-term conflict. Families that can recover from crisis tend to be more cohesive, to value unique member attributes, to noncritically support one another, and to focus on strengths rather than limitations.

Family Roles

Within the nuclear family, each family position has a number of attached roles, and each role is accompanied by expectations. After a review of the family literature, Nye (1976) identified eight roles associated with the position of spouse:

- Provider
- Housekeeper
- Child care

Box 5–9　**FAMILY STRESSORS**

Families are often challenged as they attempt to cope with a number of life events that are accompanied by seemingly insurmountable stress and grief. Family nurses can assist family members with communication skills, information, and resources needed for adaptive coping. Some of the things that test a family's coping skills include the following:

- An alcoholic member
- Divorce or separation
- Death
- Relocation
- Chronic illness
- Disability
- Shift work
- Discipline
- Drug use
- National terrorism threats or acts

Stress often involves events and our response to them, but our thoughts about the situations can be critical factors governing the ways we respond. Families differ in their coping skills and the ways they respond to stressful situations. The ways in which family members respond to stress-provoking situations affect member health. Negative stress responses and inadequate coping skills over prolonged periods of time can result in dire health consequences. Nurses focused on helping families cope with potential and/or actual stressors can enable them to live healthier lives in the present as well as avoid future long-term health risks.

- Socialization
- Sexual
- Therapeutic
- Recreational
- Kinship

Traditionally, the provider role has been assigned to the husband and the housekeeper and child care roles have been assigned to the wife. However, with societal changes and variations in family structure, the traditional enactment of these roles is not viable for many families. Consequently, more families allow some negotiation around who assumes which role and then define the expected behavioral parameters. For example, a newly married couple decides who writes the thank-you notes after the wedding. According to

Box 5–10　**COPING WITH GRIEF AND LOSS**

All families encounter times when they must cope with grief and loss. Sometimes this comes in expected ways such as the death of an aging parent who has lived a full life, but other times it is an unexpected tragedy such as the traumatic death of a teenage child in a car accident caused by drunken driving. In the case of death, most families go through usual coping strategies that often include things such as somatic or bodily distress, preoccupation with the deceased, guilt related to the deceased, hostile reactions, and lessened ability to function (Worden, 1982). A number of factors influence grief and mourning (Rando, 1993):

- The nature and meaning of the loss
- Characteristics of the mourner
- Characteristics of the death
- Social factors
- Psychological factors

many etiquette books, this is the bride's responsibility. However, a couple may decide that the bride writes thank-you notes to her kin, and the groom to his.

The ways in which decisions are made are influenced by the culture and time period in which the family lives. Many culturally prescribed behavioral expectations are situated in views of the nuclear family as the norm. When norms are not met, sanctions may occur. For instance, the bride's grandmother may express displeasure at what she perceives as a lack of respect or social grace by members of the groom's family. At other times, legal sanctions are incurred, for example, when the parents leave their children alone while they are on vacation without arranging for their care. Less-traditional family types may not have roles conventionally prescribed and may allow even greater freedom in the negotiation process. However, nontraditional family types are often subject to social sanctions just because they exist.

Idealized images about traditional roles are seen less frequently in today's marriages and partnerships, but they still exist. Today's families are continually encountering change and social influences that require a phenomenal number of life adjustments. Dating patterns of American youth are quite different today from what they were like in the past, but even early in courtship, couples often assume idealized views of behaviors and roles. Once dating subsides and a committed relationship begins, additional negotiations about roles occur and a life together is constructed. Marital quality and satisfaction are often dependent on the degree to which personal needs are met; this is greatly influenced by whether role expectations are met and are agreeable.

Various Family Roles

In every household, members have to decide the ways in which work and responsibilities will be divided and shared. Roles are negotiated, assigned, delegated, or assumed. Division of labor within the family household occurs as various members take on various roles.

Provider Role

The actual behavior demonstrated by individuals in their various roles is not necessarily congruent with member expectations. The provider role has undergone significant change in the past few decades. Although American men were once viewed as family breadwinners, the proportion of households where this is true has significantly declined over the last few decades. The proportion of families with a male living in the house, an increase in the number of families with no wage earners, a growth in multiple-earner families, and an increased number of families being solely supported by someone other than a male householder have all contributed to families' economic needs. Many families require more than one income to meet basic needs. At the same time, work conditions have become increasingly stressful for men and women and external work obligations increasingly impinge on members' abilities to meet familial role obligations.

Housekeeper and Child Care Roles

Today, many women experience a great deal of role strain in balancing provider and other familial roles. Women who work continue to be responsible for most housekeeping and child care tasks (Kalleberg & Rosenfeld, 1990; Perry-Jenkins & Folk, 1994; Pittman & Blanchard, 1996; Ward, 1993). "Many women continue to live as 'drudge wives' working full-time in the labor force and doing more than 60 percent of the housework" (Robinson & Milkie, 1998, p. 206). Husbands of employed wives spend only a small amount of additional time on housework; however, the proportion of time they spend increases because employed wives spend less time on housework (Kalleberg & Rosenfeld, 1990; McHale & Crouter, 1992). Women with children spend the most time on housework. Although husbands' roles in child care are increasing, their focus is often on playing with the children rather than on meeting basic needs. The time women spend fulfilling housekeeper and child care roles may be related, in part, to family income. Women with higher incomes spend less time on housekeeping and child care; they pay others to do it for them. Many women earn less because of familial responsibilities, and they have more familial responsibilities because they earn less. Thus, they are caught in a vicious circle.

Socialization Role

In relation to socialization of the children, the role expectations have become more egalitarian over the last few decades. Socialization includes things like the ways children learn to interact with others, care for themselves, create boundaries for relationships with extended family, peers, or others, and act as citizens of the larger society. Parents assume the major socialization roles through teaching, guiding, directing, disciplining, and counseling children. Although involvement of both parents promotes development of healthy children, the father-child relationship is qualitatively different from the mother-child relationship. Mothers assume the larger share of the responsibility for children's socialization. Men seem to take more responsibility for the socialization of boys than of girls (Harris & Morgan, 1991). Although the majority of children have little or no contact with nonresident fathers (Seltzer, 1991), many more fathers are staying involved with their children. Some fathers may choose to limit contact with children of whom they do not have custody in order to protect themselves from loss or avoid conflict.

Sexual and Therapeutic Roles

The sexual and therapeutic familial roles also require egalitarian relationships between the adult partners. In satisfactory relationships, partners or spouses need to play active roles in meeting one another's sexual and therapeutic needs. The main predictor of an egalitarian sexual relationship seems to be socioeconomic status and education. More highly educated women tend to be more assertive, whereas more highly educated men tend to be more sensitive and emotionally expressive (Francoeur, 1993). These adults are more acceptive of alternative sexual behaviors and tend to rate sexual intimacy more positively. Women and men in lower socioeconomic classes are likely to experience earlier sexual intercourse and have more traditional sexual practices.

The therapeutic role involves helping each other with intra- and extra-familial problems. This includes a willingness to share one's own concerns, listen to others, be actively involved in problem solving, and provide emotional support. The therapeutic role includes supporting family members in activities that promote health and prevent disease. Individuals are more likely to engage in health-promoting activities, such as exercise, when accompanied by a significant other. When individuals become sick, they turn to family members for validation of their symptoms. In addition to supporting each other in seeking health care, family members also play a therapeutic role in helping the sick person decide on treatment options. They frequently assist in the administration and evaluation of long-term treatments. Family support is a major determinant in rehabilitation.

Resilient families do not depend on one family member to assume this role; they share in the responsibilities. One study of family roles found that over 60 percent of husbands and wives believed that they have a duty to enact the therapeutic role (Nye, 1976). Over three-fifths disapproved of a husband or wife who refused to help a spouse with a problem. The parents included in the study thought that a family member who reacted with criticism to the person confiding the problem, who disclosed the problem to third parties, or who imposed solutions on the confider deserved verbal sanctions.

Recreation Role

Families seldom assign recreational responsibilities to particular members; the quantity and types of recreation engaged in vary with the family life cycle. When the woman works outside the home, social activities outside the family decrease, but intra-family activities and commercial recreation are not as greatly affected (Carlson, 1976). Families with a higher socioeconomic status are more active in formal, organized, and expensive activities; families with a lower socioeconomic status tend to rely more on inexpensive activities such as visiting relatives (Hawks, 1991). The major complaint about recreation is the lack of time available for it. Perceived satisfaction with leisure time is positively associated with marital sociability, marital satisfaction, marital stability, and marital intimacy (Hawks, 1991). The family's involvement in leisure activities promotes integration of the family system, but activities are often dropped when the family is under stress.

Kinship Role

Enactment of the kinship role involves maintaining contact with the extended family and friends. Women tend to function as kin keepers and maintain a higher level of interaction with the extended family than men do (Marks & McLanahan, 1993). Women generally give and receive more family help and rely on parents, children, or siblings for support. Fathers in traditional families are more likely than men in nontraditional families are to give instrumental social support to parents and children. They often provide some child care, transport family members, and do home or car repairs. Nontraditional two-parent families tend to operate in a similar manner. Whereas single fathers and mothers are more likely to receive parental support, mothers with cohabiting partners are likely to receive less. Cohabiting same-sex couples rely more heavily on friend networks. Middle-aged and elderly parents receive help from and give help to their children. A high level of exchange occurs between middle-aged and elderly parents and daughters, even when the daughter is not a caregiver (Walker & Pratt, 1991). Older adults tend to limit their help to their primary kin (Gallagher, 1994).

Role Competence

The competent performance of familial roles is a determinant of marital success. Blood and Wolfe (1960) hypothesized that the source of power in marriage was related to the comparative resources that the husband and wife bring to the marriage. Competent enactment of familial roles is a primary resource that one brings to marriage (Bahr, 1976). Role competency might be viewed as a reward to one's partner. For example, money, love, and status received from a spouse can affect the ways partners interact when differences in opinions arise. Furthermore, the more rewards one receives from a spouse, the more likely one is to be satisfied in the marriage. If the exchange is inequitable, one or both spouses may seek other alternatives. Therefore, assumption of one's familial roles and completing them competently adds to the family's overall abilities to cope, achieve goals, and make effective use of resources.

Role Strain

Lack of competence in role performance may be a result of role strain. Some have found that sources of role strain are cultural and interactional. For instance, cultures that encourage equally positive commitments to all of one's roles generate less role strain (Marks, 1994). If a culture values both work and parenting equally, little role strain occurs. However, O'Neill and Greenberger's (1994) study of patterns of commitment to work and parenting did not support Marks's hypothesis. Men experienced less role strain if they had low commitment to work and high commitment to parenting. O'Neill and Greenberger found no relationship between women's patterns of commitment to work and parenting and role strain, although women in professional-managerial jobs experienced less role strain.

Interactional sources of role strain are related to difficulties in the delineation and enactment of familial roles. Heiss (1980) identified five sources of difficulties in the interaction process:

- Inability to define the situation
- Lack of role knowledge
- Lack of role consensus
- Role conflict
- Role overload

Inability to Define Situations

These problems all place a strain on the family system. The inability to define the situation creates ambiguity about what one should do in a given scenario. Continual changes in family structures and gender roles means that members increasingly encounter situations in which guidelines for action are unclear. For example, in the 1950s, men automatically opened doors for women, but now a dating couple has to decide who opens the car door. Single parents, stepparents, nonresident fathers, and cohabiting partners deal daily with situations for which there are no norms. What right does a stepparent have to discipline the new spouse's child? Is a nonresident father expected to teach his child about AIDS? What name or names go on the mailbox of cohabiting partners? Whether or not the issues are substantive, they present daily challenges to the people involved. Some choose to withdraw from the situation and others choose to redefine the situation when they are uncertain how to act. For instance, a blended family might want to operate in the same way as a traditional family but may experience conflict when thinking about whom and whom not to include at family celebrations. When a solution cannot be found, family members suffer the consequences of role strain.

Lack of Role Knowledge

Role strain sometimes results when family members do not know a role appropriate to a situation or they have no basis for choosing between several roles that might seem appropriate. In America, most people are not clearly taught how to be parents and much learning is observational and experiential. Socialization related to caregiving of a chronically ill family member is seldom done, and many individuals are unfamiliar with and unprepared to assume the roles necessary for providing care. Whether an individual is learning how to be a parent or a caregiver, role training may be required. Knowledge may be acquired by peer observation, trial and error, or explicit instruction. Parents may have limited opportunities to observe peers, and other family members may not have the knowledge necessary to help. Thus, the family may need to seek external resources or obtain needed information using other means such as child care classes, self-help groups, or instruction from health professionals. If individuals are unable to figure out their roles in a situation, problem-solving abilities are limited.

Lack of Role Consensus

The third source of role strain is a lack of role consensus. Family members may be unable to agree about the expectations attached to a role. A family role that currently seems to be the source of family disagreement is the housekeeping role, a major problem for dual-career couples. Men who have been socialized into more traditional male roles are less inclined to accept responsibility for household tasks readily and may limit the amount of time they are willing to spend on these activities. When active participation does not meet the wife's expectations, she tends to assume responsibility for the greatest number of household tasks. If she has been socialized into thinking that women are accountable for traditional housekeeping roles, then she may feel guilty or neglectful if she asks for help. Lack of agreement about the role sometimes results in familial discord and taxes levels of satisfaction with the partner. Although persuasion, manipulation, and coercion may be used to reduce role strain, negotiation is usually required and is most likely to be effective in reaching consensus about things that can be done.

Role Conflict

A fourth source of role strain is role conflict, a phenomenon that occurs when the expectations about familial roles are incompatible. For example, the therapeutic role might involve becoming a caregiver to an elderly parent, but expectations of this new role may be incompatible with that of provider, housekeeper, and child care provider. Does one go to the child's baseball game or to the doctor with the elderly parent? Role conflict may occur when roles present conflicting demands. Individuals and families often have to set priorities. Demands of caregiver and provider roles may be conflicting and may conflict with other therapeutic familial tasks. The caregiver may withdraw from activities that, in the short term, seem superfluous but, in the long term, are sources of much-needed energy. Family nurses are likely to encounter members facing many strains due to role conflict and may need to assist by providing information and suggesting ways the family could negotiate to discover meaningful solutions.

Role Overload

A source of role strain closely related to role conflict is role overload. In role overload, the individual lacks resources, time, and energy to meet role demands. As

with role conflict, the first option usually considered is withdrawal from one of the roles. Maintaining a balance between energy-enhancing and energy-depleting roles reduces role strain (Marks & McDermid, 1996). An alternative to merely withdrawing from a role might be to add activities that are personally satisfying and energy producing—for example, the role of bridge player, artist, or tennis player. The individual who experiences either role conflict or role overload might also consider which responsibilities can be delegated to others. This requires skill in negotiation.

Distribution of Family Power and Authority

Power is one of the most important, albeit controversial, family processes. Power has been defined as "the net ability or capability of actors to produce or cause (intended) outcomes or effects, particularly on the behavior of others or on others' outcomes" (Szinovacz, 1987, p.652). Power can be identified as the way one family member holds control over other family members even when resistance from the members occurs. For example, imagine that a wife wants her spouse to attend a social function with her, and he decides to go with her despite the fact that he prefers to stay home and watch football. If he was waiting to be asked and did not resist, then no power was exerted. However, if he was talked into attending, then her power overcame his resistance. Legitimate power is authority based on position or willingness of others to be governed or directed. Conjugal power has to do with instances when one adult uses force or threat of force to get one's way. The exercise of power is a dynamic and multidimensional process.

Much discussion has occurred that differentiates power associated with gender. The class/caste system operating in American society always gives the power to the man of the family (Gillespie, 1984). "Women are structurally deprived of equal opportunities to develop their capacities, resources, and competence in competition with males" (p. 208). Three sources of men's marital power are through (1) the socialization process; (2) the marriage contract, which, in many states, legally favors men; and (3) economic resources. Men often have higher-paying jobs than women do and greater social status. Married women often have less sense of control over their personal lives than unmarried women do. If income is constant, marriage decreases a woman's sense of control (Ross, 1991). Although more women are employed and making major financial contributions to the family income, traditional views of power continue to dominate the thinking of many. However, women working full-time, especially those with higher incomes, may have a power base similar to a man's. Additionally, culture may also be a determinant, as some cultures allow women more power within the family than others do.

Blood and Wolfe (1960) were early pioneers in the study of individual and family characteristics that determine influences of power in decision-making processes. Findings indicated that economic resources, education, and organizational participation contributed to power. A family trait that tended to give power to the husband during the 1950s and 1960s was suburbanization. Suburbanization meant that husbands had the economic power to provide a home in the suburbs, a reality that often meant the isolation of the wife from her family of origin or even the isolation of the suburban family from others. While suburbanization is less common today, any form of isolation allows the stronger individual opportunity to assume more power. Findings from this study did not indicate that men have more power than women do, because 71 percent of the couples participating had egalitarian styles. However, when power differences exist, husbands are most likely to assume positions of power.

Nurturance and Care for Members

Even with the leveling off of divorce rates in the United States, marital satisfaction has continued to decline (Glenn & Weaver, 1988; Glenn, 1991). This may be related to higher expectations of marriage or to a breakdown in consensual norms. Although the research findings are contradictory, a curvilinear relationship seems to exist between marriage and the life cycle (Suitor, 1991; Vannoy & Philliber, 1992). Marital satisfaction is relatively high among newly married and older couples. The presence of children in the home reduces marital satisfaction, particularly for husbands (Vannoy & Philliber, 1992). Increased marital satisfaction in the aging may actually reflect cohort differences (Glenn, 1998). For example, older couples may experience less role strain because of their commitment to enactment of traditional familial roles. Overall, wives with nontraditional role orientations seem to experience more dissatisfaction with marriage, and wives of husbands with nontraditional role orientations seem to experience more marital satisfaction.

The quality of marital interaction is related to the spouses' involvement and responsibilities both within and outside of the household (Ward, 1993).

Satisfaction with the division of household labor has become increasingly important in the explanation of marital quality (Suitor, 1991). Indeed, the curvilinear relationship between marital satisfaction and the family life cycle also reflects wives' involvement in child care and housekeeping (Suitor, 1991). That is, newly married and aging wives have less child care and housekeeping responsibilities and are more satisfied with their marriage. Yet, the number of hours spent on household tasks was not related to marital satisfaction (Ward, 1993). Instead, wives' marital happiness was associated with the perceived fairness of household labor. Employment of the wife does not singularly affect marital satisfaction. Husbands of employed wives do not appear to experience less marital satisfaction than husbands of unemployed wives do (Vannoy and Philliber, 1992). Instead, the relative occupational attainment of the spouses seems important. Couples may be less satisfied when the wife's occupational attainment is higher than the husband's.

Time constraints are an underlying factor in the relationship between marital satisfaction and child care, household labor, and employment (Zuo, 1992). Marital interaction promotes marital happiness, and marital happiness encourages marital interaction. This holds true for both men and women throughout the life cycle. When there is less time for interaction, there is less marital happiness. Continual work or other external demands without a balance of shared leisure or recreational pursuits can threaten contentment levels and ultimately familial relationships.

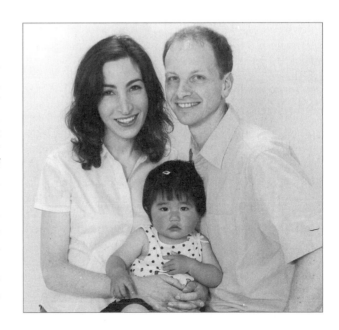

Communication Patterns

The negotiation of familial roles requires effective communication. Communication, in healthy families, occurs among autonomous individuals in an environment that is relatively free of unresolved conflicts. Healthy communication is characterized by clear, but flexible, rules governing verbal and nonverbal communication, clarity in the verbalization of feelings and thoughts, freedom to express a wide variety of feelings, and receptivity to and acknowledgment of the other person's communication (Lewis, 1986). Frequent use of psychological defense mechanisms, such as projection, denial, blaming, and scapegoating, can threaten effective verbal and nonverbal exchange.

Communication difficulties are probably the most common type of family problem and often cause members to seek external help to improve interactions. Differences in a family's cultural or developmental makeup may lead to various forms of miscommunication (Varenne, 1992). Communication difficulties may also be related to the different communication styles of men and women. Men's and women's preferences for and perceptions of communication styles vary (Hawkins, Weisberg, & Ray, 1984). Women may prefer a communication style that conveys interest in, respect for, and validation of the internal realities of self and other. Men often prefer to explore various facets of an issue. Men and women use the act of conversing differently (Tannen, 1990). For example, conflict often includes a demand-withdraw pattern where one demands conversation or attention, but the other withdraws to distance themselves (Christensen & Shenk, 1991). Same-sex families, especially lesbians, are more likely to aspire to egalitarian relationships, and conversation may be more focused on shared goals and creating an environment without imbalances (Kurdek, 1993).

Decision-Making Processes

Communication and power are basic to decision making, and family members usually have defined spheres of power. The father may choose the car; the mother, the house or kitchen; the child, their toys. In a healthy family, the balance of power resides in the parent coalition. Relationships may be complementary in that each person does the opposite or reciprocal of the other, or they may be symmetrical, that is, based on similarities rather than differences. Symmetrical participation in decision making is more likely to be satisfactory. Families are faced with making numerous decisions, including the decision to become a parent, values that are important to instill in children, discipline, use of money and other resources, and member workload.

Because the norms governing familial interactions have become outmoded, decision making has become increasingly important for identifying and attaining family goals. Family decision making is not an individual effort but rather a joint one. Each decision has at least five features (Scanzoni & Szinovacz, 1980, p. 54):

- Who raises the matter?
- What is being said?
- Supporting actions to what is being said
- Importance of what is being said to party doing the speaking
- Response of other party

For example, a two-year-old boy who refused to eat his spinach until after he had dessert involved the mother in the decision-making process. She had to decide whether the real issue was spinach, dessert, or control. If she defined the issue as the child's dislike of spinach, she could choose to omit it, substitute carrots, or coerce him into eating it. Instead, she defined the issue as control. Rather than withholding dessert until he had eaten his spinach, she decided that she did not want to get into a power struggle over this issue. She chose to let the child decide. Subsequently, he ate both his spinach and his dessert. This example emphasizes the importance of looking at the decision-making process. Parents often improve their decision-making abilities as they gain more experience within their family. If one looked only at the outcome, one could conclude that the child controlled the situation. By looking at the process, one sees that the mother made the decision to give the child control.

Decision making provides opportunity for various family members to make a contribution to the process, support one another, and jointly set and strive to achieve goals. Disagreements within a family are natural, as members often have different points of view. It is important for members to share their various viewpoints with one another. Problem solving is part of the decision-making process and frequently means that differences in opinion and emotions need to be considered.

Communication style is a strong predictor of decision-making outcomes (Godwin & Scanzoni, 1989). Certain interactional strategies disrupt problem solving, whereas others enhance it. The expression of negative emotions is a disruptive factor (Forgatch, 1989). Anger is not necessarily disruptive, but contempt, belligerence, and defensiveness are (Gottman et al., 1998). The expression of negative emotions tends to lead to conflict as an outcome of decision making. The use of "I" messages rather than blaming or accusing the other is helpful in talking through differences. Consensus, or at least continuation of negotiations, is the preferred outcome when disagreements occur. Nurses working with families can strive to help members develop communication skills that are most effective for resolving differences and making decisions.

Family Rituals and Routines

Rituals and routines have been identified in the literature as having health implications (Denham, 2003a; Fiese, 1993, 1995; Fiese & Wamboldt, 2000). Rituals are associated with celebrations, traditions, religious observances, and symbolic events, whereas routines are behaviors closely linked with daily or regular activities. Families have unique rituals and routines that provide organization and give meaning to family life. The habitual behaviors associated with rituals and routines have potential for health and illness outcomes (Denham, 1995). Family culture, context, and functional family aspects affect these rituals and routines. The importance and value of rituals in everyday life have been clearly explored in anthropological and sociological literature, but the significance of rituals is largely ignored by nurses (Denham, 2003b). Family routines are continuous behaviors, and family members use them in their roles to define responsibilities, organize daily life, and identify family characteristics or traits (Bennett, Wolin, & McAvity, 1988; Steinglass, Bennett, Wolin, & Reiss, 1987). Examples of family routines are mealtimes, bedtime routines, leisure activities, greetings and good-byes, and treatment of guests. Rituals and routines are family life processes with important consequences for individual and family health outcomes. Assessing rituals and routines related to specific health or illness needs provides a basis to envision distinct family interventions and to devise specific plans for health promotion and disease management, especially when adherence to medical regimens is critical or caregiving demands are burdensome to the family (Denham, 2003b).

NURSING IMPLICATIONS

Ideas about family structure, function, and process have broad implications for practice, education, research, and policy.

Practice

Over the last few decades, most nurses have worked in practices where patient or client contact occurs in institutional or agency settings. Educational preparation for nurses has largely assumed that professional encounters would be with single individuals, happen over several days, and take place in formal health care settings. Traditionally, nurses have been taught to provide institutional interventions that require individuals to stay long enough to receive the care prescribed. During the mid-1980s, most people stayed 5.7 to 6.5 days in hospitals, but today more than half of persons seeking health care services spend only 4 to 5 hours in the setting. Embracing the future of nursing for the 21st century means understanding that health care consumers have different needs and demands than they did in the past. More and more services are being delivered in community and home settings providing episodic interventions through short-term relationships.

We have already moved from the industrial age to the techno-informational age where consumers have access to much of the same information as health care professionals. The information and technologies are creating the demands for the future. Challenges include rethinking the work of nurses from merely provision of individual care to family-centered care. Understanding the structure, function, and process of families is becoming foundational to the delivery of care as new ways are envisioned to provide care where families live, work, and play. Health care is being revolutionized, and nurses prepared to work with families in what have been viewed as less-conventional settings will be in great demand. Orientations of disease and mortality have been transferred from focus on infectious disease and death to concerns about living with chronic illness for decades. Nurse practice in this century will entail working with consumers who have greater control and a greater demand for convenience, control, and knowledge. Nurses who understand family dynamics and are prepared to provide family-centered care will meet the changing consumer demands of those seeking health care services.

Education

Nursing education has primarily focused on the assessment, planning, implementation, and evaluation of health care services to individuals. As health care demands continue to change, it becomes more essential for nurses' education to center on individuals as part of a family context. Ideas about family are still in flux; thus, not only do nurses need basic information about family structure, functions, and processes, but also ideas need to be redefined in light of changing societal needs and a growing body of knowledge. Greater understanding about the complexities of families and the impact on individual members is needed to equip nurses to become more family-focused in their approaches to clinical care. Nurses require theoretical understandings about families, critical analysis skills, and aptitudes to synthesize information from multiple sources in order to address individual health care needs effectively. Knowledge about individual and family lifestyle behaviors, the influence of family functions and processes, and ways to redefine nursing care with diverse families, groups, and communities becomes the essential foundation for future learning.

Research

Research in the areas of family structure, function, and process has expanded over the last few decades, but there remains much work for nurses to do in all of these areas. All aspects of family need to be considered from nursing perspectives. Although the published literature identifies a large number of studies about the diverse family variables, far less study has been done about family factors and health outcomes pertinent to nurses' work. For example, studies that investigate differences in family structure often identify disparities related to differences in family type, socio-economic status, and other family variables linked to health outcomes. Although some nurses may be counselors and could use this information in practice, few can directly apply the knowledge in the work they do. Instead, family research that investigates health outcomes associated with specific diseases and tests the effects of different interventions could prove more fruitful for practice. Current understandings about family structure, function, and process are limited by the knowledge on which they are based. Additional research in all of these areas is needed to add to the body of knowledge that is distinctively in the domain of nursing.

Health and Social Policy

Health and social policies provide the standards, rules, and behaviors that the larger society deems important. Policies are dynamic and are continually challenged by contemporary ideas and societal needs. Traditional views of marriage as the accepted structure of family relationships are presently being debated by legislators and church leaders. As more American citizens choose cohabitation or decide to live openly in same-sex relationships, they are also demanding privileges and rights equal to those choosing marriage. Debates surrounding the Defense of Marriage Act will likely continue to raise questions about its place as a constitutional issue, about discrimination, and about human rights. Other questions may be related to whether a marriage remains legal if one of the partners in a heterosexual relationship has a sex change. Broad definitions of rights for those choosing varied family types are presently missing from many state and federal laws, but policies and legislation are being debated. Past and continuing changes in social policy about what constitutes a family create opportunities for public discussion and influence legislation.

Some functional roles of family are being modified as families enter the techno-informational age. Although children were once cared for by stay-at-home mothers, it is now likely that they will be placed in day care centers at early ages while mothers work. Social policy that supports family and addresses child care needs is an area where change might be expected. The health function of family is becoming greater as greater demands are placed on members to act as health providers. Legislative policies are needed to support family needs, assist with necessary health care resources, and offer health care insurance adequate to keep America's families healthy. Family processes, such as member roles, will continue to be redefined in the 21st century, and along with these changes will come needs for social and health policies pertinent to changing requirements for healthy families. Nurses who are well educated about family structure, function, and process are prepared to sit at the table where policy is decided and to become leaders in campaigns for necessary policy changes.

SUMMARY

- Family structure, function, and process provide the foundation for understanding families, the ability to analyze their many characteristics or traits, and a way to synthesize the many variables composing family.
- Patterns of family structure are being reformed as we move away from traditional ideas about the nuclear family and embrace society's demands to choose alternative family forms.
- The increase in the number of blended or cohabitating families means that the odds for

children to be raised in a household missing one of their parents have increased.

- Children are primarily socialized by the family about the values important to civil, social, and religious institutions of the larger society.
- Families serve many functional roles for household members, including procreation, nurturance, provision of a household milieu, and access to social resources.
- Families influence the ways in which members encounter sickness and cope with needs related to illness and disease.
- Nurses play important roles in helping families and their households cope with needs associated with health and illness.
- Families use a variety of dynamic and interactive processes to cope with daily stresses and make decisions affecting individual members and the family as a whole.
- Nurses can provide interventions to help family household members use roles more effectively and communication strategies to fulfill family responsibilities and meet individual needs.
- Family rituals and routines can provide nurses with the basis of planning family interventions that have health and wellness implications.
- Family structure, function, and process are not solitary entities but provide ways to understand families as dynamic systems that interact with their environment.
- Nurses who understand family structure, function, and process have a foundation for considering optimum ways to include the family as they help individuals achieve health care outcomes.

CASE STUDY ➤

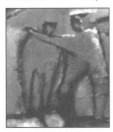

Alicia (54 years old) is a well-established professional career woman. She divorced her husband 16 years ago and has lived independently since that time. Her work schedule—technically a 40-hour week—often turns into 60 hours or more. She regularly has to travel or has long days away from home. About 8 months ago, her oldest daughter Kendra (33 years old) came to live with her because of a fractured ankle that needed elevation and rest for 6 weeks. Alicia was happy to have her daughter live with her for the prescribed time, even though she had concerns because Kendra would have to stay alone much of the time. Kendra is a single parent and has a daughter named Jenny (12 years old). Arrangements were made for Jenny to stay with her aunt Susie, who lives about 2 hours away.

Kendra has been diabetic since she was a young child and over time has developed multiple complications. She had spent a large number of her younger adult years with poor self-management of her diabetes and had indulged in risky behaviors that included alcohol and street drugs. The broken ankle resulted from tripping in a hole but was probably related to Charcot's disease. During the time it took for her ankle to heal, Kendra's vision began worsening, as did her complications of depression, gastroparesis, neuropathy, and hypertension. In fact, by the time the ankle should have healed, Kendra's condition was on a marked decline. Considerably more vision loss had occurred, and critical events of hypo- and hyperglycemia happened daily even though blood glucose levels were monitored and she complied with the prescribed diet and medications. Kendra cried continuously and became more withdrawn as she missed and worried about her daughter. Finally, the decision was made that Jenny would also come to live with Alicia so that she and her mother could be together.

Over the next few months, Kendra's condition worsened, and a serious case of pneumonia resulted in a hospitalization. During the time of the hospitalization, she completely lost the vision in her left eye. After her release from the hospital, she continued to be unable to control her blood pressure. She wound up back in the hospital, this time in a critical condition with kidney failure and severe loss of vision in her other eye. After her hospital release about 6 weeks later, she came back to live with Alicia and Jenny. She is now weak and frightened but thankful to be with her mother and happy that her daughter is with her.

Alicia is trying to continue work, as she needs her job to support herself. She finds herself getting more stressed and uncertain about how she is going to continue work and care for her daughter and granddaughter. She wants to take care of her family but is torn by the obligations she has at her workplace. Jenny is going to school and trying to help out as much as possible with her mother. She complains little about the added tasks but has a large amount of responsibility placed upon her. Kendra is having major difficulties accepting her physical and emotional status,

(continued on page 152)

CASE STUDY ➤ *(Continued)*

dealing with her blindness, wanting to mother her child, and losing her independence. Kendra is going to dialysis 3 days a week, with each of these days including a 4-hour treatment and an hour-long ride each way to the treatment center. The household mostly revolves around Kendra's needs, which tend to be around-the-clock. A community health nurse got involved, and she will be working with the family as a whole and with Kendra in particular.

1. In thinking about family structure, how does the structure of this family compromise the well-being of this family? Are there ways in which this family's structure is protective? What social structures might be important for helping this family cope with their complex problems?

2. Consider the concept of family function: what implications do you see for this family? List family strengths and limitations. If you were Kendra's dialysis nurse, what concerns would you have? What things are important to include in a plan of care?

3. Consider the concept of family process: what are the implications for this family? Think about family roles: What is going on with these family members? How are the coping skills of the family members being challenged? If you encountered this family as a home health nurse, what strengths would you build on? What risks would you address?

4. What type of interventions should the community nurse consider in working with this family?

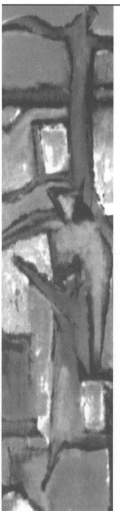

RESEARCH BRIEF

Dashiff, C. J. (2003). Self- and dependent-care responsibility of adolescents with IDDM and their parents. *Journal of Family Nursing*, *9*(2), 166–183.

Purpose of the Study
The purpose of the study was twofold. (1) Describe perceptions of the division of diabetes self- and dependent-care responsibility among young and adolescents and their parents in two-parent families. (2) Examine relationships of the perceptions about the division of diabetes self- and dependent-care responsibility among young and adolescents and their parents in two-parent families to the metabolic control of diabetes.

Methodology
A descriptive correlational study was completed with 31 adolescents with insulin-dependant diabetes mellitus (IDDM) and their parents to investigate family processes, autonomy development, and self-care. Participants were recruited through clinic waiting rooms at a children's hospital. Adolescents were between 12 and 15 years of age, diagnosed with IDDM for at least a year, and part of a two-parent intact or blended family that shared a household for at least a year. Both parents had to agree to participate.

Study data were collected through home visits scheduled at the family's convenience. An investigator-modified version of the Diabetes Family Responsibility Questionnaire (DFRQ) was used to identify the illness-related self-care responsibility of adolescents and dependent care engaged in by the parents. Metabolic control was assessed by glycosylated hemoglobin (HbA_{1c}) with one reading taken 2 months prior to administering the DFRQ and the second reading concurrent with completion of the DFRQ. Each family member completed the form separately.

Results
Moderate associations were found between mothers' and fathers' reports about adolescents' and mothers' responsibilities, and strong associations were found for reports about fathers'

(continued on page 153)

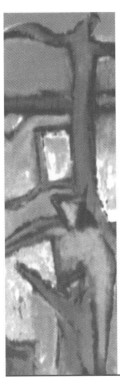

responsibilities. The correlation between adolescents' and fathers' perceptions of mothers' responsibilities was weaker. Mean scores of mothers and fathers regarding fathers' responsibilities for diabetes tasks were significant, but no significance was found between mothers' and adolescents' scores. Adolescents and mothers both viewed adolescents as having the primary responsibility for the greatest number of tasks, but fathers reported mothers as having the primary responsibility for the greatest number of tasks. Family socioeconomic status, duration of IDDM, and adolescent age and gender were not associated with the measures of HbA_{1c}. The majority of adolescents had not achieved recommended levels of metabolic control. Trends of poorer prior control of the HbA_{1c} were identified when adolescents had perceptions that their mothers had more responsibility for diabetes tasks, and the metabolic control was worse when fathers had perceptions that mothers had more responsibility.

Nursing Implications

Findings suggest that when adolescents have perceptions that mothers have greater responsibility for diabetes tasks, prior metabolic control is poorer. This might indicate that when adolescents believe themselves to be less responsible for their own care, diabetes control may be poorer. Findings from this study indicate that family members differ in their perceptions, and thus separate scores from multiple family members should be reported. Fathers were the least involved with adolescent care but may make contributions not measured by the DFRQ. Implications for practice suggested by the study indicate that parental perceptions about roles in caring for an adolescent with diabetes may need clarification. Adolescent responsibility for self-care may be a variable linked to metabolic control.

References

Allen, K. R., & Demo, D. H. (1995). The families of lesbians and gay men: A new frontier in family research. *Journal of Marriage and the Family, 57*, 111–127.

Allen, K. R., Fine, M. A., & Demo, D. H. (2000). An overview of family diversity: Controversies, questions, and values. In D. Demo, K. Allen, & M. Fine (Eds.), *Handbook of family diversity* (pp. 1–14). New York: Oxford University Press.

Amato, P. (1994). Father-child relations, mother-child relations, and offspring psychological well-being in early adulthood. *Journal of Marriage and the Family, 56*, 1031–1042.

Amato, P. (2000). Diversity within single-parent families. In D. Demo, K. Allen, & M. Fine (Eds.), *Handbook of family diversity* (pp. 149–172). New York: Oxford University Press.

Amato, P., & Booth, A. (1996). A prospective study of divorce and parent-child relationships. *Journal of Marriage and the Family, 58*, 356–365.

Annie E. Casey Foundation. (1998). *Kids count special report: When teens have sex: Issues and trends.* Baltimore, MD: Annie E. Casey Foundation.

Aquilino, W. S. (1994). Impact of childhood family disruption on young adults' relationships with parents. *Journal of Marriage and the Family, 56*, 295–313.

Bahr, S. J. (1976). Role competence, role norms, and marital control. In F. I. Nye (Ed.), *Role structure and analysis of the family* (pp. 179–189). Beverly Hills: Sage.

Bane, M. J. (1976). *Here to stay: American families in the twentieth century.* New York: Basic Books.

Barnett, R. C., Marshall, N. L., & Pleck, J. H. (1992). Men's multiple roles and their relationship to men's psychological distress. *Journal of Marriage and the Family, 54*, 358–367.

Barnett, R. C., & Shen, Y. (1997). Gender, high and low-schedule-control housework tasks, and psychological distress: A study of dual-earner couples. *Journal of Family Issues, 18*(4), 403–428.

Bell, N. W., & Vogel, E. F. (1960). *A modern introduction to the family.* Glencoe, IL: Free Press.

Bennett, L. A., Wolin, S. J., & McAvity, K. J. (1988). Family identity, ritual, and myth: A cultural perspective on life cycle transitions. In C. J. Falicov (Ed.), *Family transitions: Continuity and change over the life cycle* (pp. 211–233). New York: The Guilford Press.

Births, marriages, divorces and deaths: Provisional data for July, 2001. (2002). *National Vital Statistics Report, 59*(3), 1–2.

Blankenhorn, D. (2002). The reappearing nuclear family. *First Things: The Journal of Religion and Public Life, 119*, 20–22.

Blood, R. O., Jr., & Wolfe, D. M. (1960). *Husbands and wives: The dynamics of married living.* New York: The Free Press.

Blumstein, P., & Schwartz, P. (1983). *American couples: Money, work, sex.* New York: Morrow.

Booth, A., & Amato, P. (1994). Parental gender role nontraditionalism and offspring outcomes. *Journal of Marriage and the Family, 56*, 865–877.

Brown, S. L., & Booth, A. (1996). Cohabitation versus marriage: A comparison of relationship quality. *Journal of Marriage and the Family, 58*, 668–678.

Bulechek, G. M., & McCloskey, J. C. (Eds.). (1992). *Nursing interventions: Essential nursing treatments* (2nd ed.). Philadelphia, PA: Saunders.

Bumpass, L., Raley, R., & Sweet, J. (1994, January 20–21). *The changing character of stepfamilies: Implications of cohabitation and nonmarital childbearing* (NSFH Working Paper No. 63). Paper presented at the Rand Conference, Santa Monica, CA.

Bureau of Labor Statistics, U.S. Department of Labor. (2003a). *Mothers in the labor force.* Retrieved February 9, 2004, from http://www.infoplease.com/ipa/A0104670.html

Bureau of Labor Statistics, U.S. Department of Labor. (2003b). *Employment characteristics of families summary.* Retrieved February 9, 2004, from http://www.bls.gov/news.release/famee.nr0.htm

Carlson, J. (1976). The recreational role. In F. I. Nye (Ed.), *Role structure and analysis of the family* (pp. 131–147). Beverly Hills: Sage.

Casper, L. M., Cohen, P. N., & Simmons, T. (1999). How does POSSLQ measure up? *Historical estimates of cohabitation.* Population Division, U.S. Bureau of the Census. Retrieved January 30, 2004, from http://www.census.gov/population/www/documentation/twps0036/twps0036.html

Chambers, D. L. (1996). What if? The legal consequences of marriage and the legal needs of lesbians and gay male couples. *Michigan Law Review, 95,* 447–491.

Cherlin, A. J. (1992). *Marriage, divorce, and remarriage* (Revised and enlarged edition). Cambridge, MA: Harvard University Press.

Cherlin, A. J. (1999). *Public and private families: An introduction* (2nd ed.). Boston: McGraw Hill.

Christensen, A., & Shenk, J. L. (1991). Communication, conflict, and psychological distance in nondistressed, clinic, and divorcing couples. *Journal of Consulting and Clinical Psychology, 59,* 458–463.

Cohen, P. N., & Bianchi, S. (1999). Marriage, children, and women's employment: What do we know? *Monthly Labor Review, 122*(12), 1–2.

Cooksey, E. C., & Fondell, M. M. (1996). Spending time with his kids: Effects of family structure on fathers' and children's lives. *Journal of Marriage and the Family, 58,* 693–707.

Coontz, S. (1988). *The social origins of private life: A history of American families 1600–1900.* New York: Verso.

Coontz, S. (1992). *The way we never were: American families and the nostalgia trap.* New York: Basic Books.

Coontz, S. (1997). *The way we really are: Coming to terms with America's changing families.* New York: Basic Books.

Coontz, S. (2000). Historical perspectives on family diversity. In D. Demo, K. Allen, & M. Fine (Eds.), *Handbook of family diversity* (pp. 15–31). New York: Oxford University Press.

Darroch, J. E., Landry, D. J., & Oslak, S. (1999). Age differences between sexual partners in the United States. *Family Planning Perspectives, 31*(4), 160–167.

Dawson, D. A. (1991). Family structure and children's health and well-being: Data from the 1988 National Health Interview Survey on Child Health. *Journal of Marriage and the Family, 53,* 573–584.

Degler, C. N. (1980). *At odds: Women and the family in America from the revolution to the present.* New York: Oxford University Press.

Demo, D. H., & Allen, K. R. (1996). Diversity within lesbian and gay families: Challenges and implications for family theory and research. *Journal of Social and Personal Relationships, 13,* 415–434.

Denham, S. A. (1995). Family routines: A construct for considering family health. *Holistic Nursing Practice, 9*(4), 11–23.

Denham, S. A. (1996). Family health in a rural Appalachian Ohio county. *Journal of Appalachian Studies, 2*(2), 299–310.

Denham, S. A. (2003a). *Family health: A framework for nursing.* Philadelphia, PA: FA Davis.

Denham, S. A. (2003b). Relationships between family rituals, family routines, and health. *Journal of Family Nursing, 9*(30), 305–330.

Doherty, W. J., Kouneski, E. F., & Erikson, M. F. (1998). Responsible fathering: An overview and conceptual framework. *Journal of Marriage and the Family, 60,* 277–292.

Downey, D. B., Ainsworth-Parnell, J. W., & Dufur, M. J. (1998). Sex of parent and children's well-being in single-parent households. *Journal of Marriage and the Family, 60,* 878–893.

Edin, K., & Lein, L. (1997). *Making ends meet: How single mothers survive welfare and low-wage work.* New York: Russell Sage Foundation.

Eshleman, J. R. (1997). *The family: An introduction* (8th ed.). Boston: Allyn & Bacon.

Fiese, B. H. (1993). Family rituals in alcoholic and nonalcoholic households: Relations to adolescent health symptomatology and problem drinking. *Family Relations, 42,* 187–192.

Fiese, B. H. (1995). Family rituals. In D. Levinson (Ed.), *Encyclopedia of marriage and the family* (pp. 275–278). New York: Simon & Schuster Macmillan.

Fiese, B. H., & Wamboldt, F. S. (2000). Family routines and asthma management: A proposal for family-based strategies to increase treatment adherence. *Families, Systems & Health, 18*(4), 405–418.

Forgatch, M. S. (1989). Patterns and outcome in family problem solving: The disrupting effect of negative emotion. *Journal of Marriage and the Family, 51,* 115–124.

Francoeur, R. T. (1993). Technological change, sexuality, and family futures planning. *Marriage & the Family Review, 18*(3/40), 135–155.

Freed, S. A., & Freed, R. S. (1993). One son is no sons. In D. Suggs & A. Miracle (Eds.), *Culture and human sexuality* (pp. 166–170). Pacific Grove, CA: Brooks/Cole.

Gallagher, S. K. (1994). Doing their share: Comparing patterns of help given by older and younger adults. *Journal of Marriage and the Family, 56,* 567–578.

Ganong, L. H., Coleman, M., & Mapes, D. (1990). A meta-analytic view of family structure stereotypes. *Journal of Marriage and the Family, 52,* 287–290.

Gillespie, D. (1984). Who has the power? The marital struggle. In B. N. Adams & J. L. Campbell (Eds.), *Framing the family: Contemporary portraits* (pp. 206–228). Prospect Heights, IL: Waveland Press.

Glenn, N. D. (1991). The recent trend in marital success in the United States. *Journal of Marriage and the Family, 53,* 261–270.

Glenn, N. D., & Weaver, C. N. (1988). The changing relationship of marital status to reported happiness. *Journal of Marriage and the Family, 50,* 317–324.

Glick, P. C. (1988). Fifty years of family demography: A record of social change. *Journal of Marriage and the Family, 50,* 861–873.

Godwin, D. D., & Scanzoni, J. (1989). Couple decision making: Commonalities and differences across issues and spouses. *Journal of Family Issues, 10*(3), 291–311.

Gottman Institute. (2001). *What we've learned: What makes same-sex relationships succeed or fail?* Retrieved February 9, 2004, from http://www.gottman.com/gaylesbian/self_help/

Gottman, J. R., Coan, J., Carre, S., & Swanson, C. (1989). Predicting marital happiness and stability from newlywed interactions. *Journal of Marriage and the Family, 60*(1), 5–23.

Gove, W. R. (1973). Sex, marital status, and mortality. *American Journal of Sociology, 79,* 45–67.

Gray, J. (1992). *Men are from Mars, women are from Venus.* New York: Harper Collins.

Guttentag, M. & Secord, P. G. (1983). *Too many women? The sex role question.* Beverly Hills: Sage.

Hahn, B. A. (1993). Marital status and women's health: The effect of economic marital acquisitions. *Journal of Marriage and the Family, 55,* 495–504.

Hamilton, B. E., Martin, J. A., & Sutton, P. D. (2003). Births: Preliminary data for 2002. *National Vital Statistics Report, 51*(110), 1–20.

Hanson, T. L., McLanahan, S. S., & Thomson, E. (1996). Double jeopardy: Parental conflict and stepfamily outcomes for children. *Journal of Marriage and the Family, 58,* 141–154.

Harris, K. M., & Morgan, S. P. (1991). Fathers, sons, and daughters: Differential paternal involvement in parenting. *Journal of Marriage and the Family, 53,* 531–544.

Hauser, R. M., & Mare, R. D. (1994). *Study of American families, 1994.* Madison, WI: Data and Program Library Service [distributor]. Retrieved August 30, 2003, from http://dpls.dacc.wisc.edu/Saf/index.html

Hawkins, J. L., Weisberg, C., & Ray, D. W. (1984). Spouse differences in communication style: Preference, perception, behavior.

In B. N. Adams & J. L. Campbell (Eds.), *Framing the family: Contemporary portraits* (pp. 229–240). Prospect Heights, IL: Waveland Press.

Hawks, S. R. (1991). Recreation in the family. In S. J. Bahr (Ed.), *Family research: A sixty-year review, 1930–1990* (Vol. 1, pp. 387–433). New York: Lexington Books.

Heiss, J. (1980). Family theory 20 years later. *Contemporary Sociology, 9*(2), 201–205.

Henshaw, S. K. (1999). *Special report: U.S. teen pregnancy statistics: With comparative statistics for women aged 20–24.* Retrieved October 29, 2003, from http://www.agi-usa.org/pubs/teen_preg_sr_0699.html

Jayakody, R., Chatters, L. M., & Taylor, R. J. (1993). Family support to single and married African American mothers: The provision of financial, emotional, and child care assistance. *Journal of Marriage and the Family, 55,* 261–276.

Johnson, C., & Troll, L. (1996). Family structure and the timing of transitions from 70 to 103 years of age. *Journal of Marriage and the Family, 58,* 178–187.

Kalleberg, A. L., & Rosenfeld, R. A. (1990). Work in the family and in the labor-market: A cross-national, reciprocal analysis. *Journal of Marriage and the Family, 52,* 331–346.

Kantor, D., & Lehr, W. (1975). *Inside the family: Toward a theory of family process.* San Francisco: Jossey-Bass.

Kollock, P., Blumstein, P., & Schwartz, P. (1985). Sex and power in interaction: Conversational privileges and duties. *American Sociological Review, 50,* 34–46.

Kreider, R. M., & Fields, J. M. (2001). Number, timing, and duration of marriages and divorce: Fall 1996. *Current population reports* (pp. 70–80). Washington, DC: U.S. Census Bureau.

Kurdek, L. A. (1993). The allocation of household labor in gay, lesbian, and heterosexual parent couples. *Journal of Social Issues, 49,* 127–139.

Kurdek, L. A. (1995). Lesbian and gay couples. In A. R. D'Augelli & C. J. Patterson (Eds.), *Lesbian, gay, and bisexual identities over the lifespan: Psychological perspectives* (pp. 243–261). New York: Oxford University Press.

Lazarus, R. S., & Folkman, S. (1984). *Stress, appraisal, & coping.* New York: Springer.

Lee, G. R., Seccombe, K., & Shehan, C. L. (1991). Marital status and personal happiness. *Journal of Marriage and the Family, 53,* 839–844.

Lewis, J. M. (1986). *The birth of the family: An empirical inquiry.* New York: Brunner/Mazel.

Lytton, H., & Romney, D. M. (1991). Parents' differential socialization of boys and girls: A meta-analysis. *Psychological Bulletin, 109,* 267–296.

MacDonald, W. L., & DeMaris, A. (1995). Remarriage, stepchildren, and marital conflict: Challenges to the incomplete institutionalization hypothesis. *Journal of Marriage and the Family, 57,* 387–398.

Macoby, E. E., & Jacklin, C. N. (1974). *The psychology of sex differences.* Stanford, CA: Stanford University Press.

Manning, W., & Lichter, D. (1996). Parental cohabitation and children's economic well-being. *Journal of Marriage and the Family 58,* 998–1010.

Marks, N. F., & McLanahan, S. S. (1993). Gender, family structure, & social support among parents. *Journal of Marriage and the Family, 55*(2), 481–494.

Marks, S. R. (1994). What is the pattern of commitments? *Journal of Marriage and the Family, 56,* 112–114.

Marks, S. R., & MacDermid, S. M. (1996). Multiple roles and the self: A theory of role balance. *Journal of Marriage and the Family, 58,* 417–432.

McHale, S. M., & Crouter, A. C. (1992). You can't always get what you want: Incongruence between sex-role attitudes and family work roles and its implications for marriage. *Journal of Marriage and the Family, 54,* 537–547.

McKinnon, J. (2003). The black population in the United States: March 2002. *Current population reports* (Series P20-541). Washington, DC: U.S. Census Bureau.

McLeod, J. D., & Shanahan, M. J. (1993). Poverty, parenting, and children's mental health. *American Sociological Review, 58,* 351–366.

Measley, A. R., Richardson, H., & Dimico, G. (1989). Family stress management. In P. J. Bomar (Ed.), *Nurses and family health promotion: Concepts, assessment, and interventions* (pp. 179–196). Baltimore, MD: Williams & Wilkins.

National Center for Health Statistics. (2003). Marriage and divorce: Data for 2001. Retrieved November 2, 2003, from http://www.cdc.gov/nchs/fastats/marriage.htm

National Fatherhood Initiative. (2002). *Top ten father facts.* Retrieved October 24, 2003, from http://www.fatherhood.org/fatherfacts/topten.htm

Nelson, S., Clark, R., & Acs, G. (2001). Beyond the two-parent family: How teenagers fare in cohabiting couple and blended families. *Assessing the new federalism policy brief B-31.* Washington, DC: The Urban Institute.

Nock, S. L. (1988). The family and hierarchy. *Journal of Marriage and the Family, 50,* 957–966.

Nye, F. I. (1976). *Role structure and analysis of the family.* Beverly Hills: Sage.

O'Neil, R., & Greenberger, E. (1994). Patterns of commitment to work and parenting: Implications for role strain. *Journal of Marriage and the Family, 56,* 101–108.

Otto, H. A. (Ed.). (1970). *The family in search of a future: Alternate models for moderns.* New York: Appleton-Century-Crofts.

Parsons, T. (1951). *The social system.* New York: Free Press.

Parsons, T., & Bales, R. (1955). *Family socialization and interaction process.* New York: Free Press.

Pearlin, L. I., & Schooler, C. (1982). The structure of coping. In H. I. McCubbin, A. E. Cauble, & J. M. Patterson (Eds.), *Family stress, coping, and social support.* Springfield, IL: Charles C. Thomas.

Perry-Jenkins, M., & Folk, K. (1994). Class, couples, and conflict: Effects of the division of labor on assessments of marriage in dual-earner families. *Journal of Marriage and the Family, 56,* 165–180.

Peterson, G. W., Rollins, B. C., & Thomas, D. L. (1985). Parental influence and adolescent conformity. *Youth & Society, 16*(4), 397–421.

Pittman, J. F., & Blanchard, D. (1996). The effects of work history and timing of marriage on the division of household labor: A life-course perspective. *Journal of Marriage and the Family, 58,* 78–90.

Popenoe, D. (1999). *Life without father.* Cambridge: Harvard University Press.

Rando, T. A. (1993). *Treatment of complicated mourning.* Champaign, IL: Research Press.

Roberts, P. (2001). An ounce of prevention and a pound of cure: Developing state policy on the payment of child support arrears by low-income parents. *Alliance for Non-custodial Parent Rights.* Retrieved November 2, 2003, from http://www.ancpr.org/developing_state_policy_on_the_p.htm#STATE%20COLLECTION%20POLICIES

Robertson, A. F. (1991). *Beyond the family: The social organization of human reproduction.* Berkeley, CA: University of California Press.

Robinson, J. P., & Milkie, M. A. (1998). Back to the basics: Trend in and role determinants of women's attitudes toward housework. *Journal of Marriage and the Family, 60,* 205–218.

Rogers, R. G. (1995). Marriage, sex, and mortality. *Journal of Marriage and the Family, 57,* 515–526.

Ross, C. E. (1991). Marriage and the sense of control. *Journal of Marriage and the Family, 53,* 831–838.

Ross, C. E. (1995). Reconceptualizing marital status as a continuum of social attachment. *Journal of Marriage and the Family, 57,* 129–140.

Rutter, V., & Schwartz, P. (2000). Gender, marriage, and diverse possibilities for cross-sex and same-sex pairs. In D. Demo, K. Allen, & M. Fine (Eds.), *Handbook of family diversity* (pp. 59–81). New York: Oxford University Press.

Saul, R. (1999). Teen pregnancy: Progress meets politics. *The Guttmacher Report on Public Policy, 2*(3), 6–9.

Savin-Williams, R. C. (1998a). The disclosure to families of same-sex attractions by lesbian, gay, and bisexual youth. *Journal of Research on Adolescence, 8,* 49–68.

Savin-Williams, R. C. (1998b). Lesbian, gay, and bisexual youths' relationships with parents. In C. J. Patterson & A. R. D'Augelli (Eds.), *Lesbian, gay, and bisexual identities in families: Psychological perspectives* (pp. 75–98). New York: Oxford University Press.

Savin-Williams, R. C., & Esterberg, K. G. (2000). Lesbian, gay, and bisexual families. In D. Demo, K. Allen, & M. Fine (Eds.), *Handbook of family diversity* (pp. 197–215). New York: Oxford University Press.

Scanzoni, J., & Szinovacz, M. (1980). *Family decision-making: A developmental sex role model.* Beverly Hills: Sage.

Seltzer, J. (1991). Relationships between fathers and children who live apart: The father's role after separation. *Journal of Marriage and the Family, 53,* 79–101.

Sherman, A. (1994). *Wasting America's future: The Children's Defense Fund report on the costs of child poverty.* Boston: Beacon Press.

Simon, W., & Gagnon, J. H. (1986). Sexual scripts: Permanence and change. *Archives of Sexual Behavior, 15,* 97–120.

Smith, D. M., & Gates, G. J. (2001). Gay and lesbian families in the United States: Same-sex unmarried partner households: A preliminary analysis of 2000 United States Census data. *A human rights campaign report.* Retrieved February 7, 2004, from http://www.urban.org/UploadedPDF/1000491-gl-partner_households.pdf

Snarey, J. (1993). How fathers care for the next generation: A four-decade study. Cambridge: Harvard University Press.

Spain, D., & Bianchi, S. M. (1996). *Balancing act: Motherhood, marriage, and employment among American women.* New York: Russell Sage Foundation.

Spanier, G. B. (1989). Bequeathing family continuity. *Journal of Marriage and the Family, 51,* 3–13.

Spitze, G., Logan, J. R., Deane, G., & Zerger, S. (1994). Adult children's divorce and intergenerational relations. *Journal of Marriage and the Family, 56,* 279–293.

Steinglass, P., Bennett, L., Wolin, S., & Reiss, D. (1987). *The alcoholic family.* New York: Basic Books.

Steinmetz, S. K., Clavan, S., & Stein, K. F. (1990). *Marriage and family realities: Historical and contemporary perspectives.* New York: Harper & Roe.

Stull, D. E., & Borgatta, E. F. (1987). Family structure and prox-imity of family members. In T. H. Brubaker (Ed.), *Aging, health, and family: Long-term care* (pp. 247–261). Newbury Park, CA: Sage.

Suitor, J. J. (1991). Marital quality and satisfaction with the divi-sion of household labor across the family life cycle. *Journal of Marriage and the Family, 53,* 221–230.

Szinovacz, M. E. (1987). Family power. In M. B. Sussman & S. K. Steinmetz (Eds.), *Handbook of marriage and the family* (pp. 651–693). New York: Plenum Press.

Tannen, D. (1990). *You just don't understand: Women and men in conversation.* New York: Ballentine Books.

Teen pregnancy rates. (2003). *National Vital Statistics Report, 52*(7).

Thomson, E., McLanahan, S. S., & Curtin, R. B. (1992). Family structure, gender, and parental socialization. *Journal of Marriage and the Family, 54,* 368–378.

Umberson, D., & Slaten, E. (2000). Gender and intergenerational relationships. In D. Demo, K. Allen, & M. Fine (Eds.), *Handbook of family diversity* (pp. 105–127). New York: Oxford University Press.

U.S. Census Bureau. (1996). *Current population survey.* Retrieved January 30, 2004, from http://www.singleparentcentral.com/factstatcen5.htm

U.S. Census Bureau. (1998). Households and families. *Current population survey.* Retrieved October 31, 2003, from http://www.census.gov/population/socdemo/hh-fam

U.S. Census Bureau. (1999). *Young adults living at home: 1960 to present.* Retrieved January 30, 2004, from http://www.census.gov

U.S. Census Bureau. (2002a). *Current population survey.* Retrieved February 9, 2004, from http://www.census.gov/hhes/www/child-support/chldsu01.pdf

U.S. Census Bureau. (2002b). Annual demographic supplement. *March 2002 current population survey.* Retrieved October 25, 2003, from http://www.census.gov/Press-Release/www/2003/cb03-97.html

U.S. Census Bureau. (2003a). *Custodial mothers and fathers and their child support: 2001.* Retrieved January 30, 2004, from http://www.census.gov/prod/2003pubs/p60-225.pdf

U.S. Census Bureau. (2003b). Two married parents the norm. *Commerce News.* Retrieved October 4, 2003, from http://www.census.gov/Press-Release/www/2003/cb03-97.html

U.S. Census Bureau. (2003c). While US households contract, homes expand. Retrieved February 9, 2004, from http://www.ameristat.org/Content/NavigationMenu/Ameristat/Topics1/MarriageandFamily/While_U_S__Households_Contract,_Homes_Expand.htm

Vannoy, D., & Philliber, W. W. (1992). Wife's employment and quality of marriage. *Journal of Marriage and the Family, 54,* 387–398.

Varenne, H. (1992). *Ambiguous harmony: Family talk in America.* Norwood, NJ: Ablex Publishing.

Verbrugge, L. M. (1979). Marital status and health. *Journal of Marriage and the Family, 41,* 267–285.

Walker, A. J., & Pratt, C. C. (1991). Daughters' help to mothers: Intergenerational aid versus caregiving. *Journal of Marriage and the Family, 53,* 3–12.

Ward, R. A. (1993). Marital happiness and household equity in later life. *Journal of Marriage and the Family, 55,* 427–438.

Weitzman, L. J. (1985). *The divorce revolution: The unexpected social and economic consequences for women and children in America.* New York: The Free Press.

Williams, E., & Radin, N. (1999). Effects of father participation in child rearing: Twenty-year follow up. *American Journal of Orthopsychiatry, 69*(3), 645–647.

Women's Bureau, U.S. Department of Labor. (2003). *Women in the labor force.* Retrieved February 9, 2004, from http://www.info-please.com/ipa/A0104673.html

Worden, W. (1982). Grief counseling and grief therapy: A hand-book for the mental health practitioner. New York: Springer Publishing Company.

Yinger, J. (1995). *Closed doors, opportunities lost: The continuing costs of housing discrimination.* New York: Russell Sage Foundation.

Zuo, J. (1992). The reciprocal relationship between marital inter-action and marital happiness: A three-wave study. *Journal of Marriage and the Family, 54,* 870–878.

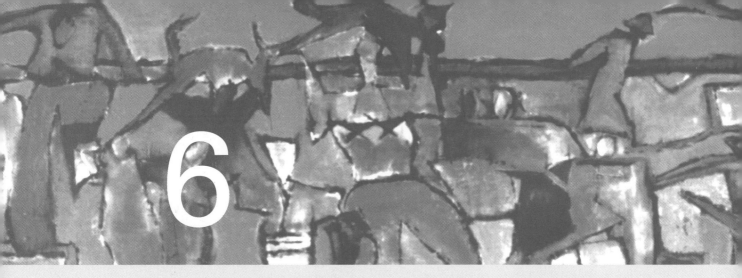

6

Families, Nursing, and Social Policy

Kristine Gebbie, RN, DrPH • Eileen Gebbie, MA

CRITICAL CONCEPTS

- The practice of nursing is always within the social and political structure of a society.

- The policy decisions made by a society or government about such things as legal relationships, support systems, financing of care, and similar matters have a profound effect on the experiences of families.

- The perspectives of nurses are influenced by those policy decisions, and those perspectives in turn affect the ways that family care will be approached.

- Nursing with families is brought to a higher level when the nurse understands a range of social and public policy perspectives relevant to families.

- The range of policy issues is so large that the nurse will have to translate these current examples to the specifics of any family or community in which care is given.

INTRODUCTION

Family is a social construct that has varied over time and across societies. At the same time that a range of family theories such as those discussed elsewhere in this text have been developed, the advances of science and evolving social and political structures have raised questions about the definition of "family" and about decision making that were neither necessary nor possible in earlier times. This chapter begins with an exploration of how social policy intersects with families in the context of health care. It will use examples from some current points of dissension to illustrate potential ways in which health can be adversely affected by social policy regarding families and present important background for the practice of nursing with families. Finally, there are multiple suggestions on when and how a nurse must use increased sensitivity to these social issues in order to provide appropriate and effective care.

This chapter includes multiple examples of situations in which patients' experiences of family appear to come into conflict with what the nurse has learned are the socially acceptable or current legal definitions of "family." It is at these points of tension that we can learn a great deal about what is important, both to individuals and to the larger social structure. The reader is encouraged to look beyond the specific examples to appreciate the enduring issue of social definition. Every existing legal definition is grounded in history and the community need for stability, particularly economic and political stability, as well as the dominant religious perspective. However, there may or may not be any genetic or biologic reason for certain definitions or restrictions; situations that on the surface may appear "illegal" or extremely unusual may in fact be extremely functional and positive for those involved. It is critical that the nurse encountering what appears to be an unusual situation be alert to the possibility that judgments based on automatically presumed "normality" can be unhealthy and limiting for the family seeking care and for the nurse. For these reasons, because "family" is so tied to women and *gender* role concerns, much attention is given to the ongoing criticism of traditional women's roles. And because issues of *sexual orientation* have continued to be the focus of extensive social and legal debate, a number of examples of how society has responded to *gay, lesbian, bisexual, and transgender* (GLBT) families have been chosen to illustrate the social and personal tensions involved.

THE INTERSECTION OF FAMILIES, HEALTH, AND SOCIAL POLICY

As discussed in earlier chapters, the dominant concept of "family" in American culture has been an idealized *normative nuclear family*. This man–woman–biological children image of "how we are" may never have been the universal standard (Coontz, 1992). The term "extended family" is commonly used to include the nuclear family and the circle of biologically and legally related grandparents, aunts, uncles, and cousins. Although we each experience "family" personally and individually, family is also socially, economically, and legally defined. Laws and social structures may attach us to individuals whom we do not like or know or whom we fear. The same structures may make it difficult to remain in touch with others for whom we have strong positive feelings. For example, despite a positive emotional tie between them, the grandparents of a noncustodial divorced parent have no continuing legal relationship to their grandchildren and may be denied access to them because of difficulties between their child (the noncustodial parent) and the custodial parent.

Neither long-standing nor emerging legal or biological definitions of "father," "mother," and "child" coincide with the actual titles or relationships of the adults most important to children. Although all humans have biological ties to at least two individuals, and many have biological ties to one or more children, these "family members" may or may not be active participants in each other's lives. Beyond issues of adoption or surrogate parenting, the separation of biologically linked individuals may be deliberate or coincident to such things as a parental death from HIV infection or the disruption of war. There are other times when a person may have no emotional or intellectual experience of others as "family," although the legal and biological relationships exist, due to isolating quarrels or divergent value judgments.

Rather than be limited by assumptions, nurses must learn to inquire of a patient in an open manner, "Who do you include in your family?" This allows the person to describe significant others and significant relationships based on personal experience and not on social expectations. Further, this opening provides some assurance to the person who may be in a nontraditional family that the nurse is truly interested in what is important to that person and prepared to hear a wide range of answers. The range of answers might come, as well, in terminology that is discomfiting to

DEFINING FAMILY RELATIONSHIPS

Terms for Describing Other Adults in the Household

Female	*Male*
Wife	Husband
Female partner	Male partner
Biological daughter	Biological son
Stepdaughter (daughter of spouse)	Stepson (son of spouse)
Adopted daughter	Adopted son
Legal ward	Legal ward
Foster child	Foster child
Partner's daughter	Partner's son
Granddaughter	Grandson
Niece	Nephew
Biological mother	Biological father
Stepmother (wife of father)	Stepfather (husband of mother)
Adoptive mother	Adoptive father
Legal guardian	Legal guardian
Parent's female partner	Parent's male partner
Grandmother	Grandfather
Aunt	Uncle
Sister	Brother
Other female relative	Other male relative
Female tenant/ boarder	Male tenant/ boarder
Other female non-relative	Other male non-relative

Source: National Survey of Family Growth, National Center for Health Statistics.

the listener. As one example, for many gays and lesbians, the term "queer" is the preferred self-label, although this may be perceived as labeling or demeaning by those unfamiliar.

There are no all-right or all-wrong descriptions of family and no universal experience of family and social policy. For example, we are increasingly aware of spousal abuse, partner abuse, child abuse, and elder abuse, in part because of laws requiring health professionals (and others) to make reports of suspected cases of abuse. These abuses and ills very likely are not new within human relationships, just newly publicized and far less tolerated than in earlier times, as evidenced by the reporting laws and the punishments meted out to the abusers. Likewise, the mythology of the older, more caring family providing services to its frail members may never have been entirely true, and social policy provided a range of assistance in the past through such community fixtures as the county home

for the elderly and the foundling hospital for children. Moreover, current families assist their members in many ways without social intervention, even when services of various kinds are publicly available (Armstrong, 1996). The wise nurse will hold assumptions about family composition and family experiences in abeyance until he or she is better acquainted with a specific family.

DEFINITIONS OF "FAMILY"

The legal rite of marriage that establishes the classic nuclear family *has* been a constant through many changes, growing from a perceived need to establish a range of "property rights," and is based in the sexual relationship seen at the heart of legal marriage (Collins, 1996). Although many couples engage in sex without benefit of a marriage license or ceremony, the relationship remains legally unrecognized unless extended over time as common-law marriage. The intersection of law and sex is illustrated by the fact that even if backed by a license, a physically "unconsummated" marriage may be annulled. Further, the modern American assumption that marriage follows romantic attachment and is based only secondarily on other considerations is being challenged by immigrant communities in which family-arranged marriages are the norm.

Images of nuclear families persist. Today's nurse, given our extremely diverse society, must be prepared to identify assumptions about family and understand that they may act to exclude some individuals from full participation in community. Whatever one's own preferred family structure or lived experience of family as positive or negative, effective nursing care requires identifying and *respecting* the meaning of "family" to each patient and each family encountered.

The book *Under the Banner of Heaven* (Krakauer, 2003) provoked extensive debates by surfacing the

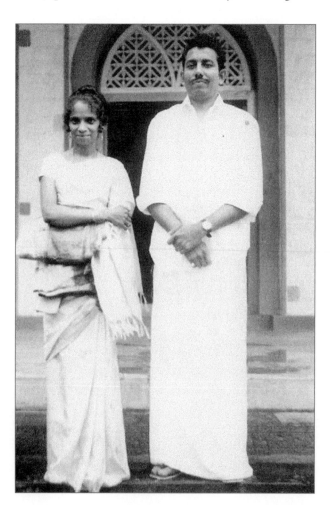

continued practice of polygamy within one conservative religious movement in the United States. The issues raised were not only those of men choosing multiple female partners, all but one without benefit of a legal relationship, but also those of child abuse, incest, and pedophilia, as many of the "wives" described were under the age of consent or were a part of the man's extended family. Although the author may have chosen an extreme example visible in only a small area of the country, the issue of overriding acceptance of a presumed religious norm at odds with the general social structure is real. The arranged marriage of an adolescent, common among European royalty centuries ago, continues for many families from India and the Middle East. Nurses must be aware of and sensitive to the occasional encounter with cases such as this and proceed carefully with questions and with choices about care.

Same-Sex Partnerships

For the most part, those partnerships established by two individuals of the same sex must be established through informal, nonlegal measures, even if they are affirmed by practical, emotional, and sexual activity. Until 2003, for example, the legal right to privacy presumed by most couples could not be claimed by same-sex partners, an example of institutionalized *heterosexism*. The most significant past case occurred in 1986 when Michael Hardwick was arrested while having oral sex with his male partner in what he thought was the privacy of his own home. When Hardwick challenged the arrest made under Georgia anti-sodomy laws, he was found to have no right to engage in oral or anal sex and no right to privacy in his bedroom (Leonard, 1997). In 2003 the U.S. Supreme Court overturned a similar "sodomy" law in Texas (Patrick, 2003), meaning that same-sex partners enjoy the same right to privacy as heterosexual couples. According to the American Civil Liberties Union (ACLU), this decision "makes it clear that states must treat gays with dignity and respect."

When asked about "family," people have listed as family members children, spouses, ex-spouses, former in-laws, children of new spouses, and friends. These people have become family by virtue of providing emotional care or because of shared responsibility combined with domesticity and/or sex (Trost, 1996). Godparents, in-laws, and the extension of family associated with adoption also illustrate the limits to our understanding of family as only "blood relations" or a

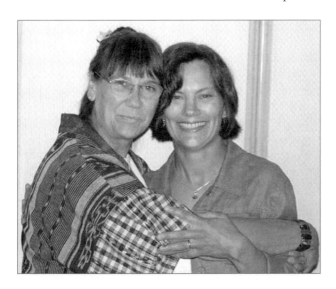

narrow legal tie. *Chosen family* is an increasingly common term in society at large, although perhaps its most extensive academic use today is within *queer theory* and social science. Whatever nurses or their patients call it, chosen families exist. One writer describes her family, their weekly meals, card playing, TV watching, house-sitting, phone calls, and choice to live in the same neighborhood: "In retrospect, the incipient trust and solidarity...combined to make Thursdays feel like family occasions" (Weston, 1996). This author does not see chosen families as *deviant* from traditional marriage-based relationships but as identical to them, apart from legality.

A moving story illustrative of the role chosen family plays in the health and illness care setting is that of Sharon Kowalski and Karen Thompson, a couple who had been living together for 4 years before the following events began. In 1983 Kowalski was paralyzed and rendered speechless in a car accident. Kowalski's parents became increasingly uncomfortable with their daughter's lesbian relationship with Thompson. When Thompson filed a suit for guardianship of her partner, the parents countered; Kowalski was then 27, a college graduate and fully independent. In mid-1985, the Kowalski parents were granted guardianship and placed their daughter in a nursing home without sufficient rehabilitation services despite Kowalski's progressing state of recovery, which had not been anticipated. Thompson and the couple's friends were denied visitation. Although she did not see Kowalski for 3 years, Thompson continued her legal battle with the help of the American Civil Liberties Union. When Thompson won a suit to have Kowalski tested

for competency (which would nullify her parents' claim), Kowalski's first request was to see Thompson. Kowalski was found to have adult-level communication skills and potential for more rehabilitation than the nursing home was providing. Her parents at this point stepped aside, and in 1991 Thompson was given custody of Kowalski, after which her continued recovery (nearly a decade after the accident) allowed her to go home. In this case, the law and tradition (apparently combined with *sexism*, *homophobia*, and *ableism*) were eventually forced to accommodate a demand for recognition that what it meant to be a *partner* and family can be based on heart, lived experience, and stubborn persistence (Griscom, 1998).

Rights of Gay Couples Growing

However marriage is defined or limited, gay men and women have been a regular presence in our communities, although in past times they were visibly invisible as the spinsters and bachelors who just happened to live together their whole lives (Armstrong, 1996). Today, in communities large and small there are gay couples living openly but quietly together, as well as the "out-and-proud" celebrities and politicians. Some state legislatures and local governments have decided that it is in society's best interests to affirm stable couples regardless of sexual orientation or sex combination even if not referring to them as "marriages." Portland, Maine, now allows queer partners to register at the city hall as a demonstration of their commitment and intention to stay coupled. Agencies that receive funding from the city and provide health insurance for straight couples must do the same for gay registered ones. In addition, those registered partners are able to work with the local school system as are any other parents, pick their children up at school functions, and access academic information on request (Associated Press, 2003a).

It is with that respect in mind that national efforts are being made to overturn Nebraska's Defense of Marriage Act (DOMA). Marriage in Nebraska is specifically—rather than by assumption—identified as available exclusively to heterosexual couples, and it legally binds the state from addressing same-sex couples in any way. Likewise, the national version of DOMA prevents the federal government from extending definitions of marriage related to immigration, taxation, or other federal programs to other than traditional married couples (Cordes, 2003). All of this was extensively debated in the 2004 presidential election campaign as a result of the 2003 Massachusetts court decision that found the gender limitation of traditional marriage in error. This interchange is further fueled by the decision of the mayor of San Francisco (himself a married, heterosexual Catholic) that issuing marriage licenses only to heterosexual couples violated the state constitution's equal-protection clause. His action was quickly followed by local elected officials in multiple jurisdictions acting on similar analyses of state law and constitutional requirements. This burst of activity has been greeted with cries of outrage from some quarters. It has also stimulated a number of thoughtful letters to the editor and columnist commentaries reminding us that there were similar tensions and outrage throughout the first half of the 20th century over questions of marriage between persons of different racial identity.

As of July 2003, gay couples working for the state of Pennsylvania received family and sick leave benefits (although not health benefits) identical to those provided to straight families in 1993's federal Family and Medical Leave Act. Also in July of 2003, the University of Illinois system extended medical and dental benefits to partners who live together and share finances. This was done in part, according to the university, to keep their system more attractive to current and potential employees (Napolitano, 2003). In October of 2003, Cook County, Illinois, began conducting domestic partnership registration from the same office that issues marriage licenses. The Chicago Commissioner said that the change would be consistent with Fortune 500 companies that already offer same-sex benefits. "So many municipalities and counties—59—have enacted same-sex partnership registries that it [being without one] is passé," he said (Pallaschm, 2003). Such moves are not universally supported, however. In June 2003 a Suffolk County,

New York, bill to give domestic partner registry to both gay and straight unmarried partnerships was defeated (Burgher, 2003).

As of June 2003 there were 20,000 registered partnerships in California (Martin, 2003). California politicians have worked to pass statewide bills of support. Assembly Bill 205 is intended to give gay and straight couples the same rights regarding "acquisition, transferring, and sharing of property; health insurance and pension coverage; and collection of government benefits" in addition to joint tax return and marriage exemptions (Jones, 2003). Furthermore, Assembly Bill 205 would safeguard gay parents' rights over their children and their right to help decide how to negotiate end of life and inheritance. In contrast, Alabama courts currently use "homosexuality" as de facto proof of a state of "unfitness," thus barring parents who "come out" after a divorce from anything but supervised visitation with their children (Bilbrey, 2002).

Research on Being Gay

It is not surprising that there has been and continues to be widespread legal discrimination on the basis of sexuality, given that homosexuality itself was classified as an illness by the American Psychiatric Association until 1973. What is surprising, though, is that the American Association for Marriage and Family Therapy did not include a nondiscrimination clause for sexuality until 1991; their accreditation commission did not follow suit until 1997.

Although gay families have had 25 years of development free of a label of pathology, GLBT people remain the focus of psychiatric research. Gay people may seek mental health treatment two to four times more than straight folks, and the treatment they

---

TELEVISION

How will current shows like *Will and Grace* and *Queer Eye for the Straight Guy* impact perceptions of gays and lesbians? At a recent in-service for university peer health educators, one author found that although enjoyed, these shows perpetuate the stereotype of gay men as beautiful, rich, and white. Although "positive" in some ways, the absence of women, disabled men, any person of color, and the real income gap between lesbians and gay men is inaccurate and limiting. Letters to the editor in many queer magazines reflect the pain of not being able to "live up" to those standards and anger at public expectation that all gay and lesbian people should. Consider the similarly mixed response to *The Cosby Show* and *All in the Family* as well as the persistent connections between media images of women and body image.

receive regarding family issues might be related to these stresses. Some data suggests that people who identify as gay (as contrasted with those who practice gay sex without altering their identity from straight) present greater risk for suicide, depression, and anxiety (Bailey, 1999). Although queer psychology journals such as the *Journal of Homosexuality* do exist, these may be read mostly by lesbian and gay people and those specifically interested in that research, not the treatment community at large. The *assimilationist* representation of GLBT families in some media may give the implication that their dynamics are identical to those of straight families, thus discouraging research into the effects of heterosexism and homophobia on the family as a whole (Clark & Serovich, 1997).

Unfortunately, research on homosexuality from an illness framework persists. In 2001 at the American Psychiatric Association's annual conference, conflicting reports of "curing" homosexuality were presented. Columbia University's Robert Spitzer conducted telephone interviews with 143 men and 57 women who had self-identified themselves as having sought help for their sexual orientation. Sixty-six percent of the men and 44 percent of the women had found what Spitzer called "good heterosexual functioning." This functioning was described as having been in a "loving and emotionally satisfying heterosexual relationship" for the year leading up to the interview, "having engaged in satisfying heterosexual sex at least monthly and having never or rarely thought of same-sex partners during heterosexual sex." Private psychiatric practitioners Ariel Shidlo and Michael Schroeder, however, found that of 202 gay individuals in their similar study, 178 reported failure in making the switch to heterosexuality, including actual harm (Goode, 2001). The aforementioned studies have been heavily criticized, and not only by GLBT community, for being more inclined to prove previously held positions rather than advancing a modern body of knowledge. The ability of nurses to communicate effectively with a wide range of individuals may mean that nurses and nursing research play a critically important part in developing a more complete understanding of gay, lesbian, bisexual, and transgendered and transsexual individuals and their families.

Defining "Parents"

The social impact of legal definitions of "family" is important to the next generation in other intriguing

ways as well. The standard birth certificate form was created many years ago with tradition in mind, with blanks for "father" and "mother," rather than "parent A" and "parent B" or some other more flexible designation. Courts in many states have affirmed adoption by gay couples, however they are labeled on the birth certificate. For all couples, the advent of newer reproductive technologies makes some of these labels even more elusive. Is "mother" the source of the ovum, the possessor of the uterus, or the person who assumes nurturance at birth? Is "father" the source of the sperm, the legal spouse of the mother, or a nurturing and caring single parent who happens to be male? How many of these mothers and fathers should be named on the permanent documentation of birth? Are they to be assured of a role throughout the child's development? Required to play a role?

Motherhood, in fact, becomes a tricky juggle of semantics, for between the genetic mother, the gestational mother, and the woman who will raise the child, the traditional definitions of "parenthood" may not be sustainable. Ragone found that when surrogates donate ova, they are attributed motherhood, but in the case of the gestational surrogate, who "simply" carries the child, she is not. In contrast, men who donate sperm, itself a kind of surrogacy, are almost never considered parents (Ragone, 1998). In these situations, *selective reduction*, in the case of multiple fertilizations, becomes even more complicated. Having asked a woman to be either a genetic or a gestational surrogate to your child for a fee, can one demand that she abort excess fetuses or abnormal ones? Our dialogue on these issues is in its infancy, pulled along by court decisions, ethical analyses, media exposés, and community exploration.

Historically, most states have made adoption records (except for those explicitly deemed open adoptions when they occur) secret, sealed under the assumption that birth parents and the children alike need to be protected from shame and derision. Adoptee advocates believe, however, that opening the records is the only way to mitigate their discomfort. Many may not have understood the slogan "Bastards of the World, Unite! You Have Nothing to Lose But Your Shame!" Following the lead of the 1980s AIDS activist group, Bastard Nation has been agitating to improve adoptees' access to records. As with the privacy gay people have demanded for their sex lives, birth parents and adoptive parents have both wanted the right to maintain their identities as they see fit and may disagree with their children on the right answer.

When, in 1998, Oregon voters granted adoptees full access to their records, affected birth mothers appealed, delaying the effect of the new law for 2 years (Silverman, 2002).

As the science of genomics advances, genetic history is emerging as an important part of a complete health history. Questions such as "Did any of your parents or grandparents have the following diseases?" apply primarily to prior generations related biologically. However, the behavioral influence of the family in which one was raised is extremely important in establishing a lifetime of health behaviors, including diet, exercise, tobacco and alcohol use, or risk taking in general. Nurses will need to remain alert to this evolving science and then carefully adjust communications to reflect the combination of desire to know with what society has allowed in the form of access to information.

Racial Identity

In our society, the specification of ethnic and racial identity has also been an important factor in family life. Birth certificates begin the process. The current standard for U.S. birth certificates allows parents to mark as many racial identity boxes as needed, a choice also available to adults in responding to the U.S. census. The infant herself is not labeled (at least by the parents). In an analysis done in 1990, 2 million youth described themselves as being of a different race than at least one of their parents, making 1 of every 35 youth mixed-race. To get an idea of what this means, think of a school with classes of 30 to 40 children, meaning that *one child in every classroom* is from a family that defies traditional racial/ethnic categorization. This dynamic, as well as a growing desire to avoid stereotyping on racial or ethnic grounds, has led to changes such as the new federal policy adding "mixed race" as an option on census and other government data collection instruments. More-recent analysis done on 2000 census data suggests that the groups most likely to find the categorizations difficult are those who identify ethnically as Hispanic, with many declining to identify a racial category at all. The challenge for medical practitioners will be moving beyond or becoming flexible in using the race-as-risk-factor emphasized in much health professional education.

Does "Having Children" Equal Family?

If the standard definition of "nuclear family" includes parents and children, does it take a child in a home to constitute a family?

> ❝When I answer that my husband, Darrin, and I have decided not to have children, the statement is usually met with bewilderment, silence, even disapproval. I can almost hear their thoughts. Why did we get married if we're not going to procreate? And it still seems far more acceptable for a man to declare he doesn't want children. How can I, as a woman, not want children? It is my duty. I have been equipped with the power to give life, and I choose not to use it. There must be something wrong with me. I have been called everything from selfish to child-hater. I actually had someone say to me, "Well, you probably abuse kids too, don't you?" I've been told that I'm "copping out on the future" by not replenishing the earth with new human beings. I used to feel embarrassed and uncomfortable, so I would lie and say that I couldn't have children (Cahill, 2003).❞

In 1998 the Current Population Survey of the U.S. Census Bureau counted 5.7 million (18.4 percent) of married women age 15 to 44 as not having children. In 1995 the National Center of Health Statistics identified 6.6 percent (4.1 million) of women as defining themselves as voluntarily "childless." That was an increase of 4.2 percent from 1982 (Paul, 2001). Leslie Lafayette is the founder of the ChildFree Network. The network links together for social activities members who do not have, cannot have, or do not want children. They advocate politically for an end to

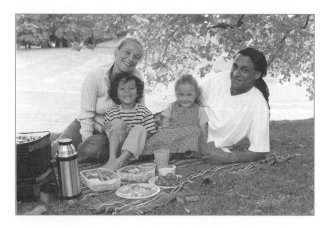

workplace inequalities, such as expectations that they will perform extra work for coworkers who are out with sick children or paying higher insurance rates because group coverage has expanded to include *in vitro fertilization* (Fost, 1996). There is some rising social awareness of the injustice and psychological damage done when a couple without children is treated as if they had neglected some important obligation or were less than complete. Some of them are infertile, with all of the social and psychological burdens that experience entails. Others are without children deliberately. In either case, respect for the individuals involves argues against leaping to any conclusions about "rightness" or "completeness" or an expectation that there will be children in the couple's future.

CHILDREN AND PARENTING

There are social policy questions around both the decision to have children and the decision that a potential fetus should not come to term. There is no way to explore the issues fully here, but some review is essential to the goals of this chapter. Just under half (48 percent) of the 6.3 million pregnancies in the United States each year are unintended. Of those unintended pregnancies, just under half (47 percent) are terminated. This means of every 10 pregnancies, four are ended. This rate has continued to decline since the 1980s because of more-successful hormonal contraception and emergency birth control. Of women who choose abortion, 21 percent report that they are not financially ready and 21 percent say they are not prepared for the responsibility. Most women asked gave more than three reasons for their decision, including relationship troubles, rape, and fetal defects. Women who have abortions represent— nearly equally—all steps of the socioeconomic ladder.

In 2000, 70 percent of abortions were performed in abortion clinics, 20 percent in another clinic, and less than 5 percent each in hospitals and in private physician offices. Nearly 60 percent of these abortions are performed before the end of the first trimester. Eighteen states provide abortion benefits under Medicaid for reasons beyond assault. However, in 32 states, minors are required to have consent, and in four states, even private insurance coverage of abortion is restricted. Counseling is required in 18 states (Physicians for Reproductive Choice and Health, 2003). Fewer physicians are performing abortions because of fear of terrorism and social marginalization. When comparing all counties in the United States, 87 percent have no abortion providers (Physicians for Reproductive Choice and Health, 2003).

In November 2003, President Bush struck one of the most significant blows against *Roe v. Wade*, the landmark Supreme Court decision validating a woman's right to privacy regarding abortion, when he signed a bill banning "partial birth abortions." The rare procedures performed in the third trimester and described by this newly coined nonmedical term constitute less than 0.8 percent of abortions performed (Physicians for Reproductive Choice and Health & The Alan Guttmacher Institute, 2003). They have been the practice only when the mother's life is at stake. As a result of this new legislation, legal grounds have been further established that many see as part of a steady push to revoke abortion access in general. The political process leading to this act included careful publicity of the procedure by a label that was never previously used by the medical community. It is very clear from the debate in Congress and in the media that this issue is a complex mix of religious values and gender role expectations and is one that will not be quickly resolved.

WHAT IS NECESSARY AND WHAT IS NOT?

In a country that does not ensure equitable health insurance coverage for all, the questions of "covered service" and "medically necessary" become critically important. Insurance companies and their utilization review staff exercise great power over the specific range of services available. For a couple in the top 20 percent of income, cash resources allow for fertility services that may require $20,000 or more in advance. A couple equally desirous of children and both emotionally and economically prepared to be excellent parents may be stopped because the only health services they are able to use are those covered under their low-end insurance plan.

Fertility Matters

On another front, research into the policies supporting and funding fertility clinics illustrates the lengths to which economically solvent straight couples are allowed to go to achieve both physically and psychologically "normal" births (Cussins, 1998). The costs are generally not covered by health insurance plans, although 14 states (Arkansas, California, Connecticut, Hawaii, Illinois, Maryland, Massachusetts, Montana, New Jersey, New York, Ohio, Rhode Island, Texas, and West Virginia at the time of writing) now ensure some coverage. According to the Centers for Disease Control and Prevention (CDC), in 2000 the cost per family of delivering one child or up to quadruplets using in vitro fertilization was $39,000 to $340,000. For those using artificial reproductive technology, the cost started at $58,865 and topped at $281,698 (Wright, Schieve, Reynolds, & Jeng, 2003). The social policy debate can be constructed around the issue of rights: if one segment of society is afforded access to this service, should it not be available to all? Putting aside the question of the very poor (that is, should public insurance pay to add to the size of a family possibly on public assistance?), is a childless assembly line worker less deserving of a chance to parent than the executive of the company, when the barrier is the question of cash in advance?

The process of producing a child to parent can profoundly challenge *and* perpetuate socially structured notions of parenthood. In Minnesota, Karen Heeney and Julia Beatty, an established, committed couple, were denied legal protection for access to artificial reproductive technologies in 1995. "The court also noted that the Minnesota parentage law on artificial insemination applied only to married couples, not single women, and that Minnesota law generally favored the institution of traditional marriage" (Moskowitz, 1995). Although the state upheld the lower court decision, the American Medical Association disagreed, stating that practicing medicine without judgment regarding sexual orientation "enhances the ability to render optimal patient care in health as well as in illness" (Harris, 2003).

Children's Rights

Social theorists Brennan and Noggle question the tendency to speak about justice *for* families instead of *within* them. This means seeing parents as the stewards of their children, "limited by children's own rights" (1997, p. 9). One law researcher believes that although our respect for the legitimacy of domestic violence charges made by adults has increased, "the unreconstructed hostility of courts (and sometimes even the same judges) toward the same battered women and domestic violence allegations, when raised in the context of custody or visitation litigation, can be stunning" (Meier, 2003). For example, having been battered, a woman may then be left without her children as they are removed because she "allowed" them to witness the violence against her. From research within social work, it appears that much of the trouble for children after divorce comes from adults' persistent need to adhere to a "homogeneous" family model, even if the family has only one parent. The family thus consists of the custodial parent and children living together in a close relationship, even though the other parent has an ongoing entitlement to a relationship with the child. For this to work, the noncustodial or visiting parent must give up the drive toward an idealized family, relinquishing control over time with her/his child (Hyden, 2001).

Foster/Adopt

Many of today's families also include the role of foster child or foster parent. This form of socially recognized family provides a legal mechanism for short-term placement of children when there are no parents or the parents have been found unfit. Foster homes are supposed to fill a temporary role, either until the original parents are once again available or until a new, permanent adoptive family is identified. Although foster parents bear all of the emotional and physical burdens of day-to-day child rearing, they are often paid only a token amount to do so and do not have the full legal custody of their charges. Legal relatives of the child (grandparents, aunts, cousins) are often

WHO IS MY PARENT NOW?

Following his mother's death, one 14-year-old boy has chosen to alternate his time between his biological father and his deceased mother's boyfriend. The men were awarded joint custody by a court recognizing the importance of choice and emotion over tradition (Arrillaga, 2003).

asked to assume this role and may feel social pressure to do so, even when their own emotional or other resources are not up to the task. Nurses encountering foster parents should be cautious about making assumptions about the motivations involved, which may range from a simple way to earn some additional income to genuine concern for children in difficult circumstances and strong, positive beliefs about family obligations.

In terms of public policy, one change in the test of best interests of a child would be to include the child's own voice in assessments regarding placement. It would also seek to prevent the need to invoke the legal standard of clear and present danger to protect children by supporting intervention while there is still a positive relationship between parent and child. They suggest education, financial assistance for single parents, universal child care, drug rehabilitation, in-home consultants such as nutritionists and housekeepers, and presumably child support enforcement. All of these are ways to provide for the nurturing of the child while respecting their right to maintain the personal relationships with their biological parents. This model could lead to such actions as reconsideration of the current nature of adoptions, which are closer to a legal transaction with children as parental property.

Over the course of recent decades, we have experienced an increased concern for the physical and emotional safety of children, arguing for rapid removal of children from potentially dangerous situations, coupled with laws requiring health and education professionals to report suspected child abuse promptly to authorities for investigation. The subsequent decisions about long-term care and rearing of the child have been complex. There is serious concern for the mental health of children moved from one foster care setting to another and of children separated from siblings in the process. The preferential use of biological family members, or members of the same ethnic/racial group, as foster parents is seen as one antidote to these problems. From time to time, there has been an associated dialogue about the economic responsibility of families to care and about whether a related foster parent should be paid as a non-relative would. Critics of this approach suggest that it is primarily a budget-saving measure rather than a well-considered policy in support of families.

The news media report with depressing regularity the problems state agencies or their contracted representatives have in providing appropriate supervision and social support to foster families. Death or severe harm seem to come to foster children all too often,

with reports such as the death of one of several children in the care of a blind 80-year-old woman, or severely malnourished foster children living side-by-side with flourishing biological siblings. Follow-up often reveals that there were indications of the problem such as abuse reports or children not visible during a social worker visit, but overworked child protective agency staff did not have the time or skill to recognize and deal with the issues. Smaller caseloads, more intense supervision, and more continuing education for both caseworkers and parents appear to be part of the mix. Finding those willing to serve as foster parents, sorting out their motives, capacities, and skills, and supporting them once they have assumed responsibilities for children who may have complex problems apparently cost more than our society is willing to pay.

Other scholars and policy makers have been more focused on questions about reestablishment of the original family group and the negative impact on children of staying in foster care for extended periods. Termination of parental rights and permanent adoption of children can take a very long time, especially when social policies keep child welfare agencies on very short staff and budget. There is some feeling that the prolonged permanent placement process is far more harmful to children than other options. The occasional widely reported death of a child known to child protective agencies but still living with the reportedly abusive parent(s) provides additional emotional fuel to the entire debate, with no tidy resolution in sight.

Transracial Foster or Adoption

In 1999, director Chi Moui Lo released the film *Catfish with Black Bean Sauce*. The story centered around two Vietnamese refugee children and their African-American adopted families. The eldest adopts a very black identity, whereas the youngest immerses herself in a community of fellow Vietnamese immigrants. In their mid-20s, their biological mother arrives for a reunion. The movie is spent in laughter and tears as each member comes to negotiate and reconcile his or her truly mixed family and identities. In most cases of transracial adoption, there have been strong pressures to place children in families of the same race or expectations that the child be given a full opportunity to learn her or his collective cultural past. The Multi-Ethnic Placement Act of 1994 (MEPA) was developed when Congress determined that historical barriers had prevented the participation of larger numbers of people of color in the foster and adoption communities. The goals of MEPA are to "decrease the length of time that children wait to be adopted; facilitate the recruitment and retention of foster and adoptive parents who can meet the distinctive needs of children awaiting placement; and eliminate discrimination on the basis of the race, color, or national origin of the child or the prospective parent" (Hollinger, 1998).

No transracial adoptions have been more contentious than those involving Native American/American Indian children. From 1969 to 1974, 25 to 35 percent of Indian children from recognized tribes were fostered or adopted out. The Indian Child Welfare Act of 1978 emerged because of "abusive child welfare practices that resulted in the separation of large numbers of Indian children from their families and tribes through adoption or foster care placement" (Brown, Limb, Munoz, & Clifford, 2001). These long-standing practices were established during periods when national policy toward Native American children included their removal to boarding schools at which use of native language and customs were punished, and every effort was made to assist in assimilation away from tribal identity into the presumed-superior dominant culture. The effect of these abuses was to deny tribes future generations and the survival of their nations (Brown, Limb, Munoz, & Clifford, 2001).

Transracial families also serve to surface several significant issues more intricate than cultural transmission. Families with members of different racial heritage may be very visible and thus targets for constant questions. Not all, but some, transracial parents considered and educated themselves on racial issues before adopting. They made mixed decisions about cultural transmission and how (or whether) to encourage the child's racial identity and contact with the community of origin. The children in these families, when interviewed, express some ambivalence about their racial identity and even anti-ethnic sentiment. The children found that other kids "require them to choose a racial identity (and loyalty)" even though their adoptive families do not (Vidal de Haymes & Simon, 2003).

Ongoing constraints on adoptions, which make a great deal of sense within the historical context of the United States, are viewed with concern by anxious-to-adopt parents who want to locate an adoptable infant regardless of cultural heritage or skin tone. Their search has led to a growth in international adoptions, almost all of them transcultural and many of them transracial. Korea has the oldest international adoption program. Korean adoption agencies are able to tell American parents about family history and how the child came to be available. These adoptive parents are also given their infants' medical records (Min, 2003). The existence of poverty and political turmoil are frequently associated with the emergence of a number of infants or children for adoption by U.S. couples. For example, Guatemala rose rapidly in the international adoption market because of privatization and an absence of government oversight until the very last stages of the process. In 2002, 2219 Guatemalan children came to the United States. The costs range from $15,000 to $20,000, with about $5000 going to the coordinating agency. In Guatemala, where families average an annual per capita income of less than $4000, some "baby factories" have emerged, as have forced pregnancies for household servants (Dellios & Rubin, 2003).

As immigrants, even older internationally adopted children are unlikely to speak English. If they have spent time in an orphanage or a refugee center, they will have more depression and even post-traumatic stress disorder. Unless arranged through the adoption agency, they may not have had immunizations or dental care and may even bring with them parasitic infections, respiratory disease, flu, pneumonia, tuberculosis, or hepatitis (Aday, 2001). One international adoption received a very high level of media attention as the frantic new parents attempted to calm a hysterical, non-English-speaking adoptee during a trans-Atlantic flight and finally resorted to force and physical restraint (Seelye, 1997). Many internationally adopted children thrive, however, and parents of these children are often reported as making extraordinary efforts to ensure that the children grow up with an appreciation for their cultural heritage and language.

Children with Disabilities

Parents with "disabled" or ill children may experience being labeled "bad parents," implying that parents are judged by the quality of their products—their children. The women in one study were effective parents according to measures of caring, nurturing, and supporting their offspring, but the situation and "cultural markers" left them feeling second-class, as if they were failing as parents. Beyond their own internal questioning as to why they and their children were made to be different, they encountered mixed social messages. One woman has described seeing a poster featuring a sick infant who resembled her own child. The poster was intended to discourage alcohol abuse during pregnancy but seemed to the woman to be accusing her, even though she had done everything "right" during her pregnancy. Women have perceived an implicit guarantee of a healthy infant if they commit to "right" behaviors such as diet, alcohol avoidance, and prenatal care. They feel indicted by society, that having a sick child is their fault.

An Australian study showed that although families of children with severe disability overwhelmingly wanted to care for their children at home, those who chose to put their kids elsewhere did so because of family "survival" (Llewellyn, Dunn, Fante, Turnbull, & Grace, 1999). In one study of families with disabled children, 50 percent of the mothers were unemployed and providing all the care for their disabled child and 48 percent of the families lived below the federal poverty levels. Thirty percent of the mothers and 24 percent of the fathers listed their own health status as "poor"; one-quarter of the fathers had a history of substance abuse. One effective service, respite care, targets families with kids with disabilities, children at environmental risk (poverty, single parents), sick infants, and those in more than one category. The care can include actual care of the child to allow a break for the primary caregiver as well as "secondary respite" in the form of training and therapy for the child. Without respite, caregivers can burn out or become a danger to the child (Cowen & Reed, 2003).

Services and monies do exist for families with disabilities:

- Title V of the Social Security Act's Maternal and Child Health and Crippled Children Services (now called the Program for Children with Special Health Care Needs) supports specialized medical care.
- The U.S. Department of Agriculture supports the Special Supplemental Food Program for Women, Infants, and Children (WIC) that can provide needed foods, including specialized formula for children with inborn errors of metabolism such as phenylketonuria.
- The U.S. Department of Education, Office of Special Education and Rehabilitative Services, supports states in giving special education and needed support services for disabled kids from birth to age 21.
- The Basic Vocational Rehabilitation Service Program supports the states to ensure that physically and mentally disabled individuals are prepared for employment, regardless of age.

- Health insurance programs, including Medicare and Medicaid, as well as supportive service programs funded through social services, mental health, maternal and child health block grants, and child welfare services, all add to the range of support available and are now required to cover the child from birth (Aday, 2001).

Negotiating all of these is daunting, however, and in some localities families sense that there is more interest in saving taxpayers money than in making life easier for families caught in difficult circumstances.

Homeless Children and Families

Popular art has given us many images of children in their safe, cozy homes. However, not every child has a home, much less a cozy one. Estimating the number of people who are homeless is difficult because the definitions vary from street living to crashing on a friend's couch. One estimate, though, is that 1 million people (of all ages) may not have a home on a given night. In 1990, a random-digit-dial telephone survey generated estimates that 14 percent of Americans (26 million) had been homeless at some point in their lifetime and 4.6 percent (8.5 million) had been so within the previous 5 years. Furthermore, 7.4 percent of Americans (13.5 million) had been at some point absolutely homeless in that they slept in shelters, abandoned buildings, or public transit stations, with 3.1 percent (5.7 million) in this position within the previous 5 years. Homeless children, a growing group, are likely to be with their young mothers. Teens often identify as runaways rather than as homeless because they have fled homes because of emotional, physical, or sexual violence. Women who are homeless have a higher prevalence of mental illness, whereas men use substances more. Women who are homeless are often striving to remain "invisible" because of their desperate need to avoid further assault (Aday, 2001).

Homeless families have not had the same level of attention from the media and academics as other homeless groups such as homeless mentally disabled adults, although these families often arrive at their situation as a direct result of public policy decisions rather than personal choices. In a New York City homeless family, the mother is typically a 20-year-old unmarried woman with one or two children age 6 or younger. She probably did not finish high school, has never worked, and had an abortion by 16. Her likelihood of having been in foster care is 1 in 5, and if she was, she is over two times as likely as other homeless moms of having an open case with child welfare agencies. Homeless kids are three times more likely to have been born to a single mother than their non-homeless counterparts are. Education is the ultimate predictor of eventual stability and success, yet education is not (or cannot be) emphasized within homeless communities. The end result is a lack of "critical skills, values, and self-esteem typically instilled in a traditional family structure" with homeless families experiencing a persistence of family ideals but lacking structure or experience to fulfill them (Nunez, 1995).

Public policies about homeless shelters (traditionally serving single men) and available housing leave these young women and their children at risk for any

Beyond the physical dangers of living on the street and the discomfort of being cold or hungry is the toll of public insensitivity told in the following letter from a homeless woman:

To the rude man I encountered Wednesday:

I was the young girl standing near the _____ station selling *the local homeless paper* when you approached me Wednesday and asked if I was homeless. As soon as I said yes, you spit on me and called me 'lazy homeless trash' and kept walking.

Lazy is one thing I do not consider myself. If I was lazy I wouldn't have been out selling homeless papers. I would have been panhandling. Instead I was trying to earn my money. Wednesday I made $3.26 working for 4 hours selling my papers. It wasn't as much as I had hoped. But it was enough to pay for one of my prescriptions I needed to fill. After selling papers, I spent a few hours at one of three local non-profits I volunteer for each week. Just because I am homeless doesn't mean that I sit around doing nothing. I try to give back to my community what they have given to me. Over the past two months I've spent my weekend volunteering for fundraiser walks for local charities. Some of the walks included the Walk for Hunger because "_____" sponsors some of the meals at the shelters I stay at. I volunteered in the pouring rain at the AIDS Walk because I know several HIV+ homeless people.

I hope you've realize by now that I'm not your 'stereotypical homeless person.' I've never done drugs, I don't drink, I don't panhandle and I shower every day. I'm smart. I have two years of college education and worked in the medical field for six years. Then why am I homeless? I may not have 'looked' it to you, but I'm disabled. I was in a car accident two years ago that left me with a broken neck, traumatic brain injury and a seizure disorder. Due to cognitive problems and other neurological problems caused by my brain injury I've had a hard time holding a job. And due to inability to keep steady income I'm currently homeless for the second time since my accident. Until I get on disability and am able to get a section 8 voucher (the waiting list is expected to be frozen for at least two years) or get into subsidized housing I will be homeless.

Every homeless person you meet is a unique individual. We each have a story of our own. We all struggle through our journeys of homelessness. Every day is a challenge for us. We have to figure out where we are going to get each meal, we have to find a shelter with an available bed each night. There are many nights when there are no available beds in the area shelters. We then have to find a safe place to sleep outside. Obtaining necessities like soap, toothbrushes, tampons and clean socks can be tough. And getting medical care isn't as simple as it sounds. It isn't an easy life. But due to circumstances like disabilities, domestic violence, fire, and loss of job we are left homeless until we can get back on our feet again or get housing assistance. Being homeless is tough. But it's more difficult when you have to face discrimination by people who don't understand what it's truly like to be homeless. It's a hard journey to go through. But it's ever harder when you have to deal with being called names, or being spit on by rude people. Homelessness could happen to anybody. All it takes is a fire, loss of a job, a sudden illness or disability and you could find yourself in my shoes. I am hoping you will read my letter, and I hope you think twice before spitting on another homeless person.

Sincerely,

The Homeless Girl

Source: Crystal. (2003, October 13). To the man who spit on me . . . [blog]. *LiveJournal.* Retrieved October 14, 2003, from http://www.livejournal.com/users/being_homeless/52934.html

number of problems, both physical and emotional (Nunez, 1995). Getting out of homelessness presents particular challenges to families, in part due to conflicting social policies. For example, a homeless mother whose several children were placed in foster care may be unable to regain custody until she has a suitable, large apartment, fulfilling the child welfare agency's mandates on safety. But under the policies of the local housing assistance agency, she may not be able to rent that much-needed apartment because her children are not living with her at the time she seeks to move out of the shelter. Nurses encounter families such as these through schools and in clinics and hospitals. Sensitive history-taking and creative use of referrals and community resources are essential to quality care.

Deliberate Abuse

Danger resides not only outside our borders but also in our own homes. According to the American Academy of Pediatrics, "child abuse is common." One in four girls and one in eight boys are sexually abused by age 18. This includes genital contact or exposure. The 1 in 20 children physically abused each year may have been burned, beaten, or broken (of limb or spirit). "Because a bruise indicates that body tissue has been damaged and blood vessels have broken, any discipline method that leaves bruises is not appropriate" (American Academy of Pediatrics, 1999). The Academy also recognizes the impact of child neglect, ranging from withholding necessities such as food and medical attention to withholding love (American Academy of Pediatrics, 1999). Severe parental child abuse includes kicking, biting, hitting with fist, and using a gun or knife on a child.

Many of the teenagers living in shelters or on the streets have experienced violence or have been dropped from the foster care system. The violence may have been physical, sexual, or emotional. Dorothy Allison's explosive and disturbing book *Bastard Out of Carolina* (1992) reflects her own childhood in extreme poverty and the physical and sexual violence she experienced. The movie version was released in 1996. Allison describes how she has "worked hard not to pass on the heritage of violence that marked my childhood." After spanking her son once (and the only time), she "hugged him tight." "He will have to be a lot older before I explain more to him, tell him that because of what was done to me as a child, I can never have children, the limp that is getting worse began then, that the reason some nights I do not sleep is not only because I like to work late" (Allison, 1999).

Abuse within families is exacerbated by poverty and social distance from peers and social institutions. Most abuse occurs between dominants and subordinates: parent to child, husband to wife, caretaker to dependent (Aday, 2001). Responding successfully to a disclosure of abuse is important. You will be worried, skeptical, and angry.

- Be sure to talk with the child in a safe place, free of physical barriers between you.
- Be on the same eye level as the child.

Health effects of domestic violence (Tacket et al., 2003):

- Injuries from assault
- Chronic health problems such as irritable bowel syndrome, backache, and headaches
- Increased unintended pregnancies, terminations, and low-birth-weight babies
- Higher rates of sexually transmitted infections, including HIV
- Higher rates of depression, anxiety, post-traumatic stress disorder, self-harm, and suicide

Advantages of routinely inquiring about domestic violence (Tacket et al., 2003):

- Uncovers hidden cases of domestic violence
- Changes perceived acceptability of violence in relationships
- Makes it easier for women to access support services earlier
- Changes health professionals' knowledge and attitudes toward domestic violence and helps reduce social stigma
- Helps maintain the safety of women experiencing domestic violence

- Thank the child for trusting you; affirm her braveness.
- Find out what the child wants you to do, making sure you outline her options.
- Let the child know exactly what you will do—even if it means going against her wishes to report the abuser—so that her trust in you will not later feel betrayed (Reilly, 1995).

While acting to report suspected child abuse, it is also important to remember the need for clear communication with parents about our community standards. There have been scattered reports, for example, of European parents comfortable with leaving a baby or small child outside a shop or cafe asleep in a stroller or pram, assuming that continuous or occasional observation through the shop window was adequate supervision. This behavior would almost always be considered negligence or endangerment in a U.S. city. Assuming no harm occurred, education rather than punishment would be the appropriate action.

Although documentation for elder abuse is limited because of the nature of that abuse, about 2 million elderly folks have experienced neglect (55 percent), physical abuse (14.6 percent), financial or material exploitation (12.3 percent), psychological or emotional abuse (7.7 percent), or sex abuse (0.3 percent). Only about 1 in 14 incidences are reported (Aday, 2001). The abuse appears to be associated with increased dependency on the part of frail elders, one of the fastest-growing segments of our society. The number of elders in regular contact with nurses in home care, in extended care, or during office and clinic visits means that nurses are critical to an effective, preventive social response.

Military Families

In 2000, about 3.3 million Americans were involved in the military, with half of those on active duty; over half of those are married, two-thirds are men, 45 percent are under 25, and 38 percent have children age 5 or younger. The numbers have only increased with U.S. action in the Middle East and involvement in peacekeeping activities around the globe. Studies of families of active-duty military report poor pay, poor health care education, poor health care reimbursement, insufficient child care, insufficient tuition assessment, and the need for more assistance for child abuse and sexual assault. Despite those struggles, the sense of community within the extended military family was strong (Mancini & Archambault, 2000).

Children and partners of service members deployed during the Gulf War reported higher levels of depression, with younger children and boys at the greatest risk (Jensen, Martin, & Watanabe, 1996). Although children whose mothers were deployed in the Gulf War did struggle during that separation, 2 years after the war, their absences were no longer a salient issue regarding behavioral problems (Pierce, Vinokur, & Buck, 1998). For the American "peacekeepers" who served in Somalia, exposure to combat was correlated with increased post-traumatic stress disorder. Their adjustment to coming home was improved by positive family support and welcome (Bolton, Litz, Glenn, Orsillo, & Roemer, 2002). The Army publicly admitted to needing to improve support services for soldiers returning home when four soldiers from Ft. Bragg killed their wives within a 3-week period in 2002. Three of the four had served in Afghanistan in Special Forces operations after September 11; all three killed themselves (Associated Press, 2003b).

When active- or reserve-duty service members are called up, families must also contend with financial strains and limited communication. The American Red Cross provides emergency communication and travel funds for service members in case of family crisis. Service members and their families can get counseling for their experiences as well (American Red Cross, 2003). One of the ironies of these services, though, is that with increased spending on wartime and postwar reconstruction, funding for social services such as these decreases.

Incarcerated Parents

The United States incarcerates individuals at a rate far higher than most other nations. Evidence suggests that many of those who are incarcerated are of childbearing age and may well leave children to be cared for by others while they "do time." Disruption of families is not only due to long sentences served by those in prisons but also due to the time that individuals spend in local jails prior to arraignment, awaiting trial, or during sentences of less than 1 year. It is even suggested that in some African-American communities, "doing time" is an expected part of moving to adulthood, an expected rite of passage. If so, this too must be understood by those providing care, whether in a corrections health program inside or to the rest of the family in the community.

Given the significant family roles filled by women, the 400 percent increase in female incarceration rate over the last 20 years is critical. This increase is primarily due to more-stringent drug sentencing (Luke, 2002). The number of inmates in general has tripled, and if trends continue, 5 percent of the total population will end up with jail experience in their lives. And despite the "three strikes and you're out" mentality expressed by legislatures recently, every year over 500,000 people are released back to their communities (Freudenberg, 2001). Their prison and jail experiences will color their approach to family thereafter.

These children "experience poverty before, during, and after their mothers' incarceration" (Luke, 2002). One 1998 estimate had 950,000 women in corrections, with responsibility for 1.9 million dependents, two-thirds of whom were under 12 (Luke, 2002). With men far more likely to be incarcerated, and to struggle to find employment afterward, more women serve as heads of households or single parents (Freudenberg, 2001). Children of color are three to nine times more likely to have a parent in the custody of the corrections system. The health outcomes include behavioral, emotional, and school problems, as well as feelings of depression, anger, sadness, guilt, anxiety, and fear. These children may also begin using substances and having sex much earlier. In some states, parents in prison quickly lose custodial rights, thus denying any hope of reunification. Although designed to help the children, such laws may be doing them harm.

Children with parents in jail are five times more likely to serve time themselves (Freudenberg, 2001). Children who survive parental incarceration best are those with positive parent-child relationships; parenting classes for incarcerated mothers help in that regard (Luke, 2002). With strong social support and positive relationships positively correlated with absence of new offenses, strengthening family ties is important for all members. The Arkansas Department of Corrections found that after 3 years of studying

their own parenting program, both mothers and children benefited from visits, letters, and classes. The benefits included improved self-esteem and more-nurturing parenting techniques. The significance of those for women who so often had histories of drug abuse and violence cannot be stressed enough (Thompson & Harm, 2000). Columbia University School of Nursing researcher Mary Byrne is working with the New York State Department of Corrections Services to study the parent-child impact of allowing women who give birth while incarcerated to raise that child for the first year of life in a supported nursery program behind bars.

EDUCATION

One of the few universal social policies in the United States is the commitment to education for all children to age 16 or to high school completion. School is an integral part of a child's life, so its structure, location, and tone have strong impact. Schools have been a part of the Americanization process for generations of immigrants. Because they have contact with almost every child, we also turn to schools as social gatekeepers. For instance, the "no shots, no school" laws enacted by states achieve a public health purpose by preventing children from attending school without certain vaccinations. This has an educational benefit as well, of course, as healthier children have better attendance and learn more. We expect schools to teach not only basic reading, mathematics, computing, and athletic skills but also human anatomy and health promotion, sexuality education, and alternatives to violence. The role of schools in educating children about values is often hotly contested at the local level, given the various views that parents and other adults have about critical values to be taught to the young. The continuing fights over the right of a school to

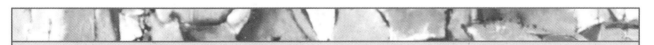

A visit to the nursery program at the maximum-security prison for women in New York State reveals healthy, happy babies; engaged mothers; and staff, inmates, and volunteers working together. Any woman entering prison receives full prenatal care and may elect to keep her baby with her for up to 1 year, after which the child goes to foster care. One of the mothers' work assignments is parenting class; other inmate workers help staff the day care center while mothers work. Older children visit on weekends, staying with volunteer families in the surrounding community. And a mother can read a book onto a tape and send both to her child, who can thus have a mother-read bedtime story.

require or offer public prayer at the beginning of the school day, to teach evolution, or to provide teens with explicit information on prevention of pregnancy suggest that this tension will not be alleviated quickly.

Isolation at School

What schools teach (overtly or covertly) about social roles, gender, and family becomes part of later adult life. Because the broader society is in conflict about sexual orientation, for example, schools have had difficulty providing appropriate support or health services (or even any explicit services) to gay, lesbian, bisexual, transgender, transsexual, and questioning teens as they struggle through adolescence. This lack of good social support during a time of self-discovery may be one of the factors leading to subsequent mental health problems or risk-taking behavior. Categorizing and social exclusion may further set the stage for problems. Whether a youth does well in school or not in practice is shaped in large part by these adolescent societies rather than school regulations (Wooden, 1996). Study of internal social structures at four California high schools found an array of cliques (as defined by members and their peers): jocks, cheerleaders, "drama freaks," punks, stoners, losers, "death rockers," brains, preppies, nerds. Each group had its own standards of style, actions, and goals (or lack thereof), and all students were expected to belong to some group.

After a 1987 group suicide at a New Jersey high school, sociologist Donna Gaines spent time with the dead teens' peer group. Outside (or in place of) school, they hung out in an abandoned building, sometimes bored, listening to music, using substances, and having sex. The teens did not lack interest in life, but they did not have any interest in the standard school activities and clubs, preferring their own company. Although the town recognized the need for greater outreach and constructive activities, "it was taken for granted that if you refused to be colonized" by such options, "you were 'looking for trouble'" (Gaines, 1996, p. 14). The blame for "failure" was bounced back to those who would be victims, leading some to describe them as "overregulated by adults, yet alienated from them . . . integrated only into the world shared with their peers" (Gaines, 1996).

Overregulation based on social values was clearly one of the biggest problems in the schools run by the missionary churches on American Indian reservations in previous centuries. Violence, denial of culture, racism, sexism, and absolute separation from blood family defined many of the children's experiences. "All I got out of school was being taught how to pray. I learned quickly that I would be beaten if I failed in my devotions or . . . prayed the wrong way, especially prayed in Indian to Wakan Tanka, the Indian Creator" (Crow Dog & Erodes, 1996). Without the religious overtones, the same abrupt separation from family and culture was the norm in schools run by the Bureau of Indian Affairs. Why is this important now? The high rate of alcohol abuse within Native American communities is attributed in part to this heritage. Although these practices have ended, the children who lived through these experiences are now the adult family members with their own responsibilities to children or the tribe. Some have become part of movements to reclaim American Indian culture and transmit it to future generations; others continue to experience *alienation* and associated personal and social pain.

Much analysis of the 1999 violence and death at Columbine High School, Littleton, Colorado, focused on the role played by preferential treatment of athletes and isolation of the black-coated "trench coat mafia" in setting the stage for violence. In Michael Moore's Oscar-winning movie *Bowling for Columbine*, he examines rates and reasons for gun violence in the United States. He finds that although Canadians have just as many guns as Americans, they have only a fraction of the shooting deaths that Americans experience. His essential argument is that we are unduly paranoid as a result of increased economic despair and media overemphasis on violent crimes. "We are being told to be afraid of this or that or whatever. And we have got to somehow find the courage, we've to find the courage to do something here . . . I don't want to be shot. Who does, right? . . . I hate to say it, I love my TV, but you got to turn it off, you got to turn it off. Because it, if you, I'm telling you, it's warping the minds of America, this non-stop, high alert, the terrorists are going to get you. It's *1984*, it's about the enemy is everywhere, the enemy is going to kill you. . . . And I want us all to draw the connections between Columbine and Iraq and everything else" (Moore, 2003). The visibility given each school-related violent event fosters a public view of young people gone wild. The fact is that juvenile violent crime has continued to fall throughout and since the 1990s, Columbine notwithstanding. The lowest year for school violence was 1996/1997, with 19 school-related deaths among 54 million children. To put this in perspective, three times more people die from lightning strikes than from school violence (Glassner, 2000).

Inequities in Education

Jonathan Kozol's landmark work *Savage Inequalities* captures the two poles of U.S. education: the college-prep schools and the inner-city wastelands. Swimming pools, computers, foreign languages, and landscaping are compared with the lack of functioning plumbing, ancient textbooks, poor teachers, and rotting insulation. One set of children has the tools and scores for entrance into the best universities and careers; the other set may see teen pregnancy and truancy as far better emotional options than the societal disregard evidenced by their education. The impact that both will have on the next generation's "parent pool" needs no elaboration. Our collective sense of community has not been extended to eliminate such a disparity of investment, although states have taken steps to set at least minimum expenditure-per-pupil equity across districts (Kozol, 1991).

Despite inequitable funding, states now require schools to administer standardized tests to prove success (Ramirez, 2002–2003). The use of such tests has grown, despite suggestions from many knowledgeable educators that they serve to limit growth rather than measure it by fostering "teaching to the test" rather than teaching to help students learn and grow. The 2002 No Child Left Behind Act includes a national requirement of annual testing as of 2005, plus the new standard that "highly qualified" teachers be in place. If that does not generate improvement, schools are required to let students transfer to better schools and to provide tutoring. If there is still no improvement in test scores in 6 years, a school can be shut down. Among the many challenges of this act, the lack of sufficient funding to accomplish the goals suggests more rhetoric than commitment to children (Masterson, 2003).

School districts may be as small as a single grade school or as large as the million-pupil New York City system; the historic expectation is that a locally elected or appointed board will determine the way in which the community's children will be educated. Federal funds—often for special education or programs for impoverished students—account for only about 7 percent of school expenditures (Ramirez, 2002–2003). The reporting about schools without texts, without modern science laboratories or computers, and cutting back on "frills" such as music, art, and gym has stimulated an active look for ways to make equitable funding available, with the expectation that standards can be established and will be met. The shift to national standards, tied to access to funds, is a move away from the long-standing local nature of education in the United States. Given the very high positive correlation between health status and level of education, this ought to be an area of concern to every nurse.

Further concern should be generated by the variability in the presence or expectations of school nurses. In some districts, there are full-time nurses in every school with both knowledge and time to work with children and parents to support or improve physical or mental health. In far too many districts, there is no nurse, a part-time nurse, or a nurse whose only role is to ensure that children with special health care needs receive their medications, catheter care, or other prescribed services. A nurse in any setting working with a family that includes school-age children should become familiar with the available school health and school nursing resources.

Head Start

Head Start is this country's clearest policy commitment to comprehensive support of child-rearing families at the low end of the income scale. This program began during the 1960s' War on Poverty and is designed to give young children in low-income families the nutrition, health services, and early learning support that makes them ready for learning. A strong bias for family involvement strengthens parents' ability to support their children, even after the completion of Head Start. Unfortunately, this program has never received appropriations sufficient to accommodate all income-eligible families.

Homeschooling

Homeschooling has become more popular, with a wide range in emphasis and nature. Such education is offered under requirements that vary by state and may in fact be minimal. Some families deciding to homeschool are motivated by faith, others by disappointment in their public schools, others by preference for personally educating their offspring. Illinois is the most open in its home school regulations. For children from 7 to 16, "as long as you are teaching the branches of education in the English language, at the proper level for your child, then you are complying with the laws of Illinois concerning education." There is no testing or oversight (Illinois Christian Home Educators, 2003). As a contrast, Washington State parents may homeschool their children only if they

HEAD START FISCAL YEAR 2002

Enrollment	912,345
Ages	
Number of 5-year-olds and older	5%
Number of 4-year-olds	52%
Number of 3-year-olds	36%
Number under 3 years of age	7%
Racial/ethnic composition	
American Indian	2.9%
Hispanic	29.8%
Black	32.6%
White	28.4%
Asian	2.0%
Hawaiian/Pacific Islander	1.0%
Number of grantees	1,570
Number of classrooms	49,800
Number of centers	18,865
Average cost per child	$6,934
Paid staff	198,000
Volunteers	1,45,000

Source: Head Start Bureau. (2003). *Head Start Program fact sheet.* Administration on Children, Youth, and Families.

have 1 hour of supervision each week from a certified instructor or they have 1 year of college, a superintendent approves them, or they have taken a course on homeschooling (Shelton, 2003). In Montana, home schools must do the following:

1. Maintain records on pupil attendance and disease immunization and make the records available to the county superintendent of schools on request
2. Provide at least 180 days of pupil instruction or the equivalent in accordance with certain regulations
3. Be housed in a building that complies with applicable local health and safety regulations
4. Provide an organized course of study that includes instruction in the subjects required of public schools as a basic instructional program
5. Notify the county superintendent of schools, of the county in which the home school is located, in each school fiscal year of the student's attendance at the school

Several districts in California provide supplies and resources to home school families. Alaska, with its huge distances and scattered population, has for decades had a distance-learning home school program (Lines, 2000). In Arizona, the state provides the Community-Assisted Schooling Alternatives Vida Home School Enrichment Center, offering some administrative support as well as teacher assessment. "In addition to networking with other home schooling parents and using the curriculum resource library, parents can consult with staff members on teaching strategies and on their home schooling curriculums. Many parents find that having a day to plan instruction for the rest of the week has a positive impact on their home instruction" (Eley, 2002). Companies such as Heritage Home School and eSylvan Online Tutoring, which sell full lesson plans, can further help with planning. However, both require online access, which is not yet in every home.

Clearly, if a child is out of the public school system, she is also out of the regular purview of school nurses, counselors, and other helpers. Although a home-schooled child may avoid the annual colds of a child in school, she may also miss out on education about such matters as vaccinations and sexual safety. School nurses are often key in spotting unrecognized health problems or signs of abuse, meaning that the nurses in other settings, such as a pediatric practice, may be in the position of early warning. It is apparently a misconception that homeschooled children will lack social skills and be unable to move smoothly to adulthood. Rather, there is strong evidence that homeschooled children survive their teen years with greater confidence and direction that those in regular schools. Home school does not equal total isolation. Many homeschooled teens attend one or more specialized classes with others or participate in athletics, music, drama, or other typical extracurricular activity.

WORK AND WELFARE

As indicated at the outset, this chapter cannot provide an exhaustive discussion of the social policies that affect families in the United States today. As with the earlier sections, this discussion of work and welfare policies is illustrative of the issues and should point the way to questions to include in a family assessment or areas of potential social advocacy.

Many European countries have family policies that support families' well-being and might even proudly describe their country as a "welfare state." Although the obvious diversity of U.S. families would make a single form of support difficult, the historic reluctance of this country to do anything that might be construed as supporting unusual relationships has worked against any sort of support at all.

The public debate on an appropriate level of support for families lacking basic housing, food, health services, or social stability is made difficult by choice of vocabulary. Socially and fiscally conservative proposals have been described in family-friendly terms, even when they appear to others to have been proposed primarily to limit public spending by pushing all responsibility onto "the family" even when the family lacks resources, a form of blaming the victim. Efforts to push all recipients of public assistance into marriage and traditional nuclear family configurations appeal to supporters of this family independence approach, with little apparent recognition of the realities experienced by individuals without regular incomes.

The problems experienced by families are made more complicated by this lack of a "coherent national policy"; research has found that the existing family programs are uncoordinated and not useful. The programs that do exist (such as Social Security, the former Aid to Families with Dependent Children, and the current Temporary Assistance to Needy Families) "are largely reactive in nature; more importantly, they are not available to all children and families" (Chung & Pardeck, 1997). Although the Family and Medical Leave Act was passed in 1993, giving people time off after the birth of an infant, an adoption, or to care for sick family members, time off does not equate to sufficient financial stability to house, clothe, and feed the family or to cover needed health services.

Poverty

Poverty in itself is a limiting and frightening experience for families. In 1969, 24.2 million Americans lived in poverty; in 1997 the number was 35.6 million, with children overrepresented in that number, and by the beginning of the 21st century one in every five children fit this definition. Also increasing are the number and proportion of these poor children with disabilities in need of special education services. The indicators of disability affiliated with poverty include asthma, environmental trauma, learning problems, and low birth weight (Fujiura, 2000). One-quarter of teens have long-term, serious health or wellness problems, including pregnancy. Since 1981, the proportion of children needing mental health help has risen 80 percent (Chung & Pardeck, 1997).

In 2002, the poverty rate rose to 12.1 percent, from 11.7 percent in 2001, meaning that 34.6 million people lived below the federal poverty guidelines (Weinberg, 2003). The Office of Family Assistance, under the Administration for Children and Families, coordinates Temporary Assistance to Needy Families (TANF). TANF came out of President Clinton's attempts to "reform" welfare because of a perception that it was overused and abused. In order to obtain assistance, recipients must be employed. College attendance no longer counts as employment, meaning that those receiving assistance are directed to whatever employment is available at their present skill levels, without the option of seeking education for subsequent employment at a higher level.

The attitudes toward welfare have been complicated by rising *xenophobia*, with legal immigrants also losing substantial social services. This appears to be a process of blaming the victims, putting the onus of social standing on the individual instead of on the social systems and institutions that perpetuate all the-isms: racism, classism, sexism, heterosexism, and ableism. "Even the use of the word 'personal' in the [Welfare Reform] act's name attests to the conviction that poverty is an individual rather than structural problem and will be solved by individual effort alone" (Schroeder & Ward, 1998).

State Assistance

Iowa initiated a TANF-like welfare system in 1993. Ten years later, Iowa's remains one of the more successful programs in removing people from public aid and maintaining quality of life. Their success is attributed in part to educating the public on the realities of living in poverty via role-play programs and allowing direct participation in decision making by welfare recipients (Garasky, Greder, & Brotherson, 2003). The relative social homogeneity of Iowa, and the heritage of social support of the Scandinavian immigrants to the area, may form part of the social history for this social policy success.

In some states, the requirement to be employed extends to women with newborns. According to one estimate, in "the absence of welfare reform, the national breast-feeding rate six months after birth would have been 5.5% higher in 2000" (Haider, Jacknowitz, & Schoeni, 2003). Women are the largest group receiving public income assistance. White women constitute the majority of those served, but a higher per capita number of women of color are enrolled. Women use welfare in four ways: in emergencies for short term, as unemployment insurance, to supplement insufficient income, and in place of work (Schroeder & Ward, 1998). One Minnesota welfare recipient "must soon complete her GED or get a job. [She] says she would love to do both, but first there's this little problem of childcare. All the openings in her neighborhood have long been filled and her children's three different schedules: preschool, p.m. kindergarten and grade school, make it near impossible to coordinate the bus route commutes for longer distance day care. As a result, [she] is afraid she will be considered uncooperative with her worker and have her welfare grant cut by 10 percent, the going rate for first-time offenses" (Rich, 1998). The overwhelmingly negative attitudes about women who remain on welfare for extended periods of time have fueled efforts to change the entire system in ways that would provide support when needed but clearly move people to independence.

In 1998, Ohio received a "failing grade" (ranked 38 out of 50) on its welfare reform efforts. "The problem in Ohio is that not enough legitimate job training programs are available. People on welfare do want to

work and grow and develop. . . . The fact that more low-income families have sought help from homeless shelters and food pantries since the new law should give us pause to reconsider some of the policies it created" (Johnson, 1998). In 1999, New York City's highest-ever number of recipients (1.1 million) went down by 400,000. However, watchdog organizations report that "little information about conditions of former welfare families and individuals is available to assess economic and social impacts and to guide the direction of policies" ("Task Force," 1999).

It is expected that several hundred thousand disabled children currently receiving funding will lose it, with more-stringent requirements of disability for establishing need in the first place. Although many of those no longer eligible for welfare are still able to participate in the Medicaid program, facilitating access to health-related services, states are not making this clear. If those previously receiving a combination of assistance and Medicaid are now receiving neither and are working in entry-level jobs with no health insurance benefit, it is likely that this will result in lowered health status for their children.

There are some who argue that governments can hurt families greatly but can help them only in limited ways ("25th Anniversary," 1996). Nevertheless, Cheryl Sullivan, director of Indiana's Family and Social Services Administration (FSSA) says, "Government alone cannot solve all the problems that families may have, but neither can it sit idly by. When families fail, everyone pays the cost." This sentiment is embodied by the Partnership for Personal Responsibility (PPR, part of "welfare reform") in which (1) participants are restricted to 2 years of assistance; (2) they do not receive additional benefits for children born after entree into the program; (3) teen parents must live with another responsible adult; and (4) everyone must sign an agreement to immunize their children, get them to school, and accept any job offered (Sullivan, 1996).

The FSSA also works with the state Department of Education to develop student educational goals. If a parent PPR member does not participate, cash benefits are reduced. Noncompliance in the PPR program includes sanctions, such as refusal of assistance for 2 to 36 months. A 1991 Indiana gubernatorial initiative known as Step Ahead organizes community councils for the creation and management of public service resources. Sixty-four of these 92 councils have begun to resolve transportation issues that keep parents from successful employment. In 1995, Indiana began a

"Most Wanted" campaign to "catch" delinquent noncustodial parents for child support payments. The amount collected that year doubled the 1989 amount. Sanctions for failure to pay include loss of driver's or professional licenses (Sullivan, 1996).

In Hartford, Connecticut, after attending the Million Man March, Executive Director John Wardlaw began the Family Reunification Program. Available for families living in housing authority facilities, the program allows fathers to live with their children and children's mother without risk of losing welfare payments. In turn, the fathers appear jointly on the lease, agree to serve as a role model by abstaining from drug activity, receive job placement, and attend support meetings and life skills classes while having their rent frozen for 18 months to enable them to break out of welfare (Callahan, 1996). In this case, public health measures have been recognized *and* facilitated by government policy. Many of the most creative and successful of these programs have operated in states with a more dispersed population and a very healthy economy. States with a concentration of poverty in inner-city neighborhoods and high rates of unemployment have a much more difficult job of overcoming systemic barriers.

Immigrants and Refugees

The newcomer image most prevalent in American culture today is probably the undocumented Mexican. However, our immigrant and refugee populations have come from all over the world, many of them fleeing persecution as much as they are seeking out better opportunity. The Khmer of Laos continue to feel the effects of Pol Pot's war; the Hmong have been forced to move between China, Vietnam, and Cambodia, and many have now arrived here. Haitian refugees bring with them the aftereffects of Papa Doc Duvalier's greed, and El Salvadorans have survived decades of civil war. The multidimensional damage of all of these groups certainly affects nursing practice (Aday, 2001).

Morone (2003) suggests that each new group of immigrants has been labeled as dirty, violent, prone to substance abuse, and oversexed. Their family habits, food choices, and child-rearing practices are subject to scrutiny and criticism, and we often demand conformity to current norms as evidence of worthiness to receive services or even simple civil attention. Judgments such as these made by a nurse are antithetical to the profession's standards and inhibit any ability to provide good care.

All issues related to immigrants and refugees have become more difficult since the terrorist events in New York City and Washington, D.C., in the fall of 2001. There have been more-aggressive searches for those who have overstayed visas, sweeps of workplaces suspected of using undocumented workers, and substantial disruption of immigrant families from the Middle East. Children who are U.S. citizens by virtue of birth may abruptly lose a parent, and families find themselves unable to speak with or learn the current standing of those in custody. As with access to other services, language barriers and lack of understanding of the U.S. legal system impede efforts to maintain family cohesion.

In terms of their health and wellness, many immigrants and refugees have never had excellent health care, regardless of the impressions of many voters. Immigrants are uninsured at twice the rate of the rest of the population and make far greater use of public or underground, illegal care, particularly for their medications. The most recent approach to welfare reform made access to care more limited, as it barred anyone arriving after 1996 from using Medicaid (Delone & Tomlinson, 2002). Some immigrants fear that enrolling in programs for which they are clearly eligible will jeopardize their own or a family member's ability to stay in the United States, despite unsuccessful efforts by the U.S. Customs and Immigration Service to advertise that this is not true. Immigrants often work in service industries and day laboring jobs, employment with few health insurance benefits.

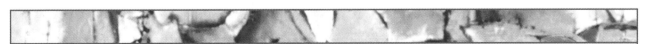

Lutheran Medical Center in Brooklyn has transformed itself since its creation to serve Norwegian immigrants to the United States in the 19th century. Now "welcome" appears in eight languages inside the front door, and community clinics with bilingual staff serve successive waves of newcomers from Europe, Asia, and Latin America.

Language barriers are significant, with the limited ability of hospitals to have translators in Russian, Khmer, Cambodian, or 100 other tongues (Ku & Freilich, 2001).

Although California's Proposition 187 was ruled unconstitutional after 3 years in effect, voters in that state continue to push for its goal: denying health care and education to illegal aliens. The court ruled that many of the law's components, including restrictions on health care and welfare benefits, were redundant; these were already covered by other federal laws and Supreme Court rulings. Initial health outcomes of the repeal of Prop 187 were decreased use of outpatient mental health services and an increased use of crisis services (Fenton, Catalano, & Hargreaves, 1996). Other results include undocumented women incurring increased costs because of troubled labors and birth outcomes (Norton, Kenney, & Ellwood, 1996) and the spread of untreated and preventable illnesses (HIV/AIDS, tuberculosis, flu) from the now-uncovered population to the general population. Nurses are on the forefront of this debate in their role of assessment and triage. "[H]ealth care groups stressed that their members could not be expected to act as 'cops,'

screening for residency status and reporting suspected illegals to federal authorities" (Anonymous, 1995).

HEALTH AND ILLNESS CARE

Ensuring access to health and illness care services is one way to improve the health of individuals and families. Although many other factors such as exposure to environmental hazards and genetic heritage are critical, it is also extremely important that children receive their immunizations and be regularly evaluated for normal growth and development. Likewise, it is important that adults be adequately immunized and screened for hypertension, diabetes, and cancer at appropriate ages and intervals. Although there is much emphasis on the roles that parents have in ensuring that their children receive needed services, many adults also have responsibilities for the health care access of aging parents. Both adults and children need dental care. And if there is an ongoing challenge to health such as asthma, early detection and comprehensive management will minimize absence from school or work and increase the likelihood of full participation in age-appropriate activities.

Coming out in medical exams can be both educational and distressing.

Nurse: *Are you sexually active?*
Patient: *Yes.*
Nurse: *Do you use birth control?*
Patient: *No.*
Nurse: *Why not?!*
Patient: *I don't have sex with men.*

At this point, the nurse pauses, fumbles, and continues with the standard list of questions.

Patient: *What I would prefer is a discussion of sexual safety between female partners. When one of my girlfriends came to me concerned that she may have exposed me to chlamydia, we went to our university health center. Her nurse practitioner began to discuss with us the importance of cleaning our dildos and vibrators, as well as using condoms. We had never used any sex toys on each other; the staff could not explain how we might transmit STDs.*

Ideally, health care providers should be prepared to ask questions and be flexible in their thinking about sex practices, such as continuing with the following:

Nurse: *Why not?*
Patient: *I don't have sex with men.*
Nurse: *How do you have sex with women?*
Patient: *Oral sex, hands, and such.*
Nurse: *Do you use dental dams or finger cots?*

The absence of a comprehensive commitment to access or assurance of universal health insurance coverage for all makes achieving the desired level of interaction with health professionals extremely difficult. At least one proposal for financing universal health care has been presented to and denied by the Congress every year since 1912 (Chung & Pardeck, 1997). Since 1994, all efforts have been piecemeal, such as the recent decision to add a drug benefit to Medicare, a benefit that many doubt is adequate or even meaningful for many seniors.

Asthma

One example of a health challenge to families that is complicated by the absence of universal payment coverage and requires the collaboration of many social institutions is asthma, whether in adults or children. According to the Centers for Disease Control and Prevention, 20.3 million people in the United States had asthma in 2001. Children of asthmatics have three to six times the risk of developing asthma than children of non-asthmatics (National Center for Environmental Health, 2003a). Although increases in the rate of asthma are leveling, the urban poor (who are overwhelmingly people of color) are most heavily impacted: "African Americans visit emergency departments, are hospitalized, and die due to asthma at rates three times higher than rates for white Americans" (National Center for Environmental Health, 2003b). Major asthma attack triggers include secondhand tobacco smoke, as well as firsthand dust, pollution, cockroaches, pets, and mold. Less-common triggers include exercise, extremes of weather, food, and hyperventilation (National Center for Environmental Health, 2003a). The objective of policy makers now is to create "asthma-friendly communities": better access to and quality of treatment for all populations but especially those in poorer communities; increased awareness of asthma and its risks for all; and environmentally safe schools and homes (Lara, Nicholas, Morton, Vaiana, Genovese, & Rachelefsky, 2002). Although the cause of asthma is not known, its worst effects are easy to prevent.

Asthma policy and research groups include Allergy and Asthma Network/Mothers of Asthmatics (AANMA) and the Department of Health and Human Services (HHS). For a family health nurse, consistent education and reeducation of patients will help reduce emergency hospitalizations and fatalities. In New York City's 22 Bureau of Child Health outpatient clinics, a combination of physician education and nurse educator oversight showed improvement in patient health outcomes (Clark et al., 1997).

Obesity

Recently brought to national attention, the rising rates of obesity and diabetes also present significant health issues for families. Although the definition of "healthy weight" has varied significantly through the last century, the current standard is the body mass index

---

In 2001, an estimated

- 31.3 million people had been diagnosed with asthma during their lifetime,
- 20.3 million people were diagnosed with asthma,
- 12 million people had experienced an asthma attack in the previous year.

In 2000, asthma accounted for

- 10.4 million outpatient visits,
- 1.8 million emergency department visits,
- 465,000 hospitalizations,
- 4487 deaths.

Source: U.S. Department of Health and Human Services. (2003). *Asthma prevalence, health care use and mortality, 2000–2001.* Centers for Disease Control and Prevention.

To calculate BMI:

$$BMI = \left(\frac{\text{Weight in pounds}}{(\text{Height in inches}) \times (\text{Height in inches})} \right) \times 703$$

$$\left(\frac{220 \text{ lb}}{(75 \text{ in}) \times (75 \text{ in})} \right) \times 703 = BMI \ 27.5$$

Alternatively, you can use the calculator at www.cdc.gov/nccdphp/dnpa/bmi/calc-bmi.htm.

Source: National Center for Chronic Disease Prevention and Health Promotion. (2003a). *BMI for adults formula*. Division of Nutrition and Physical Activity. Centers for Disease Control and Prevention.

(BMI), or the ratio of weight to height. According to the National Institutes of Health, overweight people have a BMI of 25 to 29.9; those with a BMI of 30 or higher are obese.

The rate of obesity is startling: for adults aged 20 to 74, obesity reached 27 percent in 1999. Among children and teens, around 15 percent are overweight, double the rates of the 1970s (National Center for Chronic Disease Prevention and Health Promotion, 2003b). This increase has been linked directly to greatly enlarged portion sizes, restaurant and soft drink consumption, reduced need or ability to walk to schools and services, reduced school funding for physical activity, and increased television and computer time (Nutrition, Physical Activity, and Obesity Prevention Program, 2003). In the 1990s, type 2 diabetes, which is correlated with obesity, was rare among children and teens, but now it may account for half of new diabetics (Nutrition, Physical Activity, and Obesity Prevention Program, 2003).

Excess weight leads to increased risk of heart disease, diabetes, stroke, gallstones, sleep apnea, and depression (Stunkard & Wadden, 1993). Obesity now claims $117 billion of health care costs annually; "obesity has roughly the same association with chronic health conditions as does 20 years of aging, and the costs of obesity were recently estimated to exceed the health care costs of smoking and problem drinking" (Nutrition, Physical Activity, and Obesity Prevention Program, 2003). In research on family eating patterns, children whose parents were restrictive tended to eat too much; children who were allowed to choose their own snacks ate the worst. Children who were offered food as a reward wanted that food even more; children who needed to eat a food to gain a reward wanted it even less.

Substance Abuse

Substance abuse within families impacts all members. Whether addiction is purely genetic, purely social, or some combination of both, families do "transmit" addiction and can be the source of dysfunction (Aday, 2001). In writing about her own self and family, Carolyn See argues that alcoholism in particular comes from a lack of options within our increasingly stratified society (See, 1996). Regardless, nurses must be aware of its widespread health impact. Addiction is a lasting problem that has multiple effects across generations. For teens, assertiveness, self-confidence, and healthy stress reduction have been successful in delaying the onset of using drugs and alcohol (Aday, 2001).

Most publicly funded treatment programs include residential group homes and outpatient clinics, as well as 12-step programs. People with money or insurance might opt for private inpatient or individual counseling (Aday, 2001). An early study of drug addiction treatment that included "therapeutic alliances" between the patient, family, and peers showed significant improvement in reduction of cocaine use (Glazer, Galanter, Megwinoff, Dermatis, & Keller, 2003). Unfortunately, access to services is associated with access to health insurance, as the number of publicly funded treatment services is roughly one-third of what might be needed, whereas those with private insurance coverage or personal funds are able to select from a range of service options.

WHO DECIDES?

The decisions made by a spouse on behalf of his severely impaired wife were challenged in court by his wife's parents. They were unsuccessful in the courts but later succeeded in having the court overruled by the state legislature with the encouragement of the governor. The usual spousal authority to make medical decisions in the absence of clear, written directives from the incapacitated individual provided no assurance that the wishes of the closest "family" would be supported. This particular case provides an interesting illustration of not only the complications of family relationships and decision making but also the interrelationships of the branches of government with what may be thought of as individual and personal decisions.

Access to Health Care

Any challenge to health is important for populations without access to health care. In her autobiographical book, Marion Deutsche Cohen describes how her life was reduced to "nights, lifting, and toilet" as her husband's body (but not mind) was reduced by multiple sclerosis. As academics with a way to finance health care, even the Cohens struggled to find affordable, reliable nursing and respite care (Cohen, 1996). In 2000, 40.5 million Americans under age 65 (16.8 percent) lacked health insurance; 12.4 percent of children under age 18 do not have coverage (National Center for Health Statistics, 2000). This is more than the number uninsured at the time of the last major attempt to provide universal coverage (1993–1994). The majority of those uninsured are those working in low-paying jobs that do not offer an affordable insurance policy as a benefit of employment or the families of workers who cannot afford to purchase coverage for their dependents.

The cost of insurance coverage, or of care purchased directly, continues to rise, making access ever more difficult. Those who lack insurance seek care later in an episode of illness and thus need more and more expensive care, which they cannot afford. Lacking a regular source of primary care, the emergency room becomes the caregiver of last, most-expensive resort. For example, although it is not surprising that 31.6 percent of visits to emergency rooms are for injuries and poisonings, it should be of concern that 13.3 percent of emergency room visits are for "symptoms, signs, and ill-defined conditions" (National Center for Health Statistics, 1999). The uninsured are also more likely to report not purchasing a recommended prescription for medication following a visit.

The Oregon Health Plan was created in 1989 to help cover the 14 percent of the population going without coverage ("Senator Promotes," 2003). "The Oregon Health Plan (OHP) operates under a waiver from the federal government that allows us to serve more low-income people using federal Medicaid money. We do this through an innovative system that prioritizes health care, using a list of hundreds of conditions and their treatments. Higher priority is given to conditions that can be successfully treated, and to avoiding illness through preventive care" (Office of Medical Assistance, 2003).

Half of Oregon's physicians do not take Oregon Health Plan patients because of limited reimbursement. To try to change this, the Oregon Medical Association is trying to put a cap on malpractice lawsuits for physicians who take OHP patients, thus reducing their insurance (Associated Press, 2003c). Prescription drugs account for one-quarter of OHP expenses. To reduce this amount, in 2003 Governor Kulongoski signed a bill restricting participating physicians to cheaper prescriptions, with the opportunity to get approval for needed exceptions ("Oregon Governor Backs Off," 2003). In August of 2003, Representative Ron Wyden suggested federal adoption of health services like the OHP to address national disparities.

Even with coverage, there are continuous debates about the exact services to be covered and the level of co-payment or deductible needed. These debates reflect social policies, or social conflict, including the debate about whether health and illness services are a consumer commodity to be purchased at individual preference or a social good to be made available equitably to everyone. Medicare, for example, has until now not provided coverage for prescription drugs, although doing so would probably decrease the need for hospitalization by some elderly individuals. Opposition comes from those concerned with the potential economic policy consequence of making the

U.S. government a large purchaser potentially capable of establishing price controls on drugs. Another example is the conflict between full coverage for all reproductive health services and the strong antichoice lobbying of some groups that has led to limits on funding for abortion in many public programs. An intriguing rebalance has come as the push by men to have the anti-impotence drug Viagra covered by insurance has highlighted the failure of many insurance plans to cover contraception for women.

Insurance Programs for Children

The State Child Health Insurance Program (SCHIP) enacted by Congress in 1997 represents an attempt to protect children by making affordable insurance available to them (Figure 6–1). The funds (one of the largest sums ever made available for this purpose) may be used by the states either to expand Medicaid through increased eligibility for children in families with income levels higher than those used for regular Medicaid or to create new programs. Two problems have made progress with SCHIP difficult. The process of welfare reform has removed families from Medicaid eligibility, making more children eligible for SCHIP than were contemplated when the program began. Moreover, there are at least concerns, if not documented evidence, that employers will drop dependent coverage, pushing previously insured children into this publicly supported program.

To address some of these problems, Illinois developed FamilyCare and KidCare. When he expanded the program in 2003, Governor Rod Blagojevich said, "We have thousands of working families and children who don't have decent healthcare. Often times, their only option is to go to the emergency room when they need help. . . . By signing the FamilyCare and KidCare bills into law, we are providing health care coverage in current year for 20,000 more children and 65,000 more working parents. Over the next three years, a total of 300,000 parents will receive health care" ("Governor Signs Legislation," 2003). A family of two qualifies if they earn under $1400 per month; a family of five qualifies if they earn less than $3500 per month (Illinois KidCare, 2003).

Another attempt to improve access to care for children and adolescents has been the development of comprehensive school health clinics. Schools have long been the site of some health-related services, such as screening for vision or hearing problems, dental caries, or scoliosis. They have also included at least some health education, with the most recent addition being HIV/AIDS education mandated in some or all grades in all states. School nurses have been employed to ensure evaluation of health problems that arise in the course of the school day and to oversee medications or other treatments needed by children with disabilities. It has been a natural expansion of traditional school health services to add primary health care by employing physicians, nurse

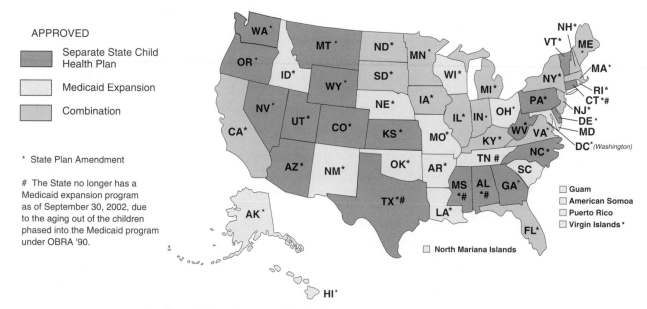

Figure 6–1 State Child Health Insurance Program plan activity.

practitioners, or physician's assistants. One rationale for placing services in the school has been the difficulties working parents have leaving work to take their children for care during ordinary daytime working hours. The first school-based clinics were for adolescents and included a strong emphasis on access to reproductive health services. Some school-based programs have considered expansion to cover the family members of the children.

Healthy People

The health of families has been improved in recent years by more than access to care. National policies regarding desirable levels of immunization and improved quality of the care are also important. *Healthy People 2010* is the current iteration of national health objectives developed by the Department of Health and Human Services (DHHS; http://web.health.gov/healthypeople/). The overall goal for the nation is increased years of healthy life and the elimination of health status disparities across racial, ethnic, sex/gender, or other lines. Developed every 10 years to cover a decade of effort, *Healthy People* has provided a national focus on important areas for investment of resources and has spurred states and localities to develop their own *Healthy People* plans as well. Public dialogue through earlier *Healthy People* efforts revealed the fact that over 50 percent of U.S. children were not fully age-appropriately immunized. This has led to significant improvements, using a combination of provider education, support for vaccine purchase, registries and recall systems, and community-wide advertising. Other areas of family health that have benefited from the comprehensive, population-focused efforts have been injury prevention, diabetes detection and management, and asthma management.

Environmental Health

Nurses have many opportunities to witness the problems created for families by the lack of health insurance, limited access to primary care, or social policies that are at odds with a family's values. Less visible are those policies about our environment that have a differential impact on families. Environmental health encompasses all those organized activities that endeavor to limit human contact with substances harmful to health by providing some form of barrier or by preventing their general release. Efforts to ensure safe drinking water, clean air, and safe disposal of waste products are all part of environmental health.

One of the signal successes of this effort is the dramatic reduction of blood lead levels in children following the removal of lead from gasoline products; additional lead control efforts focus on protection from access to old paint products or paint. As with other areas of health, those at the lowest income levels are most vulnerable to failures in our policies. This includes poor urban children living in old buildings with lead in drinking-water pipes and old, lead-based paint on the walls; rural poor children, living without benefit of a working sewer or septic tank; or the children of migrant laborers living and playing near pesticides and dangerous farm equipment. Community decisions regarding the location of waste disposal sites (both industrial waste sites and domestic waste landfills) result in those with lower income being much more likely to live in proximity to harmful waste products than those with more. The environmental justice movement has emerged as a way of bringing attention to these disparities and mobilizing action to protect all of the population.

In August of 2003, President Bush retracted the Clean Air Act's requirement that older power plants install up-to-date pollution controls. Estimates of the consequences include pollution amounts that may cause, annually, up to 400,000 asthma attacks (Wu, 2003). The top 10 states for release of lead, the leading environmental concern for children, are (in declining severity) California, Idaho, Ohio, Oregon, West Virginia, Texas, Georgia, Utah, North Carolina, and Florida. Moreover, animal waste, an increasing problem due to corporate farming, is threatening water supplies. Waste from cows and pigs (bred indoors, usually on top of drainage grates) is moved into "lagoons" to liquefy before being sprayed onto crops. What the crops cannot absorb then moves into the water system as runoff. Beyond the stench, the bacteria can kill organisms in water. Antibiotic resistance is also furthered as the massive doses the animals received become a part of the food chain (Environmental Defense, 2003). Advocacy groups attending to this issue have attempted to increase public awareness.

A group of scientists, activists, agriculturalists, and others known as "bioneers" are developing creative, safe solutions to many of these problems. Examples include farmers working only with organic materials, opening community seed banks, water treatment using solar power along the lines of existing health ecosystems, sustainable harvesting of medicinal plants (as opposed to faster clear-cutting methods that destroy sources), and retrofitting existing empty buildings for community greenhouses. One of the best-known bioneers is William McDonough, an internationally recognized architect and Dean of Architecture at the University of Virginia. His methods are remarkably simple: using more natural light in schools and business causes productivity to go up and absenteeism to go down, and it reduces electric bills. By using alleyways in neighborhoods instead of driveways, the use of pavement (which absorbs heat and impairs water runoff) goes down by half. During a project to produce a "green" upholstery, McDonough and his partners found that the wastewater coming out of their factory was cleaner than when it went in (Shea, 2000).

CAREGIVING FOR THE OLD AND THE YOUNG

One of the roles that families play within society is that of caregiver for dependent family members. These may include the ill, the young, the elderly, or those with long-term disabilities. Rates of disability have increased to 14.4 percent in 1994, from 11.7 percent in 1970 (Fujiura, 2000). The level of care needed varies widely, from those who need complete assistance with all activities of daily living and those who can manage personal hygiene and nourishment but need assistance with functional activities such as shopping or transportation to those who need regular emotional or social support while maintaining physical independence. As examples of the intersection of social policy and family health, this section will focus on issues of child care and elder care.

Child Care

First-time mothers of newborns experience better coping when their care is affirmed by a nurse, whom they "expect . . . to give them expert advice on the child's growth and development and, most importantly, on how the child's development can be promoted" (Tarkka, Paunonen, & Laippala, 1999). Today's pattern of family relocation means that professional advice may be the only advice available, as the new mother is remote from the circle of family available to at least some prior generations. Whether first-time parent, or the parent of many, paid childcare is the practical outcome of a society that is composed of individuals who both parent and work. The cost of care for even one preschooler in a family with a working mother can far exceed what is affordable on wages for a service job. Successful, affordable childcare is a persistent concern at all income levels in this country.

At the lower end of the income scale, the decision may be made to leave older, but still immature, children in charge of younger ones.

Our "leave it to the family to figure out" policy is quite different from that of some other societies such as France and the Scandinavian countries, which provide universal child care in the neighborhood or at the workplace, believing that parenting is a responsibility shared by the entire community. Overall, 73 to 95 percent of European 3- to 5-year-olds are in public day care. In this country, there has been limited support for subsidizing and organizing child care for those at the low end of the income scale, to enable those parents to participate in work training or take entry-level employment. Some businesses provide on-site child care, either as a mechanism to retain or attract skilled workers or because of labor union negotiations. Other options for parents include live-in or-out caregivers, relatives, home-based day care, center-based day care, backup adults in case of illness, mixed hours between parent work schedules, or all or any of the above. The transition of women to work outside of the home and their replacement as child caregivers with other child care options can be characterized as a "de-skilling" of the stereotypical mother (Hertz & Ferguson, 1996).

In an effort to reduce costs and rely on family, grandparents may become primary caregivers, often at significant cost in time and lost opportunities for other activities in a planned retirement or threats to their own health. In one study, grandmothers who provided care for at least 9 hours a week were at a 55 percent increased risk for heart attack (Bjerklie, 2003). As women of color, especially African-Americans, have joined the middle class, they have gained access to child care options beyond that offered by relatives at no cost. At the same time, that option raises the potential of exposing their children at a young age to experiences of racism within day care programs. Women who place children in day care report feeling less replaced as a parent, in contrast to those who bring someone into the home to provide care (Hertz & Ferguson, 1996), perhaps because they can see day care as a school, a socially positive step.

All of these child care issues are, of course, related to the work schedules given to or developed by parents. Although some may be able to organize split shifts or irregular days on/off, others must, by the nature of their work, be away from the home during regular business hours. Those families in which schedules could be juggled to accommodate more parent time in the home "push the boundaries of maintaining middle class standards. . . . [Parents] do pay career costs associated with these choices and they pay economic penalties because they earn less. Yet, they challenge conventional wisdom about what is possible in integrating work and family life: They are not waiting for the State or the workplace to implement 'family friendly' policies" (Hertz & Ferguson, 1996).

However, those parents who shift their job time and so lack full "job success" are mainly women, thus "reinforcing the old pattern of women's work ghettos" (Harrington, 1998). The most common employer approaches to accommodating parenting are leave and options to work part-time. When polled, parents suggest that flexible work hours and child care within the workplace would be preferred. Furthermore, even in places that allow sick leave and time off for family, employees who felt *stigma* or disapproval from their peers were reluctant to make use of the policies (Lee & Duxbury, 1999).

In 2001, only 28.8 percent of full-time workers had "flexible" work schedules, which allowed them to vary their start and end times. Women were less likely than men to have this schedule, and the type of occupation greatly affected this type of schedule. Of those on an alternative work shift, half were doing so because of the job itself and only 8.9 percent because of child care needs (Bureau of Labor Statistics, 2002). If shifting work schedules becomes the answer, then day care programs may need to adjust *their* hours of operation. This may also increase the participation of fathers in child care. In some studies, it was found that if a mother worked part-time, fathers were more likely to care for the child during the mother's work hours than if the mother worked full-time. But fathers' work schedules also had an impact on their availability, and those work schedules are the strongest predictor (over other socioeconomic concerns) of whether they will be child caregivers. Families with more money were also less likely to make use of fathers, although what was more important was how much the mother made relative to the father. Larger amounts of male unemployment in 1990 and 1991 resulted in a noticeable increase in paternal caregiving (Casper & O'Connell, 1998). A disturbing study by the National Institute of Child Health and Human Development found that kids' aggression, assertiveness, and defiance increased with rates of nonmaternal care (Belsky, 2002).

Sick Kids

What if the family involves a child who is critically ill? The practice of medicine within neonatal intensive care units (NICUs), where paid professionals often make decisions over or without the opinions of parents, calls into question the nature of parenting, and consequently family. Unless a family is willing to go to court, medical practitioners control care by both overt and subtle means, usually with the best of intentions. NICU doctors, nurses, aides, and the like have been trained to face the multitude of situations a sick and/or premature infant presents; most parents are not. Does this necessarily mean medicine knows best? According to Wall and Partridge, neonatologists, whose armamentarium is now so expansive, "feel culpable when they elect to limit the treatment of marginally viable infants . . . [which] may at times be either inappropriate or inhumane" (Wall & Partridge, 1997).

Even though most parents do not anticipate or consider the possibility of delivering a sick infant, does this mean they are unable to cope? They are the parents and, as such, "become the natural repositories of what little information there is about their infants' interests and are expected to act as representatives for their infants" (Heimer & Staffen, 1998). Despite this, the research interviews of NICU parents done by Ellenchild and Spielman (1996) found an ongoing "under representation" of the parents' position. Parents recalled a "general acceptance of all proffered treatments" but that "they were not informed sufficiently in the NICU." Heimer and Staffen posit that parents play only a ceremonial role, in that they get to name the infant "but do not care for it" and are irrelevant in many treatment decisions. They are told of their importance, but the actions of the NICU speak to the preeminence of medical care over parenting (Heimer & Staffen, 1998).

How does this impact the issue of family? Practitioners perceive parental education, which could promote positive parental involvement, as impossible and unwelcome. Lack of information has ethical implications: "Without information, parents are not in a strong position to be responsible decision makers. They cannot provide informed consent for any treatment of the child—a basic ethical mandate" (Ellenchild, 1996, p. 87). In Haywood's study of physician misassessment of NICU outcomes, the authors make a rather obvious statement that only with complete and cutting-edge information can practitioners *and* parents make strategic decisions (Haywood, Goldenberg, Bronstein, Nelson, & Carlo, 1994, pp. 432–439). A move toward family-centered care and full implementation of the principles on which his text is premised may provide an answer or at least a palliative that could prevent some of the clashes described hereafter.

As one example of the clash of personal values with social policy, Jehovah's Witness parents have a difficult time having their religious beliefs dominate over socially approved and medically prescribed procedures, such as blood transfusion. One family in New Zealand, having refused a liver transplant for their less than 2-year-old, very sick son, were taken to court for "unreasonableness." This decision was overturned in a higher court because the mother was acting on behalf of the family and in light of the pain and stress that would make her child's life even worse. Another family, with four children, went through a difficult and eventually further debilitating heart procedure with their oldest child. When the same procedure was suggested for their youngest, they refused. An Austrian family refused chemotherapy for a 6-year-old child's abdominal cancer in 1995. Having fled to Spain, the child was returned to Austria by state authorities and forcibly treated (Nicholson, 1997). Nurses who have not considered the issues of parental rights, parental authority, and family autonomy will not be in a good position to help families in situations such as these.

Elder Care

At the other end of life, caregiving is growing both as an inevitable family responsibility and as a profession. The Administration on Aging predicts that by 2020, 19.2 percent of the 15.2 million persons over age 65 living alone will need help with daily living. In 1998 three times the number of people had at least one member of the household caring for a friend or relative than was the case a decade earlier. Race is important in this statistic, with Asian- and African-American homes being more likely to include a caregiver than homes described as Hispanic or Caucasian (Braus, 1998).

Caregiving, both lay and professional, is facilitated both by technological advances and by need. The tools now exist for home care. More women than men are caregivers. The perception that it is women's "unique, gender-based obligation to care for others without compensation . . . restrict(s) women's choices and abilities to work, while at the same time leaving men free to be breadwinners" (Harrington, 1998). Even where policies are written to be gender neutral, as in the Family and Medical Leave Act, women experience a general expectation that they will be the care-givers of first resort regardless of the burden that places on them.

The fact that these lay caregivers are unpaid benefits greater social structures, especially Medicare and Medicaid. If we did not continue to expect home care-givers, it would cost us all a great deal more in emotional strain, earlier death, or increased taxes and fees (Schroeder & Ward, 1998). Women engaged in lay home care experienced much higher levels of stress than their other family members did, as well as more alienation from those outside of the home (Armstrong, 1996). These experiences are similar to those reported by many nurses about their workplace roles, as well (Schroeder & Ward, 1998).

End-of-Life Decisions

Related to caregiving is the process of decisions made about the end of care at the end of life. As discussed earlier, family members are frequently torn as they are asked to make decisions about continuing or discontinuing interventions when recovery from illness or injury seems remote. A unique example of a social policy in this area of family life is Oregon's Death with Dignity Act, which was voted into law in 1994, survived appeals to the Supreme Court, and was implemented in 1997 (Death with Dignity National Center, 2003). Physician aid in dying in Oregon is covered by the Oregon Health Plan but only with state funds, as is abortion, given federal policies regarding the use of Medicaid funds (Oregon Health Services Commission, 2003).

Patients eligible to use the Act must: (a) be 18 years of age or older; (b) be an Oregon resident; (c) be capable of making and communicating health-care decisions; (d) have a terminal illness with <6 months to live; and (e) voluntarily request a prescription. The patient must make one written and two verbal requests (separated by at least 15 days) of their physician. The prescribing physician and a consultant physician are required to confirm the terminal diagnosis and prognosis, determine that the patient is capable and acting voluntarily, and refer the patient for counseling if either believes that the patient's judgment is impaired by a psychiatric or psychological disorder. The prescribing physician must also inform the patient of feasible alternatives, such as comfort care, hospice care and pain control options. (Oregon Department of Human Services, 2000)

In 2001, 21 Oregonians used this law, and in 2002, 38. Five-year aggregate data show that patients' median age was 69 years; 97 percent of patients were white, 55 percent were male, 25 percent were divorced, and 38 percent had a bachelor's degree or higher. Compared with other Oregonians dying of the same underlying illnesses, those who were younger, divorced or never married, or well-educated or who had cancer or amyotrophic lateral sclerosis (Lou Gehrig's disease) were more likely to participate. Patients' major concerns over the 5 years were losing autonomy (85 percent), a decreasing ability to participate in activities that made life enjoyable (79 percent), and losing control of bodily functions (58 percent) (Widerburg, 2003).

Family-centered thinking, including in the evaluation the impact of a decision on all participating family members, is at least as appropriate in the case of adults as it is in the case of care for children. At least one observer suggests, "Our family care system is collapsing. When it worked well, it depended on the unpaid labor of women at home . . . our society has no new philosophic consensus for an economic system that would support families as care providers" (Harrington, 1998). The Hastings Center, for example, presents a case of the granddaughter of a degenerating 70-year-old woman who asks her grandmother's oncologist for help in encouraging the use of Meals on Wheels and home caregivers. The grandmother lives alone and the granddaughter, her only visitor, is not able to cope with the increasing debility. The doctor declines, as he is listening to the grandmother who is adamant about her independence and must be respected as a competent adult, a decision consistent with the best of patient autonomy approaches. The granddaughter questions whether her role as lone support is really so unimportant in the decision ("Don't I Count?" 1997). It may be that we need a reconsidered ethic of autonomy in circumstances of physical dependency such as this.

In 1965, Medicare began funding home-care services for the elderly. In 1997 the cost had gone from $46 million to $20.5 *billion*. Medicaid also contributes, paying one-quarter of those dollars for the poor and some disabled. Just under one-quarter of all home-care bills are paid by those using the service, and 4 percent are covered by insurance (Braus, 1998). In 1981, Medicaid Home and Community-Based Service Waivers were authorized, providing federal monies to home and community alternatives to nursing homes (Kennedy, 1997). By doing so, the federal government is reflecting that it values the home, whether for humanitarian or economic reasons. Some states have had active senior groups supporting similar invest-

ment of state dollars, based on the assumption that admission to an institution is only occasionally the right choice, even for an older person with serious limitations in activities of daily living.

When the family decides to use paid caregivers, it is important to realize that the family configuration is changed. Paid caregivers enter into homes influenced by their own cultural notions of their role. In the act of intimate care in the home environment, family-like relationships are creative, leading to "fictive kin" status between professional caregiver and client. At times, these chosen family members can move beyond *fictive kin* to *functional kin* status by virtue of the "substantive assistance, whether it be emotional, custodial, physical, or financial" (Karner, 1998). No assumptions should be made in advance about the relationships among identified home patients, their family members, and their caregivers, particularly ones who have been involved for some period of time. The financial relationship may or may not be associated with a well-developed emotional and social one.

Implications

The implications of understanding social policy as a context for nursing care of families are almost limitless. Social policies of all kinds surround families, define family relationships, and shape or limit the health and illness services available. Many social policies may facilitate family strength and effective child rearing. However, our failure to recognize the negative policies or the negative consequences of policies has such an enormous impact on health that this chapter has focused on those that are most challenging, or have the greatest potential for negative outcomes.

For the individual caregiver, the most critical implication is in establishing a relationship with a new patient and determining a plan of care. Assumptions about whom this patient experiences as family or assumptions about family resources available to assist in care can truncate communication or lead to decisions that are actually unhelpful. Learning to use open-ended questions that do not assume marital status, gender of partner, relationships with children, or sources of financial support will yield a much more complete description. Likewise, planning for return to the community should begin with a very open exploration of potential support or resources, without assuming that any is automatically available.

Throughout nursing education, opportunities for learning experiences in settings that have established services for particularly vulnerable populations provide the student situations in which to practice the skills previously suggested. Homeless shelters, services for gay and lesbian adolescents, shelters for victims of intimate partner abuse, outreach centers for sex workers, and street syringe and needle exchange programs all reach a disproportionate share of individuals whose family experiences are not the idealized suburban norm. Whether it is an extended clinical rotation or an opportunity to observe for an afternoon and then meet with an experienced staff member, the learning will be invaluable.

The unanswered questions about best practices in nursing care with families encountering the negative impact of social policies are too numerous to list. Nursing research has already developed useful tools and frameworks for providing nursing care across cultural barriers and under difficult circumstances. The recent development of community-based participatory research models (AHRQ, 2001) provides a methodology for studies that is more respectful of the potential different views of family in a community. This approach requires the researcher to establish a relationship with the community in which the study is to occur prior to the statement of the research question, to share all stages of research with the community, and to work collaboratively toward community improvement based on the results of the study. Adopting this level of respect for potential reshaping of any studies of "family" opens the possibility that nursing would lead in studies that not only facilitate greater health but also support families of all kinds in their striving toward health.

The inclusion of health policy as a core content area for graduate nursing education is increasing the sensitivity of nurses to social and health policy issues. Nurses understand that it is not sufficient to care in isolation from the forces that increased risk of disease or limited access to medical services. The combination of history, economics, and political science that inform our understanding of policy can be introduced in such a way that nurses at all levels are better able to understand current affairs, join nursing or other advocacy organizations, and participate in local, state, or national political processes. Those policies most relevant to the issues raised in this chapter are those that in any way limit the ability of adults to define partnerships, the ability of responsible parents to care for their children, the decisions of individuals regarding care to be acted on, or the economic and social benefits of insurance, housing, child care, or elder care to be appropriately and equitably available in a commu-

nity. Nurses are often the most familiar of the health care team with the failures of policy; they should be in the forefront of the push for corrections.

SUMMARY

- *Families are complex systems* that exist within the even more complex system of a society. They are defined by society and the material world, but many seek to change those social definitions when the definitions no longer fit.
- Nurses are educated to serve individuals within the context of their families or to provide services to families as a unit. For example, if a 19-year-old unmarried mother of two expresses the desire to work at getting a college degree so that she can fulfill her own career aspirations and improve her children's economic status, a working knowledge of the limits of welfare support, eligibility for tuition assistance, and availability of affordable child care and public transportation all should be taken into account *before* delivering a "you can do it" pep talk. *Yes, encouragement is appropriate, but it must be grounded in reality*.
- A basic ground rule both in assessing the strengths and problems and in developing interventions is *ask first*. Do not assume that you can determine by observation who the parent is, which "other" is significant, who is central to a child's well-being, or who is willing or able to be accountable for action. And when initial questions indicate that the family configuration you are exploring does not fit any category that is familiar, *admission of ignorance and a request for education is wiser than blind assumption*.
- Nurses are also in a position to act as advocates. In their day-to-day work, they see the impact that existing social systems and public policies have on families. Many of those for whom we care are not in a position to actively advocate for changes. *Nurses can give voice to the concerns of the underrepresented* and assist in devising creative alternatives to current limiting policies.
- Finally, nurses are contributors to new knowledge. Research done by nurses with and about families and about the ways to help them achieve higher levels of health within complex social systems is essential. Studies may be small or large and may focus on the newly established family, the aging family, the immigrant family, the changing family, and so on. Good studies of

social policy and family will draw on a range of disciplines and theories and will probably involve at least consultation with professionals from other disciplines. It should be clear, however, from the material in this chapter that *continuing to work indefinitely from our present level of knowledge is inadequate.*

Each of us has a biological family, the source of our genetic material. Each of us also has a birth certificate naming the individual(s) legally responsible for us. Each of us has been reared by one or more adults, who may have volunteered, inherited the process, or been hired for the job. Each of us has moved through adulthood with or without participating in a shared life that may or may not be definable as a legal marriage. Each of us will make explicit or implicit decisions about the bearing, adopting, rearing, or avoiding of children. And each of us will experience the process of aging and the search for a source of support when frail, support that may or may not come from those considered family. At each step along the way, social policy about eligibility for legal relationship, for economic and social support, and for public recognition will provide strength for or serve as a deterrent to healthy living. Nurses have multiple opportunities to support positives and to mitigate, at least by evidence of understanding, the negatives experienced today.

Doing so not only is of benefit to our patients but also can enrich our individual and personal family life as well.

STUDY QUESTIONS

1. Review the questions you typically use to identify the members of a patient's family. Are they neutral regarding legal relationships, gender, and childbearing choices? If not, identify alternatives.

2. Children as property is an old social and legal concept. Identify ways in which this has been abandoned in the 21st-century United States.

3. Describe the relationship of education to family and health.

4. What are ways in which a nurse can assist a family making decisions about care for a child with special health care needs?

5. Select one special group of families (military, homeless, those with an incarcerated member) and list at least three special challenges in providing nursing care in the home or hospital.

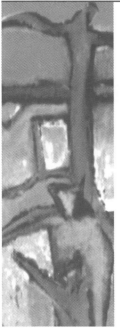

RESEARCH BRIEF

Ganzini, L., Goy, E. R., Miller, L. L., Harvath, T. A., Jackson, A., Delorit, M. A. (2003). Nurses' experiences with hospice patients who refuse food and fluids to hasten death. *New England Journal of Medicine, 349*(4), 359–365.

Purpose
The purpose of this study was to better understand those hospice patients in Oregon who voluntarily give up food and fluid as a means of hastening death, as perceived by the nurses who care for them and as compared to those who sought to use provisions of the state's physician-assisted suicide law.

Methodology
The study was conducted by a mailed survey to nurses working in Oregon hospice programs, response rate 72 percent, asking about the most recent patient cared for who refused food and fluids. Among the questions were those asking nurses to compare characteristics of the family caregivers of patients who chose to refuse food and fluids with characteristics of the family caregivers of other hospice patients on a scale from 1 to 5 (with 1 denoting much less than other hospice patients' family caregivers and 5 much more).

(continued on page 192)

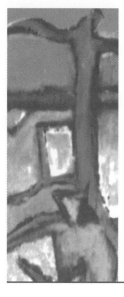

(Continued)

Results

According to the nurses, patients who chose to stop food and fluids were less likely to want to control the circumstances of their death ($P < 0.001$), less likely to fear loss of dignity ($P = 0.04$), more prepared to die ($P = 0.03$), and more likely to lack social support ($P = 0.04$) than patients who chose physician-assisted suicide.

Nursing Implications

Many nurses have been concerned that physician-assisted suicide would be used by society as a covert means of shortening the lives of those without support. This study suggests the opposite, that it is those with less social support who simply stopped eating and taking fluids and thus hastened their own deaths. Understanding patient choices at the end of life and understanding the roles that family and other social supports play are particular challenges to nurses not only in hospice but also in all long-term care and home care settings. It is critical not to make assumptions in advance but to be engaged with patients and available family as the decisions are made and then supported.

CASE STUDY ➤

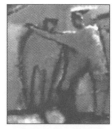

Maria, 28, has taken her girlfriend Hannah, 40, to the emergency room because of her severe abdominal pain. Because of Hannah's discomfort and anxiety, Maria has stayed right by her side throughout the admission and initial screening process. The triage nurse, who has just completed a self-study course on identification of victims of violence, begins to ask a very smart series of questions about violence and safety in her home, wanting to identify whether the abdominal pain might be either a direct result of violence or somatic evidence of high anxiety or fear of violence. She asked, among other things:

- When did your pain begin?
- Have you fallen or bumped into anything?
- Have you had other injuries in the past?

The nurse understood that a patient might not reveal concerns about violence in front of the person who had caused the injury and had begun taking the history only after asking, "Is your friend Maria the only person who is with you today?"

What this nurse forgot is that not all assaulters are male, not all adult partnerships are heterosexual, and not all victims are younger than their assaulters. Had Maria been the person involved in violence upon Hannah, she would not have been able to say so with Maria standing there looking helpful.

An improved practice would be to ask Maria to leave the room and then ask Hannah about *any* individual who has been violent or about whom she has anxieties.

Later, the examining nurse practitioner did see Hannah alone during the physical examination. Although it appeared that the abdominal pain was not due to direct physical injury, there were healing bruises on her arms and legs. The nurse practitioner asked, "Is there anything about these bruises you would like to talk about?" Hannah at first said no, then gulped deeply and said, "Yes, I guess there is." She then related that on the previous weekend, she had been kicked and punched by her younger brother, who was deeply offended by the relationship Hannah has with Maria and demanded that Maria never come to a family event in the future. Hannah had not admitted this to Maria because she was afraid of causing stress in their relationship, and in fact, this tension had contributed to the onset of pain.

With Hannah's honest admission, the nurse practitioner was able to suggest that open communication between Hannah and Maria would be appropriate and that the couple might benefit from participation in some form of supportive counseling in which they could jointly consider how to manage the relationship Hannah wanted desperately to maintain with her birth family.

References

25th anniversary: Families in a changing world. (1996). *Journal of Comparative Family Studies, 27*(2), 175–187.

Aday, L. A. (2001). *At risk in America* (2nd ed.). San Francisco: Jossey-Bass.

AHRQ. (2001). Community-based participatory research: Conference report. Retrieved June 12, 2004, from http://www.ahrq.gov/about/cpcr/cbpr/cbpr1.htm

Allison, D. (1999). Mama and mom and dad and son. In K. Kleindienst (Ed.), *This is what lesbian looks like: Dyke activists take on the 21st century.* Ithaca, NY: Firebrand Books.

American Academy of Pediatrics. (1999). *Child abuse and neglect.* The Medem Network. Retrieved October 14, 2003, from http://www.medem.com/MedLB/article_detaillb.cfm?article_ID=ZZZ3S3DRUDC&sub_cat=355

American Red Cross. (2003). *Military members and families.* Retrieved October 14, 2003, from http://www.redcross.org

Anonymous. (1995). California RNs battle moves to cut care for 'illegals.' *American Journal of Nursing, 95*(2), 75, 80.

Armstrong, P. (1996). Resurrecting 'the family': Interring 'the state.' *Journal of Comparative Family Studies, 27*(2), 221–248.

Arrillaga, P. (2003). Timmie's choice: Teen ends five-year custody battle with decision to stay in South Dakota (Domestic News) [LexisNexis]. Associated Press. Retrieved October 13, 2003.

Associated Press. (2003a). Lawsuit challenges partnership ordinance. Portland, Maine.

Associated Press. (2003b). Special Forces soldier charged in wife's slaying hangs himself. Fayetteville, NC: Associated Press State & Local Wire.

Associated Press. (2003c). Doctors' group votes for OHP damages cap. Portland, OR: Associated Press.

Bailey, J. M. (1999). Homosexuality and mental illness. *Archives of General Psychiatry, 56*(10), 883–884.

Belsky, J. (2002). Quantity counts: Amount of child care and children's socioemotional development. *Journal of Developmental and Behavioral Pediatrics, 23*(3), 167–170.

Bilbrey, S. L. (2002). Dancing Nancy: The harmful and illogical dance among Alabama courts over supervised visitation between gay parents and their children. *Law and Psychology Review, 26*(Spring).

Bjerklie, D. (2003, November 10). Hazard pay for grandma? *TIME,* p. 117.

Bolton, E. E., Litz, B. T., Glenn, D. M., Orsillo, S., & Roemer, L. (2002). The impact of homecoming reception on the adaptation of peacekeepers following deployment. *Military Psychology, 14*(3), 241–251.

Braus, P. (1998). When the helpers need a hand. *American Demographics, 20*(9), 66–70.

Brennan, S., & Noggle, R. (1997). The moral status of children: Children's rights, parents' rights, and family justice. *Social Theory and Practice, 23*(1), 1–26.

Brown, E. F., Limb, G. E., Munoz, R., & Clifford, C. A. (2001). *Title IV-B child and family services plans: An evaluation of specific measures taken by states to comply with the Indian Child Welfare Act.* Portland, OR: National Child Welfare Association and Casey Family Programs.

Bureau of Labor Statistics. (2002). *Workers on flexible and shift schedules in 2001 summary.* Washington, DC: U.S. Department of Labor.

Burgher, V. (2003, June 11). Rights rift gets personal; debate on gay registry law. *Newsday,* p. 6.

Cahill, T. (2003). *You assumed wrong* [Academic Search Elite]. Retrieved October 13, 2003.

Callahan, A. (1996). Family reunification: Bringing fathers home. *Journal of Housing and Community Development, 53*(6), 25–27.

Casper, L. M., & O'Connell, M. (1998). Work, income, the economy, and married fathers as child-care providers. *Demography, 35*(2), 243–250.

Centers for Medicare and Medicaid Services. (2003). *State child health insurance program plan activity map.* Retrieved November 13, 2003, from http://cms.hhs.gov/schip/chip-map.asp

Chung, W. S., & Pardeck, J. T. (1997). Explorations in a proposed national policy for children and families. *Adolescence, 32*(126), 426–436.

Clark, N. M., Gong, M., Schork, M. A., Maiman, L. A., Evans, D., Hurwitz, M. E., et al. (1997). Improving care of minority children with asthma: Professional education in public health clinics. *Pediatrics, 99*(2), 157–164.

Clark, W. M., & Serovich, J. M. (1997). Twenty years and still in the dark? Content analysis of articles pertaining to gay, lesbian, and bisexual issues in marriage and family therapy journals. *Journal of Marital and Family Therapy, 23*(3), 239–254.

Cohen, M. D. (1996). *Dirty details: The days and nights of a well spouse.* Philadelphia: Temple University Press.

Collins, R. (1996). Love and property. In S. J. Ferguson (Ed.), *Mapping the social landscape.* Mountain View, CA: Mayfield Publishing Company.

Coontz, S. (1992). *The way we never were: American families and the nostalgia trip.* New York: Basic Books.

Cordes, H. (2003, July 2). Rights battle turns to Nebraska: Overturning the state's defense of marriage act is a key goal. *Omaha World Herald,* p. 1a.

Cowen, P. S., & Reed, D. A. (2003). Effects of respite care for children with developmental disabilities: Evaluation of an intervention for at risk families. *Public Health Nursing, 19*(4), 272–283.

Crow Dog, M., & Erodes, R. (1996). Civilize them with a stick. In S. J. Ferguson (Ed.), *Mapping the social landscape.* Mountain View, CA: Mayfield Publishing.

Crystal. (2003, October 13). To the man who spit on me . . . [blog]. *LiveJournal.* Retrieved October 14, 2003, from http://www.livejournal.com/users/being_homeless/52934.html

Cussins, C. (1998). Producing reproduction: Techniques of normalization and naturalization in infertility clinics. In H. R. Sarah Franklin (Ed.), *Reproducing reproduction.* Philadelphia: University of Pennsylvania Press.

Death with Dignity National Center. (2003). *Death with dignity: The law.* Retrieved November 14, 2003, from http://www.deathwithdignity.org/law/

Dellios, H., & Rubin, B. M. (2003, October 4). Guatemala grapples with black market for adopted babies. *Chicago Tribune.*

Delone, S., & Tomlinson, R. (2002, October 22). *Immigrant eligibility for Medicaid and SCHIP.* Centers for Medicare and Medicaid Services. Retrieved October 14, 2003, from http://www.cms.hhs.gov/immigrants/

Don't I count? (1997). *The Hastings Center Report.*

Eley, M. G. (2002). Making the homeschool connection. *Educational Leadership, 59*(7), 54–55.

Ellenchild, W. J., & Spielman, M. L. (1996). Ethics in the neonatal intensive care unit: Parental perceptions at four years postdischarge. *Advances in Nursing Science, 19*(1).

Environmental Defense. (2003). *Scorecard.* Retrieved November 13, 2003, from http://www.scorecard.org/

Fenton, J. J., Catalano, R., & Hargreaves, W. (1996). Effect of Proposition 187 on mental health service use in California: A case study. *Health Affairs, 15*(1), 182–190.

Fost, D. (1996, April). *Child-free with an attitude* [FirstSearch]. Retrieved October 13, 2003.

Freudenberg, N. (2001). Jails, prisons, and the health of urban populations: A review of the impact of the correctional system on community health. *Journal of Urban Health, 78*(2), 214–235.

Fujiura, G. T. (2000). Trends in demography of childhood poverty and disability. *Exceptional Children, 66*(2), 187–199.

Gaines, D. (1996). Teenage wasteland: Suburbia's dead-end kids. In S. J. Ferguson (Ed.), *Mapping the social landscape.* Mountain View, CA: Mayfield Publishing.

Garasky, S., Greder, K., & Brotherson, M. J. (2003). Empowerment through involvement: Iowa's experience with welfare reform. *Journal of Family & Consumer Sciences, 95*(3), 21–26.

Glassner, B. (2000). *The culture of fear: Why Americans are afraid of the wrong things.* New York: Basic Books.

Glazer, S. S., Galanter, M., Megwinoff, O., Dermatis, H., & Keller, D. S. (2003). The role of therapeutic alliance in network therapy: A family and peer support-based treatment for cocaine abuse. *Substance Abuse, 24*(2), 93–100.

Goode, E. (2001, May 9). Study says gays can shift sexual orientation. *New York Times,* p. 24.

Governor signs legislation expanding KidCare and Family Care. (2003). *Illinois Government News Network.* Retrieved November 13, 2003, from http://www.illinois.gov/PressReleases/ShowPressRelease.cfm?SubjectID=1&RecNum=2177

Griscom, J. L. (1998). The case of Sharon Kowalski and Karen Thompson: Ableism, heterosexism, and sexism. In P. S. Rothenberg (Ed.), *Race, class, and gender in the United States.* New York: St. Martin's Press.

Haider, S. J., Jacknowitz, A., & Schoeni, R. F. (2003). Welfare work requirements and child well-being: Evidence from the effects on breast-feeding. *Demography, 40*(3), 479–497.

Harrington, M. (1998). The care equation. *American Prospect,* 39, 61–66.

Harris, C. (2003). *Can doctors refuse to treat GLBT patients?* Human Rights Campaign. Retrieved October 13, 2003, from http://www.hrc.org/issues/family/

Haywood, J. L., Goldenberg, R. L., Bronstein, J., Nelson, K. G., & Carlo, W. A. (1994, August). Comparison of perceived and actual rates of survival and freedom from handicap in premature infants. *American Journal of Obstetrics and Gynecology, 171*(2).

Head Start Bureau. (2003). *Head Start Program fact sheet.* Administration on Children, Youth, and Families. Retrieved November 14, 2003, from http://www2.acf.dhhs.gov/programs/hsb/research/2003.htm

Heimer, C. A., & Staffen, L. R. (1998). *For the sake of the children.* Chicago: University of Chicago Press.

Hertz, R., & Ferguson, F. I. T. (1996). Child care choice and constraints in the United States: Social class, race and the influence of family views. *Journal of Comparative Family Studies* (Summer), 249–280.

Hollinger, J. H. (1998). *A guide to the Multiethnic Placement Act of 1994 as amended by the interethnic adoption provisions of 1996.* Administration for Children and Families. Retrieved October 13, 2003, from http://www.acf.hhs.gov/programs/cb/publications/mepa94/

Hyden. (2001). For the child's sake: Parents and social workers discuss conflict-filled parental relations after divorce. *Child and Family Social Work, 6*(2), 115–128.

Illinois Christian Home Educators. (2003). *Homeschool law in Illinois.* Retrieved October 14, 2003, from http://www.iche.org/homeschool_law.htm

Illinois KidCare. (2003). Retrieved November 13, 2003, from http://www.kidcareillinois.com/index.html

Jensen, P. S., Martin, D., & Watanabe, H. (1996). Children's response to parental separation during Operation Desert Storm. *Child and Adolescent Psychiatry, 35*(4), 433–441.

Johnson, J. (1998, March 5). Ohio's failing grade on welfare reform. *Cleveland Call and Post,* p. 4A.

Jones, G., & Merl, J. (2003, August 17). Davis would sign domestic partners bill. *Los Angeles Times,* p. 6.

Karner, T. X. (1998). Professional caring: Homecare workers as a fictive kin. *Journal of Aging Studies, 12*(1), 69–82.

Kennedy, J. (1997). Personal assistance benefits and federal health care reforms: Who is eligible on the basis of ADL assistance criteria? *Journal of Rehabilitation, 63*(3), 40–46.

Kozol, J. (1991). *Savage inequalities.* New York: Crown.

Krakauer, J. (2003). *Under the banner of heaven.* New York: Doubleday.

Ku, L., & Freilich, A. (2001). *Caring for immigrants: Health care safety nets in Los Angeles, New York, Miami, and Houston.* Washington, DC: The Urban Institute.

Lara, M., Nicholas, W., Morton, S., Vaiana, M. E., Genovese, B., & Rachelefsky, G. (2002). *Improving childhood asthma outcomes in the United States: A blueprint for policy action.* Washington, DC: RAND.

Lee, C. M., & Duxbury, L. (1999). Employed parents' support from partners, employers, and friends. *Journal of Social Psychology, 138*(3), 303.

Leonard, A. S. (1997). Equal protection and lesbian and gay rights. In M. Duberman (Ed.), *A queer world.* New York: New York University Press.

Lines, P. M. (2000). When home schoolers go to school: A partnership between families and schools. *Peabody Journal of Education, 75*(1 & 2), 159–186.

Llewellyn, G., Dunn, P., Fante, M., Turnbull, L., & Grace, R. (1999). Family factors influencing out-of-home placement decisions. *Journal of Intellectual Disability Research, 43*(3), 219–233.

Luke, K. P. (2002). Mitigating the ill effects of maternal incarceration on women in prison and their children. *Child Welfare, 81*(6), 929–949.

Mancini, D. L., & Archambault, C. (2000, August 23). *What recent research tells us about military families and communities.* Paper read at Department of Defense Family Readiness Conference.

Martin, M. (2003, June 5). Assembly OKs expanding partners' rights. *The San Francisco Chronicle,* p. 21.

Masterson, K. (2003). Financial worries mount as states begin to comply with sweeping federal education law. Hartford, CT: Associated Press.

Meier, J. S. (2003). Symposium: Domestic violence, child custody, and child protection: Understanding judicial resistance and imagining the solutions. *American University Journal of Gender, Social Policy and the Law,* 657.

Min, S. J. (2003, August 13). Home away from Seoul. *AsianWeek,* p. 16.

Moore, M. (2003). *Bowling for Columbine: About the film.* Retrieved February 29, 2004, from http://www.michaelmoore.com

Morone, J. (2003). *Hellfire nation: The politics of sin in American history.* New Haven: Yale University Press.

Moskowitz, E. H. (1995). *In the courts: Two mothers* (March/April) [FirstSearch]. Retrieved January 7, 1999.

Napolitano, J. (2003, July 19). University enacts gay benefits. *The New York Times,* p. 10.

National Center for Chronic Disease Prevention and Health Promotion. (2003a). *BMI for adults formula.* Division of Nutrition and Physical Activity. Centers for Disease Control and Prevention. Retrieved October 27, 2003, from http://www.cdc.gov/nccdphp/dnpa/bmi/bmi-adult-formula.htm

National Center for Chronic Disease Prevention and Health Promotion. (2003b). *Defining overweight and obesity.* Division of Nutrition and Physical Activity. Centers for Disease Control and Prevention. Retrieved October 27, 2003, from http://www.cdc.gov/nccdphp/dnpa/obesity/defining.htm

National Center for Environmental Health. (2003a). *Basic facts about asthma.* Air Pollution and Respiratory Health Branch. Centers for Disease Control and Prevention. Retrieved October 27, 2003, from http://www.cdc.gov/nceh/airpollution/asthma/faqs.htm

National Center for Environmental Health. (2003b). *CDC-funded asthma activities by state and type of funding.* Air Pollution and Respiratory Health Branch. Centers for Disease Control and Prevention. Retrieved October 27, 2003, from http://www.cdc.gov/nceh/airpollution/asthma/asthmaAAG.htm

National Center for Health Statistics. (1999). National Hospital

Ambulatory Medical Care Survey: 2002 Emergency Department Summary. Retrieved from http://www.cdc.gov/nchs/data/ad/ad340.pdf

National Center for Health Statistics. (2000). *Health insurance coverage.* Centers for Disease Control and Prevention. Retrieved November 13, 2003, from http://www.cdc.gov/nchs/fastats/hinsure.htm

Nicholson, R. H. (1997, January/February). In the family's best interests. *The Hastings Center Report.* Retrieved January 7, 1999, from FirstSearch/BSSI97007267.

Norton, S. A., Kenney, G. M., & Ellwood, M. R. (1996). Medicaid coverage of maternity care for aliens in California. *Family Planning Perspectives, 28*(3), 108–112.

Nunez, R. C. (1995). Family values among homeless families. *Public Welfare, 53,* 24–32.

Nutrition, Physical Activity, and Obesity Prevention Program. (2003). *Resource guide for nutrition and physical activity interventions to prevent obesity and other chronic diseases.* Centers for Disease Control and Prevention.

Office of Medical Assistance. (2003). *Oregon Health Plan: An overview.* Oregon Department of Human Services. Retrieved November 14, 2003, from http://www.dhs.state.or.us/healthplan/overview.html

Oregon Department of Human Services. (2000). *Oregon's Death with Dignity Act: The second year.* Retrieved November 14, 2003, from http://www.dhs.state.or.us/publichealth/chs/pas/pascdsm3.cfm

Oregon governor backs off new state drug rules. (2003). NewsRx, *Health & Medicine Week.* Retrieved November 14, 2003, from http://www.NewsRx.net

Oregon Health Services Commission. (2003). *Prioritization of health services: A report to the governor and the 72nd Oregon legislative assembly.* Salem, OR: Oregon Health Services Commission.

Pallaschm, A. (2003, July 2). Cook County certifies gay couples. *Chicago Sun-Times,* p. 3.

Patrick, M. D. (2003). Immigration law, same-sex partnerships, and US immigration law. *New York Law Journal, 230,* 3.

Paul, P. (2001). *Childless by choice* (23) [Periodical Abstracts]. Retrieved October 13, 2003.

Physicians for Reproductive Choice and Health, & The Alan Guttmacher Institute. (2003, January). *An overview of abortion in the United States.* Retrieved June 12, 2004, from http://www.guttmacher.org/pubs/abslides/abort_slides.pdf

Pierce, P. F., Vinokur, A., & Buck, C. L. (1998). Effects of war-induced maternal separation on children's adjustment during the Gulf War and two years later. *Journal of Applied Social Psychology, 28*(14), 1286–1311.

Ragone, H. (1998). Incontestable motivations. In S. Franklin & H. Ragone (Eds.), *Reproducing reproduction.* Philadelphia: University of Pennsylvania Press.

Ramirez, A. (2002–2003). The shifting sands of school finance. *Education Leadership, 60*(4).

Reilly, J., & Martin, S. (1995). *Responding to a disclosure of child abuse* (Fact sheet 95–12). Reno, NV: University of Nevada Cooperative Extension.

Rich, S. (1998, October 31). Welfare to work. *The Circle,* p. 15.

Schroeder, C., & Ward, D. (1998). Women, welfare, and work: One view of the debate. *Nursing Outlook, 46.*

See, C. (1996). *Dreaming: Hard luck and good times in America* (Reprint ed.). Berkeley: University of California Press.

Seelye, K. Q. (1997, July 15). Girls were hit on flight, attendants say. *New York Times.*

Senator promotes national version of Oregon health plan. (2003).

NewsRx. *Managed Care Weekly Digest.* Retrieved November 14, 2003, from http://www.NewsRx.net

Shea, C. P. (2000). *Mimicking nature by designing out waste.* Florida Sustainable Communities Center. Retrieved November 13, 2003, from http://sustainable.state.fl.us/fdi/fscc/news/world/0008/eco-in.htm

Shelton, B. (2003). *Washington State's homeschool law.* Homeschool Oasis. Retrieved October 14, 2003, from http://www.homeschooloasis.com/art_wa_st_hs_law.htm

Silverman, B. S. (2002). The winds of change in adoption laws: Should adoptees have access to adoption records? *Family Court Review, 39*(1), 85–103.

Stunkard, A. J., & Wadden, T. A. (1993). *Obesity: Theory and therapy.* Centers for Disease Control and Prevention. Retrieved October 27, 2003, from http://www.cdc.gov/nccdphp/dnpa/obesity/consequences.htm

Sullivan, C. G. (1996). The partnership for personal responsibility. *Public Welfare, 54,* 26–30.

Tacket, A., Nurse, J., Smith, K., Watson, J., Shakespeare, J., Lavis, V., Cosgrove, K., Mulley, K., & Feder, G. (2003). Routinely asking women about domestic violence in health settings. *BMJ: British Medical Journal, 327*(7416).

Tarkka, M.-T., Paunonen, M., & Laippala, P. (1999). Social support provided by public health nurses and the coping of first-time mothers with child care. *Public Health Nursing, 16*(2), 114–119.

Task force on state welfare reform issues status report. (1999, March 10). *New York Amsterdam News,* p. 18.

Thompson, P. J., & Harm, N. J. (2000). Parenting from prison: Helping children and mothers. *Issues in Comprehensive Pediatric Nursing, 23*(2), 61–81.

Trost, J. (1996). *Family structure and relationships: The dyadic approach* [Journal]. Retrieved January 7, 1997.

U.S. Department of Health and Human Services. (2003). *Asthma prevalence, health care use and mortality, 2000–2001.* Centers for Disease Control and Prevention. Retrieved October 27, 2003, from http://www.cdc.gov/nchs/products/pubs/pubd/hestats/asthma/asthma.htm

Vidal de Haymes, M., & Simon, S. (2003). Transracial adoption: Families identify issues and needed support services. *Child Welfare, 82*(2).

Wall, S. N., & Partridge, J. C. (1997). Death in the intensive care nursery: Physician practice of withdrawing and withholding life support. *Pediatrics, 99*(1).

Weinberg, D. H. (2003). Press briefing on 2002 income and poverty measures. Washington, DC: U.S. Census Bureau.

Weston, K. (1996). Families we choose: Lesbians, gays, kinship. In S. J. Ferguson (Ed.), *Mapping the social landscape.* Mountain View, CA: Mayfield Publishing.

Widerburg, B. (2003). *Oregon Death with Dignity Act: Fifth year report.* Oregon Department of Human Services. Retrieved November 14, 2003, from http://www.dhs.state.or.us/news/2003news/2003-0305.html

Wooden, W. S. (1996). Kicking back at 'Raging High.' In S. J. Ferguson (Ed.), *Mapping the social landscape.* Mountain View, CA: Mayfield Publishing.

Wright, V. C., Schieve, L. A., Reynolds, M. A., & Jeng, G. (2003). *Assisted reproductive technology surveillance—United States, 2000* (52[SS09]). Centers for Disease Control and Prevention. Retrieved October 13, 2003, from http://www.cdc.gov/mmwr/preview/mmwrhtml/ss5209a1.htm

Wu, B. (2003). *Lethal legacy: A comprehensive look at America's dirtiest power plants.* Washington, DC: U.S. Public Interest Research Group.

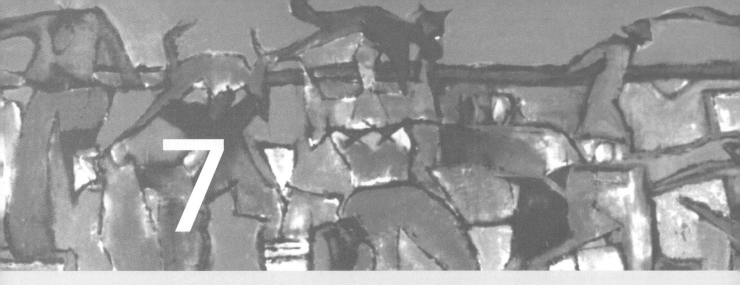

7

Sociocultural Influences on Family Health

Eleanor G. Ferguson-Marshalleck, RN, MPH, PhD • *Jung Kim Miller, RN, PhD*

CRITICAL CONCEPTS

- *Ethnicity* and *social class* are two prime molders of *family values*, family behaviors, and family structure and function.
- There is growth in ethnic diversity and the increasing disparity between *social classes* in the United States.
- There is a relationship between culture, health beliefs and practices, family health, and family coping behaviors.
- There are differences in family health status and

- health-related behaviors of families from different cultural groups.
- Ethnicity and social class and the interaction of these two variables influence family health.
- Incorporating cultural and socioeconomic assessment into the care of families is important.
- Nursing intervention strategies that enhance *cultural* sensitivity and competency improve the care of culturally diverse families.

INTRODUCTION

The influence of culture is pervasive. *Culture* intersects with all aspects of family life including family health, value systems, functions, and behavior. For the purpose of this chapter, culture is defined as sets of shared worldviews and adaptive behaviors derived from simultaneous membership in a variety of contexts such as religious background, nationality and ethnicity, social class, occupation, and political leanings. Two variables of culture and their interaction with family will be the focus of this chapter: *ethnicity* and *social class*. The family's social class plays a primary role in shaping family behavior, particularly family lifestyle, but basic to the discussion of sociocultural influences are the essential concepts of *culture, ethnicity*, and *socioeconomic status*. These influences shape family behaviors, including health behaviors.

This chapter discusses and explains some of the complex sociocultural influences on family health. It begins with a description of the growth in ethnic diversity in the United States. The chapter examines the influence of culture on the family and the extent to which health beliefs and practices, family values, and *family coping* styles influence family health. The chapter explores selected ethnic group, social class structure, and poverty as decisive factors in family health, and identifies how the health status of socially disadvantaged and minority populations differs from that of the dominant culture. These observations raise important questions for nurses and nursing students regarding social justice and the role of the family nurse as client advocate, which we discuss in the section on implications for family nursing.

COMMON THEORETICAL PERSPECTIVES

Although most family social science and nursing theories recognize culture as a significant variable in client health behaviors, these theories do not specifically focus on culture and cultural influence on family and family nursing care. This chapter introduces Madeline Leininger's culture care diversity and universality theory (Sunrise Model) as a basis for understanding culture, cultural diversity, and its influences on health and health care of the family. For more information on other theories, please refer to Chapter 2. According to Leininger (1997a), she developed her theory to address the phenomena of care and culture and to offer a comprehensive, holistic approach to "transcultural" nursing research and practice. The goals of the theory are to provide comparative dimensions that address "diversities" and "universalities" among and within cultures and to embrace care as the central concept to explain the well-being of people. Leininger formulated 13 assumptive and theoretical premises to support her position and theoretical tenets (Box 7–1).

Leininger also developed the Sunrise Model as a conceptual holistic research guide to enable researchers to discover multiple dimensions of culture care theory. Leininger's Sunrise Model summarizes the cultural and social structure that influences care expressions, patterns, and practices of individuals, families, groups, communities, and institutions. Nursing care within the model integrates generic folk care and professional systems that inform nursing care decisions and actions. Nursing care based on culture care preservation/maintenance, accommodation/negotiation, and repatterning/restructuring will ultimately lead to culturally congruent care (Leininger, 1997b, 2001). Leininger asserts that culturally based care is "the broadest holistic means to know, explain, interpret, and predict nursing care phenomena" (1997a, p. 39). This culturally congruent care approach is applied to individuals, families, groups, communities, and institutions in diverse health systems. Numerous studies have been conducted on various cultural groups using Leininger's culture care theory (Finn, 1994; Gordon, 1994; Lawrence & Rozmus, 2001; Luna, 1994; MacNeil, 1996; McFarland, 1997; Miller & Petro-Nustas, 2002). Family nursing can also apply Leininger's theory to assess family health patterns and practices, along with factors such as technology, religion and philosophy, kinship and social values, political and legal ideals, economics, and education, that influence holistic health and well-being.

Another model to consider in assessing the culture of a family is the cultural competence model developed by Larry Purnell (Purnell, 2002; Purnell & Paulanka, 1998). According to Purnell, the model is a conceptualization based on multiple theories, including family developmental theories. The schematic that depicts the model has three circles (rims), which encompass global society (outer layer/rim), community (second rim), family (third rim), and person. The inner circle is divided into 12 domains of culture, which consist of heritage, communication, family roles and organization, workforce, and so forth. The purpose of this model, according to Purnell, is to provide a framework for viewing the individual, family, or group within a unique ethnocultural envi-

Box 7–1 **THIRTEEN ASSUMPTIVE AND THEORETICAL PREMISES**

1. Care is the essence of nursing and a distinct, dominant, central, and unifying focus.
2. Care (caring) is essential for well-being, health, growth, survival, and to face handicaps or death.
3. Culturally based care is the broadest holistic means to know, explain, interpret, and predict nursing care phenomena and to guide nursing decisions and actions.
4. Nursing is a transcultural humanistic and scientific care discipline and profession with the central purpose of serving individuals, groups, communities, and institutions worldwide.
5. Care (caring) is essential to curing and healing, for there can be no curing without caring.
6. Culture care concepts, meanings, expressions, patterns, processes, and structural form of care vary transculturally with diversities (differences) and some universalities (or commonalities).
7. Every human culture has generic (lay, folk, or indigenous) care knowledge and practices and usually some professional care knowledge and practices that vary transculturally.
8. Culture care values, beliefs, and practices are influenced by and tend to be embedded in the worldview, linguistic, philosophical, religious (and spiritual), kinship, social, political, legal, educational, economic, technological, ethnohistorical, and environmental context of cultures.
9. Beneficial, healthy, and satisfying culturally based care influences the health and well being of individuals, families, groups, and communities within their environmental context.
10. Culturally congruent or beneficial nursing care can only occur when individual, group, family, community, or institutional care values, expressions, or patterns are known and used explicitly in appropriate and meaningful ways.
11. Culture care differences and similarities between professionals and client participants exist in all human cultures worldwide.
12. Cultural conflicts, imposition practices, cultural stresses, and pain reflect the lack of professional care knowledge to provide culturally congruent, responsible, and sensitive care.
13. The ethnonursing qualitative research method provides an important means to discover and accurately interpret emic and etic embedded, complex, and diverse culture care factors.

Source: Leininger, M. (1997a). Overview of the theory of culture care with the ethnonursing research method. *Journal of Transcultural Nursing, 8*(2), 32–52.

ronment and to interrelate characteristics of culture to promote congruence and facilitate the delivery of consciously competent care. This comprehensive model assists health care providers in all health disciplines in providing "holistic, culturally competent therapeutic interventions, health promotion, health maintenance, disease prevention, and health teaching across educational and practice settings" (Purnell & Paulanka, 1998, p. 7). The model also provides specific assessment guidelines for each of the 12 domains. For instance, in the family roles and organization domain, there are four specific areas that are assessed: head of household and gender role; prescriptive, restrictive, and taboo behaviors; family roles and priorities; and alternative life styles (Purnell & Paulanka, 1998).

Denham (2003) gives another perspective in the assessment of family culture. According to Denham,

"Family rituals are often culturally driven and closely associated with events that are relatively steadfast and predictable throughout family lives" (p. 306). Family rituals and routines provide the opportunity to assess similarities and differences within and between families in the ways that they utilize health information. She suggests that nurses need to determine family rituals and routines in their assessment. These family rituals and routines will also provide a basis for culturally sensitive interventions.

Leininger, Purnell, and Denham provide cultural approaches that can be a basis for understanding culture, cultural diversity, and its influences on health and health care of the family. Utilizing models/theories of culture allows one to incorporate a comprehensive inclusive conceptual framework that will guide family cultural assessment and lead to culturally competent family nursing care.

ETHNIC DIVERSITY AND GROWTH IN THE UNITED STATES

Ethnicity, a major component of culture, is defined as a group's sense of "peoplehood" based on a combination of race, religion, ancestral history, and nationality. It involves a multilayered sense of shared values and understandings within groups that fulfills a deep psychological need for identity and historical continuity (McGoldrick, 1993).

Since the 1960s and 1970s, there has been a steady growth in racial and ethnic diversity (also referred to as cultural diversity) in the United States. More than one resident in four is nonwhite or of Hispanic origin (U.S. Census Bureau, 2001). The white majority is shrinking and aging, whereas the African-American, Hispanic-American, Asian/Pacific Islander–American, and Native American populations are young and growing (U.S. Census Bureau, 2001). If the present rate of births and immigration to the United States continues, by the year 2025, national population projections suggest that Asian/Pacific Islander numbers will increase to 6.5 percent, persons of Hispanic origin to 18.2 percent, and African-Americans to 13.9 percent, and persons of European descent will decrease by 4 percent (U.S. Census Bureau, 2001).

Ethnic minorities, such as African-Americans, Asian/Pacific Islander–Americans Hispanic-Americans, and Native Americans make up a far larger proportion of the U.S. population than they did in the past. Representing 12 percent of the American population, African-Americans remain the largest minority group in the United States. This population showed a modest growth from 1990 to 2000, increasing in size from 30.5 million (12.3 percent of the total population) in 1990 to 35.3 million (12.8 percent) in 2000 (U.S. Census Bureau, 2001). African-Americans are not a homogeneous group, as is widely assumed. Although their ancestry is African and many descended from people who were enslaved, there are a number of blacks who immigrated voluntarily from Africa, Great Britain, the West Indian islands, and Central and South America, and who may not identify themselves as being African-American (Hopp & Herring, 1999; Spector, 2004). The present low rate of immigration, a high rate of infant mortality, and shorter life spans are factors that slow the rate of growth in the number of African-Americans (National Center for Health Statistics, 1992; U.S. Census Bureau, 2001).

The Asian and Pacific Islander population experienced growth from 7.5 million (3 percent of the total population) to 11.2 million (4.1 percent) in the 10-year period from 1990 to 2000. The rapid growth of this population over the past two decades is the result primarily of immigration. Asian-Americans include people from the diverse countries and cultures of Asia and the Indian subcontinent. This group consists of "at least 23 subgroups such as Asian Indian, Cambodian, Chinese, Filipino, Hmong, Japanese, Korean, Laotian, Thai, Vietnamese, and 'other Asian,' with 32 linguistic groups" (Inouye, 1999, p. 338). Despite these diversities, they share many common cultural characteristics that have been deeply influenced by Buddhism, Confucianism, and Taoism. However, many Asians are also greatly influenced by Christianity. Pacific Islanders include people from the Polynesian, Micronesian, and Melanesian groupings of islands in the North and South Pacific, such as Hawaiians, Samoans, Tongans, Tahitians, Guamanians, and Fijians. Native Hawaiians represent 57.8 percent of the U.S. Pacific Islander population (Casken, 1999).

From 1990 to 2000, people of Hispanic origin grew from 22.4 million (9.0 percent of the total population) to 32.4 million (11.8 percent). Hispanic-Americans are people or descendants of people from Mexico, Puerto Rico, Cuba, and Central and South America. Friedman (1998) explains that Hispanic-Americans are united by their common language (i.e., Spanish except for Brazilians who speak Portuguese), strong adherence to Roman Catholicism, and their common values and beliefs. The continued growth of the Hispanic population in the United States has been the result of both legal and illegal immigration and a high fertility rate (Friedman, 1998).

United States population growth today is overwhelmingly a function of growth within racial and ethnic minority populations. Some states, such as California, Florida, and New York, have become centers for immigration. Other states, particularly some in the Midwest, have more homogenous populations.

INFLUENCE OF CULTURE

All families are bearers of the culture of the society in which they live (Ablon & Ames, 1989) and of the culture with which they identify. In this sense, many families are multicultural because they are part of both the dominant culture of society and part of their particular subculture. The term *culture* refers to:

. . . those sets of shared world views and adaptive behaviors derived from simultaneous membership in a variety of contexts, such as ecological setting (rural, urban,

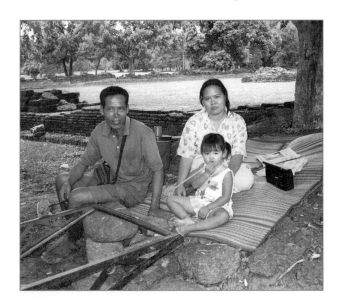

suburban), religious background, nationality and ethnicity, social class, gender-related experiences, minority status, occupation, political leanings, migratory patterns, and stage of acculturation; or values derived from belonging to the same generation, partaking of a single historical moment, or particular ideologies.
(Falicov, 1988, p. 336)

Purnell and Paulanka (1998) also define culture as "the totality of socially transmitted behavioral patterns, arts, beliefs, values, customs, lifeways, and all other products of human work and thought characteristic of a population of people that guide their worldview and decision making" (p. 2). Patterned lifeways, values, ideals, beliefs, and practices are embedded in these definitions and are transmitted from one generation to the next by the family. Leininger defines culture as "the lifeways of an individual or group with reference to values, beliefs, norms, patterns, and practices that are learned, shared, and transmitted intergenerationally" (1997a, p. 38). Spector (2004) describes culture as "the luggage" each of us carries. It is the sum of beliefs, values, norms, and practices, which is learned during the socialization of family members and is then transmitted to the next generation.

Family Acculturation

One of the factors that influences *family health* or well-being of a family in relation to culture is the family's level of acculturation. Acculturation is defined as the process of learning or adapting to a dominant host or new culture, and it occurs over time and at different rates and to different extents for different people (Marin & Gamba, 2003).

Acculturation does not necessarily mean the loss of ethnic identity or the loss of customs of one's culture (Friedman, Bowden, & Jones, 2003). Acculturation occurs on a continuum that ranges from adhering to the traditional values of an individual's homeland at the unacculturated end to adopting the mainstream values of the dominant group at the acculturated end (Kumabe et al., 1985; Locke, 1992; Spector, 2004). The process of acculturation may be influenced by factors such as time, reason for immigration, and education. Spector (2004) comments that in the United States the usual course of acculturation takes three generations.

According to Berry (2003), voluntary immigrants are likely to experience less difficulty with acculturation than those who are forced to immigrate to a new culture. Families who choose to immigrate are more open to adapting to a new culture because they are seeking educational and work opportunities as well as religious and political stability. A pilot study conducted by Friedman, Ferguson-Marshalleck, & Miller (2000) describes how some Jewish refugee families enjoyed religious and political freedom in the United States. One family member stated that "In my country, I needed to pray silently, now I can go to Temple without fear and I do not need to hide any more." Another person asserted that in America there is more personal freedom and human rights are respected.

The extent of acculturation shapes or alters the family values and health beliefs and practices that ultimately affect family health. A family's values guide the development of its norms and rules and serve as general guides to its behavior. Values involve the relationships between people, time dimension, relationship to community, perception of family roles and power, family communication, the relationship of human beings to nature (Kluckholm & Strodtbeck, 1961), and views of independence and interdependence (Lin & Liu, 1993). Some values are more central and influential than others. Given a competing set of demands, central or core values typically determine a family's priorities.

Relationships

Culturally derived values influence family health by setting priorities for making decisions and coping with life's stressors. For example, the value placed on relationships between people in part determines how the family and its members function in crisis. In some cultures, family needs and goals take precedence over individual needs and goals. Asian-Americans and Hispanic-Americans, in general, place greater emphasis than Anglo-Americans on the needs of family before the needs of individuals. Filial piety, ancestor worship, and respecting authority are important core family or central values for Asian-American families. Saving face (maintaining family honor) is another important Asian-American family value (Hong & Friedman, 1998; Friedman, 1998). Among Latino families, familism is seen as a core value (Suarez & Ramirez, 1999). *Familism* is defined as a social pattern in which family solidarity and tradition supersede individual rights and interests (Purnell & Paulanka, 1998). Members generally pull together, with primary and secondary kin supporting the family member(s) in need.

Time Dimension

Another family value that may affect family health is orientation to time. When present time is the focus rather than future time, family members may find it hard to change their lifestyle to avoid a potential health problem. For example, when family members appear to be healthy and the consequences of an unhealthy lifestyle are likely to become apparent only years later, necessary lifestyle modifications may be difficult to implement. A common example of this situation is the family in which the husband or father has essential hypertension. If the husband or father is from a culture that is primarily present oriented and he feels "well" and is able to function, he may deny the need to modify his dietary patterns and lifestyle and fail to adhere to his medication regimen (Friedman & Ferguson-Marshalleck, 1996). On the other hand, a family who is future oriented may focus more on disease prevention and health-promotion activities to avoid illness and improve its level of wellness.

Relationship to Community

The greater the congruence between a family's values and the wider community's values, the easier it is for its family members and the family to adjust to a new culture. Moreover, the greater the congruence, the greater the family's success in relating to its community (Friedman, 1998). When family values clash significantly with the values of the community and society in which the family resides, the family's rela-

tionship to its community may be strained. In such cases, families may believe they cannot obtain health and welfare services from their communities and so they "ask and receive little." Refugee families in a pilot study voiced that they first sought Armenian or Jewish community services because of ethnic and cultural similarity before they sought other public agencies. (Friedman, Ferguson-Marshalleck, & Miller, 2000). Families also may be discouraged from applying for assistance to community agencies that see them as less deserving or in some way "ineligible" for services. With diminished health or welfare services, family and individual health eventually suffers.

Family Roles, Power, and Communication

The level of acculturation also affects how family members perceive their roles and power relationships. Marin and Gamba (2003) cited several studies that focused on the impact of acculturation on gender roles in the family. For example, a study by Rosenthal, Rainieri, and Klimdis (1996) with Vietnamese adolescents found that traditional family and gender values declined as acculturation increased. Another study by Leaper and Valin (1996) with Mexican-American parents suggested that the acculturated parents tend to adopt more gender-egalitarian attitudes. Also, a study by Tang and Dion (1999) with Chinese university students showed that men held more traditional views of family hierarchy and social roles of men and women than did women.

In those families where marital partners are from the same cultural background and agree on family roles, family power distribution, and communication patterns, the common cultural understanding provides meaning, structure, and continuity. For example, in a study of 40 middle-income African-American families, J. L. McAdoo (1993) found that African-American spouses shared equally in the major decisions in the family and were satisfied with their marital lives regardless of family decision-making styles. Families in which mates are from different cultures may have differing expectations about family roles, communication, and power relationships. In these cases, family functioning may be affected negatively.

Culturally based conflicts frequently arise when family members from immigrant families have differing degrees of exposure to the wider American culture. For instance, some middle-aged immigrant Filipino parents on the West Coast do not expect to live with their children in their old age. A recent group of immigrant and native-born Filipinos, on the other hand, believe that children should take care of elderly parents (Miranda, McBride, & Spangler, 1998). Children may become more quickly acculturated to "the American way" in school. What and how they are taught in school may conflict with what and how they have been taught at home. As a result, culturally based conflicts often occur between the generations (Larrabee, 1973; Friedman, 1998). The degree of acculturation in terms of language may also cause conflicts. For instance, parents who do not speak English and children who speak only English may have conflicts or misunderstandings because of the language gap. This is evident in many Asian-American immigrant families, especially between the first generation of immigrant parents and the children born in the United States or children who immigrated when they were very young (Uba, 1994).

Family Coping Strategies

Ethnicity influences the ways in which families adapt to and cope with internal and external demands and changes. In turn, the strategies that families use to cope affect family health and family functioning.

Family coping is defined as positive problem-appropriate affective, cognitive, and behavioral responses that families and their subsystems use to solve a problem or reduce the stress produced by a problem or event (Friedman, 1992; Friedman, Bowden, & Jones, 2003). Family coping strategies develop and change over time in response to the stressors and demands experienced (Menaghan, 1983) and also differ across the family life cycle (Schnittger & Bird, 1993).

Various coping strategies are used to eliminate the stressor or demand, control the meaning of the stressor or demand, or reduce the stress or tension created by the stressor or demand. Coping strategies may be internal or external (Friedman & Ferguson-Marshalleck, 1996). Internal coping strategies rely on resources contained within the family, and external coping strategies depend on supports and resources outside of the family (McCubbin, Olson, & Larsen, 1991). Box 7–2 summarizes examples of both types of strategies.

Traditional or unacculturated ethnic families make extensive use of culturally derived, internal family coping strategies. Chinese and Vietnamese immigrant families provide a good example of ethnic differences

---

Box 7–2 TYPES OF FAMILY COPING STRATEGIES

Internal Family Coping Strategies

- Family group reliance, including delegation
- The use of humor and stress management tactics
- Increased sharing together: maintaining cohesiveness
- Controlling the meaning of the stressor/demand: cognitive refraining and passive appraisal
- Joint family problem solving
- Role flexibility
- Normalizing
- Limiting leisure time and recreational activities
- Accepting stressful events as a fact of life

External Family Coping Strategies

- Seeking information and professional help
- Maintaining active links with community groups and organizations
- Seeking and using social supports (informal and formal social support systems and self-help groups)
- Seeking and using spiritual supports
- Sharing concerns and experiences with relatives, friends, and neighbors

Adapted from Friedman, M. (1998). *Family nursing, theory, and practice* (3rd ed.). Norwalk, CT: Appleton & Lange.

in family coping patterns. Both Chinese and Vietnamese families commonly use the coping strategy of family group reliance and family cohesiveness. Consequently, in the face of family stressors, the extended family pulls together. Chinese families encourage interdependence and family loyalty and receiving and giving help between the generations (Lin & Liu, 1993).

Immigrant Vietnamese families use similar coping strategies. Gold (1993) quotes one Vietnamese family member's explanation of how his family deals with problems:

> *To Vietnamese culture, family is everything. There are aspects [coping strategies] which help us readjust to this society. . . . We solve problems because the family institution is a bank. If I need money—and my brother and my two sisters are working I tell them I need to buy a house. . . . Now I help them. They live with me and have no rent. The family is a hospital. If mom is sick, I, my children, and my brother and sister care for her. (p. 304)*

Research on ethnic differences in family coping is limited. One study conducted by Friedman (1985), looked at 55 families who had a child with cancer. Half of the families were Anglo and the other half Latino. Anglo families (mostly middle-class) reported that information seeking, the support of neighbors and friends, and the support of spouse were the most helpful coping strategies. On the other hand, Latino families (mostly working-class and lower-class Mexican-American families) reported that extended family support and spiritual support were most helpful. Latinos relied heavily on religion to cope with their children's cancer. Because culture and religion are so closely intertwined in Latin culture and most of the Latino families in this study were recent immigrants and unacculturated, the differences in coping between the two cultural groups were quite pronounced.

The Latino families in Friedman's study depended on primary and secondary kin to assist and support them with the array of demands created by childhood cancer. In those families who had recently emigrated from El Salvador and had no extended family support, family functioning was poorer. Friedman concluded that the absence of the families' natural social support system (the extended family) left a vacuum for these families and reduced their ability to cope. The inaccessibility of culturally appropriate social support and the reluctance of family members to use substitute social supports (e.g., health personnel, neighbors, friends) created personal and interpersonal difficulties in handling the stress of childhood cancer.

Family Health Beliefs and Practices

Purnell and Paulanka (1998) state that "culture is largely unconscious and has powerful influences on health and illness" (p. 2). Every cultural group possesses a system of beliefs and practices about health and illness (Helman, 1990; Spector, 2004). These include beliefs about, for instance, what a symptom is and means, when to seek help and whom to seek it from when one is ill, what symbolizes relief or cure, and who makes health care decisions. Cultures provide explanatory models of health and illness, which include the meaning, cause, process, prognosis, and treatment of illness, as well as maintenance of health (Kleinman, 1980).

Western societies typically root their explanations of disease and health in scientific findings; infection, mechanical injury, tumor growth, or stress account for many diseases. By contrast, non-Western families may have explanatory belief systems in which illness and disease are viewed as resulting from social or supernatural causes or from imbalances in the body. For instance, traditional Asian health care beliefs and practices, according to Hong and Friedman (1998), emanate from the Chinese culture, which teaches that health is a state of spiritual, psychological, and physical harmony. Violation of this harmony, or balance, causes illness and disease. For example, some Chinese individuals wear amulets—an idol or Chinese character painted in red or black ink and written on a strip of yellow paper—to ward off evil spirits and protect them from disharmony (Spector, 2004).

The view of what is an effective therapy generally stems from the beliefs about the cause of the health problem (Kleinman, 1980). If the root cause of disease is perceived as spiritual, prayer and other spiritual interventions are used. For example, spiritual interventions are sought by Mexican-Americans for certain "folk" and mental illnesses. In addition, some African-Americans believe that illness happens because of the "will of God" (Campinha-Bacote, 1998; Miranda et al., 1998) and that faith in God and prayer as a communicating link with God will bring them through their illnesses. Similarly, some Muslims perceive major illness as God's will and can find healing only through prayer (Lawrence & Rozmus, 2001).

If the root cause of disease is believed to be a problem with social interaction, individuals favor social interventions. For example, some native Hawaiians believe that there is a relationship between sickness and the breaking of social rules (Casken, 1999).

Similarly some Native Americans who believe that illness is a social phenomenon may execute elaborate, ritualized ceremonies, such as "sings" and sand paintings, for therapy (Adair et al., 1988).

Health beliefs about cause and therapy are translated into health care practices, which then affect the health status of the family and its members. Many Asian and Hispanic families use both Western and indigenous health care treatment. For example, some Asian-Americans use both Western and traditional medicine to treat chronic illness. They may undergo chemotherapy while at the same time receiving acupuncture treatments. In her study of Korean immigrants, Miller found that some Korean immigrants used traditional Eastern herbs and acupuncture for the purpose of health promotion and disease prevention. These same Korean immigrants sought Western practitioners when they needed more accurate diagnosis or fast relief from symptoms such as pain (Miller, 1988).

Most traditional health beliefs and practices, if not effective in terms of cure, are benign enough to have no negative consequences, unless they delay the decision to seek effective professional help (Helman, 1990). For example, a Hispanic family may delay seeking Western medical treatment because its members have identified a health problem as a folk illness that they expect to be alleviated by folk remedies. The folk remedies are not worsening the health problem, in all likelihood, but the delay in receiving treatment may worsen the problem.

In seeking Western health care, families may delay treatment because of the high value placed on self-control, not complaining about pain, and suppression of feelings (Hong & Friedman, 1998). African-American families who tend to be suspicious of health care professionals and who may feel socially and culturally alienated from available health care may delay seeking care. They will often withstand obvious symptoms of ill health and exhaust all home remedies known to family and friends before feeling forced to turn to the health care system for assistance (Friedman, 1998). In Asian-Indian culture, health care decisions are often discussed within the immediate family before outside help is sought because of the value placed on privacy and the desire to save face. Family input continues to play a significant role in important care decisions, even after a family member enters the health care system (Bhungalia & Kemp, 2002).

Conflicts between family members about health care beliefs and practices may adversely affect family health. These conflicts are often created by generational differences. The older generation in the family may maintain their traditional views of illness and appropriate interventions, whereas the younger generation may adopt Western health notions and health care practices. The two sets of beliefs and practices may clash, leaving the family divided and less adaptive and able to care for a family member with a major illness.

INFLUENCE OF SOCIOECONOMIC STATUS

Socioeconomic status is another cultural variable in determining how families perceive health. Because this variable is so crucial in understanding families, it is addressed explicitly. Social class has a pervasive effect on family life and each family member's life, especially within complex, heterogeneous societies such as the United States.

The terms *socioeconomic status*, *social status*, and *social class* (which are often used interchangeably in the sociological literature) are used to refer to large groups of persons who have relatively similar incomes, amounts of wealth, life conditions, life chances, and lifestyles (Ropers, 1991). A person's social class status is often determined by the family's social class; and the family's social class, in turn, is determined by occupational prestige, level of education, income, employment status, or a combination of these.

Like all other industrialized nations, the United States is stratified by class. A stratified society is marked by inequality, by differences among people that rank them as higher or lower on the scale (Gilbert & Kahl, 1987). Although social classes may be distinguished from each other, the lines of demarcation are not clear-cut. Income and wealth are indicators of social class. Available resources determine a person's or family's life conditions. The extent to which persons and families have access to and use resources reflects their social class. Power, prestige, and privilege are often manifestations of wealth and, hence, a family's social class (Ropers, 1991).

Increases in income inequality in the United States and the implications for working-class and poor families have been widely addressed in the sociological and public health literature (Braun, 1991; Gilbert & Kahl, 1987; McLaughlin & Stokes, 2002; Ropers, 1991; Wilkinson, 1996; Winnick, 1991). The rich have continued to become richer and the poor poorer (Braun, 1991; Peterson, 1993; Ropers, 1991; "Tax

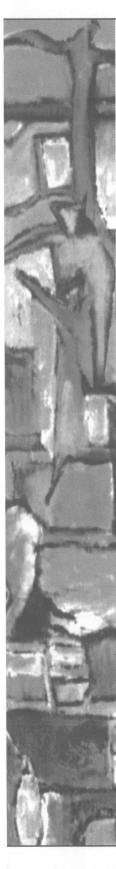

RESEARCH BRIEF

Purpose of Study

- The purposes of this study were to identify (1) the health seeking behaviors of Haitian parents for their school-aged children, (2) the barriers they experienced in obtaining desired health care services, and (3) their preventive health care practices and illness care for their children.

Methodology

- Interviews were conducted by using an interview guide and a comprehensive health access research form, which was developed by a multidisciplinary group of researchers representing nursing, psychology, education, and social work.
- An elementary school in an urban area of a southeastern state with approximately 1500 students of which 80% were of Haitian descent was selected as the setting for the study.
- Sixty-two Haitian family members with a child in the school participated in the study. Most of the participants were parents, of which 33 were mothers and 25 were fathers.
- The interview guide questions addressed the following three areas: health insurance, utilization of preventive health care services and illness care for their child, and illness care behaviors for their child when he or she was sick.

Results

- The most frequently cited reason for not receiving desired preventive health and dental care was the cost of care.
- Difficulty getting to the welfare office due to transportation problems and conflict with work were reported as a barrier for obtaining health insurance.
- Lack of knowledge on the eligibility requirements and criteria for government-supported health insurance coverage programs also served as a barrier.
- Almost all parents believed that eating good food and exercise were important for the health of their child.
- All parents believed strongly in the use of professional health services to maintain their child's health.
- Most parents rated their child's health as excellent or good.
- Parents reported the use of both traditional and nontraditional health care practices when their child was ill. Many parents reported having used tea for their child's illness; however, the use of home remedies and other ethnomedical treatments other than the use of tea was not as prevalent as expected. Also, many parents reported regularly using prayer when their child was ill.
- Generally parents held strong values regarding preventive health care.

Implications

- Educate parents and guardians about the availability of federal and state health insurance programs and eligibility requirements.
- Advocate for families in negotiating and obtaining governmental health insurance coverage.
- More extensive lobbying effort needs to be undertaken to ensure that common health problems in school-aged children are covered under state and federal insurance programs.
- Provide culturally sensitive care by understanding Haitian's attitudes, beliefs, and values toward seeking and obtaining governmental health insurance.

Source: Schantz, S., Charron, S. A., & Folden, S. L. (2003). Health seeking behaviors of Haitian families for their school aged children. *Journal of Cultural Diversity, 10*(2), 62–68.

Report Says," 1990; Wolff, 1995), a change characterized by the sociologist Winnick (1991) as a shift toward two societies, separate and unequal. The shift in the distribution of income and wealth and the consequent growing gap between rich and poor began in the early 1970s but accelerated during the Reagan administration in the 1980s because of the reduction of social programs serving poor people.

The increase in income inequality has adversely affected access to education and employment, particularly for lower-class and working-class families. This economic disparity and reduction of social programs has also affected the health and health care of families.

Poverty, Underclass, and Homelessness

Families with incomes below the poverty line make up an increasing proportion of families in the United States today. The overall percent of Americans living in poverty in 2002 increased to 12.1 percent, up from 11.7 percent in 2001 (Protor & Dalaker, 2003). The percent of persons living in poverty continued to differ significantly by race and ethnicity in 2002. Regardless of age, a higher percent of Hispanic- and African-American persons than non-Hispanic white persons were poor or near poor. The individuals and families who have suffered most from deterioration or stagnation in the economy and reductions in the level of governmental assistance are children, young families, older adults, and poorly educated and unskilled persons (Chilman, 1991; U.S. Census Bureau, 2001). Other individuals and families heavily affected by the economic conditions are African-American men, illegal immigrants, families headed by women, and residents of inner cities and economically depressed small towns and rural areas

There are two groups of poor families: those in temporary poverty and those in persistent poverty. The majority of those who are in temporary poverty escape it by obtaining jobs with wages sufficient for living or by joining extended family units to gain a combined income that will ameliorate the worst effects of poverty. Those in persistent poverty, primarily women and children, have a much more difficult time escaping from it (Friedman & Ferguson-Marshalleck, 1996).

Underclass is a term used to describe people in persistent poverty with attitudes, values, and lifestyles that do not conform to the values of mainstream American society (H. R. McAdoo, 1993). Because of the clash in values and behaviors between underclass families and the mainstream dominant culture, these families have a strained relationship with the wider community. This conflict makes it difficult for underclass families, who are stigmatized by the wider society, to obtain the resources needed to function at even a minimally acceptable level. Poor persons, particularly those in the underclass, are a vulnerable population who are living in poverty conditions with multiple, persistent stressors that undermine the physical, psychological, and economic health of the family and its members (Chilman, 1991).

Homelessness is another growing, significant family stressor for poor people. In a status report titled "Hunger and Homelessness in America's Cities," requests for emergency shelter by homeless families with children increased in 88 percent of the 25 cities that were surveyed in the United States (United States Conference of Mayors, 2002). This report also cited the fact that 82 percent of the cities reported an increase in the length of time people are homeless.

Homelessness is defined as losing one's possessions, living with relatives during hard times, or simply having no home. In the latter instance, families or individuals may or may not have temporary housing in a shelter. In the 1950s through the 1970s, most homeless persons had some form of shelter: "flophouses," single room–occupancy hotels, or mission shelters. However, many contemporary homeless people are literally sleeping on the streets. Being homeless subjects family members to a myriad of physical and psychosocial stressors.

Homeless families are likely to be socially isolated, with no regular or strong ties to family, friends, or other social networks. Their lack of social support magnifies their vulnerability to disabilities and deprivations (Rossi et al., 1987). Compared with those who have homes, the prevalence of mental illness is greater among the homeless, as is the prevalence of alcoholism and other forms of substance abuse (Aday,

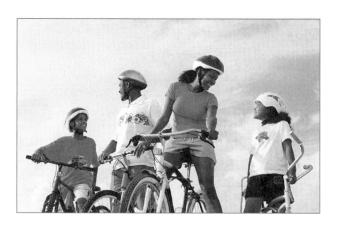

2001; U.S. Department of Health and Human Services, 1998).

> 66 Because of numerous stressors, poor people find it difficult to be future-oriented and concerned about healthy lifestyles. 99

Socioeconomic Status Effects on Health

A family's social class affects the family's lifestyle—or where and how the family lives—family members' health status and longevity, their educational and occupational opportunities, and a multitude of other life conditions (Lee & Estes, 1997). For example, Hussey (1997) in a study using data from the National Longitudinal Mortality Study found that injury mortality in young persons was closely linked with family income, education, household structure, and residential location. This study supports the evidence linking socioeconomic differential to inequality in life chances.

The more affluent an individual or family, the better their life conditions, the greater their access to preventive and therapeutic health care services, and the better their health status. Further, families from the upper and middle classes, regardless of ethnic background, tend to have better self-care behaviors. Because of numerous stressors, poor people find it difficult to be future-oriented and concerned about healthy lifestyles.

The correlation between social class and health holds true for both adults and children. For example, Starfield (1992) found that poor children are more likely to become ill and to have serious illnesses than children from higher-income families. The higher rates of serious health problems and the increased death rates from disease in children from poor families reflect exposure to environmental hazards, poor nutrition, inadequate preventive care, and poor access to medical care, all of which are a part of social class inequalities in life conditions and life chances. Research findings since the 1930s have demonstrated consistently that lower-class, economically distressed families are more likely to have poorer family health, less family stability, poorer marital adjustment, greater problems in family coping, and troubled family relationships (Voydanoff & Donnelly, 1998).

Socioeconomic status is linked to health status through multiple pathways including distribution of health care, psychosocial condition, health behaviors, and access to and quality of health care (Institute of Medicine, 2001; Seccomb, 2000). Being poor is a major barrier to obtaining access to the health care system (Spector, 2004). And, among the working poor and near-poor the lack of health insurance is a major hurdle according to a recent national survey of health care and health insurance coverage. Uninsured children and non-elderly adults are substantially less likely to visit health care facilities than their insured counterpart (National Center for Health Statistics, 2003).

THE INTERACTION OF ETHNICITY AND SOCIAL CLASS

While the separate influences of ethnicity and social class on family health are considerable, the influence of these two variables together may be profound. Certain ethnic and racial groups in the United States have become entrenched in poverty. Institutional racism often locks families into a state in which social class mobility is practically nonexistent. Therefore, these families tend to pass on their "inherited" class disadvantages from one generation to the next.

Gordon (1964) described the pronounced association between ethnic group membership and social class as *ethclass*. This intersection of ethnicity and social class produces identifiable dispositions and behavioral patterns in families and individuals. Social class and ethnicity in interaction define the basic conditions of life and simultaneously account for differences among ethnic groups with different social class positions. For instance, important commonalities are created among families because of their common cultural heritage and by virtue of being black in America. Despite these important commonalities, lifestyles and life chances vary drastically between affluent African-American families and poor African-American families.

Being from an ethnic family of color and being poor poses greater hazards to family and individual health than being either from an ethnic family of color that is not poor or from a poor white family. African-American and Hispanic children are nearly four times more likely than Anglo-American children to live in poverty, and indicators of poorer health status are clustered among these poor minority children (U.S. Census Bureau, 1997; U.S. Department of Health and Human Services, 2002).

In fact, race and ethnicity have a significant negative impact on health status primarily because ethnically and racially diverse families are more frequently disadvantaged socioeconomically (Cockerham, 1987). Hence, even though cultural background is linked to differences in individual health status, social class is more important in producing such variation. One glaring indication of this is the difference in infant mortality rates between socioeconomic classes. Babies of poor families, regardless of ethnic or racial background, die at twice the rate of babies of families who are not poor (Boone, 1989; Kramer, 1988; Lee & Estes, 1997).

The interaction of culture and social class may also substantially influence health care practices. For example, de la Torre (1993) speculates that ethnic families in the United States who are poor use folk medicine and home remedies more often, simply because they lack access to professional health care. Evidence to support this idea comes from a large survey of Mexican-Americans in Southern California (Keefe, 1981). Among Keefe's sample of Mexican-Americans, it was only the unacculturated, poor Mexican-American families who still used folk medicine to any great extent. Among the middle-class and more affluent Mexican-American families, the use of folk medicine had practically disappeared.

Contrary to Keefe's sample of Mexican Americans, Korean immigrants relied on Eastern herb and acupuncture treatment, regardless of their income and education. Miller (1990) in her study of 102 Korean immigrants reported that respondents with higher income ($40,000 and higher) made more visits to the Eastern doctors' offices for herbal medicines than their poor counterparts. This may have been because most herbs are rather expensive and poorer Korean immigrants could not as easily afford to buy them.

IMPLICATIONS FOR FAMILY NURSING PRACTICE, RESEARCH, EDUCATION, AND POLICY

The family's sociocultural background is central in shaping family values, beliefs, and behaviors, and in shaping specific health beliefs and practices. Social class and ethnic background (ethclass), both singly and in combination, affect families' health status. Because

of the centrality of sociocultural influences on family life and health, sensitivity to ethnicity, social class, and culture are imperative to nurses who are working with families. This section addresses implications for family nursing practice, research, education, and policy as it pertains to culture.

Practice

To effectively assist in the care of families from diverse cultures, ethnic groups, and social classes, family nurses must have a clear understanding of their own ethnic and social class identification and recognize their own potential and real biases (H. R. McAdoo, 1993). Health professionals are repositories of their own ethnic, religious, racial, and social class subcultures. They often believe that they can nullify their biases. However, it is only with continuing self-exploration and awareness of their preconceptions, attitudes, values, and beliefs that health professionals can develop an understanding and sensitivity to different cultures and social classes. One's awareness and sensitivity are never complete. Interpretations continue to arise that have cultural or social class connotations that may interfere with the process of providing services to clients (H. R. McAdoo, 1993).

In the words of De Vore and London (1993), "practice skills and techniques must be adapted to respond to the needs or dispositions of various ethnic [and class] groups" (p. 324). Further, cultural and socioeconomic assessments must be an integral component of family assessments (Table 7–1).

In addition, Purnell's Model for Cultural Competence is another assessment tool that could be used in the assessment of the family functions and family health. When caring for an immigrant family, it is important to assess not only their ethnic background but also the level of acculturation of each family member, because acculturation does not occur uniformly.

Research

Although some progress has been made in nursing research using Leininger's theory of Culture Care in studying various ethnic groups, the studies have been focused primarily on individuals within a group. A paucity of research still exists in studies directed at sociocultural influences focusing on the family and family health. More research studies are needed in the area of acculturation and family relations/functions

Table 7–1 SOCIOECONOMIC ASSESSMENT GUIDELINES

Assessment Criteria	*Questions*
Family composition and educational level	How many members compose this family's constellation? Who is the head of the household? How many members are under 18 years of age and over 65 years of age? What are the educational levels of family members?
Family perceptions of their housing and finances	How do family members feel about the adequacy of their housing arrangements and their finance situation?
Family financial resources	How many are gainfully employed full-time and part-time? What are their occupations? What is the household annual income? Who are the breadwinner(s) in the family? What are other financial resources (e.g., government, public funds, or assistance)? How does the family pay for health services? How well is the family managing financially?
Family expenses	How much is spent, on average, per month for the following? Rent or mortgage Food Child and/or elder care Health and dental care Recreational and leisure activities Transportation Utilities Other

Adapted from Friedman, M. (1998). *Family nursing, theory, and practice* (3rd ed.). Norwalk, CT: Appleton & Lange.

PRACTICAL TIPS FOR PROVIDING CULTURALLY COMPETENT CARE

- Be aware of one's own cultural and spiritual values and beliefs.
- Know one's own cultural bias and its influence on one's attitudes and behaviors.
- Learn about and respect values and beliefs of families from different ethnic and sociocultural backgrounds.
- Listen attentively and show respect.
- Avoid stereotyping of families from socioculturally diverse backgrounds.
- Recognize and accept common customs and behaviors of families.
- Understand and attend to the family's needs in the total context of their situation.
- Negotiate conflicts in ethnocultural health beliefs and practices.
- Recognize and commend immigrant families for their strengths and achievements.
- Link families to one another and to relevant resources in the community.
- Partner with families to create culturally appropriate intervention strategies.

and structural changes, such as the impact of migration on family functions and structures, and the levels of acculturation and families' health beliefs and health practices. Research studies are also needed in the area of programs and policy that take into account the context in which families of different ethnic and social class are functioning.

Education

As culturally diverse populations increase, nurses are faced with caring for families from cultures that are totally foreign to their own. Nurses cannot hope to achieve cultural competency unless culture and culturally competent nursing care directed to families are at the core of the nursing curriculum at the undergraduate and graduate levels. To prepare nurses to be more competent in caring for families from diverse ethnocultural backgrounds, students should be exposed to theoretical content as well as to practical experience in their programs of study. Culture-appropriate experiential learning opportunities must be included and teaching-learning strategies should feature role play, games, and activities that facilitate assessment of one's own cultural bias.

The nursing curriculum must also focus on the preparation, knowledge, and proficiency of nurses in the advocacy role for families of diverse backgrounds. Nurses are frequently required to assist families with diverse backgrounds in negotiating the health care and social services system, which requires knowledge of the advocacy role and social policy. Culture specific programs and services that support families from socioculturally diverse backgrounds need to be incorporated in nursing education.

Policy

Nurses should engage in planning coalitions to improve the health status of families from ethnic and socioeconomically diverse backgrounds by creating media support, organizing the community, lobbying legislatures, and presenting testimony at all levels of government: local, county, state, and federal. Nursing must take the leadership role in developing and implementing culturally appropriate and competent health care programs and services for families from socioculturally diverse backgrounds. It is imperative that nurses become aware of and are actively involved in the policy decision making process.

SUMMARY

- The influence of culture is pervasive. Ethnicity and socioeconomic or social class are two major variables of culture that are prime molders of family values and beliefs, family behaviors, and family lifestyle.
- The health status of individuals in the United States differs dramatically across ethnic groups and social classes. Major indicators show that the health status of minority Americans compared with whites is substantially poorer. The same is true in terms of social class differences: Health status is worse among poor Americans.
- The separate influences of ethnicity and of social class on family health are considerable, and the influence of the interaction of social class and culture (ethclass) may have a much more profound effect.
- The major implications for nursing include the following:
  1. Nurses must be knowledgeable about the socioeconomic and cultural factors that can be modified to facilitate the desired health-related behavioral change.
  2. Nurses must be sensitive and competent in working with families from the various ethnic and social classes. To do this, nurses need to assess their own cultural and class biases.
  3. Nurses must advocate for socioculturally diverse families.
  4. Nurse researchers need to focus on the influences of sociocultural factors and the intersection of ethnicity and socioeconomic status or social class (ethclass) on family and family health.

CASE STUDY ➤

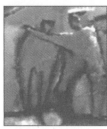

The Lindero family consists of Pedro, age 28; Margarita, his 23-year-old wife, three children, and Mrs. Josefina Lindero, Pedro's mother. Margarita delivered an infant boy, Ernesto, 6 weeks ago. He is currently experiencing upper respiratory distress. Margarita calls the nurse at the doctor's office to determine what to do for her baby. The nurse urges Margarita to bring the infant into urgent care. Pedro, who has just returned home from work, is informed by Margarita of her need to take Ernesto into urgent care. Josefina Lindero tells Pedro and Margarita that it is not necessary to take Ernesto to the hospital. She believes that it will do more harm to take the infant out of the house. Pedro agrees with his mother. Margarita calls the nurse back and informs her that she will not be bringing the baby to urgent care.

Case Study Discussion Questions
1. How would the nurse assist this family to resolve the situation?
2. What cultural factors need to be considered?
3. What family structure and functions need to be assessed?
4. What family nursing interventions would be culturally appropriate?
5. How would you apply the assessment instruments that appear in this chapter?

References

Ablon, J., & Ames, G. M. (1989). Culture and family. In C. L. Gilliss et al. (Eds.), *Toward a science of family nursing* (pp. 129–145). Menlo Park, CA: Addison-Wesley.

Adair, J., et al. (1988). *The people's health: Anthropology and medicine in a Navaho community*. Albuquerque: University of New Mexico Press.

Aday, L. A. (2001). *At risk in America: The health and health care needs of vulnerable populations in the United States* (2nd ed.). San Francisco: Jossey-Bass Publishers.

Berry, J. W. (2003). Conceptual approaches to acculturation. In K. M. Chun, P. B. Organista, & G. Marin (Eds.), *Acculturation: Advances in theory, measurement, and applied research* (pp. 17–37). Washington, DC: American Psychological Association.

Bhungalia, S., & Kemp, C. (2002, January). (Asian) Indian health beliefs and practices related to the end of life. *Journal of Hospice and Palliative Nursing, 4*(1), 54–58.

Boone, M. S. (1989). *Capital crime: Black infant mortality in America*. Newbury Park, CA: Sage.

Braun, D. (1991). *The rich get richer*. Chicago: Nelson-Hall.

Campinha-Bacote, J. (1998). African-Americans. In L. D. Purnell & B. Paulanka (Eds.), *Transcultural health care: A cultural competent approach* (pp. 53–73). Philadelphia: FA Davis.

Casken, J. (1999). Pacific Islander health and disease: An overview. In R. M. Huff & M. V. Kline (Eds.), *Promoting health in multicultural populations: A handbook for practitioners* (pp. 397–417). Thousand Oaks, CA: Sage.

Chilman, C. (1991). Working poor families: Trends, causes, effects, and suggested policies. *Family Relations, 40,* 191–198.

Cockerham, W. L. (1987). *Medical sociology* (2nd ed.). Englewood Cliffs, NJ: Prentice-Hall.

de la Torre, A. (1993, March 31). Access is vital in health care reform. *Los Angeles Times,* p. B7.

Denham, S. (2003). Relationships between family rituals, family routines, and health. *Journal of Family Nursing, 9*(3), 305–330.

De Vore, W., & London, H. (1993). Ethnic sensitivity for practitioners. In H. R. McAdoo (Ed.), *Family ethnicity: Strength in diversity* (pp. 317–331). Newbury Park, CA: Sage.

Falicov, C. J. (1988). Learning to think culturally. In H. A. Liddle, D. C. Breunlin, & R. C. Schwarts (Eds.), *Handbook of family therapy, training, and supervision* (pp. 335–357). New York: Guilford.

Finn, J. (1994). Culture care of Euro-American women during childbirth: Applying Leininger's theory to transcultural nursing discoveries. *Journal of Transcultural Nursing, 5*(2), 25–30.

Friedman, M. (1985). *Family stress and coping among Anglo and Latino families with childhood cancer*. Unpublished doctoral dissertation, University of Southern California, Los Angeles.

Friedman, M. (1992). *Family nursing: Theory and practice* (3rd ed.). Norwalk, CT: Appleton & Lange.

Friedman, M. (1998). *Family nursing, theory, and practice* (3rd ed.). Norwalk, CT: Appleton & Lange.

Friedman, M., & Ferguson-Marshalleck, E. (1996). Sociocultural influences on family health. In S. Hanson & S. Boyd (Eds.), *Family health care nursing: Theory, practice, and research* (pp. 81–100). Philadelphia: FA Davis.

Friedman, M., Bowden, V. R., & Jones, E. G. (2003). *Family nursing: Research, theory, and practice* (5th ed.). Upper Saddle River, NJ: Prentice Hall.

Friedman, M., Ferguson-Marshalleck, E., & Miller, J. K. (July, 2000). *Refugee families: The migration experience and family impact*. Paper presented at the International Family Nursing Conference, Chicago.

Gilbert, D., & Kahl, J. A. (1987). *The American class structure: A new synthesis* (3rd ed.). Chicago: Dorsey.

Gold, S. J. (1993). Migration and family adjustment: Continuity and change among Vietnamese in the United States. In H. R. McAdoo (Ed.), *Family ethnicity: Strength in diversity* (pp. 300–314). Newbury Park, CA: Sage.

Gordon, M. M. (1964). *Assimilation in American life*. New York: Oxford University Press.

Gordon, S. M. (1994). Hispanic cultural health beliefs and folk remedies. *Journal of Holistic Nursing, 12*(3), 307–322.

Helman, C. G. (1990). *Culture, health, and illness: An introduction for health professionals*. London: Wright.

Hong, G., & Friedman, M. (1998). The Asian-American family. In M. M. Friedman (Ed.), *Family nursing: Research, theory, and practice* (4th ed.) (pp. 547–566). Stamford, CT: Appleton & Lange.

Hopp, J., & Herring, P. (1999). Promoting health among Black American populations: An overview. In R. C. Huff & M. V. Kline (Eds.), *Promoting health in multicultural populations: A handbook for practitioners* (pp. 201–221). Thousand Oaks, CA: Sage.

Hussey, J. M. (1997). The effects of race, socioeconomic status, and household structure on injury mortality in children and young adults. *Maternal and Child Health Journal, 1*(4), 217–227.

Inouye, J. (1999). Asian American health and disease: An overview of the issues. In R. C. Huff & M. V. Kline (Eds.), *Promoting health in multicultural populations: A handbook for practitioners* (pp. 337–356). Thousand Oaks, CA: Sage.

Institute of Medicine. (2001). *The future of the public's health in the 21st century: Committee on assuring the health of the public in the 21st century, Board on Health Promotion & Disease Prevention, Institute of Medicine of the National Academics.* Washington, DC: The National Academies Press.

Keefe, S. E. (1981). Folk medicine among Mexican-Americans: Cultural persistence, change and displacement. *Hispanic Journal of Behavioral Science, 3*, 41–48.

Kleinman, A. (1980). *Patients and healers in the context of culture. An exploration of the borderland between anthropology, medicine, and psychiatry.* Berkeley: University of California Press.

Kluckholm, E., & Strodtbeck, E. (1961). *Variations in value orientations.* New York: Row, Peterson.

Kramer, J. M. (1988). Infant mortality and risk factors among American Indians compared to black and white rates: Implications for policy change. In W. A. Van Home & T. V. Tonnesen (Eds.), *Ethnicity and health* (pp. 89–115). Milwaukee: University of Wisconsin Institute on Race and Ethnicity.

Kumabe, K. I., et al. (1985). *Bridging ethnocultural diversity in social work and health.* Honolulu: University of Hawaii School of Social Work.

Larrabee, E. (1973). *Comments to Loretta Ford's Research. An Ethnic Perspective. Community Nursing Research: Collaboration and Completion.* Denver, CO: Western Institute of Higher Education Commission.

Lawrence, P., & Rozmus, C. (2001, July). Culturally sensitive care of Muslim patient. *Journal of Transcultural Nursing, 12*(3), 228–233.

Leaper, C., & Valin, D. (1996). Predictors of Mexican American mothers' and fathers' attitudes toward gender equality. *Hispanic Journal of Behavioral Sciences, 18*, 343–355.

Lee, P. R., & Estes, C. (Eds.) (1997). *The nation's health* (5th ed.). Sudbury, MA: Jones & Bartlett.

Leininger, M. (1997a). Overview of the theory of culture care with the ethnonursing research method. *Journal of Transcultural Nursing, 8*(2), 32–52.

Leininger, M. (1997b). Transcultural nursing research to transform nursing education and practice: 40 years. *Image: Journal of Nursing Scholarship, 29*(4), 341–347.

Leininger, M. (2001). *Culture care diversity and universality: A theory of nursing.* Boston: Jones and Bartlett.

Lin, C., & Liu, W. T. (1993). Relationships among Chinese immigrant families. In H. R. McAdoo (Ed.), *Family ethnicity: Strength in diversity* (pp. 271–286). Newbury Park, CA: Sage.

Locke, D. C. (1992). *Increasing multicultural understanding: A comprehensive model.* Newbury Park, CA: Sage.

Luna, L. (1994). Care and cultural context of Lebanese Muslim immigrants: Using Leininger's theory. *Journal of Transcultural Nursing, 5*(2), 12–20.

MacNeil, J. (1996). Use of culture care theory with Baganda women as AIDS caregivers. *Journal of Transcultural Nursing, 7*(2), 14–20.

Marin, G., & Gamba, R. (2003). Acculturation and changes in cultural values. In K. M. Chun, P. B. Organista, & G. Marin (Eds.), *Acculturation: Advances in theory, measurement, and applied research* (pp. 83–93). Washington, DC: American Psychological Association.

McAdoo, H. R. (1993). Ethnic families and conclusions. In H. R. McAdoo (Ed.), *Family ethnicity: Strength in diversity* (pp. 3–14, 332–334). Newbury Park, CA: Sage.

McAdoo, J. L. (1993). Decision making and marital satisfaction in African-American families. In H. R. McAdoo (Ed.), *Family*

ethnicity: Strength in diversity (pp. 109–119). Newbury Park, CA: Sage.

McCubbin, H. I., Olson, D., & Larsen, A. (1991). F-COPES: Family crisis oriented personal evaluation scales. In H. I. McCubbin & A. Thompson (Eds.), *Family assessment inventories for research and practice* (pp. 203–216). Madison: University of Wisconsin-Madison.

McFarland, M. (1997). Use of culture care theory with Anglo and African American elders in a long-term care setting. *Nursing Science Quarterly, 10*(4), 186–192.

McGoldrick, M. (1993). Ethnicity, cultural diversity and normality. In E. Walsh (Ed.), *Normal family processes* (2nd ed.) (pp. 331–360). New York: Guilford.

McLaughlin, D. K., & Stokes, S. (2002). Income in equality & mortality in the US counties: Does minority racial concentration matter? *American Journal of Public Health, 92*(1), 99–104.

Menaghan, E. G. (1983). Social stress and the family: Individual coping efforts and family studies. Conceptual and methodological issues [Special issue]. *Marriage and Family Review, 6*(112), 113–135.

Miller, J. E., & Petro-Nustas, W. (2002, July). Context of care for Jordanian Women. *Journal of Transcultural Nursing, 13*(3), 228–236.

Miller, J. K. (1988). Health beliefs and health utilization patterns of Korean immigrants. Unpublished doctoral dissertation. University of Southern California, Los Angeles.

Miller, J. K. (1990, October). Use of traditional health care by Korean immigrants to the United States. *Sociology and Social Research, 75*(1), 38–48.

Miranda, B. F., McBride, M. R., & Spangler, Z. (1998). Filipino-Americans. In L. D. Purnell & B. J. Paulanka (Eds.), *Transcultural health care: A cultural competent approach* (pp. 245–272). Philadelphia: FA Davis.

Murray, R. B., & Zentner, J. R (1993). *Nursing assessment and health promotion: Strategies across the life span* (5th ed.). Norwalk, CT: Appleton & Lange.

National Center for Health Statistics. (1992). *Health: United States, 1991.* Hyattsville, MD: U.S. Public Health Service.

National Center for Health Statistics. (2003). *Health, United States, 2003.* Hyattsville, MD: U.S. Public Health Service.

Peterson, J. (1993, April 11). Life in the United States, graded on the curve, *Los Angeles Times*, pp. Al, AI6.

Protor, B. D., & Dalaker, J. (2003). *Poverty in the United States: 2002* (U.S. Census Bureau, Current Population Reports, P60–222). Washington, DC: U.S. Government Printing Office.

Purnell, L. D. (2002, July). The Purnell model for cultural competence. *Journal of Transcultural Nursing, 133*, 193–196.

Purnell, L. D., & Paulanka, B. (1998). *Transcultural health care: A cultural competent approach.* Philadelphia: FA Davis.

Ropers, R. H. (1991). *Persistent poverty.* New York: Plenum.

Rosenthal, D., Rainieri, N., & Klimdis, S. (1996). Vietnamese adolescents in Australia: Relationships between perceptions of self and parental values, intergenerational conflict, and gender dissatisfaction. *International Journal of Psychology, 31*, 81–91.

Rossi, R. H., et al. (1987). The urban homeless: Estimating composition and size. *Science, 235*, 1136–1341.

Schantz, S., Charron, S. A., & Folden, S. L. (2003). Health seeking behaviors of Haitian families for their school aged children. *Journal of Cultural Diversity, 10*(2), 62–68.

Schnittger, M. H., & Bird, G. W. (1993). Coping among dual-career men and women across the family life cycle. *Family Relations, 39*, 199–205.

Seccomb, K. (2000). Families in poverty in the 1990s: Trends, causes, consequences, and lessons learned. *Journal of Marriage and the Family, 62*, 1094–1113.

Spector, R. E. (2004). *Cultural diversity in health and illness* (6th ed.). Upper Saddle River, NJ: Pearson Prentice Hall.

Starfield, B. (1992). Child and adolescent health status measures. In Center for the Future of Children. *The Future of Children. The David and Lucille Packard Foundation, 2,* 24–39.

Suarez, L., & Ramirez, A. (1999). Hispanic/Latino health and disease: An overview. In R. C. Huff & M. V. Kline (Eds.), *Promoting health in multicultural populations: A handbook for practitioners* (pp. 115–136). Thousand Oaks, CA: Sage.

Tang, T., & Dion, K. (1999). Gender and acculturation in relation to traditionalism: Perceptions of self and parents among Chinese students. *Sex Roles, 41,* 17–29.

Tax report says rich gained, poor lost during the 80s (1990, February 6), *Los Angeles Times,* p. A4.

Uba, L. (1994). *Asian American: Personality, patterns, identity, and mental health.* New York: Guilford.

United States Conference of Mayors (2002). *A status report on hunger & homelessness in America's cities 2002.* Retrieved from http://www.usmayors.org

U.S. Census Bureau. (1997). *Age, sex, household relationship, race, and Hispanic origin and selected statuses: Ratio of income to poverty level in 1996.* Retrieved October 3, 1997, from http://ferret.bls.census.gov/macro/03197/pov/2_001–3.htm.

U.S. Census Bureau. (2001). *Statistical abstracts of the United States.* Washington, DC: U.S. Government Printing Office.

U.S. Department of Health and Human Services. (1998). *Profile of homelessness.* Retrieved June 9, 1999, from http://aspe.os.dhhs.gov/progsys/homeless/profile.htm.

U.S. Department of Health and Human Services. (2002). *Child health USA.* Health Resources and Services Administration, Maternal Child Health Bureau. Rockville, MD: U.S. Department of Health and Human Services.

Voydanoff, P., & Donnelly, B. W. (1998) *Economic distress, family coping and quality of family life.* In P. Voydanoff & L. C. Le Majka (Eds.), *Families and economic distress* (pp. 97–115). Newbury Park, CA: Sage Publications.

Wilkinson, R. G. (1996). *Unhealthy societies: The afflictions of inequality.* London: Routledge.

Winnick, A. J. (1991). *Toward two societies.* New York: Praeger Press.

Wolff, E. N. (1995). How the pie is sliced: America's growing concentration of wealth. *The American Prospect, 22*(Summer), 58–64.

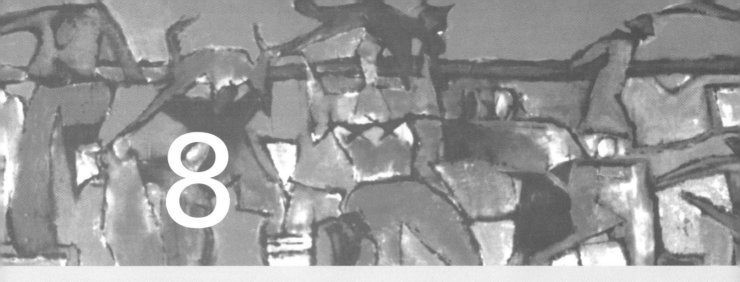

8

Family Nursing Assessment and Intervention

Joanna Rowe Kaakinen, RN, PhD • *Shirley May Harmon Hanson, RN, PMHNP, PhD, FAAN, CFLE, LMFT*

CRITICAL CONCEPTS

- Nursing practice requires the ability to use nursing knowledge and reason through details to make skilled judgments while not losing sight of the whole client picture and desired outcomes of care.

- Nurses decide what data to collect and how, when, and where that data is collected.

- Each family has a story about how the potential or actual health issue influences the individual members, the family functioning, and how they manage the problem.

- Nurses determine through which lens the family health problem will be best addressed: from a family-as-context perspective, family-as-client perspective, or family-as-community perspective.

- Nurses work with families to determine realistic outcomes based on the ability of each family to adapt successfully to the health issue, given the strengths of the family, the pattern of family response in similar situations, and the trajectory of the family health care problem.

- Nurses build on their expertise by reflecting on client stories and their practice with each family. Self-reflection and self-evaluation are critical thinking strategies that advance nursing practice from the novice to expert designation.

- Selection of appropriate and sensitive assessment tools is important, as the information collected serves as the foundation for the development of client specific plans.

INTRODUCTION

As families are complex social systems, the use of logical, systematic approaches to the family client are essential. Nurses use a variety of assessment models to collect information about a family. This information is used to frame or structure the interventions nurses and families develop to help the family manage the current issues or stressors. Some tools are based on theoretical models and some are developed using a psychometric approach to tool development. The purpose of this chapter is to explore assessment and intervention models nurses use while working with families.

Nurses are encouraged to use sophisticated assessment instruments in providing nursing care to family clients. The selection of appropriate and sensitive assessment tools is important, as the information collected serves as the foundation for the development of client-specific plans. In this chapter, suggestions are offered on how to select appropriate tools. Family genograms and ecomaps are demonstrated. The nursing process approach described for family nursing is the Outcome Present State Testing (OPT) model (Pesut & Herman, 1999). Three family assessment and intervention models developed by nurses will also be discussed. A case study of the OPT model appears at the end of the chapter. A case study of the Family Systems Stressor-Strength Inventory (FS³I) (Hanson, 2001) can be found in Appendix C.

Selection of Family Assessment and Measurement Tools

Because there are approximately 1000 family-focused instruments that have been developed and used in assessing family-related variables (Touliatos, Perlmutter, & Straus, 2001), it is imperative that the assessment and measurement tools that nurses select render information pertinent to the purpose of working with the family. At times a simple tool that can be administered and completed in a few minutes can provide insight into planning and intervention, such as a tool that addresses the discipline of children or attitudes about spanking. Other times, more comprehensive family assessment tools are necessary, such as use of the Family Systems Stressor-Strength Inventory (FS³I) (Hanson, 2001; Kaakinen, Hanson, & Birenbaum, 2004). For example, the FS³I can be used to explore ways of helping a family adapt to having an elderly grandmother move in with her son's family. No matter which tool the nurse is using, families should always be informed of how the information provided from the tool will be used by the health care provider.

In order to select the most appropriate tool, nurses need to understand the distinction between assessment and measurement and between qualitative and quantitative assessment strategies. *Assessment* is a continuously evolving process of data collection whereby the nurse draws on the past and the present in order to plan and predict for the future (Hanson, 2001). *Measurement* is the process of assigning numbers or symbols to variables upon which we perform statistical operations (Vogt, 1999). Measurement involves a formal instrument that gives numerical values or *quantifies* the traits being measured. Such instruments generally give a quantitative result when a particular attribute is examined. Measurement is often considered a narrower aspect of assessment that focuses on more specific concepts or traits.

The following suggestions will help the nurse select the most appropriate short assessment instrument:

- The tools should be written in uncomplicated language at a sixth grade level.
- These tools should be able to be completed in 10–15 minutes.
- The tool should be relatively easy to score and should provide valid data on which to base decisions.
- The tools should be sensitive to gender, race, social class, and ethnic background.
- Genograms and ecomaps are two short easy tools to use that supply valuable family data.

Note: Do not confuse a genogram with a pedigree. A pedigree, described in Chapter 17, is specific to genetics assessments, whereas a genogram has broader uses for nurses.

GENOGRAMS AND ECOMAPS

The genogram and ecomap are essential components of family assessment. The genogram provides a quick snapshot of the family members from an intergenerational perspective, such as how they are related, health or genetic trends, and potential sources of support for the family. The ecomap provides information about systems outside of the family that are sources of support or stressors to the family. Sometimes these tools reveal valuable sources of support that are not currently being used or accessed by the family. Both tools should be used concurrently with all family assessment models, as they are easy to conduct and provide a wealth of information in a visual format that can be placed in the chart for use by multiple health care providers.

Genogram

The *genogram* is a format for drawing a family tree that records information about family members and their relationships over at least three generations (McGoldrick, Gerson, & Schellenberger, 1999). Basically the genogram is a diagram, a skeleton, or a constellation that depicts the structure of intergenerational relationships. Genograms are used in both genealogy and genetics and are now being used in family therapy and in health care settings. They offer a rich source of information for planning intervention strategies because they display the family visually and graphically in a way that provides a quick overview of family complexities.

❝The genogram and ecomap are essential components of family assessment. They should be used concurrently with all family assessment approaches.❞

The genogram was developed primarily out of the family systems theory of Murray Bowen (Bowen, 1985; Bowen & Kerr, 1988). According to Bowen, people are organized into family systems by generation, age, sex, and similar variables. How a person fits into the family structure influences the person's functioning, relational patterns, and type of family he or she will form in the next generation. Bowen incorporated Toman's (1976) ideas about the importance of sex and birth order in shaping sibling relationships and characteristics. According to Bowen (1985), families repeat themselves over generations in a phenomenon called the transmission of family patterns. What happens in one generation repeats itself in the next, so the same issues are played out from generation to generation. These include both psychosocial and health issues.

Figure 8–1 provides a basic genogram from which the nurse can start plotting family members over the first, second, and third generations (McGoldrick, Gerson, & Schellenberger, 1999). Figure 8–2 shows symbols used to describe basic family membership and structure, family interaction patterns, and other family information of particular importance, such as ethnic background, religion, education, health, drug and alcohol use, occupation, military service, and nodal events, such as retirement, trouble with the law, and family relocations (McGoldrick, Gerson, & Schellenberger, 1999, p. 192).

The health history of all family members (e.g., morbidity, mortality, and onset of illness) is very important information for family nurses and can be the focus of analysis of the family genogram. An example of a family genogram developed from one interview is contained in the OPT case study in Figure 8–9.

During the assessment interview, the nurse asks the family for background information and then completes the genogram together with the family; it is a joint nurse and family endeavor. An outline for a brief genogram interview is given in Box 8–1 (McGoldrick, Gerson, & Schellenberger, 1999, pp. 193–197). Most families are cooperative and interested in completing their genogram, which becomes a

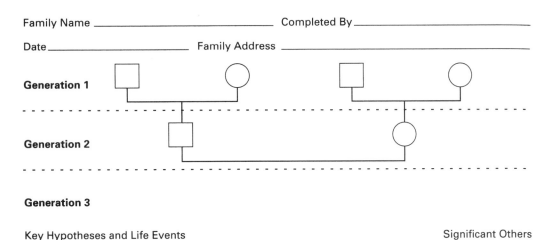

Figure 8–1 Basic genogram format.
Source: McGoldrick & Gerson (1985).

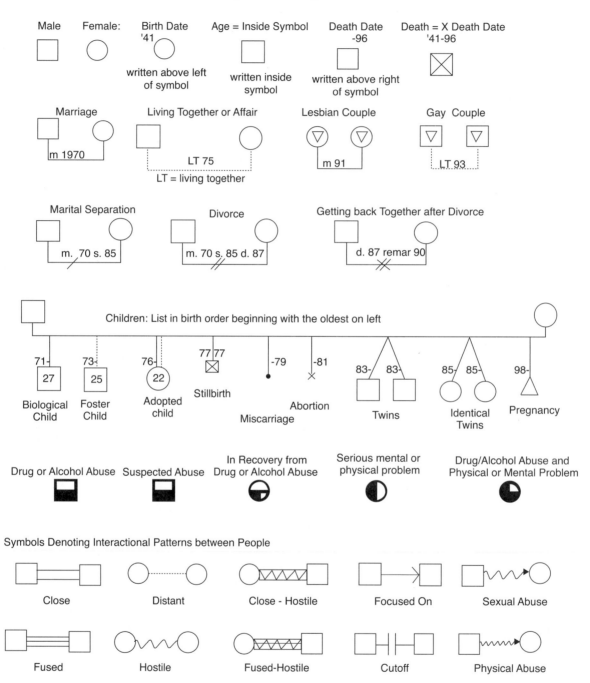

Figure 8–2 Genogram symbols.
Source: McGoldrick, Gerson, & Shellenburger (1999, p. 192).

part of the ongoing health care record. The genogram does not have to be completed at one sitting. As the same or a different nurse continues to work with the family, data can be added to the genogram over time in a continuing process.

Ecomap

An *ecomap* provides information about systems outside the family that are sources of support or that are stressors to the family (Hartman & Laird, 1983;

Box 8–1 **OUTLINE FOR A BRIEF GENOGRAM INTERVIEW**

Index Person, Children, and Spouses

Name? Date of birth? Occupation? Are they married? If so, give names of spouses and the name and sex of children with each spouse. Include all miscarriages, stillbirths, and adopted and foster children. Include dates of marriages, separations, and divorces. Also include birth and death dates, cause of death, occupations, and education of the above family members. Who lives in the household now?

Family of Origin

Mother's name? Father's name? They were which of how many children? Give name and sex of each sibling. Include all miscarriages, stillbirths, and adopted and foster siblings. Include dates of the parents' marriages, separations, and divorces. Also include birth and death dates, cause of death, occupations, and education of the above family members. Who lived in the household when they were growing up?

Mother's Family

The names of the mother's parents? The mother was which of how many children? Give name and sex of each of her siblings. Include all miscarriages, stillbirths, and adopted and foster siblings. Include dates of grandparents' marriages, separations, and divorces. Also include birth and death dates, cause of death, occupations, and education of the above family members.

Father's Family

The names of the father's parents? The father was which of how many children? Give name and sex of each of his siblings. Include all miscarriages, stillbirths, and adopted and foster siblings. Include dates of grandparents' marriages, separations, and divorces. Also include birth and death dates, cause of death, occupations, and education of the above family members.

Ethnicity

What are the ethnic and religious backgrounds of family members and the languages they speak, if not English?

Major Moves

Tell about major family relocations and migrations.

Significant Others

Add others who lived with or were important to the family.

For All Those Listed, Note Any of the Following

- Serious medical, behavioral, or emotional problems
- Job problems
- Drug or alcohol problems
- Serious problems with the law

(continued on page 220)

Box 8–1   **OUTLINE FOR A BRIEF GENOGRAM INTERVIEW** *(Continued)*

For All Those Listed, Indicate Any Who Were

- Especially close
- Distant or conflictual
- Cut off from each other
- Overly dependent on each other

Source: McGoldrick, M., Gerson, R., & Shellenburger, S. (1999). *Genograms in family assessment* (2nd ed., pp. 193–195). New York: W.W. Norton.

McGoldrick, Gerson, & Shellenburger, 1999; Ross, 2001; Friedman, Bowden, & Jones, 2003; Hanson, 2001). The ecomap is a visual representation of the family unit in relation to the community; it shows the nature of the relationships between family members and between family members and the world around them. The ecomap is thus an overview of the family in its situation, picturing both the important nurturant and stress-producing connections between the family and the world (Hanson, 2001).

The blank ecomap form consists of a large circle with smaller circles around it (Figure 8–3). To complete the ecomap, the genogram of the family is placed in the center of the large circle. This circle marks the boundary between the household and its external environment. The smaller outer circles represent significant people, agencies, or institutions in the family's context. Lines are drawn between the circles and the family members to depict the nature and quality of the relationships and to show what kinds of resources are going in and coming out of the family. Straight lines show strong or close relationships; the more pronounced the line, the stronger the relationship. Straight lines with slashes denote stressful relationships and broken lines show tenuous or distant relationships. Arrows show the direction of the flow of energy and resources between individuals and between the family and the environment. See case study for an example of a completed family ecomap (Figure 8–10).

The ecomap organizes factual information to provide the nurse with a more integrated perception of the family situation. Ecomaps not only portray the present but also can be used to set goals, for example, to increase connections and exchanges with individuals and agencies in the community.

NURSING AND CLINICAL REASONING

It is imperative in any discussion of nursing that critical thinking be recognized as an essential underlying element. Critical thinking is the "cognitive engine" driving the process of professional nursing judgment (Facione & Facione, 1996). Paul (1993) stated that critical thinking is the "intellectually disciplined process of actively and skillfully conceptualizing, applying, synthesizing, or evaluating information gathered from, or generated by, observation, experience, reflection, or communication, as a guide to belief or action" (p. 110). Nurses are able to direct the intellectual process in a way that is disciplined and effective in the recognition of and subsequent solving of client problems. Each "comprehension" of the family client needs, and nursing interventions, must be adjusted to the unique family story.

Each step of working with families, whether applied to the individual within the family as context or to the family as client, requires a thoughtful deliberate clinical reasoning process. Nurses decide what data to collect and how, when, and where that data is collected. The nurse determines the relevance of each new piece of information and how it fits into the emerging family story. Before moving forward, nurses decide whether sufficient information has been obtained on problem and strength identification or whether gaps exist that require additional data gathering. Each situation evolves as it is analyzed, and each item of new information must be judged in terms of accuracy, clarity, and relevance.

The nurse must always be aware that the "common" interpretation of the data may not be the "correct" interpretation in a given situation, and the commonly expected signs and symptoms or cues may not appear

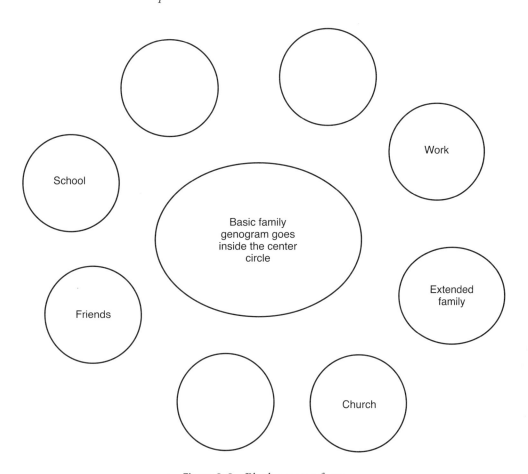

Figure 8–3 Blank ecomap form.

in every case or in the same configuration. The ability to be open to the unexpected, to be alert to the unusual or different response, is critical to the identification of the keystone problem confronting the family client. As each new nurse-client interaction begins, creative thinking allows access to any or all the possibilities. Nurses are able to see that which is not obvious or clearly drawn and to understand how this family story is similar or different from others. In the context of nursing, the creative nurse thinker must be open to the universe of possibilities in any given situation, be able to recognize the new and the unusual, decipher unique and complex situations, and be inventive and imaginative in designing approaches to problem solving.

Development of Family Nursing Process

Yura and Walsh (1988) initially defined the *nursing process* using four steps: (1) assessment, (2) planning,

(3) implementation, and (4) evaluation. Nurses used to write problem lists for a client in the order of priority of client needs; the medical model heavily influenced these problem lists. A list of common patient problems led to the groundbreaking work of the classifications of nursing diagnosis in 1973 (Gebbie & Lavin, 1975). At that time, nursing diagnoses were focused on the individual client.

The second generation of the nursing process occurred from 1970 to 1990, during which time several processes developed. The linear four-step process evolved into an information-processing and decision-making five-step process, which included assessment, diagnosis, planning, implementation, and evaluation. The family nursing process described by Ross (2001) entailed family assessment, analysis, planning, implementation, evaluation, and reassessment steps. This model of family nursing process is depicted in Figure 8–4.

Gordon (1982, 1994) described a six-step process:

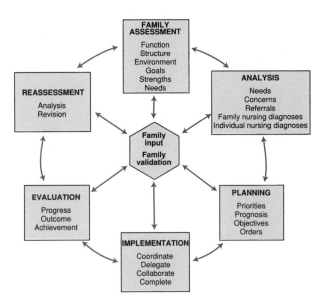

Figure 8–4 Family nursing process. *Source:* Ross (2001).

assessment, analysis, outcome projection, planning, implementation, and evaluation. Carnevali and Thomas (1993) included diagnostic reasoning, nursing prognosis, and testing concepts along with the traditional five-step nursing process model.

The classic work of Benner (1988) and Benner, Tanner, and Chesla (1996) demonstrated that novice and expert nurses use different critical thinking processes. They found that expert nurses make clinical judgments and decisions based on pattern recognition of client problems and therefore arrive at decisions more rapidly than novice nurses. They suggested that expert nurses use a more abstract thinking process that simultaneously considers multiple aspects of a client issue; they termed this thinking process "nursing intuition." However, they only described this process via individual nursing exemplars and qualitative research. They did not diagram how nurses begin to think in this fashion.

The shift of health care from a process goal–oriented approach to an outcome-oriented approach requires nursing to develop a dynamic third generation nursing process that reflects current practice. Building on the traditional nursing process model, the OPT model by Pesut and Herman (1999) is a third generation nursing process approach that emphasizes clinical reasoning and is outcome oriented and client centered (Kaakinen, Hanson, & Birenbaum, 2004). Table 8–1 shows how the two models interact.

Outcome Present State Testing Model

The OPT model (Pesut & Herman, 1999) builds on the previous nursing process steps and includes the use of nursing classification systems. Therefore, it can be used in all settings. The authors of this model felt that it was critical to develop a new model, with new language to assist nurses to think about clients in a more dynamic interactive thinking process. See Figure 8–5 for an adaptation of the OPT model; note that the nurse enters this model from the right side, beginning with the client story. Brief descriptions of the elements

Table 8–1 COMPARISON OF OUTCOME PRESENT STATE TESTING (OPT) MODEL WITH TRADITIONAL NURSING PROCESS

Traditional Nursing Process Components	*OPT Components*
Assessment	Client story
	Framing
	Cue logic
Nursing Diagnosis	Cue logic
	Keystone issue
Planning	Framing
	Present state
	Outcome state
	Testing
Implementation	Decision making
Evaluation	Judgment
	Reflection

in the model are described later; more detailed explanations follow in this chapter.

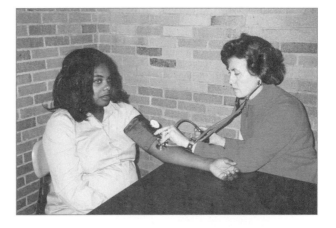

- The *client story* represents the assessment aspect of the OPT process relative to the current health issue the family is encountering.
- The *frame* is the lens the nurse uses to gather and cluster data into appropriate groupings. This step is critical because the nurse filters data gathered in the story through different lenses, which may include the trajectory of the illness or problem, the place of care, and client beliefs.
- *Cue logic* is the process of clustering data into meaningful groups so that the relationships between the issues can be identified.
- The *keystone issue* is the main primary problem the client is presently experiencing.
- The *present state* of the client includes the most relevant or pressing issues confronting the family client.
- Desired *outcomes* are developed for each present state.

- To determine if the outcome is being achieved or not, the nurse identifies tests or measures that provide information about the resolution of the problems.
- Nurses *make decisions* about which nursing interventions are most appropriate for the family.
- A major component of the process is nursing

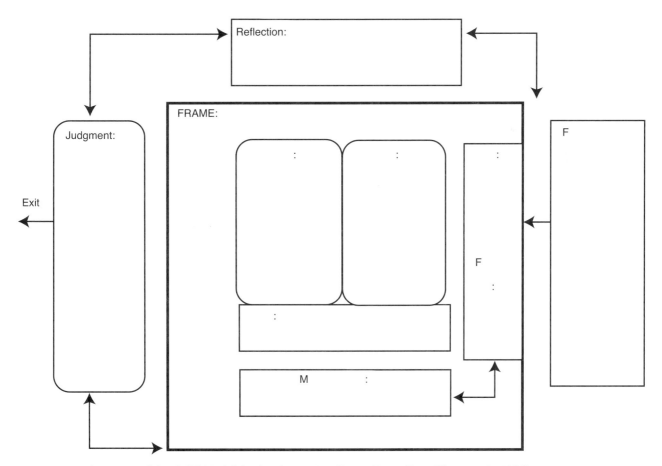

Figure 8–5 Adaptation of the OPT Model for family nursing. From (Pesot, P., & Herman, A., 1999).

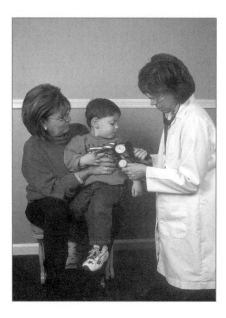

judgment, which evaluates client progress toward the outcomes.

- The last aspect of the OPT model is *reflection* strategies nurses use to review and learn from clients that enhance and expand their practice base.

The following sections explain how to use the OPT model in the nursing of families.

Family Client Story

Nurses encounter families in diverse health care settings for a myriad of issues. Each family has a story about how the potential or actual health issue influences its individual members, family functioning, and their management of the problem. The specific questions nurses will ask depend on the reason for the visit. The nurse is challenged in getting the family story not only to focus on the medical aspect of the issue but also to include how the family members are involved or affected by the issue.

Data collection involves both subjective and objective data, or data verbally shared with the nurse by the client and data obtained by direct observation and examination or in consultation with other health care providers. This section of the OPT model is similar to the assessment step in the traditional nursing process approach. Family data collection begins when the family is identified by a source, which may include the family, the physician, a school nurse, or a caseworker. Several examples include the following:

1. A family is referred to the home health agency for wound care to the foot of a diabetic client.
2. A family calls the Visiting Nurse Association to request assistance in providing care to a family member with increasing dementia.
3. A school nurse is asked to conduct a family assessment by the school psychologist who is investigating potential child neglect issues.
4. A physician requests a family assessment with a child who has nonorganic failure to thrive.

As soon as the case is identified, nurses begin to collect data about the family story. Sources of data that can be collected prior to contacting a family for an appointment are listed in Box 8–2. Specifically, the nurse needs to know the following:

- The reason for the referral or requested visit
- If the family knows about the visit or referral
- Specific medical information about the family member with the health issue
- What has been tried before
- Insurance sources
- Family issues that the other health providers have expressed concern about.

Before contacting the family to arrange for the initial appointment, the nurse decides if the most appropriate place to conduct the appointment is in the family's home or the clinic/office. The type of agency may dictate this decision. For instance, home health agencies provide nursing in the home, or mental health agencies require family meetings to occur in

---

Box 8–2 SOURCES OF FAMILY PRE-ENCOUNTER DATA

- Referral source: includes data that indicated a problem for this family, as well as demographic information
- Family: includes family members' views of the problem, surprise that the referral was made, reluctance to set up the meeting, avoidance in setting up the appointment
- Previous records: in the health care systems or that are sent by having the client sign a release for information form, such as process logs, charts, phone logs, or school records

Table 8–2 ADVANTAGES AND DISADVANTAGES OF HOME VISITS VERSUS CLINIC VISITS

Home Visit	*Clinic Visit*
ADVANTAGES	ADVANTAGES
• Opportunity to see the everyday family environment. • Observe typical family interactions as the family members are likely to feel more relaxed in their physical space. • More family members may be able to attend the meeting. • Emphasizes that the problem is the responsibility of the whole family and not one family member	• Conducting the family appointment in the office or clinic allows for easier access to consultants. • The family situation may be so strained that a more formal, less personal setting will facilitate discussions of emotionally charged issues.
DISADVANTAGES	DISADVANTAGES
• Home may be the only sanctuary or safe place for the family or its members to be away from the scrutiny of others. • The nurse must be highly skilled in communication, specifically setting limits and guiding the interaction, or the visit may have a more social tone and not be efficient or productive.	• May reinforce a possible culture gap between the family and the nurse.

the neighborhood clinic office. Advantages and disadvantages of a home setting or clinic setting are listed in Table 8–2.

Contacting the family for the appointment provides valuable information about the family. It is telling if the family acts surprised that the referral was made, is reluctant to set up the meeting, or is eager to work with the nurse on the problem. The family likewise gathers information about the nurse from the phone call to arrange the meeting. Therefore it is imperative that the nurse be confident and organized when making the initial contact. Box 8–3 outlines steps to follow when making an appointment with a family.

Nurses investigate the health issue using a typical history and physical approach. However, family nursing is more than medical care for the individual with the health issue. When the nurse meets with the family, it is important to investigate how all members of the family are affected by the issue. The person with the health problem or reason for the referral may not be the family member who is experiencing the most difficulty. An important question to ask is, "If

Box 8–3 SETTING UP FAMILY APPOINTMENTS

- Introduce yourself.
- State the purpose of the requested meeting, including who referred the family to the agency.
- Do not apologize for the meeting.
- Be factual about the need for the meeting, but do not provide details.
- Offer several possible times for the meeting, including late afternoon or evening.
- Let the family select the most convenient time that allows the majority of family members to attend.
- Confirm date, time, place, and directions.

there is one question that you would like answered or issue addressed while I am here today, what would that be?" This keeps the focus on the family's needs and will help the nurse to understand what is most important to the family. Family roles should be assessed. For example, how are the roles of the family members being altered by the health issue, how long are family members expected to take on additional roles, and is there role stress or overload. Other important areas to investigate are how receptive the family is to having others help them, who should be involved, and what is the best way to mobilize support for this family (Hanna & Brown, 2004). By using the family OPT clinical reasoning web described in the keystone issue section below, the nurse will collect data using a family holistic approach. Later in this chapter, family nursing assessment instruments (which can be used to collect more data than in a normal family OPT) are described in detail.

> ❝Family nursing is more than simple medical care for the individual with the health issue. When the nurse meets with the family, it is important to investigate how all members of the family are affected by the issue.❞

Frame

The frame provides an outline for thinking about the family problem that clusters data into meaningful groups, develops the desired outcomes, and suggests appropriate family nursing interventions. The nurse filters data gathered in the story through different lenses, which may include the trajectory of the illness or problem, the place of care, and client beliefs. The frame of reference for the family influences how nurses ask questions and collect data about the family. For example, if the problem is one that is life threatening for a family member, the issues the family experiences will be different from the issues they will experience if the problem is time limited with complete recovery expected by the family member. Another example is if the person affected is the primary child care person. Then the other members of the family are more significantly affected by the illness than if the person ill is less central to the functioning of the entire family.

In addition to the above filters, the nurse determines through which lens the problem will be termed, such as is this issue best addressed from a family-as-context perspective, family-as-client perspective, or family-as-community perspective. See Chapter 1 for approaches to nursing of families and specific questions that elicit different information depending on the family nursing lens or frame.

Cue Logic

The purpose of cue logic is to consolidate the data into meaningful patterns or groups so that the nurse and family can see more easily the relationships between and among the patterns of how the family is managing the problem. Diagramming the family and the relationships between the data clusters assists in the identification of the keystone issue. The keystone issue is the problem that, if and when solved, will positively affect the majority of other areas of family functioning.

This family OPT step is similar to the analysis step in the traditional nursing process. The nurse can draw a family clinical reasoning web to assist in an understanding relationship between and among the data elements. The organizational structure of the family web assists nurses to think holistically about a family experiencing a health-related issue, which is similar to a family ecomap except this web looks at the internal and external family structure. The components of this organizational structure have been pulled from various theoretical concepts, such as family structure and function, family developmental stage, family stress theory, and family health promotion models. Refer to Figure 8–6 for a generic template of a family clinical reasoning web. The elements include the following:

1. Family routines of daily living, i.e., sleeping, meals, child care, exercise
2. Family communication
3. Family supports and resources
4. Family roles
5. Family beliefs
6. Family developmental stages
7. Family health knowledge
8. Family environment
9. Family stress management
10. Family culture
11. Family spirituality

Clustering data into a clinical reasoning web is a pictorial representation of the relationships between the clusters. Arrows are drawn between group clusters showing the direction of influence if the data in one cluster influences the data in another cluster. The nurse systematically diagrams the relationships between each of the categories. The family keystone

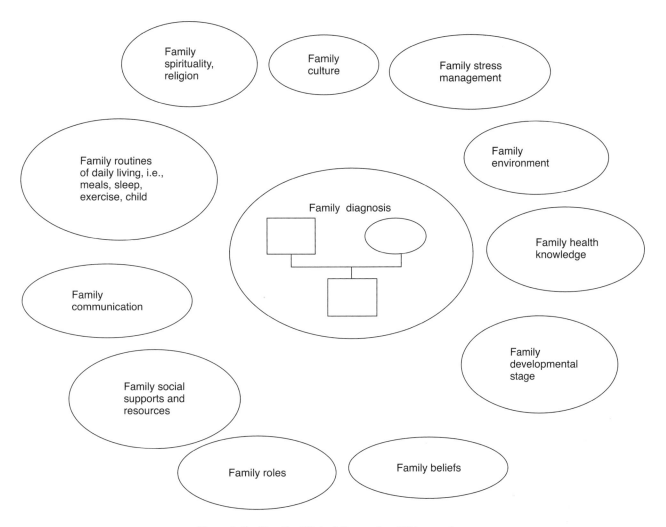

Figure 8–6 Family Clinical Reasoning Web template.

issue is the group with the most arrows or has the strongest relationship to all other areas of family functioning. If the keystone family issue is not accurately identified, the family and the nurse will collect data, design interventions, and implement plans of care that do not meet the most pressing needs for that family.

Once the data have been clustered, a family nursing diagnosis is determined for each set of data. Nursing diagnoses create the links between collecting information and care planning (Gordon, 1994). The North American Nurses Diagnosis Association (NANDA; 2003) is the most global nursing classification system. NANDA nursing diagnoses that are specific to families are listed in Box 8–4. If the keystone issue does not fall under one of these accepted NANDA nursing diagnoses, nurses are encouraged to write the family nursing diagnosis in a NANDA format. Nurses should forward the most common, unlisted family nursing

diagnoses to the North American Nursing Diagnosis Association to be considered for inclusion in the diagnosis list.

> ❝If the keystone family issue is not accurately identified, the family and the nurse will collect data, design interventions, and implement plans of care that do not meet the most pressing needs for that family.❞

Other diagnostic classification systems that can be used with families include the Omaha System for use in the community (Martin & Scheet, 1992), the Diagnostic and Statistical Manual of Mental Disorders (DSM; American Psychiatric Association, 2000), and the International Classification of Disease (ICD-9; American Medical Association, 2004). See Table 8–3 and Table 8–4, respectively, for examples of

Box 8–4 **NANDA NURSING DIAGNOSES RELEVANT TO FAMILY NURSING**

- Risk for impaired parent/infant/child attachment
- Caregiver role strain
- Risk for caregiver role strain
- Parental role conflict
- Compromised family coping
- Disabled family coping
- Readiness for enhanced family coping
- Dysfunctional family processes: alcoholism
- Readiness for enhanced family processes
- Interrupted family processes
- Readiness for enhanced parenting
- Impaired parenting
- Risk for impaired parenting
- Relocation stress syndrome
- Ineffective role performance
- Ineffective family therapeutic regimen management

Source: Ackley, B. J., & Ladwig, G. B. (2004). *Nursing diagnosis handbook: A guide to planning care* (6th ed.). St. Louis: Mosby.

Table 8–3 **SELECTED FAMILY-CENTERED DIAGNOSES FROM DSM-IV-TR™**

V61.9 Relational problem related to a mental disorder or general medical condition
V61.20 Parent-child relational problem
V61.10 Partner relational problem
V61.8 Sibling relational problem
V71.02 Child or adolescent antisocial behavior
V62.82 Bereavement
V62.3 Academic problem
V62.4 Acculturation problem
V62.89 Phase of life problem

Source: American Medical Association. (2004). *International classification of diseases: Clinical modifications (IDC-9CM)* (10th ed.). Dover, DE: American Medical Association.

outcomes need to be based on the ability of the family to successfully adapt to the health issue, given the strengths of the family, the pattern of family response in similar situations, and the trajectory of the family health care problem. The type of outcomes possible depends on the frame of the problem for the family. The outcome may be directed at preventing a poten-

Table 8–4 **SELECTED FAMILY-CENTERED DIAGNOSES/ THERAPEUTIC PROCEDURES FROM ICD-9-CM 2004**

313.3 Relationship problems
313.8 Emotional disturbances of childhood or adolescence
V61.0 Family disruption
V25.09 Family planning advice
V61.9 Family problem
94.41 Group therapy
94.42 Family therapy

Source: American Psychiatric Association. (2000). *Diagnostic and statistical manual of mental disorders (DSM-IV-TR™)* (4th ed.). Washington, DC: Author.

selected family diagnoses from the DSM and ICD-9 sources. After the keystone family diagnosis has been identified and verified with the family, the next step is determining the present state, the outcome, and the testing evaluation criteria that will be used to determine if the outcomes have been achieved.

Present State, Outcome State, Testing

The relevant characteristics in the keystone issue that nursing can influence make up the present state of the client by ascertaining what is important to the client and is vital to successful planning. By prioritizing the data in the keystone issue, the nurse and family focus on the relevant aspects of the priority nursing diagnosis. Those concerns, considered most crucial at a given point in time, must be dealt with first. Keep in mind that as conditions change, priorities may change. This aspect of the family OPT model is similar to the planning step of the nursing process.

The nurse works with the family to determine realistic outcomes for each aspect of the present state. The tial problem, minimizing a problem, stabilizing a problem, or recognizing that a deteriorating problem exists. The outcome statement should be stated positively and in measurable terms. See Box 8–5 for examples of family outcome statements. To establish realistic, attainable family outcomes, the nurse determines both the probable outcome and the best possible recovery or state of health, given the family frame, and includes a time frame for achievement.

From experience and information known about the family, the nurse predicts what tests or assessment processes will be used to analyze the course of events or the pattern of change expected to occur. Testing is the process of juxtaposing the family present state with projected family outcomes in order to determine what progress the family has made toward achieving the outcome.

Decision Making

Nurses make decisions about which interventions are the most client specific, cost effective, and efficient to achieve the desired outcome. The more specific the family intervention, the more positive the influence on client outcomes will be. This part of the family OPT model is similar to the implementation step of the nursing process because the nurse develops nursing interventions specific to the family problem and puts the plan into action.

While making decisions about interventions, it is important for nurses to recognize that the family has the right to make its own health decisions. The role of the nurse is to offer guidance to the family, provide information, and assist in the planning process. The nurse may assist the family by (1) providing direct care, (2) removing barriers to needed services, and (3) improving the capacity of the family to act on its own behalf and assume responsibility.

Nurses must also make these decisions with an eye toward available resources, including time, support systems, and financial resources. It is essential that nurses not recommend courses of action, equipment, and placements that clients cannot afford and that the family system cannot accommodate.

Judgment

In making clinical judgments, nurses engage in critical thinking to determine whether or not and to what extent an outcome is successfully met. During this step, nurses use judgment and perform a comparative analysis to determine how well this gap between pres-

---

| Box 8–5 | **EXAMPLES OF OUTCOME STATEMENTS** |

- Identify realistic perception of role.
- Acknowledge problems contributing to inability to carry out usual role in the family.
- Describe a decrease in the difficulties of managing medications for family member.
- Express feelings and perceptions regarding impacts of illness, disability, or hospitalization on parental role.
- Verbalize internal resources to help deal with the family situation.
- Identify need for and seek outside support.
- Express realistic understanding and expectation of family member.
- Treat impaired family member as normally as possible to avoid overdependence.

---

ent state and outcome state is being filled. When a family outcome is partially met or not successfully achieved, the nurse and the family work together to determine the barriers that may be preventing the outcome. This element in the family OPT model is similar to the evaluation step in the nursing process.

Throughout the judgment phase, data gathering continues. The nurse obtains new information with each contact with the client and incorporates this additional information into the current database, analyzes it for relevance and importance, and makes decisions as to whether to proceed as originally planned, to modify the plan of care, or to revisit the client story in total. As indicated previously, the family OPT nursing process is not linear. In practice, there is a constant flow between the components of the model.

In assessing reasons for not achieving outcomes, the nurse should consider whether family apathy and indecision are the barriers. Family apathy may occur because of value differences between the nurse and the family. The family may be overcome with a sense of hopelessness, may view the problems as too overwhelming, or may have a fear of failure. Nurses should also consider whether they themselves imposed barriers. A more detailed list of possible barriers can be found in Box 8–6.

Aside from evaluating outcomes, another important part of the judgment step is the decision when to terminate the relationship with the family. Sometimes termination with a family occurs suddenly. In this case, it is important for the nurse to determine the forces bringing about the closure. The family may be initiating the termination prematurely, which may require a renegotiating process. The insurance or agency requirements may be placing a financial constraint on the amount of time the nurse can work with a family. Other times, the termination arrives more naturally, as when the nurse and family together determine that the family has achieved the intended outcomes.

Building termination into the interventions will benefit the family by providing for a smooth transition process. Strategies often used in termination include decreasing contact with the nurse, extending invitations to the family for follow-up, and making referrals when appropriate. If possible, the termination process should include a summary evaluation meeting where the nurse and family put formal closure to their relationship. Following up the family client termination with a therapeutic letter encourages families to continue positive adaptation. The therapeutic letter should include recognition of the family achievement, a summary of the actions, commendations to each family member, and an insightful rhetorical question that may provide the family a future direction (Wright, Watson, & Bell, 1996). An example of a therapeutic family letter is found in Box 8–7.

Reflection

The final step in the OPT clinical reasoning model is for nurses to engage in critical, creative, and concur-

rent reflection about the family and their work with the family. This step has three distinct parts. One is to reflect on the success of the family outcome. The second purpose of reflection is to build the nurse's mental file or library of knowledge about similar family cases. The third purpose of reflection is to engage in self-evaluation (Pesut & Herman, 1999).

Reflection entails thinking about your thought process relative to this family client. Nurses can link ideas and consequences together in logical sequences using an "if . . . then . . . " mental exercise. Nurses can use a comparative analysis approach to the family problem by analyzing the strengths and weaknesses of competing alternatives. The nurse may decide to reframe the family client problem or keystone issue by attributing a different meaning to the content or context of the family situation based on testing, judgment, or changes in the context or content of the family story (Pesut & Herman, 1999).

The second purpose of reflection is for nurses to build on their expertise by reflecting on client stories and their practice with each family. In essence, the nurse creates a library of family stories so that each time a nurse comes upon a similar family story, the nurse can pull ideas from previous experience. This aspect of reflection assists the nurse with pattern recognition.

The third purpose of reflection is to engage in self-reflection and self-evaluation. By using this critical thinking strategy, nurses learn from mistakes and cement patterns of actions that assist them to advance in their nursing practice from novice to expert family nurse.

OPT is an outcome-oriented assessment and intervention strategy for working with families. It can be used in any setting for a variety of family problems. In the next section, three family assessment models that were developed by family nurses specifically for working with families are presented.

FAMILY NURSING ASSESSMENT MODELS AND INSTRUMENTS

Family nurses have developed three family nursing assessment models. The Family Assessment and Intervention Model and the Family Systems Stressor-Strength Inventory (FS³I) were developed by Berkey-Mischke and Hanson (1991). Friedman developed the Friedman Family Assessment Model (Friedman, Bowden, & Jones, 2003). The Calgary Family Assessment Model (CFAM) and Calgary Family

---

Box 8–6	**BARRIERS THAT MAY INTERFERE WITH ACCOMPLISHING FAMILY CLIENT OUTCOMES**

- Family apathy
- Family indecision about the outcome or actions
- Nurse-imposed ideas
- Negative labeling
- Overlooking family strengths
- Neglecting cultural or gender implications
- Family perception of hopelessness
- Fear of failure
- Limited access to resources and support
- Limited finances
- Fear and distrust of health care system

Intervention Model (CFIM) were developed by Wright and Leahey (2000). These three approaches vary in purpose, unit of analysis, and level of data collected. Table 8–5 has a detailed comparison of the essential components of the three assessment models.

Family Assessment and Intervention Model

The *Family Assessment and Intervention Model*, originally developed by Berkey-Mischke and Hanson (1991), is theoretically based on Betty Neuman's health care systems model. Figure 8–7 depicts the Family Assessment and Intervention Model based on Neuman's health care systems model (Hanson, 2001; Hanson & Mischke, 1996; Neuman, 1995; Reed, 1993). Neuman's theoretical constructs were extended by Mischke and Hanson to focus on the family rather than on the individual.

According to the Family Assessment and Intervention Model, families are subject to tensions when stressors, in the form of problems, penetrate

---

Box 8–7   EXAMPLE OF THERAPEUTIC LETTER

Dear W, H, and T,

First I want to thank all of you for allowing me the opportunity to get acquainted with your family. I appreciated your openness and willingness to talk with me.

During our time together, we discussed several issues that were important to your family. One of these issues was the ongoing possibility of H losing his job due to the seasonal nature of his work. We explored the effects of potential job loss on a personal and family level.

H, you expressed some concern about your ability to adequately provide for your family. You indicated a personal constraining belief that a lack of steady employment meant that you were letting your family down and not providing for them. We discussed the idea that a paying job is only one part of the entire family support system that you provide. We explored some examples of non-economic means of support, such as specific tasks related to farm chores, household management, and child care. If your job situation changes again, I hope you will find some of these suggestions helpful.

W, I was so impressed with your ability to juggle your nursing job with home, farm, kids, and spouse. I can't think of many women who could handle all of that with such strength and grace. With all that you do, it's not surprising that there isn't much time left over for your own personal endeavors. We discussed your constraining belief that you had to be responsible for everything. You envisioned the possibility of letting go of certain tasks and suggesting ways to share other tasks more equitably among family members. If you and your family choose to implement some tasks-sharing ideas, I sincerely hope this will work for all of you.

T, you have mapped out a path to higher education and a future career. You have every reason to expect success. We briefly touched upon what "success" might mean for you and whether success depends on the university attended. I hope you will consider my thoughts in this regard. Whatever the outcome, you have the love and support of your parents.

Finally I would like to commend all of you for your deep devotion to each other and for putting family first. You value family time and you strive to communicate in a way that sustains your close relationship with each other.

I would like to invite W and H to consider a suggestion regarding making time for just the two of you. "Couple time" is easy to overlook when you are focused on creating a loving, stable home for E and helping to launch T into higher education. Please remember that you two are the solid foundation of your family; the stronger your relationship, the stronger your whole family can be.

As a result of our time spent together, I came away with the feeling that your family is exceptionally strong, deeply committed to one another, and fully capable of adapting to any of life's challenges. Thank you again for your time.

Best wishes to you and your family,
Suzanne Ahn, R.N., UP_ FNP Student

Table 8–5 **COMPARISON OF ASSESSMENT APPROACHES DEVELOPED BY FAMILY NURSES**

Name of Model	Family Assessment and Intervention Model and the Family System Stressor-Strength Inventory (FS³I)	Friedman Family Assessment Model	Calgary Family Assessment and Intervention Model (CFAM/CFIM)
Citation	Berkey-Mischke & Hanson (1991) Hanson (2001)	Friedman, Bowden, & Jones (2003)	Wright & Leahey (2000)
Purpose	Concrete focused measurement instrument that helps families identify current family stressors and builds intervention based on family strengths	Concrete global family assessment interview guide that looks primarily at families in the larger community in which they are embedded	Conceptual model and multidimensional approach to families that looks at the fit among family functioning, affective, and behavioral aspects
Theoretical Underpinnings	Systems: Family systems Neuman Systems Model: Stress-coping theory	Developmental Structural-functional Family stress-coping Environmental	Systems: Cybernetics Communication Change theory
Level of Data Collected	Quantitative: Ordinal and interval Qualitative: Nominal	Qualitative: Nominal	Qualitative: Nominal
Settings in Which Primarily Used	Inpatient Outpatient Community	Outpatient Community	Outpatient Community
Unit of Analysis	Family as context Family as client Family as system Family as component of society	Family as client Family as component of society	Family as system
Strength	Brief Easy to administer Yields data to compare one family member	Comprehensive list of areas to assess family	Multiple theoretical approach

(continued on page 233)

	with another family member Assess and measure focused presenting problem		
Weakness	Narrow variable	Large quantities of data that may not relate to the problem No quantitative data	Not concrete enough to be useful as a guideline unless you study this model and approach in detail

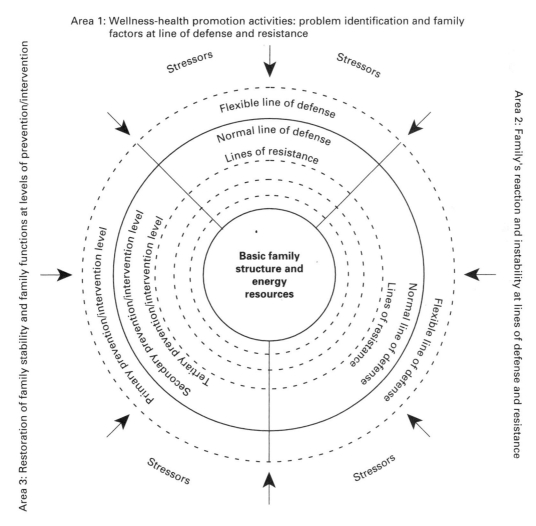

Figure 8–7 Family Assessment and Intervention Model.
Source: Hanson (2001).

their defense system. The family's reaction depends on how deeply the stressor penetrates the family unit and how capable the family is in adapting to maintain its stability. The lines of resistance protect the family's basic structure, which includes the family's functions and energy resources.

The core contains the patterns of family interactions and unit strengths. The basic structure must be protected at all costs, or the family ceases to exist. Reconstitution or adaptation is the work the family undertakes to preserve or restore family stability after stressors penetrate the family lines of defense, altering usual family functions. The model addresses three areas: (1) health promotion, wellness activities, problem identification, and family factors at lines of defense and resistance; (2) family reaction and instability at lines of defense and resistance; and (3) restoration of family stability and family functioning at levels of prevention and intervention. The basic assumptions of this family-focused model are listed in Box 8–8.

The *Family Systems Stressor-Strength Inventory* (FS³I) is the assessment and intervention tool that accompanies the Family Assessment and Intervention Model. The FS³I is divided into three sections: (1) family systems stressors—general, (2) family stressors—specific, and (3) family system strengths. An updated copy of the instrument, with instructions for administration and a scoring guide, can be found in Appendix C.

Box 8–8   BASIC ASSUMPTIONS FOR FAMILY ASSESSMENT AND INTERVENTION MODEL

Though each family as a family system is unique, each system is a composite of common, known factors or innate characteristics within a normal given range of response contained within a basic structure.

Many known, unknown, and universal environmental stressors exist. Each differs in its potential for disturbing a family's usual stability level, or normal line of defense. The particular interrelationships of family variables—physiological, psychological, sociocultural, developmental, and spiritual—at any time can affect the degree to which a family is protected by the flexible line of defense against possible reaction to one or more stressors.

Over time, each family or family system has evolved a normal range of response to the environment, referred to as a "normal line of defense," or usual wellness or stability state.

When the cushioning, accordion-like effect of the flexible line of defense is no longer capable of protecting the family or family system against an environmental stressor, the stressor breaks through the normal line of defense. The interrelationships of variables—physiological, psychological, sociocultural, developmental, and spiritual—determine the nature and degree of the system reaction or possible reaction to the stressor.

The family, whether in a state of wellness or illness, is a dynamic composite of the interrelationships of variables—physiological, psychological, sociocultural, developmental, and spiritual. Wellness is on a continuum of available energy to support the system in its optimal state.

Implicit within each family system is a set of internal resistance factors, known as "lines of resistance," which function to stabilize and return the family to the usual wellness state (normal line of defense) or possibly to a higher level of stability after an environmental stressor reaction.

Primary prevention is general knowledge that is applied in family assessment and intervention for identification and mitigation of risk factors associated with environmental stressors to prevent possible reaction.

Secondary prevention is symptomatology following reaction to stressors, appropriate ranking of intervention priorities, and treatment to reduce their noxious effects.

Tertiary prevention is the adjustive processes taking place as reconstitution begins and maintenance factors move the client back in a circular manner toward primary prevention.

The family is in dynamic, constant energy exchange with the environment.

Source: Hanson, S. M. H. (2001). Family nursing assessment and intervention. In *Family health care nursing: Theory, practice, and research* (2nd ed., p. 174). Philadelphia: FA Davis.

Family stability is assessed by gathering information on family stressors and strengths (Curran, 1983, 1985). The assessment of general, overall stressors is followed by an assessment of specific problems. The assessment of general, overall stressors is followed by an assessment of specific problems, such as birth of first child, loss of job, and divorce. Family strengths are identified to give an indication of the potential and actual problem-solving abilities of the family system. For the three problems cited above, family strengths could include supportive extended family, savings or high employability, and family counseling with a divorced family.

Family strengths are identified to give an indication of the potential and actual problem-solving abilities of the family system. Nurses have a history of asking people about their problems (stressors), but often nurses have not identified the strengths and resources the family possesses to deal with its problems.

The FS³I is intended for use with multiple family members, who may be assessed collectively or individually. This tool helps to identify both stressful situations that occur in families and the strengths families use to maintain healthy functioning, despite their problems. Individual members can complete the FS³I or the entire family can sit together and complete the assessment. The nurse meets with family members and interviews them to clarify perceived general stressors, specific stressors, and family strengths as identified by family members. This information is used by the nurse and family to develop a plan of care.

After the interview, the nurse completes the quantitative summary through which each participant's score is rated on the graph. This comparison visually shows the representation of family health perceptions. Variations in how individuals and the nurse view the situation are easily compared across stressors and strengths. The nurse completes the qualitative summary that synthesizes the interview information gleaned from all family participants. A family care plan with intervention strategies is developed and shared with the family. A case study using the FS³I with scoring and a plan of care are located in Appendix C.

A strength of the FS³I approach is that both quantitative and qualitative data are used to determine the level of prevention and intervention needed: primary, secondary, or tertiary (Pender, Murdaugh, & Parsons, 2001). Primary prevention focuses on moving the individual and family toward a state of improved health or toward health promotion activities. *Primary interventions* include providing families with information about their strengths, supporting their coping and functioning capabilities, and encouraging movement toward health through family education. *Secondary interventions* attain system stability after stressors or problems have invaded the family system. *Secondary interventions* include helping the family to handle its problems, helping family members to find and use appropriate treatment, and intervening in crises. *Tertiary prevention* is designed to maintain system stability through intervention strategies that are initiated after treatment has been completed and may include, for example, coordination of care after discharge from the hospital or rehabilitation services.

In summary, the *Family Assessment and Intervention Model* extends the Neuman Health Care Systems Model to focus on the family as client. The FS³I was developed as one way of assessing families using this model. This assessment approach focuses on family stressors and strengths and provides the nurse with data useful for nursing interventions.

The Friedman Family Assessment Model

The *Friedman Family Assessment Model* (Friedman, Bowden, & Jones, 2003) is based on the structural-functional framework and developmental and systems theory. This assessment model takes a macroscopic approach to family assessment by viewing families as subsystems of the wider society, including institutions devoted to religion, education, and health. Family is considered an open social system and focuses on the family's (1) structure, (2) functions (activities and purposes), and (3) relationships with other social systems. The Friedman model is commonly used when the family-in-community is the setting for care (e.g., in community and public health nursing). This approach enables family nurses to assess the family system as a whole, as a subunit of the society, and as an interactional system. The general assumptions of this model are delineated in Box 8–9 (Friedman, Bowden, & Jones, p. 100).

Structure refers to how a family is organized and how the parts relate to each other and to the whole. The four basic structural dimensions are role systems, value systems, communication networks, and power structure. These dimensions are interrelated and interactive, and they may differ in single-parent and two-parent families. For example, a single mother may be the head of the family, but she may not necessarily take on the authoritarian role that a traditional man might in a two-parent family. In turn, the value

Box 8–9 **UNDERLYING ASSUMPTIONS OF FRIEDMAN'S FAMILY ASSESSMENT MODEL**

- A family is a social system with functional requirements.
- A family is a small group possessing certain generic features common to all small groups.
- The family as a social system accomplishes functions that serve the individual and society.
- Individuals act in accordance with a set of internalized norms and values that are learned primarily through socialization.

Source: Friedman, M. M., Bowden, V. R., & Jones, E. G. (2003). *Family nursing: Research, theory & practice* (5th ed.). Upper Saddle River, NJ: Prentice Hall/Pearson Education.

systems, communication networks, and power structures may be quite different in the single-parent and two-parent families as a result of these structural differences.

Function refers to how families go about meeting the needs of individuals and meeting the purposes of the broader society. In other words, family functions are what a family does. The functions of the family historically are discussed in Chapter 1, but the following specific family functions are considered in this approach:

- Pass on culture, religion, ethnicity.
- Socialize young people for the next generation (e.g., to be good citizens, to be able to cope in society through education).
- Exist for sexual satisfaction and reproduction.
- Provide economic security.
- Serve as a protective mechanism for family members against outside forces.
- Provide closer human contact and relations.

The Friedman Family Assessment Model form consists of six broad categories of interview questions: (1) identification data, (2) developmental stage and history of the family, (3) environmental data, (4) family structure (i.e., role structure, family values, communication patterns, power structure), (5) family functions (i.e., affective functions, socialization functions, health care functions), and (6) family stress

and coping. Each category has several subcategories and can be found in the most recent book by Friedman, Bowden, and Jones (2003).

Friedman's assessment (short and long form) was developed to provide guidelines for family nurses who are interviewing a family. The guidelines categorize family information according to structure and function. Friedman's Family Assessment Form exists in both a long form and a short form. The long form is quite extensive, and it may not be possible to collect all of the data in one visit. Moreover, all the categories of information listed in the guidelines may not be pertinent for every family. Like other approaches, this model has its strengths and weaknesses. One problem with this approach is that it can generate large quantities of data with no clear direction as to how to use all of the information in diagnosis, planning, and intervention. The short form, which can be found in Appendix D, outlines the types of questions the nurse can ask. The long form is quite extensive, providing 13 pages of questions.

The Calgary Family Assessment Model

The *Calgary Family Assessment Model* (CFAM) by Wright and Leahey (2000) blends nursing and family therapy concepts that are grounded in systems theory, cybernetics, communication theory, change theory, and a biology of recognition. The following concepts from general systems theory and family systems theory make up the theoretical framework for this model (Wright & Leahy, 2000, pp. 38–44):

- A family system is part of a larger suprasystem and is also composed of many subsystems.
- The family as a whole is greater than the sum of its parts.
- A change in one family member affects all family members.
- The family is able to create a balance between change and stability.
- Family members' behaviors are best understood from a perspective of circular rather than linear causality.

Cybernetics is the science of communication and control theory; therefore, it differs from systems theory. Systems theory helps change the focus of one's conceptual lens from parts to wholes. By contrast, cybernetics changes the focus from substance to form. Wright and Leahey (2000, p. 45) pull two useful concepts from cybernetics theory:

- Families possess self-regulating ability.
- Feedback processes can simultaneously occur at several system levels with families.

Communication theory in this model is based on the work of Watzlawick and colleagues (1967, 1974). Communication represents the way that individuals interact with one another. Concepts derived from communication theory used in the Calgary Family Assessment Model are listed below (Wright & Leahey, 2000, pp. 46–49):

- All nonverbal communication is meaningful.
- All communication has two major channels for transmission: digital (verbal) and analogical (nonverbal).
- A dyadic relationship has varying degrees of symmetry and complementarity.
- All communication has two levels: content and relationship.

Helping families to change is at the very core of family nursing interventions. Families need a balance between change and stability. Change is required to make things better, and stability is required to maintain some semblance of order. A number of concepts from change theory are important to this family nursing approach (Wright & Leahey, 2000, pp. 49–59):

- Change is dependent on the perception of the problem.
- Change is determined by structure.
- Change is dependent on context.
- Change is dependent on coevolving goals for treatment.
- Understanding alone does not lead to change.
- Change does not necessarily occur equally in all family members.
- Facilitating change is the nurse's responsibility.
- Change occurs by means of a "fit" or meshing between the therapeutic offerings (interventions of the nurse) and the biopsychosocial-spiritual structures of family members.
- Change can be the result of a myriad of causes.

Figure 8–8 shows the branching diagram of the Calgary Family Assessment Model (Wright & Leahey, 2000, p. 68). The assessment questions that accompany the model are organized into three major categories: (1) structural, (2) developmental, and (3) functional. Nurses examine a family's structural components to answer these questions: Who is in the family? What is the connection between family members? What is the family's context? Structure includes family composition, gender, sexual orientation, rank order, subsystems, and the boundaries of the family system. Aside from interview and observation, strategies recommended to assess structure include the genogram and the ecomap.

> 66 Change is required to make things better, and stability is required to maintain some semblance of order. 99

The second major assessment category in the Calgary approach is family development, which includes assessment of family stages, tasks, and attachments. For example, nurses may ask, "Where is the family in the family life cycle?" Understanding the stage of the family enables nurses to assess and intervene in a more purposeful, specific, and meaningful way. There are no actual tools for assessing development, but nurses can use developmental tasks as guidelines.

The third area for assessment in the CFAM is family functioning. Family functioning reflects how individuals actually behave in relation to one another, or the "here-and-now aspect of a family's life" (Wright & Leahey, 2000, p. 128). Aspects of family functioning include activities of daily life, such as eating, sleeping, meal preparation, and health care, as well as emotional communication, verbal and nonverbal communication, circular communication, problem solving, roles, influence and power, beliefs, and alliances and coalitions. Wright and Leahey indicate that nurses may assess in all three areas (i.e., structural, developmental, functional) for a macroview of the family or they can use any part of the approach for a microassessment.

Wright and Leahey developed a companion model to the CFAM, the Calgary Family Intervention Model (CFIM) (2000). This intervention model provides concrete strategies by which nurses can promote, improve, and sustain effective family functioning in the cognitive, affective, and behavioral domains. More detail about this assessment model and intervention is available in Wright and Leahey's book, *Nurses and Families: A Guide to Family Assessment and Intervention* (2000).

These three family assessment approaches and instruments offer options to the family nurse. Table 8–5 compares these family approaches and instruments.

SUMMARY

- The selection of appropriate and sensitive assessment tools is important, as the information

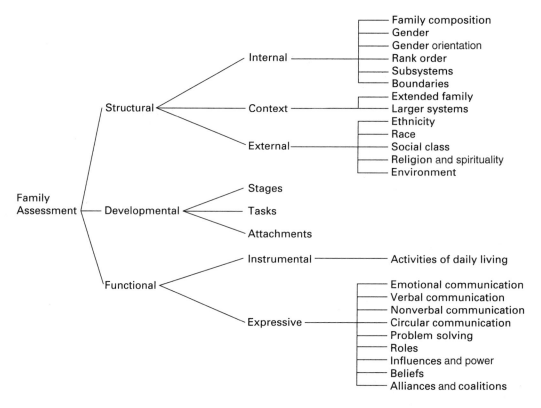

Figure 8–8 Diagram of the Calgary Family Assessment Approach.
Source: Wright & Leahey (2000).

collected serves as the foundation for the development of client-specific plans.

- The genogram provides a quick snapshot of the family members from an intergenerational perspective, such as how they are related, health or genetic trends, or potential sources of support for the family.
- The ecomap provides information about systems outside the family that are sources of support or that are stressors to the family.
- Both the family genogram and family ecomap should be used concurrently with all family assessments.
- Each step of working with families, whether applied to the individual within the family as context or to the family as client, requires a thoughtful, deliberate clinical reasoning process.
- The nurse must always be aware that the "common" interpretation of the data may not be the "correct" interpretation in a given situation, and the commonly expected signs and symptoms or cues may not appear in every case or in the same configuration.

- Each family has a story about how the potential or actual health issue influences its individual members, family functioning, and their management of the problem.
- Family nursing is more than simple medical care for the individual with the health issue. When the nurse meets with the family, it is important to investigate how all the members of the family are affected by the issue.
- If the keystone family issue is not accurately identified, the family and the nurse will collect data, design interventions, and implement plans of care that do not meet the most pressing needs for that family.
- Hanson's Family Systems, Stressor, Strength Intervention (FS³I) is used to measure specific family-identified issues. It is an assessment and measurement instrument that yields both qualitative and quantitative data.
- Friedman's Family Assessment Model (both the long and the short form) is a broader, more general assessment instrument, and is particularly useful for viewing families in the context of

their community. It does not have a measurement component.

- Wright and Leahey's CFAM and CFIM provide both assessment and intervention, though this method is less specific than the other two approaches. The CFAM is broad in perspective, and it focuses on internal relations within the family rather than the interface between the family and community.

CASE STUDY ➤

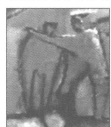

LB is a 35-year-old mother recovering from a cesarean-section delivery 7 days ago. She is coming into the mother-baby clinic office with her newborn daughter HB, 2-year-old daughter SB (also a cesarean delivery), and husband MB for a verbal assessment of the mother and physical assessment of the newborn. LB expresses some concerns with effectiveness in her breast-feeding techniques but proves to be efficient upon demonstration.

LB usually acts as the child-rearer, events planner, disciplinarian, and health expert. However, her surgical recovery is inhibiting her. LB has a Master's degree in elementary education and typically teaches third grade. She has taken 3 months off for maternity leave. The strong ties and responsibility she feels toward her school and teaching career has made this change difficult. However, LB feels extremely validated as both a mother and teacher. LB does not have any existing health problems.

MB works for Frito Lay in sales and distribution. His primary functions at home are as the decision-maker, maintenance person, pioneer, and information provider. These roles have altered in that he is additionally acting as the listener and mediator for the needs of his wife and daughter and the grandparents who inevitably add fuel to this conflict. He feels little attachment to his occupation and welcomes this new birth and the change in routine/opportunity to leave work. His current medical problems include DM Type II and mild HTN; both are well managed and controlled by oral diabetic and antihypertensive medications. Presently he is on the Atkins diet to reduce his weight and the extent of symptomatology experienced from his health conditions.

SB is a healthy 2-year-old girl who is developmentally appropriate. Psychologically SB is in the autonomy-versus-shame-and-doubt developmental stage. Her parents report that she often attempts to try new things on her own, and they frequently praise her efforts to promote independence. Piaget would place SB in the preoperational and preconceptual phase of cognitive development. She demonstrates egoism, a marked trait of this phase, and concrete thinking. In fact, her extent of egoism will be further explored, as it is a major family concern. She has yet to become interested in potty training. She is in Kohlberg's moral developmental stage of punishment and obedience orientation. According to the Denver Developmental Model, she should be able to wash and dry hands, and brush teeth with help, start to put on clothes, build a town of six cubes, speak with two words that are half-understandable, throw a ball, and jump up. Based on observation and parental reports, SB is able to complete all of these tasks. Her immunizations are current. She normally goes to a day-care center that is close to her mother's school during the work week. This past week she has stayed home to become acquainted with her sister. Her most noteworthy health history includes frequent ear infections. SB is somewhat unsure about her new sister and still continues to demonstrate an increased need to be close to her father. Adjusting to having a baby sister in the family has been extremely difficult for SB and is the main concern for the family today.

HB was delivered after 42 weeks gestation and was proved to be AGA (10–90th percentile), 53.75 cm and 3966 g, with APGARs of 8 at 1 minute and 9 at 5 minutes. HB shows normal development. Her weight is back to original birth weight with an additional 2 ounces. HB nurses approximately eight to ten times in a 24-hour period and requires six to seven diaper changes daily.

Support available: Today LB's incision line evidences marked healing with rapid approximation at the site and no signs of infection. LB does report occasional discomfort in the regions when she "overdoes it." When this happens, she calls on family support to resume tasks at hand and rests until feeling better. They have been able to help without requiring the usual "guest" protocols. MB's parents have been in town the past week, but will be returning home. This may perpetuate SB's interpretation of unimportance

(continued on page 240)

CASE STUDY ➤ *(Continued)*

and being ignored. LB's parents will remain in town for the next several weeks. LB is well aware of activity restrictions suggested for cesarean delivery.

Throughout the examination of HB, the parents demonstrate overwhelming signs of bonding by talking with the infant and bragging about her beauty and temperament. However, during this time, SB throws toys and attempts to crawl onto her mother's lap while her mother is nursing, but wants nothing to do with her otherwise. SB insists on remaining in her father's arms the rest of the time. The parents report that she has been very temperamental and inconsolable at day care. She often suggests bringing the baby back to the hospital or putting her back in her mother's womb. SB is entirely avoidant with her mother. When MB attempts to coddle or praise the baby, SB becomes extremely displeased with her father.

Frame: Healthy Caucasian nuclear family with two developmentally appropriate children. The 2-year-old daughter is evidencing adjustment difficulties with the addition of the new infant.

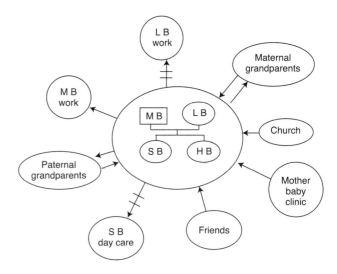

Figure 8–10 Case study ecomap of the B family.

Keystone Issue: Altered parent/child/infant attachment newborn needs are conflicting with needs and routine of toddler sibling, resulting in increased attachment and regression of toddler.

Present State:

1. SB regresses and fails to maintain normal developmental behaviors causing concern and stress for parents feeling conflicted about which child to console.
2. Family reports anxiety concerning ability to provide for both children, meeting their needs of attention, affection, and affirmation.
3. Parents express concern regarding environmental supports for assistance with increased demands of parenting when newborn and sibling seeking additional attention.

Outcome State:

1. Family will verbally report SB's demonstration of behavior appropriate for developmental age and regain baseline level of functioning prior to entrance of newborn within 1 week.
2. Family will report confidence in ability to provide sufficient and appropriate attention for both children by end of the checkup.
3. Parents will fully develop a list of resources including family, community resources, peers, church, and friends to assist in caring for children

Testing:

1. Observe sibling behavior on follow-up appointment for marked improvement in coping ability

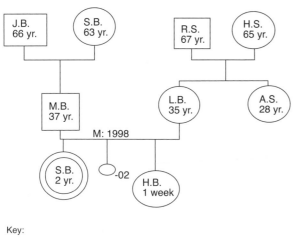

Key:

Male = ☐

Female = ◯

Married = ⌐_⌐

Children = |

Miscarriage = ◯ Year

Family member with health problem = Double circle or square

Figure 8–9 Case study genogram of the B family.

and adaptation to newborn and through the parents gauging and verbal reporting.
2. Verbally assess parents' anxiety level to ensure achievement of manageable level of concern
3. Have parents identify resources they have been able to tap into for assistance.

Interventions:

- Find out what about SB's behavior stresses the family the most and what their major concern is about her difficult adjustment.
- Explore with family how they have been dealing with SB's behavior, what works and what they have found does not work.
- Assist parents in recognizing behaviors used by SB to communicate avoidance/stress and approach/engagement.
- Support parents' ability to alleviate SB's distress by allowing participation in providing care for newborn.
- Assist parents to find a way to spend time alone with each child.
- Assist parents in developing new care-giving practice competencies by revisiting and extending old ones.
- Validate parents' concerns for providing for the needs of both children and provide written handouts to affirm teaching of this new parenting demand.
- Provide appropriate pain management routine for mother to increase activity level and ability to care for the children.
- Encourage family members to support mother through recovery and openly praise both siblings.
- Discuss change and how it affects toddlers. Assist family not to change too many routines and rituals that are specific to SB and to establish some new routines and rituals with HB.

Judgment

1. Outcome 1 was partially met though instruction and suggestions were provided. Observation and feedback are necessary at a future appointment.

2. Outcome 2 was fully met. Parents were able to decrease overall anxiety and feel empowered by suggestions and resources to deal with sibling rivalry.
3. Outcome 3 was fully met. Plans have been arranged to utilize other resources, including grandparents and peers in the upcoming weeks and the list of other possibilities for relief of care remains close at hand.

Reflection:

1. In caring for this family, I did an excellent job empathizing and validating the family's concern for the added stresses of a newborn. I was actually able to follow this family from post-partum to a clinic setting and found that the latter truly allowed for greater analysis of family dynamic. Though health-focused concerns were addressed on the unit, the clinic setting presented an ideal time to improve parenting techniques and ease fears concerning adjustment post-discharge. Learning how to shift focus from the more medical concern to family dynamic was the most challenging aspect.
2. Really watching how the rest of the family copes with newborns in the future will allow me to see this often-overlooked piece more readily. Perhaps working through this in a more detailed manner in the clinic will increase my efficiency in attacking this issue on the labor and delivery unit.
3. Providing outside contact numbers, brainstorming about parenting techniques, sending home fliers about parenting, and acting as a sounding board for this adjusting family truly empowered their overall ability to cope.
4. Little was done in the clinic setting in regard to spirituality. I would address more than "Who is available in your place of worship to assist in adjusting and care?".
5. I learned that both parents were adopted. I really empathized and actively listened to their concerns and family story.

References

Ackley, B. J., & Ladwig, G. B. (2004). *Nursing diagnosis handbook: A guide to planning care* (6th ed.). St. Louis: Mosby.

American Medical Association. (2004). *International classification of diseases: Clinical modifications (IDC-9CM)* (10th ed.). Dover, DE: American Medical Association.

American Psychiatric Association. (2000). *Diagnostic and statistical manual of mental disorders (DSM-IV-TRtm)* (4th ed.). Washington, DC: Author.

Benner, P. (1988). *From novice to expert.* Menlo Park, CA: Addison-Wesley.

Benner, P., Tanner, C., & Chesla, C. (1996). *Expertise in nursing practice.* New York: Springer.

Berkey-Mischke, K. M., & Hanson, S. M. H. (1991). *Pocket guide to family assessment and intervention.* St. Louis: Mosby Year Book.

Bowen, M. (1985). *Family therapy in clinical practice.* Norvale, NJ: Jason Aronson.

Bowen, M., & Kerr, M. (1988). *Family evaluation: An approach based on Bowen's Theory.* New York: W.W. Norton.

Carnevali, D., & Thomas, M (1993). *Diagnostic reasoning and treatment decision making in nursing.* Philadelphia: J.B. Lippincott Company.

Curran, D. (1983). *Traits and the healthy family.* Minneapolis: Winston Press.

Curran, D. (1985). *Stress and the healthy family.* Minneapolis: Winston Press.

Facione, N., & Facione, P. (1996). Externalizing the critical thinking in knowledge development and clinical judgment. *Nursing Outlook, 44*(3), 129–136.

Friedman, M. M., Bowden, V. R., & Jones, E. G. (2003). *Family nursing: Research, theory & practice* (5th ed.). Upper Saddle River, NJ: Prentice Hall/Pearson Education.

Gebbie, K., & Lavin, M. (1975). *Classification of nursing diagnosis: Proceedings of the first national conference.* St. Louis: Mosby.

Gordon, M. (1982). *Nursing diagnosis.* New York: McGraw-Hill.

Gordon, M. (1994). *Nursing diagnosis: Process and application.* New York: McGraw-Hill.

Hanna, S. M., & Brown, J. H. (2004). *The practice of family therapy, Key elements across models* (3rd ed.). Belmont, CA: Thompson/Brooks/Cole.

Hanson, S. M. H. (2001). Family nursing assessment and intervention. In *Family health care nursing: Theory, practice, and research* (2nd ed., pp. 170–195). Philadelphia: FA Davis.

Hanson, S. M. H., & Mischke, K. M. (1996). Family health assessment and intervention. In P. J. Bomar (Ed.), *Nurses and family health promotion: Concepts, assessment and interventions* (2nd ed.) (pp. 165–202). Philadelphia: WB Saunders.

Hartman, A., & Laird, J. (1983). *Family-centered: Social work practice.* New York: Free Press.

Kaakinen, J., Hanson, S. M. H, & Birenbaum, L. (2004). Family development and family nursing assessment. In M. Stanhope & J. Lancaster (Eds.) *Community health nursing: Promoting health of aggregates, families and Individuals* (pp. 562–593). St. Louis: Mosby.

Martin, K. S., & Scheet, N. J. (1992). *The Omaha System: Applications for community health nursing.* Philadelphia: WB Saunders.

McGoldrick, M., & Gerson, R. (1985). *Genograms in family assessment.* New York: WW Norton.

McGoldrick, M., Gerson, R., & Shellenburger, S. (1999). *Genograms in family assessment* (2nd ed.). New York: W.W. Norton.

Neuman, B. (1995). The Neuman systems model. In *The Neuman systems model* (3rd ed.) (pp. 3–44). Norwalk, CT: Appleton & Lange.

North American Nursing Diagnosis Association. (2003). *Nursing diagnosis: Definitions and classifications.* Philadelphia: Author.

Paul, R. (1993). *Critical thinking.* Santa Rosa, CA: Foundation for Critical Thinking.

Pender, N. J., Murdaugh, C. L., & Parsons, M. A. (2001). *Health promotion in nursing practice* (4th ed.). Upper Saddle River: Prentice Hall.

Pesut, D., & Herman, J. (1999). *Clinical reasoning: The art and science of critical and creative thinking.* Boston: Delmar.

Reed, K. S. (1993). *Betty Neuman: The Neuman systems model.* Newbury Park, CA: Sage.

Ross, B. (2001). Nursing process and family health care. In S. Hanson, *Family health care nursing: Theory, practice and research* (2nd ed.) (pp. 146–169). Philadelphia: FA Davis.

Toman, W. (1976). *Family constellation: Its effect on personality and social behavior,* (3rd ed.). New York: Springer Publishing.

Touliatos, J., Perlmutter, B., & Straus, M. (2001). *Handbook of family measurement techniques.* Newbury Park, CA: Sage.

Vogt, W. P. (1999). *Dictionary of statistics and methodology: A nontechnical guide for the social sciences* (2nd ed.). Thousand Oaks, CA: Sage.

Watzlawick, P., et al. (1967). *Pragmatics of human communication.* New York: W.W. Norton.

Watzlawick, P., et al. (1974). *Change: Principles of problem formulation and problem resolution.* New York: W.W. Norton.

Wright, L. M., & Leahey, M. (2000). *Nurses and families: A guide to family assessment and intervention* (3rd ed.). Philadelphia: FA Davis.

Wright, L. M., Watson, W., & Bell, J. (1996). *Beliefs: The heart of healing in families and illness.* New York: Basic Books.

Yura, H., & Walsh, M. (1988). *The nursing process: Assessment, planning, implementation, and evaluation* (5th ed.). Norwalk, CT: Appleton & Lange.

Bibliography

Carter, B., & McGoldrick, M. (1999). *The expanded family life cycle: Individual, family, and social perspectives* (3rd ed.). Boston: Allyn & Bacon.

Clemen-Stone, S., et al. (1991). *Comprehensive family community health nursing* (3rd ed.) St. Louis: Mosby.

Feetham, S. (1983). Feetham Family Functioning Survey. Available from Suzanne Feetham, National Center for Nursing Research, Office of Planning Analysis Evaluation, Building 31, Room 5BO9, Rockville Pike, Bethesda, MD 20882.

Herrick, C. A., & Goodykoontz, L. (1989). Neuman's Systems Model for nursing practice as a conceptual framework for a family assessment. *Journal of Child Adolescent Psychiatric Mental Health Nursing, 2,* 61–67. [Also reprinted in Wegner, G. D., & Alexander, R. J. (1999). *Readings in family nursing* (2nd ed.). Philadelphia: Lippincott.]

Nurse, A. R. (1999). *Family assessment: Effective uses of personality tests with couples and families.* New York: John Wiley & Sons.

Polit, D. F., Beck, C. T., Hungler, B. P. (2001). *Essentials of nursing research: Methods, appraisal, and utilization.* Philadelphia: Lippincott.

Reed, K., & Tarko, M. (2004). Using the nursing process with families. In P. Bomar (Ed.), *Promoting health in families: Applying family research and theory to nursing practice* (3rd ed.) (pp. 257–273). Philadelphia: Saunders.

Vaughan-Cole, B., et al. (1998). *Family nursing practice.* Philadelphia: WB Saunders.

Walsh. F. (2002). *Normal family processes: Growing diversity & complexity* (3rd ed.). New York: The Guilford Press.

Waltz, C. F., & Jenkins, L. S. (Eds.). (2003). *Measurement of nursing outcomes. Vol. 1: Measuring nursing performance in practice, education, and research* (2nd ed.). New York: Springer Publishing.

Wegner, G. B., & Alexander, R. J. (Eds.). (1999). *Readings in family nursing.* Philadelphia: J.B. Lippincott.

Werth, E., & Conoley, J. C. (1995). *Family assessment (Buros-Nebraska Series on Measurement and Testing).* Lincoln, NE: University of Nebraska Press.

Yingling, L. C., Miller, W. E., McDonald, A. L., & Galewaler, S. T. (1998). *GARF assessment sourcebook: Using the DSM-IV global assessment of relational functioning.* Washington, DC: Brunner/Mazel/Taylor & Francis.

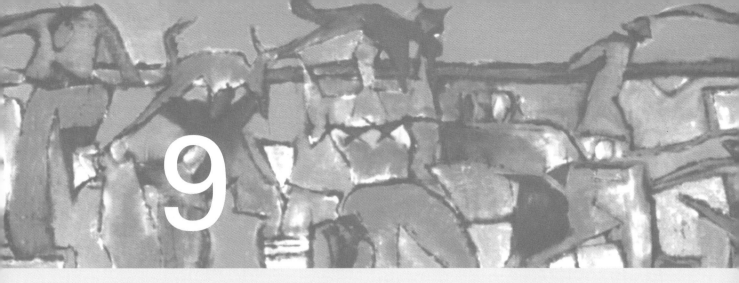

9

Family Health Promotion

Perri J. Bomar, RN, PhD

CRITICAL CONCEPTS

- Fostering the health of the family as a unit and encouraging families to value and incorporate health promotion into their lifestyle are essential components of family nursing practice.

- Health promotion is learned within families, and patterns of health behaviors are formed and passed on to the next generation.

- The role of the family nurse is to help families attain, maintain, and regain the highest level of family health possible.

- Family health is a holistic, dynamic, and complex state. It is more than the absence of disease in an individual family member or the absence of dysfunction in family dynamics. Instead it is the complex process of solving, negotiating day-to-day family life events and crises, and providing for a quality of life for its members.

- Health and family policies at all governmental levels affect the quality of individual and family health.

- Health promotion advertisements have generally targeted the more health-conscious middle class, rather than the vulnerable and underserved who are often the targets for alcohol and tobacco advertising campaigns.

- Families who are flexible and able to adjust to change are more likely to be involved in health-promoting activities. Vulnerable families are often coping with a pileup of stressors and may be unable to focus on activities to enhance family health. Low-income families may focus less on health promotion and more on basic needs such as obtaining shelter, adequate food, and health care.

- Through verbal and nonverbal communication, parents teach behavior, share feelings and values, and make decisions about family health practices.

- Different cultures define and value health, health promotion, and disease prevention differently. Clients may not understand or respond to the family nurses' suggestions for health promotion because the suggestions conflict with their health beliefs and values.

- The goal of the family nurse is to facilitate family adaptation by empowering the family to promote resilience, reduce the pileup of stressors, make use of resources, and negotiate necessary change to enhance the family's ability to rebound from stressful events or crises.

- Family health promotion should become a regular part of taking a family history and a routine aspect of nursing care.

INTRODUCTION

Fostering the health of the family as a unit and encouraging families to value and incorporate health promotion into their lifestyle are essential components of family nursing practice. Health promotion is learned within families, and patterns of health behaviors are formed and passed on to the next generation. The family is primarily responsible for providing health and illness care, being a role model, teaching self-care and wellness behaviors, providing for care of members across their life course and during varied family transitions, and supporting each other during health-promoting activities and acute and chronic illnesses. A major task of the family is to teach health maintenance and health promotion, regardless of age. The case study at the end of the chapter describes a family scenario in which lifestyle changes would improve the mother's and the whole family's health. The role of the nurse is to help families attain, maintain, and regain the highest level of family health possible.

What Is Family Health?

Definitions of *family health* have evolved from anthropological, biopsychosocial, developmental, family science, religious, cultural, and nursing paradigms. They vary depending on their origin (Anderson & Tomlinson, 1992; Bomar & McNeeley, 1996; Doherty & Campbell, 1988). Family scientists define healthy families as resilient (McCubbin & McCubbin, 1993) and as possessing a balance of cohesion and adaptability that is facilitated by good communication (Olson et al., 1989). Family therapy definitions often emphasize optimal family functioning and freedom from psychopathology (Bradshaw, 1988). Within the developmental framework, healthy families complete developmental tasks at appropriate times (Duval & Miller, 1985).

Taking a sociological view, Pratt (1976) describes a healthy family as an *energized family*, a family that responds to the needs and interests of all its members, copes effectively with life transitions and problems, is flexible and egalitarian in distribution of power, interacts regularly among its members and with the community, and encompasses a health-promoting lifestyle of individual members and the family unit.

❝The role of the nurse is to help families attain, maintain, and regain the highest level of family health possible.❞

Other definitions include the totality, or *gestalt*, of the family's existence and include the internal and external environment of the family. A holistic definition of family health encompasses all aspects of family life, including interaction and health care function. Family health care function includes family nutrition, recreation, communication, sleep and rest patterns, problem solving, sexuality, use of time and space, coping with stress, hygiene and safety, spirituality, illness care, health promotion and protection, and emotional health of family members (Bomar, 2004a; Friedman, Bowden & Jones 2003). A healthy family has a sense of well-being and is free from dysfunction. In summary, *family health* is a holistic, dynamic, and complex state. Family health is more than the absence of disease in an individual family member or the absence of dysfunction in family dynamics. Instead, it is the complex process of solving and negotiating day-to-day family life events and crises and providing for a quality life for its members (Bomar, 2004a) (see Table 9–1).

❝*Family health promotion* is defined as achieving maximum family well-being throughout the family life course and includes the biological, emotional, physical, and spiritual realms for family members and the family unit (Bomar, 2004a; Loveland-Cherry & Bomar, 2004).❞

COMMON THEORETICAL PERSPECTIVES

There are many models and theories applicable to family health and family health promotion (See Box 9–1). This section briefly describes the several models of family health and family health promotion.

Models of Family Health

Building on Smith's (1983) models of health, Loveland-Cherry (1986) suggests that there are four views of family health:

1. The *clinical model.* Examined from this perspective, a family is healthy if its members are free of physical, mental, and social dysfunction.
2. The *role-performance model.* This view of family health is based on the idea that family health is the ability of family members to perform their routine roles and achieve developmental tasks.

Table 9–1   TRAITS OF A HEALTHY FAMILY

Unity

COMMITMENT

- Develops a sense of trust
- Teaches respect for others
- Exhibits a sense of shared responsibility

TIME TOGETHER

- Shares family rituals and traditions
- Enjoys each other's company
- Shares leisure time
- Shares simple and quality time

Flexibility

ABILITY TO DEAL WITH STRESS

- Displays adaptability
- Sees crises as a challenge and opportunity
- Shows openness to change
- Grows together in crisis
- Seeks help with problems

SPIRITUAL WELL-BEING

- Encourages hope
- Shares faith
- Teaches compassion for others
- Teaches ethical values
- Respects the privacy of one another

Communication

POSITIVE COMMUNICATION

- Communicates and listens effectively
- Fosters family table time and conversation
- Shares feelings
- Displays non-blaming attitudes
- Is able to compromise and disagree
- Agrees to disagree

APPRECIATION AND AFFECTION

- Cares for each other
- Exhibits a sense of humor
- Maintains friendship
- Respects individuality
- Has a spirit of playfulness

Source: Curran, D. (1983). *Traits of a healthy family* (pp. 23–24). Minneapolis, MN: Winston Press; Olson, D., & DeFrain, J. (2003). *Marriage and the family: Diversity and strengths* (4th ed.). New York: McGraw-Hill.

Box 9–1   HISTORICAL PERSPECTIVES OF FAMILY HEALTH PROMOTION

Although the majority of health care professionals continue to focus their activities on prevention and treatment of illness in individuals and dysfunctional families, key social forces, including the wellness and self-care movement of the past 30 years, continue to stimulate the nursing profession to focus on health promotion for families. The 1980 White House Conference on Families pointed out the need to improve family functioning and encourage healthy family lifestyles. The conference brought to light the importance of disease prevention and health promotion for improving the quality of family life in the United States. Three documents from the U.S. Department of Health and Human Services—*Healthy People: The Surgeon General's Report on Health Promotion and Disease Prevention* (1979); *Promoting Health/Preventing Disease: Objectives for the Nation* (1980); and *Healthy People 2000: National Health Promotion and Disease Prevention Objectives* (1990)—provided overall goals for the nation regarding health promotion for individuals and families.

(continued on page 246)

Box 9–1   **HISTORICAL PERSPECTIVES OF FAMILY HEALTH PROMOTION** *(Continued)*

Although there are many improvements in the health status of the nation as a whole, the newest document, *Healthy People 2010* (U.S. Department of Health and Human Services, 2000), builds on the lessons learned from the three previous initiatives. The goals for the year 2010 are to eliminate health disparities and to increase the quality and years of life. Major objectives for the millennium include promoting healthy behaviors, promoting healthy and safe communities, improving systems for personal and public health, and preventing and reducing diseases and disorders. Reference Chapter 15, Families and Community/Public Health Nursing.

Since the first report by the surgeon general in 1979 and the continued national interest in health promotion in the 1990s, health professionals, family scientists, sociologists, psychologists, religious leaders, and social workers have made considerable strides in understanding and intervening to improve the quality of family health. Members include health professionals with special interest in the health and illness of families across the life span. Another example of this continuing national interest in health promotion is the increasing use of parish nurses, who provide health care and health promotion to individuals and families in faith communities (Solari-Twadell, McDermott, & Matheus, 1999).

3. The *adaptive model.* In this model, families are adaptive if they have the ability to change and grow and possess the capacity to rebound quickly after a crisis.

4. The *eudaimonistic model.* Professionals who use this model as their philosophy of practice focus on efforts to maximize the family's well-being and to support the entire family and individual members in reaching their highest potential.

According to Loveland-Cherry and Bomar (2004), these family health models are useful in three ways: (1) they provide frameworks for understanding the level of health that families are experiencing; (2) they may be useful in designing interventions to assist families in maintaining or regaining good health or in coping with illness; and (3) they may facilitate organization of the family nursing literature and serve as a focus for family research. There are numerous models that incorporate the stages of wellness and illness and explain the impact of illness on individuals and families.

Family Cycle of Health and Illness

Danielson, Hamel-Bissell, and Winstead-Fry (1993) synthesize the previous work of Doherty and McCubbin (1985) and of Coe (1970) in their model of the family cycle of health and illness. Table 9–2 outlines this model, which depicts the dynamic movement between the phases of illness and wellness. Families do not always progress sequentially from one phase to another; some phases may be bypassed. For

example, if an illness is transitory and brief (such as influenza), the family rapidly passes from a healthy state to experiencing symptoms, the sick role, medical consultation, adaptation, and then back to a healthy state. In transitory illness, the process takes about 10 days. On the other hand, in the case of a chronic disease, the stages are longer and require more permanent family adjustments and adaptations. During each phase of the cycle, the family and its members engage in activities to foster family health and attain optimal levels of functioning.

PHASES OF FAMILY CYCLE OF HEALTH AND ILLNESS

1. During the *family health promotion and risk reduction* phase, the family engages in a variety

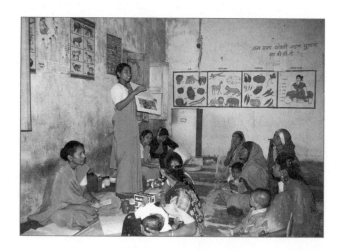

Table 9–2   PHASES OF THE FAMILY CYCLE OF HEALTH AND ILLNESS

PHASE	DESCRIPTION
Family health (family health promotion and risk reduction)	The family develops and instills beliefs, values, and patterns that promote a healthy lifestyle and reduce the risk of disease or family dysfunction.
Family vulnerability and experience symptoms of illness	Members vulnerable to disease or the family unit vulnerable to dysfunction, stress, or crisis. The awareness that illness or dysfunction is present.
Sick role assumed/family illness appraisal	The meaning the family gives to the illness or situation. Also, includes initial role changes that give evidence of illness.
Contact with the health care system and diagnosis of the problem/illness	Seeking legitimating of the sick role or problem. Family acceptance of the diagnosis or solution.
Family acute response	Adjustments the family makes in response to an illness or situation. This includes making such adjustments as making arrangements in the family to care for the ill member, temporary role changes, and financial management.
Family adaptation to illness and recovery	Incorporation of the illness/event into family lifestyle while attempting to return to normalcy in family roles, structures, functions, and interactions.
Death of a member and family reorganization	Family adjustments and adaptations to the death of a member. This includes the period of grief and role adjustments involved in recovery to a healthy family of a different type.

Source: Doherty, W. J., & Campbell, T. L. (1988). *Families and health.* Newbury Park: Sage; Danielson, C., Hamel-Bissell, B., & Winstead-Fry, P. (1993). *Families in health and illness* (pp. 65–91). St. Louis: Mosby.

of activities to improve and maintain the health of individual members and promote family functioning. For example, one health-promoting behavior is spending an evening together as a family.

2. The second phase in the health and illness cycle is the *family vulnerability and symptom experience* phase, when the family perceives that its members are vulnerable and takes action to reduce the risk of illness of a member or the risk of family dysfunction. Examples of risk reduction behaviors include routine breast self-examination and immunizations for individuals and regularly scheduled family meetings to problem solve for family risk reduction. During this phase, some families may use folk and home remedies for illnesses and consult their network for advice. If symptoms persist or adequate resources are not available, the family

may then decide to make contact with a health professional.

3. During phase 3, *family illness appraisal/sick role*, the family accepts the sick role of the family member, evaluates potential threats or loss from the illness, and makes adjustments in family activities and the family lifestyle to accommodate the illness (Danielson, Hamel-Bissell, & Winstead-Fry, 1993).

4. In the fourth phase, *family medical contact and diagnosis*, the family consults the health care system for diagnosis of the illness and to assist the family in understanding the health problem. The level of family communication contributes significantly to family understanding and adjustment in this phase.

5. After the illness is diagnosed, the family begins the fifth phase, which is called *family acute response.* The illness may progress to become

acute or chronic or may result in death. If the ill member is cured and gives up the sick role, the family returns to the first phase, family health. If the illness continues, the family becomes a family with a chronically ill family member.

6. The sixth phase is the period of *recovery and rehabilitation*, in which the major tasks are relinquishment of the sick role, establishment of new patterns of family life, and return to phase 1. Long-term chronic diseases or severe disabilities bring a separate sixth phase: *chronic adjustment adaptation*. The family's ability to cope with the illness is influenced by its resources and its ability to adapt during crisis (McCubbin & McCubbin, 1993).

7. After the death of a family member, the family enters phase 7, *death and family reorganization*, which includes the stressful processes of family grieving and reorganization of both family and extra-familial roles and functions. After completing reorganization, the family unit returns to phase 1 of the cycle.

Models for Family Health Promotion

Family health promotion occurs in phase 1 of the family health and illness cycle. In the past, most of the attention of health professionals focused on individuals, family subsystems (marital and parent-child dyads), and community health problems. There is a great need to encourage health promotion of the whole family unit because health behaviors, values, and patterns are learned within a family context. Family health promotion activities are crucial both during wellness and during illness of a family member. Family health promotion increases family unity and quality of life. According to Pender (1996), family health promotion involves the family's lifelong efforts to nurture its members, to maintain family cohesion, and to reach the family's highest potential in all aspects of health. Overall, family health promotion refers to activities families engage in to strengthen the family as a unit.

❝Family health promotion increases family unity and quality of life.❞

Preliminary Health Promotion Model

Most models of health promotion focus on the individual. Adapting Pender's (1996) health promotion

model, Loveland-Cherry and Bomar (2004) presented a preliminary family health promotion model. In this model, the likelihood of a family engaging in health-promoting behaviors is influenced by the following general, health-related, and behavioral specific factors:

1. *General influences*
   • Family systems patterns such as values, communication, interactions, and power
   • Demographic characteristics such as family size, structure, income, and culture
   • Biological characteristics
2. *Health-related influences*
   • Family health socialization patterns
   • Family definition of "health"
   • Perceived family health status
3. *Behavior-specific influences*
   • Perceived barriers to health-promoting behavior
   • Perceived benefits to health-promoting behavior
   • Prior related behavior
   • Family norms regarding health-promoting behavior
   • Intersystem support for behavior
   • Situational influences
   • Internal and environmental family cues

For example, a family who lives in poverty would be less likely to be involved in health promotion. In addition, if a family defines "health" as the absence of disease, they are also less likely to engage in a health-promoting lifestyle.

All of these variables are interrelated and affect the quality of family health-promoting outcomes. Although there are similarities in families in each of these variables, families also have unique differences that affect health outcomes. For example, family health beliefs, religion, social support, and gender roles affect health promotion. Clinicians are encouraged to assess each of these categories to determine how it contributes to the family's health-promoting outcomes. Ongoing research is needed to determine the relationship between the concepts in the model and family health promotion outcomes.

Developmental Model of Health and Nursing

The Developmental Model of Health and Nursing (DMHN) constructed by Canadian scholar F. Moyra Allen in the mid-1970s and 1980s (Allen, & Warner, 2002) has a goal of collaborating and increasing the capacity of families and individuals in health promotion in everyday life situations. In this interaction model, the nurse's role changes at each phase of the health promotion process, thereby empowering clients toward improving their health status. Examples of the nursing functions include the following:

- Focuser, stimulator, and resource producer who involves the client in such tasks as clarifying concerns and goals and thinking about his/her learning style
- Integrator and awareness raiser who assists clients with analyzing the situation, identifying additional resources, and seeking potential solutions
- Role model, instructor, coach, guide, and encourager as clients make decisions on alternatives and try new behavior
- Role re-enforcer and reviewer as clients review and evaluate outcomes (Allen & Warner, 2002, p. 122)

Ford-Gilboe (2002) summarized six studies that tested the propositions of Allen's DMHN. The studies tested four concepts: health potential, health work, competence in health behavior, and health status. Results indicated significant relationships between health potential and health work. Also noted was a significant prediction of family functioning by level of family health potential, health work, and health competence. Although in the past decade family health promotion has received considerable emphasis in nursing, reports on the effectiveness of family-focused health promotion continue to be scanty. Therefore, continued research is required using family health promotion models to evaluate the effectiveness of interventions to promote family health.

Pearsall (1990) presented a lay model for family health promotion in which families are encouraged to use their inner resources to strengthen, comfort, and heal family relationships (see Box 9–2 for strategies to promote family health).

ECOSYSTEM INFLUENCES

Family health promotion is a multidimensional construct that is the by-product of family interactions with both factors outside the home and internal family processes (Bomar, 2004a). The following section describes the ecosystem influences on family quality of life.

External Influences

External ecosystem influences include such things as the national economy, family and health policy, socie-

tal and cultural norms, media, and environmental hazards such as noise, air, soil, crowding, and chemicals.

Economic Resources

The national economy directly affects the family's ability to promote health. The availability of jobs directly affects the quality of a family's lifestyle. Clear disparities exist between health promotion initiatives geared toward middle-class families and toward low-income families. Until the mid-1980s, little attention was given to the health of minorities and people of low income (U.S. Department of Health and Human Services [USDHHS], 1985). The U.S. Office of Minority Health was created in 1985 to address the specific health needs of African-Americans, Asians and Pacific Islanders, Hispanics, and Native Americans. With the adoption of *Healthy People 2000* and *Healthy People 2010*, the health promotion and disease prevention focus has moved more toward alleviating the clear health disparities between socioeconomic classes (USDHHS, 1990, 2000).

Likewise, when a family has economic health, it has the resources needed for family health promotion. Adequate family income contributes to emotional well-being and supplies resources for adequate family space, recreation, and leisure. Socioeconomic class is a crucial ingredient in family health promotion. Middle- and upper-class families are more likely than poor families to engage in health-promoting and preventive activities. The cost of buying recreational and exercise equipment, for example, is often beyond the means of low-income families. The activities of low-income families are often directed toward meeting basic needs—providing for food, shelter, and safety and curing acute illness—rather than prevention or health promotion.

Health and Family Policies

Health and family policies at all governmental levels also affect the quality of individual and family health. Many of the objectives in *Healthy People 2000* and *Healthy People 2010* are couched in terms of the individual; many of these objectives, however, can be attained only by providing access to health care and changing family health lifestyles (Shi & Singh, 1998). Local communities provide water and monitor its quality, maintain sanitation, develop and maintain parks for recreation, and provide health services to low-income and elderly families. Such local services

Box 9–2 **STRATEGIES TO PROMOTE FAMILY HEALTH**

Families are encouraged to consider the following strategies to promote family health:

- **Family *rituals*** are the receptive behaviors or activities between two or more family members that occur with regularity in the day-to-day activities of daily living. Examples are a hug when a member leaves or returns, saying grace at meals, bedtime stories for children, and so forth. Rituals provide security and attachment to oneness (unity) of the family system.
- **Family *rhythm*** is learning to do things together. This is a calm moving together in harmony during the family activities of daily living.
- **Family *reason*** is being reasonable during irrational times. Is there fairness and effort on everyone's part to reduce conflict? Recognition that family health is created not by being an actor but rather by interaction with others.
- **Family *remembrance*** is keeping of the family heritage, respect for family history, and learning from the conflicts of members from the previous generation.
- **Family *resilience*** is the process of staying together through the stresses of life, to tolerate and grow as a unit with family spirit.
- **Family *resonance*** is making good family vibes. It is a sense of the family as a unit of energy rather than as a group of individuals. Family members are free to self-actualize as well as work together for family unity.
- **Family *reconciliation*** is the process of getting back together again after conflict. This includes always forgiving, tolerating, and loving no matter what the family problem. It involves not allowing anything to destroy the family because unforgivingness leads to a life of regret.
- **Family *reverence*** is protecting the dignity of the family unit by concern for "us." It involves having a pride and respect for the uniqueness of the family unit and an "enduring commitment to the eternal unity of the family."
- **Family *revival*** is quick recovery from family conflicts, arguments, and feuds.
- **Family *reunion*** is the process of bringing together the family for the purpose of celebrating life together, maintaining family cohesion, comforting one another, learning from each other, and loving.

Source: Pearsall, P. (1990). *The power of the family: Strength, comfort, and healing.* New York: Doubleday.

enhance the health of individuals and enhance family health. At the state level, services include assistance with medical care through Medicaid, the maintenance of state recreational areas and parks, health promotion and prevention programs, and economic assistance for low-income families and children (Hagen, 1999).

Additional federal level policies and fiscal support are needed to improve the quality of family health; in particular, there is a need for policy supporting the following:

1. Primary care for individuals across the life span
2. Child care
3. Economic support for vulnerable families
4. More national parks and recreation areas
5. Research on families and family health-promoting lifestyle practices

Because of the number of different government agencies involved in health care and family issues, there is a need for collaboration among these policy-making bodies. Chapter 6 discusses national policies related to caregiving, child care, education, and welfare.

Environment

According to Bomar (2004c), awareness of the quality of family living environment is crucial because the family and its members are exposed to public, occupational, and residential hazards. Environmental health is one of the areas of emphasis of the *Healthy People 2010 Objectives*. Box 9–3 lists the major objectives specific to families. Many environmental hazards are not monitored consistently by families or organiza-

Box 9–3   *HEALTHY PEOPLE 2010* ENVIRONMENTAL OBJECTIVES SPECIFIC TO FAMILIES

Number	Objective Short Title
Outdoor Air Quality	
8–1	Reduce harmful air pollutants
8–2	Increase alternative modes of transportation
8–3	Increase the use of cleaner alternative fuels
Water Quality	
8–5	Increase access to safe drinking water
8–6	Reduce waterborne disease outbreaks
8–7	Increase water conservation
8–8	Reduce surface water health risks
8–10	Reduce human consumption of contaminated fish
Toxics and Waste	
8–11	Reduce elevated blood lead levels in children
8–12	Reduce risks posed by hazardous sites
8–13	Reduce pesticide exposures
8–14	Reduce toxic pollutants in the environment
Healthy Homes and Healthy Communities	
8–16	Reduce indoor allergens
8–17	Improve office building air quality
8–18	Increase homes tested for radon
8–20	Implement school policies to protect against environmental hazards
8–21	Increase disaster preparedness plans and protocols
8–22	Increase lead-based paint testing
8–23	Reduce the number of occupied substandard housing
Others Environmental Objectives Specific to Children	
24–2a	Reduce asthma-related hospitalizations of children under 5
27–9	Reduce the percentage of children regularly exposed to secondhand smoke

Source: U.S. Department of Health and Human Services. (2000). *Healthy people 2010.* Washington, DC: U.S. Government Printing Office.

tions. Therefore, it is imperative to increase the capacity of families to recognize environmental hazards and to teach strategies to prevent, remove, or cope with environmental hazards such as pollution of air, water, food, and soil from numerous chemicals, occupational hazards, and violence (Bomar, 2004c; Sattler & Lipscomb, 2003). For instance, to prevent exposure to lead and pesticides, families could be taught to wash fruits and vegetables well prior to eating. Workers should be taught to monitor chemicals and infectious materials that might be transmitted to themselves and their families on work clothing and/or their skin. In addition, paint of older homes and outside play areas of children should be inspected for lead contamination. Families with young children and workers who work around metals and chemicals need to be especially cautious of lead poisoning and should consult Websites such as the one for the Centers for Disease Control for additional information.

Media

Another influence on family health is the visual and print media. Many advertisements advocate drinking alcohol, using tobacco products, and consuming foods that are high in sugar, salt, and fat. Health promotion advertisements have generally targeted the more health-conscious middle class, rather than the vulnerable and underserved who are often the targets for alcohol and tobacco advertising campaigns. Relatively recent tobacco advertising regulations take a small step in the right direction toward promoting healthier families. For example, in the 1990s, laws were passed that prohibit tobacco advertisements near schools, on tee shirts, and in magazines for teens. Many states require that cigarettes not be in the reach of minors in retail stores.

Science and Technology

Advances in science and technology have increased the life span of Americans, decreased the length of hospital stays, and contributed to our understanding of how to prevent, reduce, and treat disease. The development of more effective medications and advanced medical equipment technology has greatly increased the feasibility of home health care for chronically ill family members of all ages. Families are often the caregivers for ill members, and they provide the majority of care to older adults. There are now many valuable sources of information on health promotion for families and individuals. The Internet and the use of the World Wide Web is one forum that has come of age in the areas of family life education and health promotion (Elliot, 1999). Other technological advan-ces are also changing how we provide health care. Telemedicine technology, for instance, permits families to transmit heart rates via telemedicine to health care providers and for specialists to consult with family physicians, making it easier for individuals to access health care and for practitioners to provide it.

Internal Influences

Internal ecosystem influences include family type and developmental stage, family lifestyle patterns, family processes, the personalities of family members, power structure, family role models, coping strategies and processes, resilience, and culture.

Family Type and Development

Family type, whether healthy or dysfunctional, affects the health and well-being of the family (McCubbin & McCubbin, 1993). Families who are flexible and able to adjust to change are more likely to be involved in health-promoting activities. Vulnerable families are often coping with a pileup of stressors and may be unable to focus on activities to enhance health (Hertz & Ferguson, 1997). When families experience transitions, changes in their health-promoting lifestyles are often required (Faux, 1998). Thus, when a family member becomes ill, the health-promoting activities of the caretakers are generally curtailed. Often, the well-being of the family and caregiver is compromised, beginning with phase 3 of the family health and illness cycle and continuing to the end of phase 7 (from the sick role and family appraisal to the chronic illness phase or death and reorganization phase). The stage of family development, including childbearing, school-age launching, retirement, and the accomplishment of developmental tasks, also significantly influences a family's ability to be healthy.

Family Structure

Families in this millennium are quite different from the families of the 1970s. Family structures are more diverse; there are more dual-career/dual-earner families, blended families, same-gender couples, and single-parent families. The number of vulnerable families has also increased, including low-income traditional families, low-income migrant families, homeless families, and low-income older adults. Included in the vulnerable population are low-income, single-parent families and single-parent teen families. Health promotion for these different families presents various challenges. For example, a single, working parent may lack parent-child time, experience role stress, and have poor lifestyle patterns and poor life satisfaction (Loveland-Cherry, 1986; Wijnberg & Weinger, 1998). As stated earlier, low-income families may focus less on health promotion and more on basic needs of obtaining shelter, adequate food, and health care.

Family Processes

Family processes are continual actions, or series of changes, that take place in the family experience. Essential processes of a healthy family include functional communication (Crawford & Tarko, 2004) and family interaction (Denham, 2003). Through both verbal and nonverbal communication, parents teach behavior, share feelings and values, and make decisions about family health practices. Summarizing four studies of Appalachian families, Denham (2003) reported that mothers are the primary people in the family to teach and provide health care. It is through communication that families adapt to transitions and develop cohesiveness (Olson, 2000). Positive, reinforcing interaction between family members leads to a healthier family lifestyle. In order for optimal health promotion to take place, families must utilize their natural support systems (McGoldrick and Giordano, 1996: Bullock, 2004).

Culture

Different cultures define and value health, health promotion, and disease prevention differently (Huff & Kline, 1999; Leininger & McFarland, 2002). There is a mounting trend toward a global society with ever-increasing diversity among the populations. An expanded worldview is necessary for health care students and providers (Purnell & Paulanka, 1998). Clients may not understand or respond to the family nurse's suggestions for health promotion because the suggestions conflict with their health beliefs and values. Hence, it is crucial to assess and understand the family culture and health beliefs before suggesting changes in health behavior (Spector, 2000).

Family Lifestyle Patterns

Lifestyle patterns affect family health. In North America there are hundreds of thousands of unnecessary deaths each year that can be directly attributed to unhealthy lifestyles. These deaths can be traced back to heart disease, hypertension, cancer, cirrhosis of the liver, diabetes, suicide, and homicide. When family members engage often in leisure activities, recreation, and exercise, they are better able to cope with day-to-day problems (Fomby, 2004). In addition, time together often promotes family closeness. Healthy lifestyle practices such as good eating habits (James, 2004), good sleep patterns (Kick, 1996; Langford, 2004), proper hygiene, and positive approaches to stress management (Boss, 2003; McCubbin & McCubbin, 1993) are passed from one generation to another. In addition, when one family member initiates a health behavior change, other family members often make a change too. For example, when an individual family member changes eating patterns, perhaps by going on a diet, other family members often change their eating patterns. Moreno (1975) calls this process *vertical diffusion*.

Role Models

Family members provide both negative and positive role models (Friedman, Bowden, & Jones, 2003). For example, smoking, use of drugs and alcohol, poor nutrition, and inactivity are often intergenerational patterns (Crooks, Iammarino, & Weinberg, 1987; Loveland-Cherry, 1996). Stress management, exercise, and communication are learned from parents, siblings, and extended family members such as grandparents (Duffy, 1986). By health teaching in the community, faith-based centers, homes, and the workplace, nurses promote positive role modeling.

Religion and Spirituality

Another factor that influences the quality of family life is religion and spirituality (Friedemann, 1995; Wright, 1997). Although often used interchangeably, the terms are different. Religion tends to relate to the expression of beliefs and includes a relationship with God or some supernatural power (Warner & Bomar, 2004). Religiosity is a component of spirituality. Spirituality provides transcendence, meaning, and compassion for others. Pivotal life events such as births, marriage, life-threatening illness, tragedy, and death provide situations that may spark a family's interest in spirituality (Ingersoll-Dayton, Krause, & Morgan, 2002).

Family spirituality provides the basis for harmony, communication, and wholeness among family members (Warner & Bomar, 2004). Two common nursing diagnoses related to family spiritual health are spiritual well-being and spiritual distress (Johnson, Bluchek, McCloskey-Dochterman, Mass, & Moorehead, 2001). Spiritual well-being is transcendence and connection with self, others, nature, life, and the universe. Spiritual distress is a disruption in the harmony of life and pervades the entire person or family's universe. Religion is a significant factor in family resilience, health, and healing (Walsh, 1999). Religion shapes family health values, practices, and beliefs and may be a positive force in family life because it does the following:

1. Provides a source of social support and belonging
2. Encourages family togetherness through family activities and recreation
3. Provides a sense of meaning in family life
4. Promotes love, hope, faith, trust, forgiveness, forbearance, goodness, self-control, morality, justice, and peace

5. Encourages a belief in divine assistance during times of family stress and crisis
6. Teaches reverence for family life (Warner & Bomar, 2004)

The social support of religion and the clergy is often particularly helpful during family transitions (Warner & Bomar, 2004). Many faith communities sponsor support groups that are a valuable resource for single parents, stepfamilies, single adults, the bereaved, widows and widowers, the unemployed, and parents of young children. Religion aids in family coping responses (Friedman, Bowden, & Jones, 2003) and is reported to provide support for selected caregivers (Picot, Debanne, Namazi, & Wykle, 1997). To provide holistic care, clinicians should assess a family's spiritual health (Dunn & Dawes, 1999), in a nonjudgmental manner support the family's spiritual beliefs, assist families to meet their spiritual needs, provide spiritual resources for family transitions and lifestyle changes, and assist families to find meaning in their circumstances (Carson & Koenig, 2002; Solari-Twadell, McDermott, & Matheus, 1999). Lastly, to foster a family's spiritual well-being, the health professional should listen, be encouraging and empathetic, show vulnerability, and demonstrate commitment. Research on the dimensions of religion and spirituality and family health are sparse. Sample topics for research on religion and family life include punitiveness, coping and family stress, religion and family life satisfaction, and marital satisfaction.

THE NURSING PROCESS FOR FAMILY HEALTH PROMOTION

Family nurses have a crucial role in facilitating health promotion and wellness within the family context across the life span. Enhancing the well-being of the family unit is essential during periods of wellness, as well as during illness, recovery, and stress. A primary goal of nursing care for families is empowering family members to work together to attain and maintain family health. Family nursing that focuses on health promotion should be logical and systematic and include the client(s). The family nursing process for health promotion includes the following:

- Family assessment
- Intervention and empowerment for health promotion
- Evaluation
- Follow-up

The reader is encouraged to consult Chapter 8 for additional discussion of aspects of family nursing process and family assessment.

When working with families in the realm of health promotion, the nurse makes assumptions about families and self-responsibility for their health. According to Bomar (2004b), the following assumptions are a useful guide for family health promotion and nursing practice:

1. Families are ultimately responsible for their own health.
2. Families have the capacity to change in constructive as well as destructive directions.
3. Families have a right to health information in order to make informed decisions about behaviors and lifestyle choices.
4. The health-seeking process occurs in the context of interpersonal and social relationships.
5. Families will employ only health behaviors that they find relevant and compatible with their family lifestyle and structure.
6. Families have the potential for improvement in their health, and a nurse who is caring and culturally competent can enhance this.

Family health promotion needs and interventions, which differ for each family, will be influenced by the nurse's assumptions and actions.

Assessment

As discussed in Chapter 8, nurses are encouraged to base family assessment on scientific models of family health developed by family scientists or family nurses. As explained in Chapter 3, models that nurses use to assess family health vary. A holistic nursing model for family health promotion includes structural and functional, health promotion, and health protection components of the family system. The purpose of assessment is to determine a family's health status by thorough examination of family interaction, development, coping, health processes, and integrity (Anderson & Tomlinson, 1992).

Through assessment, nurses identify family strengths that foster health promotion and stressors that impede health promotion (Pender, Murdaugh, & Parsons, 2002). Integration of the family perspective into assessment and planning facilitates more effective plans for health promotion (Papenfus & Bryan, 1998). It also assists the nurse to identify areas for intervention. Readers are encouraged to consult Pender,

Murdaugh, and Parsons (2002) and review the Health Promotion and Protection Plan. The plan includes assessment of family demographics, values, family strengths, family self-care patterns, and family goals. The health care provider empowers the family to prioritize goals, to select specific behaviors to change, and to create approaches to facilitate family change within a specified time frame.

Interventions

There are a myriad of strategies or interventions that facilitate family health promotion, such as family contracting, empowerment, education, promotion of family integrity, maintenance of family process, exercise promotion, environmental management, mutual goal setting, parent education, confluence, and anticipatory guidance and teaching (Denham, 2003; Hulme, 1999).

Once the nurse and family have identified family strengths and areas for growth or change, the family should prioritize its goals. The commitment of all family members to achieving a goal is crucial to the family's success in reaching it. Nurses negotiate and implement contracts with families or encourage families to use self-care contracts. In the contracting process, the roles of the nurse include health teacher, motivator, resource finder, and evaluator of the family's health promotion plan (Allen & Warner, 2002).

Family nurse scholars (Bomar, 2004b; Denham, 2003; Leininger & McFarland, 2002) identified the following areas in which nurses can provide family support, anticipatory guidance, family education, and family enrichment:

- Coping with family transitions (such as births, acute and/or chronic illnesses, separations, launching children, divorce, death, and retirement)
- Family and individual dietary patterns
- Family and individual recreation and exercise
- Family sexuality
- Family sleep and rest patterns
- Family environmental practices
- Transition from illness to wellness
- Socialization and rearing of children
- Risk reduction and socialization of individual family members in health care practices (prevention and promotion)
- Encouraging a balance between togetherness and individuation

- Providing for family systems and household maintenance
- Encouraging family spirituality

Although beginning family nurses may not be skilled in all these areas, they can seek out community resources such as Websites for well families and individual members.

Family needs and nursing interventions differ with varying family structures and stages in the family life course. For example, in a nuclear family, health promotion includes promotion of a healthy marriage as well as the health of each individual. Family legacy is a living tradition that is developed through dialogue between families of origin and past generations. It is reshaped over time and influenced by family, culture, and society. According to Plager (1999), exploring and acknowledging family legacy recognizes a rich part of family life. This view enhances the nurse's and the family's understanding of family health and related practices, activities, and habits. Specific selected nursing interventions are discussed in the following sections.

Family Contracts

Contracting with a family to change or initiate an activity to strengthen family health increases the likelihood of attaining desired goals (Hill & Smith, 1990; Gray, 1996; Pender, 1996). A health *contract* outlines a set of goals mutually agreed on by a health care provider and an individual or a family (Hill & Smith, 1990; Friedman, 1998) and secures agreement by all parties to take steps to meet the goals. A contract may be oral or written. There are three types of contracts. The first is a *nurse/client contract*, which is an agreement between the nurse and client (family) to work together to attain goals that are determined by the client. The second type is a *contingency contract*. This type of contract includes the process of setting a goal and identifying costs and rewards of goal attainment with a health professional or other support person. The purpose of the contingency contract is to reinforce the behaviors needed to reach a goal. The third type of contract is the *self-care contract*. The client develops this type of contract to improve a health behavior, independently of a health professional.

Contracts are useful for making lifestyle changes, reframing attitudes, and modifying unhealthy interaction patterns. Table 9–3 provides components and sample items of a family self-care contract. They are most effective when the components are negotiated and signed by all family members. The disadvantages of contracts are that they are often time-consuming to develop and that they require commitment by the health professional and all family members involved (particularly in completing a self-care contract). In addition, periodic reevaluation and renegotiations may be necessary. Swain and Steckle (1981) reported improvement in health-promoting behaviors in clients with hypertension, diabetes, and arthritis who followed their contracts. However, recently, there are few reports on the success rate of family contracting.

Family Empowerment

Reciprocal trust is a cornerstone of effective family nursing care (Robinson, 1998). For successful outcomes, the family and the nurse collaborate to make changes in the family's lifestyle that will enhance the family's health. The nurse collaborates with the

Table 9–3   COMPONENTS OF A FAMILY SELF-CARE CONTRACT

COMPONENT OF THE CONTRACTING PROCESS (MUTUALLY AGREED ON BY FAMILY MEMBERS AND HEALTH PROFESSION OR BY FAMILY ALONE)	EXAMPLE OF ITEM IN A FAMILY CONTRACT
Family *assessment* of wellness and identification of area for improvement	Our family feels a sense of always being hurried with no time to relax, and we are irritable with each other.
Set the goal, environmental planning, and reinforcement	We want to have more relaxing time together as a family and to enjoy our time together.
Develop a plan	Have a family meeting to evaluate barriers and create a plan. The outcome might be to reduce sports activities for children. Specify a family fun night/afternoon.
Assign responsibilities	Plan an evening game night with no television or phone calls allowed. All members agree on the game or recreation activity. No one else but the family should participate. Evaluate the budget for games. The family nurse will assist the family to create the plan. Family members will agree to take part in the family fun time.
Determination of time frame	We plan to do this for 2 months one night a week on Sunday evening from 4:00 P.M. to 7:00 P.M.
Evaluate the outcomes	After each week, we will spend 5 minutes talking about what was good and what could be improved. How are we relating to each other the remainder of the week?
Modify, renegotiate, or terminate	We will evaluate the family fun time after 2 months and mutually agree on changes.

Adapted from Hill, L., & Smith, N. (1990). *Self-care nursing*. Englewood Cliffs, NJ: Prentice Hall.

family and provides information, encouragement, and strategies to help the family make lifestyle changes. This process is termed *empowerment.*

According to Hulme (1999), empowerment can be viewed as a process (becoming empowered), an outcome (being empowered), and an intervention (empowering others). In order to be most effective in empowering a family, the nurse should have theoretical knowledge, education, and training opportunities in empowerment (Valentine, 1998). A family's goal may be to reframe a situation, strengthen behaviors that enhance coping with stress or crisis, or incorporate health-promoting activities in family behavior patterns. A family with a member who is dying of AIDS, for example, can be empowered by teaching family members how to cope with feelings of isolation and how to obtain resources and social support in the family and the community. The primary emphasis in family empowerment is involvement of the family in goal setting, planning, and acting, not on having the nurse do this for the family.

A key role of nurses in health promotion for families is to empower family members to value their "oneness," to appreciate family togetherness (Denham, 2003; Friedemann, 1995; Bradshaw, 1988), and to plan activities to foster their unity. One way to enhance family bonding would be to encourage shared meals together when possible. This gives families an opportunity to be together and to enhance communication. A family could also negotiate a family contract for scheduled weekly family time. Each member would make that family time a priority and let no other activity interfere with it. The nurse could help by consulting local newspapers, family magazines, and community agencies for activities that might interest the entire family and afterward encouraging them to continue these activities themselves.

Families may need help in meeting both the needs of the family as a whole and members' individual needs. In order to find a balance, each family member should have time alone to develop a sense of self and to focus on spiritual growth. Friedemann calls this *individuation.* The family also needs to plan "family time," when the sense of belonging and "oneness" or "togetherness" can be experienced. Healthy families have both kinds of time (Olson & DeFrain, 2003; Friedemann, 1995).

> ❝The primary emphasis in family empowerment is on involvement of the family in goal setting, planning, and acting, not on having the nurse do this for the family. ❞

During their life course, families inevitably experience crises and stress. The family's resilience, unity, and resources influence how they cope with crisis and stress (Boss, 2003). The goal of the family nurse is to facilitate family adaptation by empowering the family to promote resilience, reduce the pileup of stressors, make use of resources, and negotiate necessary changes to enhance the family's ability to rebound from stressful events or crises. The nurse can teach families to anticipate life changes, make the necessary adjustments in family routines, evaluate roles and relationships, and cognitively reframe events. For example, in military families, changes occur in family decision making, roles, responsibilities, communication patterns, and power when the military member is deployed. Anticipatory guidance by health professionals could help military families anticipate economic changes, maintain the household, maintain communication, and parent the children long-distance.

Confluence

Another intervention to improve family well-being is confluence. *Confluence* is the process of combining activities to promote togetherness; it fosters family unity and closeness (Friedemann, 1995). For example, Fomby (2004) suggested that planning routinely to prepare and eat most meals as a unit, having regularly scheduled family time for recreation, and going to bed and waking up at the same time foster family togetherness.

Health Teaching and Anticipatory Guidance

Nurses working with well families can teach family awareness, encourage family enrichment, and provide information on community agencies and Websites that are resources for strengthening and enriching families. The family could be encouraged to agree on a goal to attend or find out more about such a program. In some cases, the nurse may need to review Websites, call an agency, or visit and observe an agency in action to determine its appropriateness.

The beginning family nurse is prepared to intervene by teaching about healthy processes (e.g., basic nutrition, exercise routines, hygiene, preventive health practice). Awareness of family life education, family enrichment, and marriage enrichment are interventions that are more appropriate for advanced practice nurses.

Some communities have family enrichment programs for well families. In the 1980s, "ministers of health" were first appointed in faith communities. For example, in the early 1980s, a national multidisciplinary organization, the Health Ministries Association, was formed with the goal of promoting a healthy body, mind, and spirit for all persons in religious congregations. Members include pastors, health educators, health professionals, and concerned congregation members. With the development of such health ministries, many nurses are assuming positions as *parish nurses*, in which the role of the community or family nurse is combined with spiritual counseling from a holistic perspective (Solari-Twadell, McDermott, & Matheus, 1999).

Activities of a health ministry program often include the following:

- Education on health promotion, wellness, disease prevention, and other topics for families and individuals across the life span
- Coordination of volunteers to provide social and network support to members with lifestyle and health problems
- Personal counseling
- Monitoring and screening for health promotion, disease prevention, and treatment of chronic diseases
- Parenting and fatherhood classes
- Service as a health resource and referral agent
- Support groups for single parents, older adults, and remarried families
- Promotion of the integration of faith and individual and family health

Many communities provide resources such as couple communication workshops, family retreats, family magazines, parenting classes for young and adolescent families, support for stepfamilies, lesbian and gay support groups, and so forth. A list of selected family agencies, resources, and Websites appears in the appendix.

Preparation for Termination

As the individual or family approaches its goal, the nurse sees the client less frequently (Wright & Leahey, 2000). Pender (1996) called this the step-down phase. During this phase, the family takes on more responsibility for planned activities and becomes more self-reliant in problem solving and evaluating its progress toward goals. When the goal is met, the nurse and client negotiate for the time for termination of the relationship. Throughout the nursing process,

regular, frequent reviews of goals and progress may eliminate problems with termination.

Evaluation and Follow-Up

During this phase, the nurse reviews the progress of the client/family toward the health promotion goals, and if the family did not meet the goals, the nurse and family discuss why they are not getting their desired outcomes and, if necessary, plan other options. After incorporating the desired change into the family lifestyle, the nurse discontinues family appointments. Providing an opportunity for families to follow-up with the nurse by appointments, calls, or periodic visits increases the likelihood of the family sustaining the health promotion changes.

IMPLICATIONS OF HEALTH PROMOTION IN FAMILY NURSING

Family health promotion is an important component of nursing practice, nursing education, family policy, and nursing research.

Nursing Practice

As resources changed in the 1990s and into the new millennium, individuals and families assumed more responsibility for the care and support of their families in the area of health promotion. Major tasks of nursing with families are to (1) work in partnership with families, (2) empower and increase the capacity of families to find ways to achieve their lifestyle and health care goals, (3) illuminate the importance of family health promotion, (4) serve as a family advocate, and (5) be an expert in family health promotion matters. The goal is for families to attain, maintain, or regain the highest possible level of family health.

The advanced practice nurse, particularly the family nurse practitioner who practices in a primary care setting, has the opportunity to interact with the family, initiate family health promotion, and assist families to identify risks to their well-being. The continuing shift in health care from the hospital to community settings means that nurses will have more direct interactions with families in ambulatory health care settings and homes. The increase in family empowerment for providing care for ill family members requires in-depth evaluation and creative interventions to focus on family health, family protection, and family health promotion. At all stages of the family health and illness cycle, the goal is to return the family, as a whole, to its highest health potential. To do so, nurses provide programs for family health promotion and reducing risks for dysfunction in a variety of settings. Selected topics include parenting from infancy to old age; role changes during family and individual transitions such as retirement, birth of a new baby, bereavement, and so forth; and coping with individual and family stressors.

Single-parent and blended families often need anticipatory guidance, family enrichment activities, and parenting and stepparenting education. The nurse can encourage all family members to monitor their family for its unity, strengths, and a sense of belonging. In any setting, nurses can advocate for families by writing and voting on family issues, supporting a philosophy of practice that encourages family nursing, volunteering in community activities for families, and supporting family programs. In general, health promotion assessment should become a regular part of taking a family history and a routine aspect of nursing care.

Nursing Education

In addition to traditional content on family theoretical frameworks, illness, stress and coping, and crisis, curricula at the undergraduate and graduate level should include content on family health promotion. At the present time, however, few students are prepared in family health promotion. Most curricula continue to focus primarily on acute and chronic physical illness, psychosocial problems, and community nursing; the primary focus is on the individual in the context of the family. Limited attention is paid to groups of families in the community or to healthy families.

If nurses are to be a part of the efforts to meet the national health goals for the year 2010, undergraduate and graduate curricula in schools of nursing will need to include content on the family as the unit of care and on family health promotion and disease prevention. Although the individual might be the patient, students should be taught that assessments and interventions should include the family. For example, diabetic teaching should include all family members, particularly the person who prepares meals. Schools of nursing will need to use learning-service community partnership models and create innovative sites for clinical practice where students can provide nursing care to well families (Kataoka-Yahiro, Cohen, Yoder, & Canhan, 1998). Such sites might include a nursing clinic in a low-income housing project, a senior center, a family exercise center, a faith community, a work site, a rural health clinic, or a school or nurse-managed primary care clinic.

Family Policy

The document *Healthy People 2010* and the current emphasis on eliminating disparities in health care for all citizens will help shape local, state, and national policies geared toward improving family health. The passage of the 1993 Family Medical Leave Act marked a beginning in the effort to implement policies to improve the quality of family health. In order to reach the goals for the nation by the year 2010, families must be empowered to assume more responsibilities in the realm of health promotion and disease prevention for family members. Family issues most frequently reviewed by policy makers include marriage, divorce, family violence, abortion, child care, child health care, and family health insurance coverage. Continuing 21st-century family health policy issues are family poverty and economic well-being (Bogenschneider, 2002; Hildebrandt, 2002). The family nurse needs to be aware of policies advancing family health throughout the family life course and should support them. Nurses can support family policy legislation by keeping informed about issues, voting, communicating with policy makers about family needs, giving expert testimony, maintaining membership in and supporting professional nursing organizations, and financially supporting the political advocacy activities of health professional organizations (Briar-Lawson, Lawson, Hennon, & Jones, 2001). Examples of U.S. congressional legislation reviewed in 2003 include Family Medical Leave Act enhancement, family life span respite care, and tax credits for family caregivers, adult stem cell research, and genome research. Such policies would support families and would improve the quality of family life.

Family Nursing Research

Many regional and national nursing research societies and organizations sponsor family research interest groups; however, research on family health promotion is still needed. The National Institute of Nursing Research (NINR) agenda for nursing research includes developing and testing community-based programs to promote family health using nursing models and assessing the effectiveness of nursing intervention for families during the chronic illness of a family member. Specific research for family health promotion that needs to be explored includes the following:

- Design of research that strengthens family health promotion, well-being, economic development, and environment
- Creation, testing, and dissemination of intervention and evidence-based family-focused studies
- Testing and development of family health promotion theories on diverse families and their issues, processes, and challenges
- Design of international research intervention evidence-based, qualitative studies to illuminate and provide solutions to improve the health of families and their members
- Family factors that are important in health promotion for families from diverse cultures
- Design of intervention research that tests family-centered health promotion strategies to reduce obesity, violence, substance abuse, smoking cessation, and so forth
- Research focused on vulnerable families and individuals
- Design of intervention research to assess issues of health care technology and telehealth with ethnic families (Bomar, 2004b, p. 646)

SUMMARY

- *Family health* is defined as a dynamic process that includes the activities a family uses to promote and protect the well-being of the family as a unit and the individual family members.
- Promoting and protecting the health of the family unit is in the formative stages; therefore, health professionals have challenging opportunities to develop and test interventions in family health promotion.
- The Family Health Promotion Model illustrates that complex multiple factors influence a family's health-promoting outcomes.
- The Developmental Model of Health and Nursing has a goal of collaborating with families and increasing the capacity of families in health promotion in everyday situations.
- Continuing research is needed to test family health promotion models and interventions to empower diverse families in health-promoting lifestyle practices.
- Advanced practice nurses in primary care are in the best position to foster family health given the fact that a major aspect of primary care is health promotion.
- The role of the nurse in family health promotion includes assessing and collaborating with families, collaborating with groups and other professionals, and building the capacity of and strengthening families. The nurse's role as a scholar of family nursing includes researching and building a knowledge base for family health promotion and disseminating family nursing outcomes and research findings.

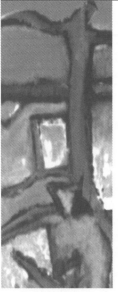

RESEARCH BRIEF

Monteith, B., & Ford-Gilboe, M. (2002). The relationships among mother's resilience, family health work, and mother's health-promoting lifestyle practices in families with preschool children. *Journal of Family Nursing, 8*(4), 383–407.

Purpose of the Study
The purpose of the study was to test the relationships among the mother's resilience, family health work, and the mother's health-promoting lifestyle practices in families with preschool children. The conceptual model used for the study was Allen and Warner's Developmental Model of Health and Family.

Methodology
The study was a descriptive correlation survey of a convenience sample of 67 mothers (ages 27 to 44) with preschool children (3 to 5 years of age) in southern Ontario, Canada. The sample was recruited from three nursery schools. Research instruments used were a demographic survey, Wagnild and Young's Resilience Scale, Ford-Gilboe's Health

(continued on page 261)

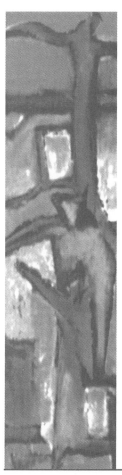

Options Scale, and Walker and Hill-Polerecky's Health-Promoting Lifestyle II. Four hypotheses were tested. Data were analyzed using the Pearson's *r* correlation coefficients and hierarchical multiple regression analysis.

Results

The mean scores for the mothers' resilience, health work, and health-promoting lifestyle practices were high to moderate. Family income, mothers' education, and employment status were significantly related to the key study variables. Results of the hypotheses tested were (1) significant positive relationship between the mother's resilience and family health work, (2) significant positive relationship between health work and the mother's health-promoting lifestyle, and (3) a moderate positive correlation between the mother's resilience and health-promoting lifestyle practices. Results from the hierarchical multiple regression were as follows: (1) family income was related to health-promoting lifestyle practices, (2) family income significantly predicted 11 percent of the variance in the mother's health-promoting lifestyle practices, (3) the mother's resilience explained 17 percent of the variance, and (4) 24 percent of the variance in health-promoting lifestyle practices was explained by health work.

Implications

Study findings suggest that nurses should support activities that strengthen family resilience and health work, which could enhance family health-promoting lifestyle practices. Finally, nurses should create programs to educate and increase the capacity of mothers and families of all socioeconomic and ethnic groups in health-promoting lifestyles. Further research is needed to explore the relationships between resilience, health work, and health-promoting lifestyle practices in families of varied developmental stages, ethnic groups, socioeconomic status, cultural backgrounds, family structures and functioning, and health issues. In addition, research to develop a measure specific to family health-promoting lifestyle practices is needed.

CASE STUDY ➤

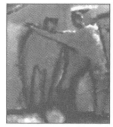

THE BUDD FAMILY

James (age 38) and Eleanor (age 36) have two sons, Derek (age 8) and Dustin (age 10). James is a full-time engineer who also teaches part-time at a community college. Eleanor has a full-time position as a professor of education, and her classes are scheduled in the evenings two nights a week. James teaches Monday and Wednesday evenings and Eleanor teaches Tuesday and Thursday evenings. On the weekends and the other evenings, the couple are doing household chores, preparing for classes, or grading papers in their spare time. Meals are usually rushed and often eaten at different times in front of the television, so that the family rarely eats meals together. While their parents are reading, working, or grading papers, the boys watch television, play video games, or do their homework. Except for family vacations and holidays, the Budds rarely spend time together enjoying each other's company. Eleanor was seen by a nurse in the family practice clinic for complaints of fatigue, lingering fluid and pain in her ears, vertigo, and nausea for 2 months. She was given antibiotics and nasal cortisone for her ear infection, after which her ear condition improved gradually.

However, her complaint of extreme fatigue lingered. Laboratory tests revealed no physiological reason for the continuing fatigue. A nursing assessment of the family and Eleanor was completed using Pender, Murdaugh, and Parsons' (2002) framework for individual health assessment and Hanson and Mischke's (1996) *Family Systems Stressors-Strength Inventory.*

(continued on page 262)

CASE STUDY ➤ *(Continued)*

Major Family Stressors Insufficient "me" time, Eleanor's illness, decreased housekeeping standards, insufficient couple and family play time, television, inadequate time with the children, over-scheduled family calendar, and lack of shared responsibility.

Family Strengths Shared religious core, respects privacy of one another, values work satisfaction, financial security, encouragement of individual values, affirmation and support of one another, and trust between members.

Lifestyle Changes Indicated Increased individual time for parents, improved family recreation and couple time, revision of family calendar, and increased sharing of household tasks.

Discussion What would the role of the family nurse be with this family? (1) List some of the roles, and (2) describe how the nurse might use the role to improve family well-being.

1. Examples: Focuser, awareness raiser, identifying additional resources, teacher, coach, encourager, empowerment agent, reinforcer, and reviewer
2. Help the family focus on the family strengths and encourage them to evaluate family priorities. Encourage the family to begin a regular meal-time together at least on the weekend and, if possible, during the week. Encourage them to plan a family recreation time where they relax together. In addition, create time for Eleanor to relax on the weekend by having each family member assume chores that are appropriate for his or her age. James and Eleanor need to plan for couple time by establishing a regular date without the children.

SQ STUDY QUESTIONS

1. Review the traits of a healthy family and describe the traits of this family and areas for growth. What strategies would you use to empower this family to develop more healthy traits?

2. What activities could empower this family to reslove the crisis so that James does not feel alone and the rest of the family does not feel avoided?

References

Allen, F. M., & Warner, M. (2002). A developmental model of health and nursing. *Journal of Family Nursing, 8*(2), 96–135.

American Nurses Association. (1995). *Nursing: A social policy statement.* Kansas City, MO.

American Nurses Association. (1998). *Scope and standards of parish nursing practice.* Washington, DC: American Nurses Pub.

Anderson, K. H., & Tomlinson, P. S. (1992). The family health system as an emerging paradigmatic view for nursing. *Image: Journal of Nursing Scholarship, 24,* 57–63.

Bogenschneider, K. (2002). *Family policy matters: How policymaking affects families.* Mahwah, NJ: Lawrence Erlbaum Associates.

Bomar, P. J. (Ed.). (1996). *Nurses and family health promotion: Concepts, assessment and intervention.* Philadelphia: WB Saunders.

Bomar, P. J. (2004a). Introduction to family health nursing and promoting family health. In P. J. Bomar (Ed.), *Promoting health in families: Applying family research and theory to nursing practice* (3rd ed., pp. 3–37). Philadelphia: WB Saunders.

Bomar, P. J. (Ed.). (2004b). *Promoting health in families: Applying family research and theory to nursing practice* (3rd ed.). Philadelphia: WB Saunders.

Bomar, P. J. (2004c). Family environmental health. In P. J. Bomar (Ed.), *Promoting health in families: Applying family research and theory to nursing practice* (3rd ed., pp. 534–580). Philadelphia: WB Saunders.

Bomar, P. J., & McNeeley, G. (1996). Family health nursing role: Past, present, and future. In P. J. Bomar (Ed.), *Nurses and family health promotion: Concepts, assessment and intervention* (2nd ed.). Philadelphia: WB Saunders.

Boss, P. (Ed.). (2003). *Family stress: Classic and contemporary readings.* Thousand Oaks, CA: Sage.

Bradshaw, J. (1988). *Bradshaw on family.* Deerfield Beach, FL: Health Communications.

Briar-Lawson, K., Lawson, H. A., Hennon, C. B., & Jones, A. R. (2001). *Family-centered policies and practices.* New York: Columbia University Press.

Bullock, K. (2004). Family social support. In P. J. Bomar (Ed.), *Promoting health in families: Application of research and theory to nursing practice* (3rd ed.). Philadelphia: WB Saunders.

Carson, V. B., & Koenig, H. G. (2002). *Parish nursing.* Philadelphia: Templeton Foundation Press.

Coe, R. (1970). *Sociology of medicine.* New York: McGraw-Hill.

Crawford, J., & Tarko, M. A. (2004). Family communication. In P. J. Bomar (Ed.), *Promoting health in families: Applying family research and theory to nursing practice* (3rd ed.). Philadelphia: WB Saunders.

Crooks, C., Iammarino, & Weinberg. (1987). The family's role in health promotion. *Health Values, 2,* 7–12.

Curan, D. (1983). *Traits of a healthy family.* Minneapolis, MN: Winston Press.

Danielson, C. B., Hamel-Bissell, B., & Winstead-Fry, P. (1993). *Families in health and illness.* St. Louis, MO: Mosby.

DeFrain, J., & Stinnett, N. (1992). Building on the inherent strengths of families: A positive approach for family psychologists and counselors. *Topics in Family Psychology and Counseling, 1,* 15–26.

Denham, S. A. (2003). *Family health: A framework for nursing.* Philadelphia: FA Davis.

Doherty, W., & Campbell, T. (1988). *Families and health*. Newbury Park, CA: Sage Publications.

Doherty W. J., & Carlson, B. Z. (2002). *Putting family first*. New York: Owl Books.

Doherty, W., & McCubbin, H. I. (1985). Families and health care: An emerging arena of theory, research, and clinical interventions. *Family Relations, 34*, 5–10.

Duffy, M. E. (1986). Primary prevention behaviors: The female-headed, one-parent family. *Research in Nursing and Health, 9*, 115–122.

Duffy, M. E. (1988). Health promotion in the family: Current findings and directives for nursing research. *Journal of Advanced Nursing, 13*, 109–117.

Dunn, A. B., & Dawes, S. H. (1999). Spirituality-focused genograms: Keys to uncovering spiritual resources in African American families. *Journal of Multicultural Counseling and Development, 27*(4), 240–255. Retrieved December 31, 2003, from http://web5epnet.com.citation via EBSCO host.

Duval, E. M., & Miller, B. C. (1985). *Marriage and family development* (6th ed.). New York: Harper & Row.

Elliot, M. (1999). Classifying family life education on the World Wide Web. *Family Relations, 48*, 7–13.

Faux, S. (1998). Historical overview of responses of children and their families to chronic illness. In K. Knafl (Ed.), *Children and families in health and illness* (pp. 179–195). Thousand Oaks: Sage Publications.

Fomby, B. W. (2004). Family routines, rituals, recreation, and rules. In P. J. Bomar (Ed.), *Promoting health in families: Application of research and theory to nursing practice* (3rd ed., pp. 450–475). Philadelphia: WB Saunders.

Ford-Gilboe, M. (2002). Developing knowledge about family health promotion by testing the developmental model of health and nursing. *Journal of Family Nursing, 8*(2), 140–156.

Friedemann, M. L. (1995). *The framework of systemic organization: A conceptual approach to families and nursing*. Thousand Oaks: Sage Publications.

Friedman, M. M. (1998). *Family nursing: Research, theory and practice* (4th ed.). Norwalk, CT: Appleton & Lange.

Friedman, M. M., Bowden, V. R., & Jones, E. G. (2003). *Family nursing: Research, theory and practice* (5th ed.). Upper Saddle River, NJ: Prentice Hall.

Gilliss, C. L., & Davis, L. L. (1992). Family nursing research: Precepts from paragons and peccadillos. *Journal of Advanced Nursing, 17*, 28–33.

Gray, R. (1996). Family self-care. In P. J. Bomar (Ed.), *Nurses and family health promotion: Concepts, assessment, and intervention* (2nd ed.). Philadelphia: WB Saunders.

Hagen, J. L. (1999). Public welfare and human services: New directions under TANF: Families in Society. *The Journal of Contemporary Human Services, 80*, 1.

Hanson, S. M. H., & Mischke, K. (1996). Family health assessment and intervention. In P. J. Bomar (Ed.), *Nurses and family health promotion: Concepts, assessment, and intervention*. Philadelphia: WB Saunders.

Hertz, R., & Ferguson, I. T. (1997). Kinship strategies and self-sufficiency among single mothers by choice: Postmodern family ties. *Qualitative Sociology, 20*(2), 187–208.

Hildebrandt, E. (2002). The health effects of work-based welfare. *Journal of Nursing Scholarship, 34*(4), 363–368.

Hill, L., & Smith, N. (1990). *Self-care nursing*. Englewood Cliffs, NJ: Prentice-Hall.

Huff, R. M., & Kline, M. V. (1999). *Promoting health in multicultural populations*. Thousand Oaks, CA: Sage.

Hulme, P. A. (1999). Family empowerment: A nursing intervention with suggested outcomes for families of children with a chronic health condition. *Journal of Family Nursing, 5*(1), 35–50.

Ingersoll-Dayton, B., Krause, N., & Morgan, D. (2002). Religious trajectories and transitions over the life course. *International Journal of Aging and Human Development, 56*(1), 51–70.

James, K. (2004). Family nutrition. In P. J. Bomar (Ed.), *Promoting health in families: Applying family research and theory to nursing practice* (3rd ed.). Philadelphia: WB Saunders.

Johnson, M., Bluchek, G., McCloskey-Dochterman, J., Mass, M., & Moorehead, S. (Eds.). (2001). *Nursing diagnosis, outcomes, and interventions*. St. Louis: Mosby.

Kataoka-Yahiro, M., Cohen, J., Yoder, M., & Canhaim. (1998). A learning-service community partnership model. *Nursing and Health Care Perspectives, 19*, 274–277.

Kick, E. (1996). Sleep and the family. In P. J. Bomar (Ed.), *Nurses and family health promotion: Concepts, assessment and intervention* (2nd ed.). Philadelphia: WB Saunders.

Langford, D. (2004). Family health protection. In P. J. Bomar (Ed.), *Promoting health in families: Applying family research and theory to nursing practice* (3rd ed.). Philadelphia: WB Saunders.

Leininger, M., & McFarland, M. (2002). *Transcultural nursing: Concepts, theories, research, and practice* (3rd ed.). New York: McGraw-Hill.

Loveland-Cherry, C. J. (1986). Personal health practices of single-parent and two-parent families. *Family Relations, 35*, 133–139.

Loveland-Cherry, C. J. (1996). Family health promotion and protection. In P. J. Bomar (Ed.), *Nurses and family health promotion: Concepts, assessment and interventions* (2nd ed.). Philadelphia: WB Saunders.

Loveland-Cherry, C. J., & Bomar, P. J. (2004). Family health promotion and health protection. In P. J. Bomar (Ed.), *Promoting health in families: Applying research and theory to nursing practice* (3rd ed., pp. 61–89). Philadelphia: WB Saunders.

Ma, G. X., & Wenk, D. (1997). A holistic family wellness program focusing on family strengths. *Practicing Anthropology, 19*, 30–34.

McCubbin, M. A., & McCubbin, H. I. (1993). Families coping with illness: The resilience model of family stress adjustment and adaptation. In C. B. Danielson, B. Hamel-Bissell, & P. Winstead-Fry (Eds.), *Families in health and illness* (pp. 21–63). St. Louis: Mosby.

McGoldrick, M., & Giordano, J. (1996). Overview: Ethnicity and family therapy. In M. McGoldrick et al. (Eds.), *Ethnicity and family therapy* (pp. 1–30). New York: Guilford Press.

Mischke, K. B., & Hanson, S. M. H. (1996). Family health assessment and intervention. In P. J. Bomar (Ed.), *Nurses in family health promotion: Concepts, assessment and interventions* (2nd ed.). Philadelphia: WB Saunders.

Moreno, P. R. (1975). Vertical diffusion effects within black and Mexican-American families participating in the Florida parent education model. *Dissertation Abstracts International, 36*, 1358.

National Institute of Nursing Research. (1999). Research directions: Capsule descriptions of selected studies. Retrieved March 26, 1999, from http://www.nih.gov/ninr/ResDir.htm

Olson, D. H. (2000). Circumplex model of marital and family systems. *Journal of Family Therapy, 22*(2), 144–167.

Olson, D. H. L., & DeFrain, J. (2003). *Marriage and the family: Diversity and strengths* (4th ed.). New York: McGraw-Hill.

Olson, D. H., McCubbin, H. I., Barnes, H., Larsen, Muxen, M., & Wilson, M. (1989). *Families: What makes them work* (2nd ed.). Beverly Hills, CA: Sage Publications.

Papenfus, H., & Bryan, A. A. (1998). Nurses' involvement in interdisciplinary team evaluations: Incorporating the family perspective. *Journal of School Health, 68*(5), 184–195.

Pearsall, P. (1990). *The power of the family: Strength, comfort, and healing*. New York: Doubleday.

Pender, N. J. (1996). *Health promotion in nursing practice* (3rd ed.). Norwalk, CT: Appleton & Lange.

Pender, N. J., Murdaugh, C. L., & Parsons, M. A. (2002). *Health promotion in nursing practice* (4th ed.). Upper Saddle River, NJ: Prentice Hall.

Perez, M. (1999). Quincenera. *New Moon, 6*(3), 184–195.

Picot, S. J., Debanne, S. M., Namazi, K. H., & Wykle, M. L. (1997). Religiosity and perceived rewards of black and white caregivers. *The Gerontologist, 37*(1), 89–101.

Plager, K. (1999). Understanding family legacy in family health concerns. *Journal of Family Nursing, 5*(1), 51–71.

Pratt, L. (1976). *Family structure and effective health behavior and the energized family*. Boston: Houghton Mifflin.

Purnell, L. D., & Paulanka, B. J. (1998). *Transcultural health care: A culturally competent approach*. Philadelphia: FA Davis.

Robinson, C. (1998). Women, families, chronic illness and nursing interventions: From burden to balance. *Journal of Family Nursing, 4*(3), 271–291.

Sattler, B., & Lipscomb, J. (Eds.). (2003). *Environmental health and nursing practice*. New York: Springer.

Shi, L., & Singh, D. A. (1998). *Delivering health care in America: A systems approach*. Baerrien Springs, MI: Aspen.

Smilkstein, G. (1978). The family APGAR: A proposal for family function test and its use by physicians. *Family Practice, 6*, 1231–1239.

Smith, J. (1983). The idea of health: Implications for the nursing profession. New York: Teachers College Press.

Smith, S. D. (2003). *Parish nursing: A handbook for the new millennium*. Binghamton, NY: Harworth Press.

Solari-Twadell, P. A. (1999). The community as clients: Assessment of assets and the needs of the faith community and the parish nurse. In P. A. Solari-Twadell & M. McDermott (Eds.), *Parish nursing: Promoting whole person health within faith communities* (pp. 83–92). Thousand Oaks: Sage Publications.

Solari-Twadell, P. A., McDermott, M., & Matheus, R. (1999). Educational preparation. In P. A. Solari-Twadell & M. McDermott (Eds.), *Parish nursing: Promoting whole person health within faith communities*. Thousand Oaks: Sage Publications.

Spector, R. E. (2000). *Cultural diversity in health and illness* (5th ed.). Upper Saddle River, NJ: Prentice Hall.

Swain, M. S., & Steckle, S. (1981). Contracting with patients to improve compliance. *Hospitals, 51*, 81–84.

Umar, K. B. (2003, August). Health care headaches: Accessing safety net services. *Closing the gap* (p. 12). Office of Minority Health, U.S. Department of Health and Human Services. Retrieved December 21, 2003, from http://www.omhrc.gov/ctg/CTG%20August%202003.pdf

U.S. Department of Health and Human Services. (1979). *Healthy people: The surgeon general's report on health promotion and disease prevention* (U.S. Public Health Service, Pub. No. PHS 79–55071). U.S. Department of Health, Education, and Welfare. Washington, DC: U.S. Government Printing Office.

U.S. Department of Health and Human Services. (1980). *Promoting health/preventing disease: Objectives for the nation*. Washington, DC: U.S. Government Printing Office.

U.S. Department of Health and Human Services. (1985). *Report of the secretary's task force on black and minority*. Washington, DC: U.S. Government Printing Office.

U.S. Department of Health and Human Services. (1986). *The 1990 health objectives: A midcourse review*. Rockville, MD: Office of Disease and Health Promotion, Public Health Service. Washington, DC: U.S. Government Printing Office.

U.S. Department of Health and Human Services. (1990). *Healthy people 2000: National health promotion and disease prevention objectives* (Department of Health and Human Services, Publication No. PHS 91–50213). Washington, DC: U.S. Government Printing Office.

U.S. Department of Health and Human Services. (1996). *Report of final natality statistics*. Retrieved February 17, 1999, from http://www.hhs.gov

U.S. Department of Health and Human Services. (2000). *Healthy people 2010* (Vol. 1). Washington, DC: U.S. Government Printing Office. Retrieved from http://www.health.gov/healthy-people/Document/tableofcontents.htm

Valentine, F. (1998). Empowerment: Family-centered care. *Pediatric Nursing, 10*, 24–27.

Walsh, F. (1999). Religion and spirituality: Wellsprings for healing and resilience. In F. Walsh (Ed.), *Spiritual resources in family therapy* (pp. 3–27). New York: Guildford.

Warner, C. G., & Bomar, P. J. (2004). Family spirituality. In P. J. Bomar (Ed.), *Promoting health in families: Applying research and theory to nursing practice* (3rd ed.). Philadelphia: WB Saunders.

Weaver, A. J., Samford, J. A., Morgan, V. J., Koenig, H. G., & Flannelly, K. J. (2002). A systematic review of research on religion in six marriage and family journals: 1995–1999. *The American Journal of Family Therapy, 30*, 293–309.

White House Conference on Families. (1980). *Listening to America's families: Action for the 1980s*. Washington, DC: U.S. Government Printing Office.

Wijnberg, M., & Weinger, S. (1998). When dreams wither and resources fail: The social support system of poor single mothers. *Families in Society: The Journal of Contemporary Human Services, 79*(2), 212–219.

Wright, L. (1997). Suffering and spirituality: The soul of clinical work with families. *Journal of Family Nursing, 3*, 3–14.

Wright, L. & Leahey, M. (2000). *Nurses and families: A guide to family assessment and intervention* (3rd ed.). Philadelphia: FA Davis.

Zimmerman, S. (2001). *Family policy: Constructed solutions to family problems*. Thousands Oaks, CA: Sage.

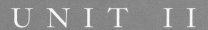

UNIT II

Family Nursing Practice

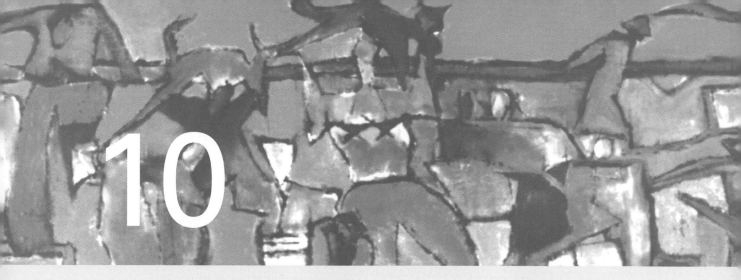

10

Family Nursing with Childbearing Families

Louise Martell, RN, PhD

CRITICAL CONCEPTS

- While giving direct physical care, teaching patients, or performing other traditional modes of maternity nursing, childbearing family nurses focus on family relationships and the health of all members of the childbearing family.

- Family systems, transition, and family development theories help nurses understand and plan care for childbearing families.

- Even though the *family life cycle theory* was developed for two-parent nuclear families, it can guide health promotion for contemporary childbearing families.

- When a mother or a newborn has serious threats to health, family nurses act to maintain and promote family relationships.

- Family nurses can be leaders in practice, policy development, and education related to childbearing families.

- Nurses will be leaders in research about the impact of new reproductive technologies on childbearing families.

INTRODUCTION: WHAT IS CHILDBEARING FAMILY NURSING?

Before the onset of professional nursing in North America during the late 19th century, caregivers for childbearing were primarily female networks of midwives, neighbors, friends, servants, and relatives (Wertz & Wertz, 1989). Most caregiving activities were carried out in families' homes during the birth and the *postpartum periods*. Care was not solely for births but included maintaining family functions of the household, tending to new babies and mothers' other children, and providing postpartum physical care. Today, more and more, health care providers for women are recognizing the impact of reproductive events on all family members and consequently are including family concepts in their care. Childbearing family nursing is not synonymous with obstetrical nursing. Rather, it considers the family as client and/ or the family as context for the care of its members. Family nursing with childbearing families covers the period before conception, pregnancy, labor, birth, and the postpartum period. It focuses on health and wellness rather than on procedures and medical treatment.

Childbearing family nursing traditionally begins when families are considering whether to start having children and continues until parents have achieved a degree of relative comfort in their roles as parents of infants and have ceased adding babies to their families. Often family nursing expands to include the periods between pregnancies and other aspects of reproduction such as family planning and sexuality. Decisions and changes surrounding childbearing vary for families according to their cultural and psychological needs; therefore, the beginning and end point of the reproductive cycle may be different for each family.

Nurses have known for a long time that social support, family functioning, family structure, and life events are related to pregnancy outcomes (Norbeck & Tilden, 1983; Ramsey, Abell, & Baker, 1986; Tilden, 1983). For example, women living with their spouses or other family members were more likely to have healthy, full-term babies than were women living alone (Norbeck & Tilden, 1983; Ramsey, Abell, & Baker, 1986; Tilden, 1983). Women whose families were sources of stress, rather than protectors from stress, had smaller babies (Norbeck & Tilden, 1983; Ramsey, Abell, & Baker, 1986; Tilden, 1983). Mercer and Ferketich (1990) found that antepartal hospitalization was stressful to women and their partners and that negative (or stressful) life events had a negative impact on family functioning.

Nurses involved with childbearing families use family concepts and theories as part of developing the plan of action for nursing care. At any one time, family members may have related but different health needs pertaining to the same family health concern. Thus, childbearing family nursing practice uses all the traditional components of nursing, such as direct physical care, patient teaching, and referral to other health care providers, but orients this knowledge to the entire childbearing family.

In this chapter, family nursing for all nurses involved with childbearing will be explored. Theoretical perspectives that guide nursing practice with childbearing families will be presented in the chapter. Most of the chapter focuses on health promotion for the childbearing family, with consideration for threats to health, which are akin to "acute" and "chronic" illness. The chapter ends with implications for nursing practice, education, research, and policy.

COMMON THEORETICAL PERSPECTIVES

Several theories, especially those from the family social science genre, contribute to nurses' understanding

---

HISTORICAL PERSPECTIVE

Late 1800s—Industrialization

- Families moved to more urban areas; household size and functions diminished.
- Traditional networks of women were not always available, and mothers needed to replace care previously carried out in the home.
- Childbearing still occurred at home for many middle-class families (Leavitt, 1986; Wertz & Wertz, 1989).

(continued on page 269)

First Third of the 20th Century

- The hospital became the place for labor, birth, and early postpartum recovery for middle-class families.
- Many immigrant and working-class urban families continued to have babies at home with their traditional care providers.
- An impetus to the development of public health nursing was concern for the health of urban mothers and babies.
- Realizing that the health needs of all the family members were intertwined, early public health nurses considered families, not individuals, as their clients.

1930s through the "Baby Boom" of the 1950s

- With the dramatic shift of births to hospitals, family involvement with childbearing diminished (Leavitt, 1986).
- Concerns about infection control contributed to separation of family members.
- Family members were forbidden to be with women in the hospital.
- Babies were segregated into nurseries and brought out to their mothers only for brief feeding sessions.
- Nurses focused on the smooth operation of postpartum wards and nurseries through the use of routine and orderliness.
- Despite these inflexible conditions, families tolerated them because they believed that hospital births were safer for mothers and babies.

1960s to 1970s

- Some women and a few physicians began to question the need for heavy sedation and analgesia for childbearing and embraced natural childbirth.
- A feature of natural childbirth was the close relationship between the laboring woman and a supportive person serving as a coach, and in North America, husbands assumed this supportive role (Wertz & Wertz, 1989).
- Expectant parents actively sought out physicians and hospitals that would best meet their expectations for father involvement, and the control over childbearing began to shift from health care professionals to families.
- Some nurses were skeptical about the changes families demanded, but others were enthusiastic about increased family participation.
- Many hospital-based maternity nurses began to consider themselves mother-baby nurses rather than nursery or postpartum nurses, and labor and delivery nurses often collaborated with family members in helping women cope with the discomforts of labor.

1980s to the Present

- The research of Klaus and Kennell (1976) served as the impetus for the growth of family-centered care (American College of Obstetricians and Gynecologists & Interprofessional Task Force on Health Care of Women and Children, 1978).
- Today promotion of family contact is becoming the hallmark of childbearing care.
- Many hospitals have renamed their obstetrical services, using names such as Family Birth Center to convey the importance of family members in childbearing health care even though obstetrical care is becoming more dependent on technology.
- With the trend for shorter hospital stays after birth, postpartum care is becoming family-based with nursing guidance.

of how families grow, develop, function, and change during childbearing. Application of theory to family health situations during childbearing can guide family nurses in making more-complete assessments and planning interventions congruent with the predictable consequences of events during childbearing. The theories presented in Chapter 3 that are especially applicable to childbearing families include general systems theory, change (transition), and developmental theory. A brief summary of their application follows.

General Systems Theory

Even though much of the classic work on general systems theory for childbearing families was done more than a decade ago, this theory still applies to childbearing family nursing. General systems theory focuses on both family processes and outcomes. The central idea of general systems theory is that a family functions in such a way as to maintain balance between stress from within and outside its boundary. The technical name for this balance is homeostasis. Through adaptation, homeostasis is maintained or regained. Because a family is considered an open system, it is affected by exchanges with its outside environment. The outside environment includes the community and its institutions such as the health care system. The degree of openness is regulated by the family boundary that may impede or facilitate a family's interaction with social systems outside itself (Broderick, 1993; Mercer, 1989). Individuals within a family are interdependent on one another, which contributes to a family's ability to adapt and maintain homeostasis even when responding to stress and strains from both inside and outside itself.

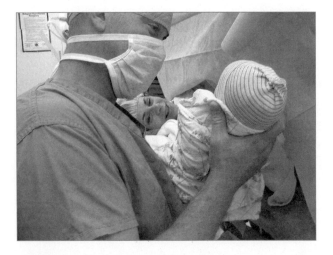

Becoming parents or adding a child brings stress to a family by challenging family homeostasis not only for the nuclear and extended family systems but also for the individual members and subsystems of the family. As new subsystems are created or modified by pregnancy and childbirth, there is a sense of disequilibrium until a family adapts to its new member, hence achieving homeostasis. For example, changes in the husband-wife subsystem occur as a response to development of the new parent-child subsystems.

Imbalance, or disequilibrium, occurs while adjustments are still needed and new roles are being learned. Families with greater flexibility in role expectations and behaviors tend to experience these periods of disequilibrium with less discomfort. The greater the range or number of coping strategies available to the family, the greater the ability to engage in various family roles, and the more effective the family's response will be to both internal strains and external stress associated with childbearing. External stresses may be important in predicting disequilibrium in pregnant women, and nurses should assess the effect of stress on family homeostasis.

The general systems theory is especially effective for childbearing family nurses when they consider that a family, while in a state of change and readjustment, has more-permeable boundaries or is more open to the outside environment because the family becomes aware of resources beyond itself. Consequently, the family is apt to be engaged in more interactions with systems outside the family. Families become more receptive to interventions such as health teaching than they may be at other times in the family life cycle. This openness of family boundaries allows nurses more access to the family for health promotion.

Very closed or enmeshed families have nonpermeable boundaries and reject outside influences such as nursing. Families can become closed because they interpret the outside environment and systems as hostile or difficult to cope with. An example would be a family who is culturally diverse and non-English speaking. These families may not allow stress or energy to diffuse out from the family and tend not to interact with the social community beyond the family. Consequently, they do not obtain the help they need even though childbearing may put them at higher risk for poor childbearing outcomes than are more open families (Ramsey, Abell, & Baker, 1986). These families are challenging for nurses because they are less readily accessible or responsive to family nurses.

Transition Concepts

The concept of transition is similar to change theory, discussed in Chapter 2, but it differs because it focuses on the processes involved with second-order change as families move from non-childbearing to childbearing entities. Inherent in transition is a period of upheaval as the family moves from one state to another. Historically, "transition to parenthood" was thought to be a crisis by early family researchers (LeMasters, 1957; Steffensmeier, 1982). The notion of transition to parenthood as a crisis is now being abandoned. More recent work focuses on the transition processes associated with change in families. In a more contemporary approach, transition to parenthood has been defined as a long-term process that results in qualitative reorganization of both inner life and external behavior (Cowan, 1991). Reorganization occurs in three phases:

- First is disbelief in the reality of the change.
- Second is frustration over not being able to cope in the old ways.
- Third is accommodation, when a new identity as parents is claimed and role expectations consistent with being parents are learned.

Nurse researchers have focused on transition to motherhood. Even though other family members have transitions, concepts related to motherhood give nurses insight into family transition. For example, Nelson (2003) described the primary process as "engagement," or opening one's self to the opportunity to grow and be transformed. Opening of self relates to making a commitment to mothering, experiencing the presence of a child, and caring for her child. This notion of transition gives foundation to nursing interventions that promote parenting because opening of self involves the real experience of being with and caring for her child. A nurse could use this theory by realizing that the mother may be frustrated over not being able to cope in her old ways. This would be a sign of her readiness to accept parenting education by a nurse.

Developmental Theories

Developmental theories focus on predictable changes and growth that occur throughout life. Changes occur in stages during which there is upheaval while adjustments are being made. What occurs during these stages is generally referred to as *developmental tasks.* Duvall's (Duvall & Miller, 1986) family life cycle theory describes tasks and processes for different stages during a family's life. In this theory, the family childbearing stage is defined as the period from the beginning of the first pregnancy until the oldest child reaches 18 months of age. Many nurses think that the tasks of this stage of the family life cycle do not end when the oldest child reaches 18 months of age and that family life stages can overlap. Some tasks reoccur as other children are added during a family's life cycle, whereas others are more salient for first children. The tasks during the childbearing stage are listed in Table 10–1. The family life cycle theory guides nurses in assessment of family achievement of developmental tasks and interaction aspects such as roles and relationships. In addition, they set the stage for anticipatory teaching addressing normal family events and stresses. However, nurses must consider that the family life cycle theory was developed decades ago. Many present-day families do not precisely fit into the stages and tasks, such as when one or both partners have children from previous relationships, parents are unmarried or single, couples are of the same sex, or children were born later in life. Even though families may have more diversity now, the family life cycle still has relevance for present-day families. This theory can help nurses think about families and assess the similarities and differences of families. The section on health promotion in this chapter is an illustration

---

Table 10–1 DEVELOPMENTAL TASKS FOR CHILDBEARING FAMILIES

- Arranging space (territory) for a child
- Financing childbearing and child rearing
- Assuming mutual responsibility for child care and nurturing
- Facilitating role learning of family members
- Adjusting to changed communication patterns in the family to accommodate a newborn and young children
- Planning for subsequent children
- Realigning intergenerational patterns
- Maintaining family members' motivation and morale
- Establishing family rituals and routines

Adapted from Duvall, E. M., & Miller, B. C. (1986). *Marriage and family development.* New York: Harper & Row.

of how nurses can use the family life cycle theory in their care.

An Eclectic Use of Theories for Childbearing Family Nursing

Just as no one theory covers all aspects of the nursing of families, no theory described in this chapter will work for every situation experienced with childbearing families. General systems theory emphasizes the need to maintain balance and counteract change. With childbearing, change is inevitable and may be in conflict with homeostasis, the goal of a family system. The concept of change or transition may imply a negative response to a new situation, which may not be the case with childbearing. Family life cycle theory is rooted in change, but it has been criticized for not being applicable to many contemporary family situations because it was based on the typical experiences of mainstream North American families in the middle of the 20th century. Nevertheless, the ideas gleaned from these theories of systems, change, and family development can help nurses organize assessments and manage predictable and unpredictable events during childbearing.

The following concepts derived from general systems, transition, and family developmental theories are highly relevant for guiding childbearing family nursing:

- Changes will occur in a family during the child-bearing cycle.
- Changes that occur during childbearing are not necessarily negative.
- Change in one member or one aspect of a child-bearing family induces changes in other members and aspects of a family.
- Families are usually open to influence of the environment during the childbearing cycle.
- Becoming parents involves experiences with the child.
- Environmental influences, such as social support and family nursing, can have a positive impact on a childbearing family.
- Developmental tasks for pregnancy and child-bearing families are predictable and lead to new ways of functioning for individuals and families.

Nurses may not even be aware that they use these concepts with childbearing families. For example, most maternity inpatient units encourage families to initiate care of the baby soon after birth. In this way,

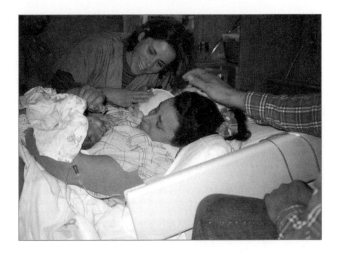

nurses use the concept "Becoming parents involves experiences with the child."

HEALTH PROMOTION FOR THE CHILDBEARING FAMILY

The developmental tasks of the childbearing family identified in the family life cycle theory (Duvall & Miller, 1986) guide health promotion in the childbearing family. This theory is helpful because it addresses the patterns of adaptation to parenthood that are typical for many families of Western cultures. Family nurses will find that many of these tasks are similar for families of different configurations and cultures. The developmental tasks with appropriate nursing actions are discussed in the following sections.

Arranging Space (Territory) for a Child

Typically, during the third trimester of pregnancy, families make space preparations for their babies. Often families move to a new residence during pregnancy or the first year after birth to obtain more space, or they modify their living quarters and furnishings to accommodate new babies.

Nurses are not usually involved in actually arranging or providing space for childbearing families; however, families' concerns about space are of interest to nurses. By asking about the living space and physical preparation for the baby, nurses can assess whether these developmental tasks are being met. If a family has not made physical preparations for the baby, nurses should investigate the reasons.

Busy families may inadvertently delay space preparations. Nurses' inquiries about material and physical preparation for the baby may prompt parents to arrange space. Lack of preparation may have other causes. Nurses need to be aware of families' cultural practices regarding preparation for the baby. For some groups, preparation for a baby's material needs during pregnancy is not acceptable; it may mean bad luck or misfortune for the baby if space is changed (Lewis, 2003). Families who fear or have actually experienced perinatal loss often delay preparations. These families may fear that their babies may not live and do not wish to again experience the heartbreak of dismantling nurseries that will not be used. Nurses can help these families explore and manage their fear about survival of the baby. By recognizing and managing fears, a family's coping can be mobilized and family development can continue. Lack of space preparation may be due to the parents having not accepted the reality of the coming baby, perhaps because stress has diverted their attention. Stress affecting childbearing families needs to be recognized and, if possible, dealt with promptly. Nurses should be especially concerned if adolescent parents have not made arrangements. It could be from denial of the pregnancy or fear about repercussions from their families if pregnancy is revealed. Nurses could help adolescents address ways to communicate with their families and make plans for the future of the baby and the adolescent parents. Failure to prepare space may be due to inadequate, unsafe housing or homelessness, which may be real threats to the safety of some childbearing families. Nurses should refer these families to appropriate resources for obtaining safer housing or for further investigation of their living situations.

Financing Childbearing and Child Rearing

Childbearing family nurses recognize the impact of finances on childbearing families. Health care providers may not be able to accept patients who are not insured or who cannot pay for obstetrical services. The nurse's role is to help families find needed resources, such as nutrition programs and prenatal clinics that fit with the financial resources of the family. For most present-day families, childbearing results in both additional expenses and lower family income because most employed women will miss some employment and forgo possible career advancement during childbearing. Even with legislation to protect women from loss of jobs during childbearing, maintaining earnings and opportunities for advancement may be difficult for women returning to work after birth. These financial stresses can be extremely emotional for mothers without partners or for women who provide most of the income for their families.

Families cope with threats to income in a variety of ways. It is not uncommon for new and expectant fathers to work more hours at their current jobs or to change jobs, which may be a source of more anxiety and stress for the family. Women often alter their employment situations to be more compatible with life with a new baby. Families may fall back onto savings, increase their debt, or alter their lifestyles to match changing levels of income. Adolescents are especially prone to financial difficulties. Childbearing may disrupt their education, which sets them up for future poverty because they may not be able to obtain jobs that pay well enough to support a family.

Child care should be considered long before families need it. Last-minute scrambling to obtain safe and adequate child care is extremely stressful for families and often results in less-than-satisfactory arrangements for both parents and babies. By directing families to information and resources, nurses help them choose safe and appropriate child care. A less obvious but equally important role is to help families overcome nonfinancial barriers for needed resources and care. Such barriers to prenatal care often include lack of transportation and child care, hours of service that conflict with family employment, and cultural insensitivity.

Assuming Mutual Responsibility for Child Care and Nurturing

Besides additional expenses, the care and nurturing of infants bring sleep disruptions, demands on time and energy, additional household tasks, and personal discomfort for caretakers. Most people would not consider these aspects of parenting pleasant. Why, then, do adults voluntarily assume responsibility for a helpless infant? Explanations range from the biological drive to reproduce, the idea of producing a new generation, and fulfillment of personal expectations to social desirability and acceptance. The affectionate bonds or *attachment* that develops between parents and their children may be one of the driving forces for engaging in infant care and nurturing even under difficult circumstances or when the baby is adopted. The process of parent-infant attachment at the time of birth is well described in up-to-date maternity nursing texts.

Promotion of family integrity, feeding management, and risk identification for poor attachment are particularly important interventions for nurses whose goals are to enhance nurturing among all family members. The rest of this section will focus on these interventions.

Family Integrity Promotion

Throughout the childbearing cycle, nurses assist families to understand and respond to the impact of a new baby on existing children. No matter what age siblings are, the addition of a new baby affects the position, role, and power of older children, thereby creating stress for both parents and children. Teaching parents to emphasize the positive aspects of adding a family member helps them focus on sibling "relationships" rather than "rivalry." Parents may need help recognizing that *all* the children, not just the new baby, have needs. Parents may be concerned whether they have "enough" energy, time, and love for additional children. Practical ideas for time and task management can alleviate some of their concerns.

Once a baby has been born, opportunities for children to visit their mothers and new siblings in health care settings can enhance sibling relationships. Older children feel special when nurses express warmth and hospitality by recognizing their new roles as "big brother" or "big sister." Availability of age-appropriate toys, furnishings, and educational materials help children feel part of the experience. Sibling visitation offers an opportunity to explain older children's expected or unexpected behavior to parents. For example, crying by a 2-year-old may be the child's way of expressing stress over the strange environment rather than rejection of the new baby. Although parents may want to discourage children's visits because of crying, nurses can use the situation to discuss the needs of children in adapting to new siblings, including ongoing contact with their mothers.

During pregnancy, nurses should inquire about logistics of care for other children at the time of birth and during mothers' hospital stay. Usually it is less stressful for children to be cared for in their homes instead of going somewhere else. What is important for children at the time of birth and during postpartum hospital stay is that they be cared for and supported by a responsible adult whom they trust.

All family members experience household upheaval during the first few days and weeks that a new baby is in the home. Assisting parents to be realistic in their expectations about themselves, each other, and their children helps them to plan ahead by identifying appropriate support resources, such as help with household chores.

Feeding Management

Feeding tends to be synonymous with love and nurturing. Success in feeding their babies induces feelings of competency in mothers and love toward their babies. A family's comfort with its infant feeding method is as crucial for the physical, emotional, and social well-being of an infant as the food itself. Regardless of the parents' choice of feeding method, nurses' instructions need to emphasize the development of relationships between infant and parent through feeding. Being held during feeding enhances social development whether a baby is being breast-fed or bottle-fed. Parents should take the time during feedings to enjoy interacting with their babies. When the infant is adopted, social interaction with feeding is a special opportunity for developing attachment.

Even though the act of breast-feeding is a strictly female function, fathers need not be excluded from the feeding experience. Nurses can promote paternal-infant attachment by encouraging fathers to be involved with feeding. For example, the father can comfort the baby while the mother is getting ready to breast-feed or can burp the baby during and after feedings. Another way to involve fathers is to have them give the breast-fed baby an occasional bottle of expressed breast milk or formula. Early involvement of fathers in feeding is especially beneficial later when infants are being weaned or mothers are preparing to return to employment.

Risk Identification for Poor Attachment

Risk identification involves identifying families and individuals who are likely to have difficulty with attachment. Attachment difficulties may be related to the health of either the parents or the infant or to the parents' inability to carry out their role as parents. Unrealistic expectations about the baby may be another factor in difficulty with attachment. Examples are adolescents thinking that a baby will fulfill their needs for love and status, or parents feeling that a baby will strengthen a failing marriage. Usually women do not volunteer information about their depression. Therefore, the nurse needs to ask appropriate questions to determine moods, sleep, appetite, energy, fatigue level, and ability to concentrate. Beck (1998a, 2002) developed the Postpartum Depression

Predictor Inventory. The Edinburgh Postnatal Depression Scale by Cox, Holden, and Sagovsky (1989) has been found to be valid for several cultures (Eberhard-Gran, Eskild, Tambs, Opjordsmoen, & Samuelsen, 2001).

Extreme stress, health risk factors, and illness can interfere with parent-newborn contact that is needed for the development of attachment. Stressful conditions that pull parents' energies and attention away from their newborns can be detrimental to attachment. Nurses can be instrumental in ensuring contact between families and supportive networks in these situations. In extremely stressful family situations, such as drug dependency, childbearing family nurses may refer these families for appropriate therapy. Postpartum depression negatively affects a mother's interactions with her baby (Beck, 1995, 1998b). Mood disorders are the most common mental health issues

in the postpartum period (American Psychiatric Association, 2000). Women with postpartum depression are unable to be emotionally available to their children. Nurses need to be aware of the negative impact of postpartum depression. Early identification and referral for treatment of women with postpartum depression can reduce the risk of adverse parent-infant interactions.

Families are at risk for poor attachment if a parent has suffered abuse, neglect, or abandonment during childhood. Nurses can help these parents gain a perspective on the poor parenting they experienced and help them develop awareness that they can choose to not repeat these behaviors with their own children. Family nurses convey to these families a sense of caring and concern that may have been missing in their own childhoods. Family nurses help parents develop new skills in caregiving and interacting with

POSTPARTUM DEPRESSION AND THE FAMILY

Research on postpartum depression is especially important for family nurses because it affects others in their client families. Postpartum depression affects 10 to 15 percent of all childbearing women (Beck, 1995). Consequently, a large number of children and other adults, especially fathers, are affected by postpartum depression.

Beck, a nurse-researcher, conducted a meta-analysis of 19 research studies on the effects of postpartum depression on mother-infant interaction. Depressed women and their babies show consistent patterns of maternal-infant interaction (Beck, 1995). Depressed mothers display less affectionate contact behavior, less responsiveness to infant cues, a flattened affect, and withdrawal from or hostility toward their infants. Infants of depressed mothers behaved differently from infants of nondepressed women. They were fussier, had more avoidant behaviors, and made fewer positive vocalizations and facial expressions. Statistically, the meta-analysis indicated that postpartum depression had a moderate to large effect on maternal-infant interaction during the infants' first year. The adverse effects of postpartum depression may have long-term effects on children's cognitive and emotional development (Beck, 1998b).

The impact of postpartum depression on women's partners is drawing more interest. A team of nurse-researchers (Meighan, Davis, Thomas, & Droppleman, 1999) studied the experiences of eight men whose spouses had postpartum depression. These fathers' lives and relationships with their wives were disrupted. They felt fear, confusion, and concern for their spouses, yet they were frustrated by not being able to do anything to alleviate the depression. They made sacrifices to hold the family together. They were uncertain about the future with their wives, who seemed very different from the way they were before the birth.

Nurses, through recognizing postpartum depression and promptly referring women for treatment, not only help affected women but also enhance the social and emotional environment for infants and promote the survival of family relationships.

Beck, C. T. (1998). The effects of postpartum depression on child development: A meta-analysis. *Archives of Psychiatric Nursing, 12,* 12–20; Beck, C. T. (1995). The effects of postpartum depression on maternal-infant interaction: A meta-analysis. *Nursing Research, 44,* 298–304; Meighan, M., Davis, M. W., Thomas, S. P., & Droppleman, P. G. (1999). Living with postpartum depression: The father's experience. *MCN: The American Journal of Maternal/Child Nursing, 24,* 202–208.

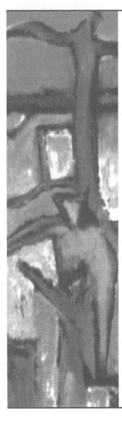

RESEARCH BRIEF

Purpose
To study whether fatigue is a predictor of early postpartum depression.

Methods
Researchers studied a convenience sample of 38 healthy women that were within 24 hours of an uncomplicated birth. They used a Modified Fatigue Symptom Checklist with the women on the day of birth and 7, 14, and 28 days after birth. On day 28 after infant birth, they also administered the Center for Epidemiological Studies Depressive Symptomatology Scale.

Results
A significant correlation was found between fatigue and postpartum depression for days 7, 14, and 28.

Implications for Nursing
Within the first 2 weeks after birth, nurses on a home visit or in the mother-baby clinic could screen for fatigue using a simple scale. As most women will not volunteer feelings of depression with health care workers, it is incumbent on the nurse to be aware of the possibility of postpartum depression.

Source: Bozoky, I., & Corwin, E. (2002). Fatigue as a predictor of postpartum depression. *Journal of Obstetric, Gynecologic, and Neonatal Nursing, 31,* 436–443.

their babies, such as ways for soothing a fussy baby (Solchany, 2001). In these situations, nurses work with social workers, psychotherapists, and developmental specialists to help these parents care for and nurture their children.

Nurses often identify families at risk for poor attachment through listening to what parents say about their babies and observing parent behaviors. At-risk families may have misconceptions about infant behavior such as believing that babies cry just to annoy their parents. Other concerns for nurses to address include verbal expressions of dissatisfaction with the baby, comparison of the baby to disliked family members, failure to respond to the infant's crying, lack of spontaneity in touching the baby, and stiffness or discomfort in holding the baby after the first week. Isolated incidences of these behaviors are probably not detrimental to attachment, but persistent trends and patterns could foreshadow relationship difficulties. An important step is for the nurse to evaluate whether the parent-infant relationship is progressing positively. The enjoyment and love of children grow over time. If the parents' enjoyment of the baby as a unique individual and commitment to the baby are not progress-

ing, the family needs continuing education, role modeling, encouragement, and realistic appraisal. Childbearing family nurses may need to refer these families who do not demonstrate these nurturing behaviors to other professionals who can provide more-intensive intervention.

Facilitating Role Learning of Family Members

Learning roles is particularly important for childbearing families. For many couples, taking on the role of parents is a dramatic shift in their lives. Difficulty with adaptation to parenthood may be related to the stress of learning new roles as well as to role conflicts. Role learning involves expectations about the role, developing the ability to assume the role, and taking on the role.

Expectations about the Parent Role

Expectations about parent roles are part of the transition to parenthood. Mothers often compare their actual experiences with their expectations. Expectations about partners' role also influence the transition to parenthood. For example, men are seen as helpmates, supports, and bystanders during childbearing rather than as parents. If women are regarded as the "real" parents, men are not encouraged to grasp the reality of fatherhood (Jordan, 1990). These role expectations can interfere with men believing that they have the knowledge, support, or skills to become involved parents.

In North America, societal expectations about the parent role, especially motherhood, are unrealistic and may set up parents to feel inadequate. The media support the myth of motherhood and are full of images of new mothers clad in luxurious lace while they feed glowing, contented babies in immaculate homes. The reality of early motherhood is that prepregnancy clothes do not fit, babies periodically become demanding malcontents, and houses are messy because family members are too exhausted to clean. Traditional nursing and medical textbooks reinforce this myth of the mother role by implying that at 6 weeks after birth, when healing of the reproductive system is complete, women are ready to resume all their previous activities. In reality, it takes longer for women to resume their roles. Studies of postpartum women showed that virtually no woman had regained full functioning 6 weeks after birth (Smith-Hanrahan & Deblois, 1995; Tulman, Fawcett, Groblewski, & Silverman, 1990). Incongruence between the ideal and the real parent role may result in frustration, turmoil, and loss of confidence. Unrealistic expectations about being parents and about children's development are often present in angry, abusive families. Unrealistic expectations about the impact of a baby on adolescent parents' lives will affect their parent roles.

Adoptive parents have many of the same feelings and fears as those of birth mothers. Regardless of the way in which a family is formed, parents react with the same intense feelings and emotions that range from happiness to distress when they first meet their child. Even though the child is not biological or the parental relationship may not be established immediately at birth, bonding can be just as strong and immediate for adoptive parents and children (Hockenberry, Wilson, Winkelstein, & Kline, 2003).

Nurses can help parents discuss and face their ideals and bridge the gap between the idealized and actual roles. One nursing intervention is to have expectant parents, before their baby's birth, describe what they think being parents will be like. By assessing these responses, nurses can tailor education for parents about the realities of parenting. For example, nurses can help expectant parents see themselves in very real situations with interrupted sleep and little free time. By presenting a realistic but balanced view of parenthood, nurses help parents shift from a totally positive view to a more realistic parent role. Encouraging contact with others who are in the process of taking on the parenting role may be more effective than any information that nurses can give. Contact with other parents is especially helpful for parents who are isolated, adolescent, or culturally diverse and living apart from traditional networks.

Nurses assist pregnant couples to explore their attitudes and expectations about the role of their partners. For instance, a woman may not realize that she is placing her partner in a role subordinate to her role as the primary parent or the "expert." Nurses should encourage expectant women to bring their partners into the experience by sharing their physical sensations and emotions of being pregnant. Men may need to be encouraged to think about how they expect to enact their role as fathers. Being relegated to a subordinate role can be discouraging to men and ultimately may result in their becoming less involved in parenting. If women expect their partners to be fully involved parents, they need to provide opportunities for them to become skilled infant caregivers. For example, when her mate assumes infant care responsibilities, a woman should not rush in to correct her mate's "mistakes" such as a loose diaper or a shirt that is on backward.

Developing Abilities for the Parent Role

Expectant mothers and fathers develop parenting abilities and skills through their own childhood experiences and contact with other parents, friends, family members, and health care providers. Nurses in all childbearing care settings teach parenting skills. Prospective parents and parents often turn to guidebooks on parenting. The position found in more current parenting books is one that is less rigid, thereby emphasizing satisfactory physical and emotional well-being for parents and children. Parents are reassured that they will not be "perfect parents" and that they will make mistakes. The approaches of these guidebooks vary, with some more descriptive of development and some more specific to family issues, for example, single parenting. The parenting books that nurses recommend should be appropriate for the specific family, as well as developmentally appropriate for the age of the child. The nurse should encourage parents to review several recommended books and select at least two for support and various ideas (Hockenberry, Wilson, Winkelstein, & Kline, 2003). When planning educational strategies for parents, nurses must consider expectant parents' past experiences and the range and diversity of their information sources.

The role of parent is a dynamic one because children's needs change as children develop. Fortunately, parents' skills grow and change along with their children. Nurses can continue to help families develop the abilities they need for the parent role beyond the childbearing stage. This is especially important for teenage parents and parents with limited experience with children.

Taking On the Role of Parent

Becoming parents requires not only learning to perform caretaking tasks but also developing the feelings and problem-solving abilities associated with parenting. Praising parents in their early efforts and modeling the feelings associated with the parental role are likely to encourage a pattern of positive parenting. Specific behaviors to model include displaying warmth toward the baby and expressing pleasure over care of the baby. This is especially important, as depressed parents often do not experience pleasure in caring for their babies (Beck, 1996, 1999).

As parents take on their roles, they tend to use problem-solving strategies that they are familiar with and that suit their own life situations and needs (Martell, 2001). As parents meet their babies' needs consistently and successfully under a variety of conditions, positive feelings about being parents grow. Hospital-based nurses can help by discussing how to perform parenting tasks at home with their own baby-care equipment. A useful strategy for nurses is to apply the parents' typical problem solving in teaching parenting skills. An example would be suggesting books on child care to parents who consult printed sources for information for making decisions. Astute childbearing family nurses evaluate the current popular works on child rearing and help families determine the most appropriate approaches for their family. Some families tend to defer major decisions to older and "wiser" family members such as mothers or grandparents. In this situation, it is helpful for nurses to identify which family members are consulted regularly on child care issues. Even if the advice from family members is not the same as that of health care providers, nurses should not contradict it unless the advice is harmful. By contradicting long-held family values and customs, nurses will erode the trust of families.

By being knowledgeable of normal growth and development of infants, nurses can provide guidance to help families understand what is developmentally appropriate behavior for their baby so that parents do not misinterpret the infant's behavior or use inappropriate actions. Much of parenting involves being able to empathize with the baby. If the baby is thriving and the parents are becoming skilled caregivers with warmth, concern, and affection for their baby, then they are clearly taking on the parent role.

Adjusting Communication Patterns to Accommodate a Newborn

As parents and infants learn to interpret and respond to each other's communication cues, they develop effective, reciprocal communication patterns. Infant cues may be so subtle, however, that parents may not be sensitive to cues until nurses point them out (Schiffman, Omar, & McKelvey, 2003; Sumner, 1990). Educating parents about different infant temperaments so that they can interpret their baby's unique style of communication is another way to promote better communication patterns (Brazelton, 1992). For example, many babies respond to being held by cuddling and nuzzling, but others respond by arching their backs and stiffening. Parents may interpret the latter as rejecting and unloving responses, and these negative interpretations may adversely affect the parent-infant relationship.

Nurses can help families relate to these difficult babies in several ways. Nurses can point out that the baby is not rejecting the parents but has a unique temperament. Such babies need time to "warm up" to interacting with others. The parents should be encouraged to talk to and engage in eye contact with the baby. Interacting with the baby without tactile stimulation at first will give the baby the opportunity to interact with gazing and cooing. These responses can boost parents' positive feelings about the baby.

Nurses need to be aware of interaction styles of depressed mothers and take steps to improve the quality of parent-infant interaction through facilitating treatment of depression. Mothers who are depressed are less attuned to their infants, which may lead to poorer cognition later in infants' lives (Murray, Fiori-Cowley, Hooper, & Cooper, 1996). Depressed mothers may withdraw socially from their infants and act like robots in their everyday activities with their babies (Beck, 1996). Referral for appropriate care for depressed mothers will profoundly affect the babies' future (Lowdermilk, Peters, & Bobak, 2000).

Communication between parents changes with the transition to parenthood. During the years of childbearing, many men and women devote considerable time to career development. Present-day families may have to work more than 40 hours per week to have adequate income. The time demands of work may affect a couple's relationship. While taking on the everyday aspects of rearing children, parents often do not give their couple relationship the attention needed to sustain it. Parents need to recognize the importance of being a couple because families thrive with a strong, sustained couple relationship (Jordan, Stanley, & Markman, 1999).

Couple communication should be incorporated into care and education of expectant parents. Expectant parents will need to communicate with each other long after they have used labor coping skills that are the essence of traditional expectant parent preparation programs. An innovative expectant parent education program that is based on evidence from research incorporates a communication program that uses information, building of skills, and support (Jordan, 2002). The anticipated outcome of this program is stronger, longer-lasting couple relationships. Nurses can promote more-effective couple communication by encouraging the partners to listen to each other actively, using "I phrases" instead of blaming the other. An example of an "I message" is "I feel useless when you take over baby care without asking me" instead of "You're so bossy about the baby." The "I message" gives the recipient feedback and clarification about the partner's response to a behavior. Such feedback and clarification can give a couple the opportunity to discuss and problem-solve a troublesome situation. Another way to promote couple communication and stronger relationships is to encourage them to set aside a regular time to talk and enjoy each other as loving partners, not as parents (Ross, Channon-Little, & Simon-Rosser, 2000).

Planning for Subsequent Children

Some parents with their first baby have definite, mutually agreed-upon plans for additional children, whereas others have definitely decided not to have more children. Families who have definite plans primarily need information about family planning options so that they can carry out their plans. Nurses will also encounter parents who are uncertain about having more children. In this situation, nurses can help couples through education, assistance with clarifying their values, and discussion about decision making.

Nurses always need to consider a family's cultural background in considering sensitive reproductive matters. When discussing childbearing decisions, nurses must consider the power structure and locus of decision in the family. Mutuality in making decisions implies that both members of a couple have equal power and status. It is counterproductive for nurses not to consider the male partner in families with male-dominated power structures. In such a family, the woman may acquiesce in her partner's decisions even when she does not agree.

Realigning Intergenerational Patterns

The first baby adds a new generation in the family lineage that carries the family into the future. Expectant parents change from being children of their parents to becoming parents themselves. Childbearing may signify the onset of being an adult for adolescent parents and some cultural groups.

Childbearing changes relationships within extended families. The parents' siblings become aunts and uncles, children from previous relationships become stepsiblings, and their own parents become grandparents. Nurses working with pregnant women can promote development of grandparent-parent relationships in several ways (Martell, 1990). Nurses may encourage discussion by saying, "Tell me how things are going between you and your mother." From the pregnant woman's response, nurses assess the quality of the relationship and, when appropriate, consider interventions that may enhance their relationship.

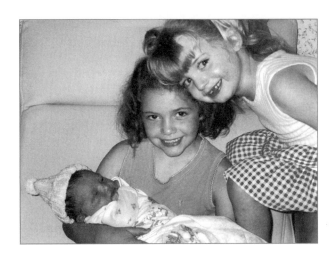

This approach is especially important for adolescents and their mothers because adolescents often have very stormy relationships with their mothers. For example, nurses may suggest that the pregnant woman ask her mother to tell her about her own pregnancy and birth experiences. Sharing these experiences offers a sense of continuity. If conflict exists between the expectant mother and the family, nurses can help by teaching pregnant women communication strategies that open discussions with their mothers and have the potential to resolve conflicts.

Potential areas of conflict between generations include infant feeding methods, dealing with crying babies, and other aspects of child rearing. Current recommendations for infant care and feeding are not the same as what grandparents did with their own children a generation ago. Consequently, new parents may receive conflicting information from health care providers and members of their extended families. New parents may find it stressful to confront their parents on an adult-to-adult level, especially when their parents genuinely want to be helpful. Nurses can suggest tactful ways for expectant parents to confront their own parents who have outmoded advice and information. Ideally, conflict can be prevented prior to the arrival of the baby through information sharing and open discussion about what would be helpful. Nurses can educate new and expectant grandparents about recommendations by helping them compare their experiences with present-day practices, giving them tours of hospital facilities, and providing up-to-date educational materials (Starn, 1993; Polomeno, 1999, 2000).

Parents and grandparents may have different expectations about the role of grandparents. For example, a traditional expectation of grandmothers is that they are willingly available for child care. This expectation is not realistic for present-day families. Contemporary grandmothers have life situations as varied as those of younger women. They may be career women, homemakers, caretakers of other grandchildren, and care providers for their aging parents. Many grandparents live geographically distant from their children, which affects the development of their role as a grandparent.

Roles of grandparents are on a continuum from purely symbolic to actively instrumental (Kornhaber, 1996). Nurses more often see the more practical roles, such as role model for their children and nurturer. The nurturing role often comes into play with adversity, such as being the main support for a pregnant daughter undergoing a divorce. A growing trend in the United States is grandparents assuming parenting of the newborns when their own adult children are unable to care for their children. An example of this situation is the incarceration of parents ("Mothers in Prison . . . Children in Crisis," 2000; Bullock, 2001). Nurses need to be aware of the grandparent roles their midlife clients are assuming because these roles can be a source of joy or of stress.

Reliance on health care professionals for childbearing and child-rearing guidance is primarily a middle-class phenomenon. For other socioeconomic and some cultural groups, nurses may not be as esteemed as the older women in families are on matters relating to childbearing. In these situations, nurses may feel frustrated when new parents more readily accept the advice of other family members, such as their own mothers, rather than the health care providers' recommendations. If the advice from non–health care providers is not safe, the nurse needs to provide information that supports current practice so that the new mother can make an informed health care decision. In all such situations, it is more important for nurses to maintain a professional relationship with these families instead of being "right."

Maintaining Family Members' Motivation and Morale

The care, feeding, and comforting of infants demand time, energy, and personal resources. Women may be fatigued for months from the physical exertion and blood loss of birth compounded by the demands of infant care (Troy, 1999, 2003). Some women have little chance to be well rested before they are expected to return to their jobs (Killien, 1993). In addition, maternal exhaustion can contribute to postpartum depression. The demands of early parenting tend to draw mothers and fathers away from the couple relationship.

Nurses can help family members maintain motivation and morale and avoid becoming overwhelmed by the transition to parenthood. Before new mothers are discharged from nurses' care, both parents need to know ways to promote their rest and sleep (Troy & Dalgas-Pelish, 1997). For example, helping new mothers with comfort measures for a sore perineum or uterine cramps makes it easier for them to rest and cope with fatigue, which in turn improves morale.

Families need to be realistic about infant sleep patterns. Typically, infants will need nighttime feedings for several months, no matter how parents modify the timing and content of feedings. Time-honored ways to promote parental rest while a baby needs nighttime feedings are to alternate who responds to the baby and feeding the baby in the parents' bed. Infant crying seems to be more irritating if parents are fatigued, and it can exacerbate sleep loss. Thus, helping parents cope with crying helps boost family morale. Being able to soothe a fussy baby increases confidence for new parents and allows them to get additional sleep.

In present-day North American families, the postpartum period can be lonely. Many young families live in communities far from their extended families. Some families have recently moved into a new neighborhood and have not established friendships or a sense of community. Many ethnically diverse groups had special support and recognition of the postpartum period in their countries of origin, but in North America there may not be replacements for traditional postpartum care. Counseling families about the duration of postpartum recovery and making suggestions for adaptation will decrease their feelings of isolation.

Frequently, new parents find support from friends, family members, organized parent groups, and work colleagues. When young families find that their parenting experiences are similar to those of others, their morale tends to improve. Nurses and other health professionals can also boost morale by educating families about parenting and providing positive feedback. Often new parents want to appear self-sufficient and are reluctant to accept offers of help. They may be vague about their needs or not recognize what they need. In such cases, nurses assist them to articulate their needs and find help in ways that support their self-esteem as new parents.

Couples need to be aware of potential changes in their sexual relationship with the arrival of a baby. Sensitive nurses counsel couples about changes in sexuality after birth and help them develop mutually satisfying sexual expression (Ross, Channon-Little, & Simon-Rosser, 2000). Often couples need to be encouraged to take time for themselves apart from the baby. The physical separation from the baby is not as important in itself as the fact that it allows parents to interact with each other and enjoy each other's company outside of the parenting role. This can be done even in very brief periods of conversation and physical closeness when the baby is asleep.

Most parents need activity, companionship, and interests beyond the family for improved quality of their lives. For example, a study on postpartum well-being showed that women who had more vigorous exercise had more confidence in tasks of mothering, more satisfaction with motherhood and their partner's participation in child care, and higher quality of relationship with their partners (Sampselle, Seng, Yeo, Killion, & Oakley, 1999). Nurses work with families to develop strategies that maintain their couple activities, adult interests, and friendships.

Establishing Family Rituals and Routines

Rituals develop as children come into a family, and these rituals become a source of comfort as well as part of the uniqueness and identity of a family (Fomby, 2004). The predictability of rituals helps babies develop trust. Family rituals include bedtime and bathing routines, baby's special possessions such as a treasured blanket, and nicknames for body functions. For some families, rituals have special cultural meanings that nurses should respect. When families are disrupted or separated during childbearing, nurses can help them deal with stress by encouraging them to carry out their usual routines and established rituals related to their babies and other children.

THREATS TO HEALTH DURING CHILDBEARING

For the majority of families, childbearing is a physically healthy experience. For some families, health during childbearing is threatened, and the childbearing experience becomes an illness experience. In such cases, concern for the physical health of the mother and the fetus tends to outweigh other aspects of pregnancy, and rather than eagerly anticipating the birth and baby, family members experience fear and apprehension. Moreover, the family's functioning and developmental tasks are disrupted as the family focuses its attention on the health of the mother and the survival of the fetus or baby. Families with threats to health have additional needs for maintaining and preserving family health.

Acute and Chronic Illness during Childbearing

For this chapter, "acute" will be defined as health threats that come on suddenly and may have life-threatening implications. Examples are fetal distress during labor and pulmonary embolism for postpartum women. "Chronic" conditions are those that occur during pregnancy that persist, linger, or need control to avoid becoming acute. Examples are pregnancy-induced hypertension, gestational and preexisting diabetes, and postpartum depression. Some threats to health vacillate between acute and chronic. Preterm labor can be acute and result in a preterm birth. However, if preterm labor contractions are suppressed, it becomes "chronic" with regimens to keep contractions from reoccurring.

Impact of Threats to Health on Childbearing Families

Even though gestational diabetes and suppression of preterm labor are managed at home, these threats to childbearing health are disruptive for childbearing families. According to systems theory, a health threat to a member of the childbearing family will affect the other members. The functioning and structure of the family that keep the family system stable are upset. The family strives to regain balance, which is stressful on all family members.

Although nurses may not be directly involved in care of a family beyond prescribed management and health care settings, understanding a family's experiences can contribute to the effectiveness of care. The following are some issues faced by childbearing families with threats to health and nursing implications.

Assuming Household Tasks

Other family members must assume household and family tasks so that the expectant mother or a sick baby can stay on prescribed regimens. Shifting of these tasks may be stressful and may affect the family's functioning (Bomar, 2004). Expectant fathers, especially, find that *all* their time and energy are consumed by employment and household management, which were previously shared or done solely by their partners. Children's lives change when mothers have to limit activities. Toddlers do not understand why their mothers cannot pick them up or run after them. The resulting frustration for children can manifest itself in behavior changes such as tantrums and lapses in toilet training. When bed rest is part of medical management, the demands of families may make bed rest a stressful experience for expectant mothers and fathers (Gupton, Heaman, & Ashcroft, 1997; McCain & Deatrick, 1994). Because of their frustration and the burdens of family tasks, women may not be fully compliant with the regimens to control threats to health (Josten, Savik, Mullett, Campbell, & Vincent, 1995).

Nurses need to understand how changes in daily living create stress for all family members (Bomar, 2004). Helping families find ways to streamline and prioritize household tasks contributes to stress reduction and adherence to medical regimens. For example, having the adults list household management tasks and determine who does what when will help a family be more efficient and effective in managing these tasks. Another way nurses can help with stress reduction is by educating families about the impact of parents' health difficulties on children and by providing practical, age-appropriate suggestions for managing children. For example, hiring a teenager after school for active play with young children may replace activities they had before their mothers' restricted activity. Providing ways for young children to have some quiet one-on-one time with their mothers can reduce stress for both mothers and children.

Managing Changes in Income and Resources

The at-risk pregnancy is stressful in terms of the family's financial and other resources. Time away from paid employment may result in loss of income. Medical expenses may rise due to the need for increased care, including possible neonatal intensive care. Personal expenses may increase because of the need for changes in diet, medications, alterations in transportation, and help with household tasks. If a family is in debt, threats to health can increase the burden of debt.

The impact on nonmonetary resources, such as energy and social networks, cannot be measured as easily as money. Often, others outside of the nuclear family can assume various household tasks such as meal preparation, laundry, and cleaning. Not all families have social networks or extended families in the immediate vicinity. Isolation can increase a family's burden. Changes in employment may cause separation from persons and activities that were stimulating.

Although nurses are not directly involved in changes to family income, they need to recognize the stress related to changes in finances and resources (Bullock, 2004). Nurses can help a family identify and use resources by drawing a family ecomap, which may include home health agencies and parents' groups in the community that will assist with household management, thus boosting their morale (see Chapter 8). Reducing the sense of isolation can restore energy to families. For families with the necessary resources, using a computer to connect with other at-risk families can prevent or decrease feelings of isolation. Nurses can direct families to appropriate Internet sites such as the ones listed in the "Selected Resources" section at the end of this chapter.

Facing Uncertainty and Separation

Because of the unpredictable nature of high-risk childbearing, planning for the future becomes more difficult. Family adaptation to preterm infants or high-risk infants is different from family adaptation when the baby is a term and normal child (Holditch-Davis & Miles, 2000). With pending preterm birth, expectant parents, especially employed women, may not be able to determine accurately when to begin and end parental leave because the family may have to cope with sudden hospitalization. Small children may become extremely anxious over their mother's sudden departure, especially if they are unprepared or unable to comprehend what is happening to their mother and the new baby.

Nurses should acknowledge the difficulties of uncertainties associated with difficult perinatal situations. Being honest and informative about the condition and prognosis can be reassuring. Health care providers often use terms not understood by family members. Explanations to all family members should be accurate, thorough, and tailored to families' anxiety levels.

Transfer to a distant perinatal center is not uncommon for families in remote rural areas. Such transfers separate family members for days or weeks and make it difficult to maintain and develop family relationships. Even if the logistical problems are solved and a family can be together, coping with basic tasks of living is challenging in these high-tech settings. For instance, a family may not know where to stay, how to find reasonably priced meals, how to obtain transportation, or where to park a car.

Nurses are pivotal in promoting family relationships in high-risk situations. Electronic communication, such as e-mail, facilitates contact between family members and health care professionals. Calling families about their members' progress and sending photographs help families cope with uncertainty and enhance relationships of physically separated family members.

A family's absence from where the family member is being cared for should not be interpreted as poor relationships or indifference. Nurses should investigate and reduce the barriers that families encounter at the distant perinatal center, such as lack of transportation, other responsibilities, employment, and the threatening environment of the setting. For example, social interactions, such as greeting family members by name, help them feel welcomed and recognized. Encouraging family members to participate in care helps family relationships. In neonatal settings, nurses who include families in care of their infants promote development of parenting skills. Pointing out a baby's unique characteristics and cues cement the parent-child relationship (VandenBerg, 1999).

Coping

With threats to health, the coping strategies of families may be inadequate for the level of stress/crisis or may be exhausted. Before having an at-risk pregnancy, many young families have not experienced situations of threatened health, drained financial resources, uncertainty, or separation from loved ones. The family's coping strategies can be compromised further by unrealistic perceptions of their situation. In these situations, the nurses' role is to help childbearing families develop appropriate coping strategies such as exercise and sharing their experiences with other families in similar situations. Some families benefit from the support of others even though they may be reluctant to ask for help.

Nurses can help them realistically appraise threats to health and identify their strengths and resources for coping. Family strengths may include positive ways they have coped with stressful situations in the past; resources include available helpful persons, financial assistance, and informational sources. Finally, nurses can assist families in the longer term by teaching them to problem-solve and by developing new resources and strategies for healthy, effective coping. See Box 10–1 for tips on healthy coping.

IMPLICATIONS FOR NURSING

The concerns of childbearing family nursing go beyond care of the individual family. Nurses are participants in guiding nursing practice and education, developing and using research, and setting and implementing policy.

Practice

Family-centered care is prevalent in North America. In a survey of 50 hospital obstetric units across the United States, 90 percent had implemented or were in the process of developing mother/baby care while 10 percent still had separate postpartum and nursery units (Bajo, Hager, & Smith, 1998). The incorporation of the word "family" in the names of health care institutions may make nurses complacent about the state of family nursing practice in their settings. Serious examination of institutional policies could

Box 10–1   **TIPS FOR COPING**

"How Can I Help?"

Often, childbearing families are reluctant to ask for help when they have a new baby, a tired mother, and sleep-deprived family members. The following are ways family members and friends can help a childbearing family cope:

- Provide nutritious meals and snacks.
- Do errands, household chores, shopping, and laundry.
- Ask a new mother to go for a walk or another form of outdoor exercise.
- Encourage the family not to make other major life-changing decisions during pregnancy and the first few months after birth.
- Make an appointment with a health care professional if the mother has symptoms of postpartum depression.
- Encourage partners of new mothers to accompany her to appointments so that they know what is going on with her health.
- Accept new mothers' feelings as valid and important.
- *Do not* tell new mothers to "stop crying." Instead, listen to her and ask what she wants.
- Instead of asking, "What can I do?" make specific suggestions such as offering to take the older children to their activities or run an errand.

help nurses determine whether the word "family" is part of a catchy name for marketing purposes or reflects a strong influence on philosophy, policies, and nursing standards.

Nurses may find barriers in their practice settings that interfere with promoting family development. For example, lack of privacy, complex machinery, and location of a neonatal intensive care unit may stifle interaction between family members and babies. To some nurses "mother/baby" means that the family members will assume all the care for the baby with nurses periodically "checking in" and renewing baby care supplies. In such situations, families feel ignored or burdened with too much independence (Martell, 2001, 2003). This was not the original intent of *family-centered care*. The role of nurses for family-centered care is thought to be primarily teaching. Direct care and assistance can be just as effective in promoting family care. For example, in those rare situations when breast-feeding newborns need feeding supplements, nurses could give the supplements. This would free families for rest and make them feel more cared about. Some other suggestions for making family-centered care a reality include identifying physical, psychological, and nursing staff requirements for family-centered care; developing a clear vision of family-centered care units; and involving nurses in planning and implementation of change (Martell, 2003).

In settings other than hospitals, changing the focus of care from individuals to families is the most important step in promoting family care. In-home care will be more effective when family members are included in care.

Education

The education needs to be specific to issues of families and individual family members in the childbearing stage. The most important aspect of education for all childbearing families, including families with high risk, is health promotion. Advances in technology continue in areas such as fertility treatment, gene therapy, fetal surgery, and obstetrical critical care units. These advances have enabled a wider range of families to bear children. Therefore, the education must cover current evidence-based nursing of childbearing situations. Many of the women in childbearing years are immigrants from various countries and cultures. It is imperative that nurses be educated to provide culturally sensitive and competent care. As well as culture, nurses need to be aware of ways of interacting with various alternative family situations and types.

Research

Technological advances such as gene therapy in human reproduction are rapidly increasing and becoming more commonplace. The scientific knowledge about the impact of these technologies on families still needs investigation. Because nurses focus on the full range of human experiences, nursing could be the leader in launching such studies. Areas for study include the most effective ways to counsel or interact with clients around infertility, genetic counseling, in vitro surgeries, and other medical advances.

Childbearing families represent the increasing diversity of families. The content of this chapter is partially based on study of two-parent, middle-class North American families. Research on the childbearing experience of ethnic and blended families is increasing, but more is needed on the full range of present-day families. In addition to studying various family cultures and types, it is critical to advance the studies relative to multiple births. One aspect that needs study is how alternative families adjust to miscarriages, stillbirths, and infertility issues. Adoption issues for the childbearing family need further study.

Research on family nursing interventions and outcomes for childbearing families needs to be supported for the development of evidence-based nursing practice. Evaluation of the effectiveness of family nursing interventions is especially critical when health care costs are under close scrutiny. Third-party payers need to be convinced that family nursing interventions result in improved outcomes of childbearing and that they are cost-effective (Cook, 1997).

Policy

Much of the chapter titled "Families, Nursing, and Social Policy" (Chapter 6) addresses important issues for childbearing families. The legal definitions of "family," official recognition of the diversity of families, access to health care, alternatives to traditional childbearing such as cross-cultural adoption, and growing needs of poverty-stricken families are just a few of the policy areas vital to childbearing family nursing.

Nurses need to be aware of the impact of legislation on childbearing families. One example is family leave for childbirth, which can profoundly affect the health and development of childbearing families. The Family Medical Leave Act entitles family members to take unpaid time away from employment without penalizing them, to care for a family member, such as a newborn, with health care needs. Unfortunately, many families cannot take advantage of this act because it applies only to businesses of a certain size and employers are not obligated to pay on-leave employees. Unlike the citizens of many developed nations, parents in the United States are not entitled to government benefits for childbearing.

In the United States, the Newborns' and Mothers' Health Protection Act of 1996 sets standards for minimal length of inpatient hospital stay for mothers and newborn infants. Many states now have legislation addressing postpartum care (Ferguson & Engelhard, 1997). Through active involvement with legislation, nurses can promote improved welfare of childbearing families.

All types of policies affect family nursing every day. Hospitals often have policies that form barriers to family welfare and relationships. In these situations, family nurses often are advocates for families. Often nurses think of policies as entities beyond their control. In actuality, nurses have a voice and power in forming and changing policies. Beginning steps include close scrutiny of their practice and settings for issues related to the welfare of families and their members.

SUMMARY

- While giving direct physical care, teaching patients, or performing other traditional modes of maternity nursing, family nurses focus on family relationships and health of all members of the childbearing family.
- Theories help nurses understand childbearing families and structure care.
- Even in extreme threats to health, family nurses do not ignore the whole of the family.
- Nurses can have a powerful influence on practice, education, policy, and research on childbearing families.

STUDY QUESTIONS

1. Discuss ways that childbearing family nurses can enhance an expectant father's role as a parent.
2. A new mother and her mother do not agree on how to handle a newborn's persistent crying. Discuss nursing actions that would help them resolve their differences.
3. Describe how postpartum depression can affect the developmental tasks of the childbearing family.
4. Write a care plan to help parents and older children develop a relationship with their baby in a special-care nursery.

CASE STUDY ➤

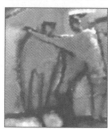

THE JOHNSONS: A FAMILY WITH A PRETERM BIRTH

The Johnson family illustrates the impact of threats to health on a childbearing family. Tom and Mary Johnson's first child, Jenny, was born at full term. Mary had no health problems with the pregnancy. At that time, the Johnsons lived in a large city in the western part of the United States, near their parents, siblings, and childhood friends. Two years later, the Johnsons moved to a small town 500 miles away from their friends and families to find better professional opportunities for Tom and more affordable housing. A month after the move, they discovered that Mary was about 3 months pregnant. Even though it would strain family finances, Mary decided to postpone seeking employment as a secretary until after the birth and concentrate on fixing up the old two-story house they had bought.

Unexpectedly, Mary had health problems with this pregnancy. At 27 weeks of pregnancy, her obstetrician diagnosed gestational diabetes and she had to modify her diet to keep her blood glucose under control. At 29 weeks she began to have preterm labor. To stop the contractions, her physician insisted that Mary stay on bed rest around the clock except for a very brief daily shower and use of the bathroom. Tom had to take over meal preparation, house cleaning, and caring for Jenny. He arranged the living room so that Mary could lie on the couch and Jenny could play near her mother while he was at work. Because he had not yet accrued vacation or sick time, Tom could not take off time from his job to help Mary and take care of Jenny without sacrificing pay.

High-risk childbearing is especially stressful when a family has a limited social or family network to assume family tasks such as meal preparation, child care, and household maintenance. Mary's premature labor occurred before the Johnsons had developed a social network in their new community. Had they had a supportive network, some of the burden of household management may have been eliminated.

Mary found it difficult to follow her diet and stay on bed rest. She was frustrated because she had to stop her house renovation and Tom's cooking and house-cleaning were not up to her standards. She was tempted to run the vacuum cleaner, wash dishes, and eat sweets while Tom was at work. The medication to suppress contractions made her so anxious and tremulous that she could not amuse herself with crafts, sewing, or puzzles. She was lonely for her mother and friends, 500 miles away; she longed for companionship but found herself complaining and nagging Tom when he was home. Jenny frequently had tantrums because she could not play outside with her mother and began to have lapses in toilet training.

As the description of the Johnson family shows, shifting of these tasks may be stressful and affect the family's functioning. Certainly Mary's anxiety was in part a response to feeling unable to handle family demands, and her nagging and complaining were probably expressions of her anxiety. With adequate support, Mary may not have felt so lonely and perhaps someone could have taken Jenny out to play. In other families, both parents' jobs may be affected by the unpredictability of the course of their pregnancy.

Interventions for health promotion need to be modified for the family with high-risk pregnancy. For example, a nurse managing Mary's care for preterm labor would see that the prescribed regimen of bed rest was disrupting family morale and plans to arrange space for the new baby, that Tom was suffering role overload, and that the mother-child relationship between Mary and Jenny was strained. Lacking a local social network, the Johnson family had little exchange with outsiders, and consequently stress could not diffuse out from this family. Nurses might help a family identify and use resources such as home health agencies and parents' groups in the community for assistance with household management and morale. Nurses could help Tom and Mary discuss the frustration of Mary's bed rest and diet changes, Tom's role overload, and the ways in which stress was affecting their relationship. Information about the impact of change on a 2-year-old child could help Tom and Mary understand and better manage Jenny's behavior.

At 32 weeks of pregnancy, Mary's membranes ruptured, and her physician sent her to a perinatal center 100 miles away from home because it had better facilities to care for preterm babies. Jenny went with her parents to the perinatal center to wait until one of her grandmothers could come and take care of her. Jason was born 28 hours after the Johnsons arrived at the perinatal center hospital.

When Jason needed to remain at the perinatal center, neonatal nurses with a family focus would recognize the impact of having a preterm baby in a regional neonatal intensive care unit on the develop-

(continued on page 287)

ment of attachment to the baby, role learning, and family morale. Interventions for the Johnson family would include creating ways for them to have contact with Jason through telephone or e-mail updates on his condition and photographs even when they could not be with him physically.

When the Johnsons could visit, encouraging them to do normal infant care tasks for Jason would enhance their attachment and parenting skills. The baby's siblings should be especially welcomed. Often the communication cues of preterm infants are difficult for parents to interpret. Pointing out Jason's responses to their interactions would help the parents interpret his cues. In turn, Jason's responses would make parent-child interactions more rewarding. Often nurses encourage parents to develop a support system with other parents of intensive care infants.

Mary was discharged from the perinatal center within 24 hours after birth. At home, she felt extremely weak and was overwhelmed by household tasks and caring for Jenny. She was disappointed that she was unable to breast-feed the baby. Two weeks later, she was weeping frequently, felt very sad, had no appetite, and had difficulty sleeping. Being with their new son was difficult because each visit required a 200-mile round-trip, Tom had a full-time job, and Mary cared for Jenny during the day. Jason, the new baby, remained at the perinatal center in the special-care nursery until he was mature and stable enough to go home 4 weeks later. At her 6-week postpartum checkup, she told the office nurse that she did not enjoy caring for her new baby and that she had difficulty with her sleep.

Parents' concerns about themselves may be overlooked after birth. Mary Johnson's postpartum recovery was long and difficult because of her bed rest during pregnancy. After bed rest during pregnancy, postpartum women have reduced muscle strength, leaving them weak and vulnerable (Maloni, 1993). Even though Jason was healthy, a preterm birth experience can be disappointing because of unmet expectations. Consequently Mary developed symptoms of postpartum depression. Astute nurses would continue care for the family after the birth. Families need to be informed about the realities of a prolonged postpartum physical recovery after pregnancy bed rest. Mary may have been able to breast-feed Jason through a program of breast pumping to stimulate lactation while separated from him and through the support of nurses who are enthusiastic about and capable of helping women breast-feed their preterm babies. Mary could have been referred to a lactation consultant, a breast-feeding support group, and home nursing services. Nurses need to counsel families about postpartum depression and help them obtain expert care for postpartum depression.

References

American College of Obstetricians and Gynecologists (ACOG) & Interprofessional Task Force on Health Care of Women and Children. (1978). *Joint statement on the development of family centered maternity/newborn care in hospitals.* Chicago: ACOG.

American Psychiatric Association. (2000). *Diagnostic and statistical manual of mental disorder* (4th ed.). Washington, DC: American Psychiatric Association Press.

American Society for Reproductive Medicine. (2002). *Frequently asked questions about infertility.* Retrieved October 1, 2002, from http://www.asrm.org

Anderson, A. M. (2001). Fathering promotion. In M. Craft-Rosenberg & J. Denehy (Eds.), *Nursing interventions for infants, children, and families* (pp. 77–97). Thousand Oaks, CA: Sage.

Applegarth, L. (2000). Individual counseling and psychotherapy. In L. Burns & S. Covington (Eds.), *Infertility counseling: A comprehensive handbook for clinicians.* New York: Parthenon Publishing Group.

Bajo, K., Hager, J., & Smith, J. (1998). Clinical focus: Keeping moms and babies together. *AWHONN Lifelines, 2*(2), 44–48.

Beck, C. T. (1995). The effects of postpartum depression on maternal-infant interaction: A meta-analysis. *Nursing Research, 44,* 289–304.

Beck, C. T. (1996). Postpartum depressed mothers' experiences interacting with their children. *Nursing Research, 45,* 98–104.

Beck, C. T. (1998a). A checklist to identify women at risk for developing postpartum depression. *Journal of Obstetric, Gynecologic, and Neonatal Nursing, 27,* 39–46.

Beck, C. T. (1998b). The effects of postpartum depression on child development: A meta-analysis. *Archives of Psychiatric Nursing, 12,* 12–20.

Beck, C. T. (1999). Maternal depression and child behaviour problems: A meta-analysis. *Journal of Advanced Nursing, 29,* 623–629.

Beck, C. T. (2002). Revision of the postpartum depression predictors inventory. *Journal of Obstetric, Gynecologic, and Neonatal Nursing, 31,* 394–402.

Boivin, J., Appleton, T. C., Baetens, P., Baron, J., Bitzer, J., Corrigan, E., et al. (2001). Guidelines for counseling in infertility. *Human Reproduction, 16,* 1301–1304.

Bomar, P. (Ed.). (2004). *Promoting health in families: Applying family research and theory in nursing practice* (2nd ed.). Philadelphia: Saunders.

Bozoky, I., & Corwin, E. (2002). Fatigue as a predictor of postpartum depression. *Journal of Obstetric, Gynecologic, and Neonatal Nursing, 31,* 436–443.

Brazelton, T. B. (1992). *Touchpoints: Your child's emotional and behavioral development.* Reading, MA: Addison-Wesley.

Broderick, C. B. (1993). *Understanding family process.* Newbury Park, CA: Sage.

Bullock, K. (2001). Healthy family systems? The changing role of grandparents in rural America. *Education and Ageing, 16,* 163–178.

Bullock, K. (2004). Family social support. In P. Bomar (Ed.), *Promoting health in families: Applying family research and theory in nursing practice* (2nd ed.). Philadelphia: Saunders.

Cook, S. S. (1997). Configuring childbirth education to survive managed care. *Advanced Practice Nursing Quarterly, 2,* 22–26.

Cowan, P. A. (1991). The individual and family life transitions: A proposal for a new definition. In P. A. Cowan & M. Hetherington (Eds.), *Family transitions* (pp. 3–30). Hinsdale, NJ: Lawrence Erlbaum Associates.

Cox, J., Holden, J., & Sagovsky, R. (1989). Edinburgh Postnatal Depression Scale. *British Journal of Psychiatry, 150,* 782–786.

Duvall, E. M., & Miller, B. C. (1986). *Marriage and family development.* New York: Harper & Row.

Eberhard-Gran, M., Eskild, A., Tambs, K., Opjordsmoen, S., & Samuelsen, S. O. (2001). Review of validation studies of the Edinburgh Postnatal Depression Scale. *Acta Psychiatrica Scandinavica, 104,* 243–249.

Eliason, M. J. (2001). Perinatal substance abuse treatment. In M. Craft-Rosenberg & J. Denehy (Eds.), *Nursing interventions for infants, children, and families* (pp. 221–240). Thousand Oaks, CA: Sage.

Ferguson, S. L., & Engelhard, C. L. (1997). Short stay: The art of legislating quality and economy. *AWHONN Lifelines, 1,* 16–23.

Fomby, B. W. (2004). Family routines, rituals, recreation and rules. In P. Bomar (Ed.), *Promoting health in families: Applying family research and theory in nursing practice* (2nd ed.). Philadelphia: Saunders.

Fowles, E. R. (1998). The relationship between maternal role attainment and postpartum depression. *Health Care for Women International, 19,* 83–94.

Gupton, A., Heaman, M., & Ashcroft, T. (1997). Bed rest from the perspective of the high-risk pregnant woman. *Journal of Obstetric, Gynecologic, and Neonatal Nursing, 26,* 423–430.

Harvey, M. G. (1992). Promoting parenting: The obstetric patient in an intensive care unit. *Critical Care Nursing Clinics of North America, 4,* 721–728.

Hockenberry, M. I., Wilson, D., Winkelstein, M. L., & Kline, N. E. (2003). *Wong's nursing care of infants and children* (7th ed.). St Louis: Mosby.

Holditch-Davis, E., & Miles, M. (2000). Mothers' stories about experiences in the neonatal intensive care unit. *Neonatal Network, 19,* 13–21.

Jordan, P. (1990). Laboring for relevance. *Nursing Research, 13,* 11–16.

Jordan, P. (2002). *Becoming parents program* (#RO1 NR 004912). Washington, DC: National Institute of Nursing Research.

Jordan, P., Stanley, S., & Markman, H. (1999). *Becoming parents: How to strengthen your marriage as your family grows.* San Francisco: Jossey-Bass.

Josten, L. E., Savik, K., Mullett, S. E., Campbell, R., & Vincent, P. (1995). Bed rest compliance for women with pregnancy problems. *Birth, 22,* 1–14.

Kalmus, D., Davidson, A., & Cushman, L. (1992). Parenting expectations, experiences, and adjustment to parenthood: A test of the violated expectations framework. *Journal of Marriage and the Family, 54,* 516–526.

Killien, M. G. (1993). Returning to work after childbirth: Considerations for health policy. *Nursing Outlook, 41,* 73–78.

Klaus, M. H., & Kennell, J. H. (1976). *Maternal-infant bonding.* St. Louis: Mosby.

Klock, S. (2000). Psychosocial evaluation for the infertile patient. In L. Burns & S. Covington (Eds.), *Infertility counseling: A comprehensive handbook for clinicians.* New York: Parthenon Publishing Group.

Kornhaber, A. (1996). *Contemporary grandparenting.* Thousand Oaks, CA: Sage.

Leavitt, J. W. (1986). *Brought to bed: Childbearing in America 1750–1950.* New York: Oxford University Press.

LeMasters, E. E. (1957). Parenthood as crisis. *Marriage and the Family, 31,* 352–355.

Lewis, J. A. (2003). Jewish perspectives on pregnancy and childbearing. *MCN: The American Journal of Maternal/Child Nursing, 28,* 306–311.

Lowdermilk, D., Peters, S., & Bobak, I. (2000). *Maternity and gynecological care* (7th ed.). St. Louis: Mosby.

Maloni, J. A. (1993). Bedrest during pregnancy: Implications for nursing. *Journal of Obstetric, Gynecologic, and Neonatal Nursing, 22,* 422–426.

Martell, L. K. (1990). The mother-daughter relationship during daughter's first pregnancy: The transition experience. *Holistic Nursing Practice, 4*(3), 47–55.

Martell, L. K. (2001). Heading toward the new normal: A contemporary postpartum experience. *Journal of Obstetric, Gynecologic, and Neonatal Nursing, 30,* 65–72.

Martell, L. K. (2003). Postpartum women's perceptions of the hospital environment. *Journal of Obstetric, Gynecologic, and Neonatal Nursing, 32,* 478–485.

McCain, G. C., & Deatrick, J. A. (1994). The experience of high-risk pregnancy. *Journal of Obstetric, Gynecologic, and Neonatal Nursing, 23,* 421–427.

Meighan, M., Davis, M. W., Thomas, S. P., & Droppleman, P. (1999). Living with postpartum depression: The father's experience. *The American Journal of Maternal/Child Nursing, 24,* 202–208.

Mercer, R. T. (1989). Theoretical perspectives on family. In C. L. Gilliss, B. L. Highley, B. M. Roberts, & I. M. Martinson (Eds.), *Toward a science of family nursing* (pp. 9–36). Menlo Park, CA: Addison-Wesley.

Mercer, R. T., & Ferketich, S. L. (1990). Predictors of family functioning eight weeks following birth. *Nursing Research, 39,* 76–82.

Miller, S. R., & Winstead-Fry, P. (1982). *Family systems theory in nursing practice.* Reston, VA: Reston Publishing.

Mothers in prison . . . children in crisis. (2000). *Justice Works Community.* Brooklyn, NY.

Murray, L., Fiori-Cowley, A., Hooper, R., & Cooper, P. (1996). The impact of postpartum depression and associated adversity on early mother-infant interactions and later infant outcome. *Child Development, 67,* 2512–2526.

Nelson, A. M. (2003). Transition to motherhood. *Journal of Obstetric, Gynecologic, and Neonatal Nursing, 32,* 465–477.

Newton, C. (2000). Counseling the infertile couple. In L. Burns & S. Covington (Eds.), *Infertility counseling: A comprehensive handbook for clinicians.* New York: Parthenon Publishing Group.

Nichols, F. H. (Ed.). (1993). Perinatal education. *Clinical Issues in Perinatal and Women's Health Nursing, 4,* 1–159.

Norbeck, J., & Tilden, V. P. (1983). Life stress, social support and emotional disequilibrium in complications of pregnancy: A prospective multivariate study. *Journal of Health and Social Behavior, 24,* 30–46.

Peterson, K. J., & Peterson, F. L. (1993). Family-centered perinatal education. *Clinical Issues in Perinatal and Women's Health Nursing, 4,* 1–4.

Polomeno, V. (1999). Perinatal education and grandparents: Creating an interdependent family environment. *Journal of Perinatal Education, 8,* 1–11.

Polomeno, V. (2000). Evaluation of a pilot project: Preparenthood and pregrandparenthood education. *Journal of Perinatal Education, 9,* 27–38.

Ramsey, C. N., Abell, T. D., & Baker, L. C. (1986). The relationship between family functioning, life events, family structure, and the outcome of pregnancy. *Journal of Family Practice, 22,* 521–527.

Ross, M., Channon-Little, L., & Simon-Rosser, B. (2000). *Sexual health concerns: Interviewing and history taking for practitioners* (2nd ed.). Philadelphia: FA Davis.

Sampselle, C. M., Seng, J., Yeo, S., Killion, C., & Oakley, D. (1999). Physical activity and postpartum well-being. *Journal of Obstetric, Gynecologic, and Neonatal Nursing, 28,* 41–49.

Schiffman, R. F., Omar, M. A., & McKelvey, L. M. (2003). Mother-infant interaction in low-income families. *MCN: The American Journal of Maternal/Child Nursing, 28,* 246–251.

Smith-Hanrahan, C., & Deblois, D. (1995). Postpartum early discharge: Impact on maternal fatigue and functional ability. *Clinical Nursing Research, 4,* 50–66.

Solchany, J. E. (2001). *Promoting maternal mental health during pregnancy.* Seattle: NCAST Publications.

Starn, J. (1993). Strengthening family systems. *Clinical Issues in Perinatal and Women's Health Care Nursing, 4,* 35–43.

Steffensmeier, T. H. (1982). A role model of the transition to parenthood. *Journal of Marriage and the Family, 44,* 319–334.

Sumner, G. (1990). *Keys to caregiving.* Seattle: NCAST Publications.

Tilden, V. P. (1983). The relation of life stress and social support to emotional disequilibrium during pregnancy. *Research in Nursing and Health, 6,* 167–174.

Troy, N. W. (1999). A comparison of fatigue and energy at 6-weeks and 14-to-19 months postpartum. *Clinical Nursing Research, 8,* 135–152.

Troy, N. W. (2003). Is the significance of postpartum fatigue being overlooked in the lives of women? *MCN: The American Journal of Maternal/Child Nursing, 28,* 252–257.

Troy, N. W., & Dalgas-Pelish, P. (1997). Development of a self-care guide for postpartum fatigue. *Applied Nursing Research, 8,* 92–96.

Tulman, L., Fawcett, J., Groblewski, L., & Silverman, L. (1990). Changes in functional status after childbirth. *Nursing Research, 39,* 70–75.

VandenBerg, K. (1999). What to tell parents about the developmental needs of their babies at discharge. *Neonatal Network, 18,* 57–59.

Wertz, R. W., & Wertz, D. C. (1989). *Lying-in: A history of childbirth in America.* New Haven, CT: Yale University Press.

Bibliography

Ainsworth, M. D. S. (1973). The development of infant-mother attachment. In B. M. Caldwell & H. N. Riccuiuti (Eds.), *Review of infant research* (Vol. 3). Chicago: University of Chicago Press.

Brazelton, T. B. (1989). *The earliest relationship: Parents, infants, and the drama of early attachment.* Reading, MA: Addison-Wesley.

Callister, L. C. (2001). Culturally competent care of women and newborns: Knowledge, attitude, and skills. *Journal of Obstetric, Gynecologic, and Neonatal Nursing, 30,* 209–215.

Carter, E., & McGoldrick, M. (1980). *The family life cycle: A framework for family therapy.* New York: Gardner Press.

Cowan, C. P., & Cowan, P. A. (1992). *When partners become parents: The big life change for couples.* New York: Basic Books.

Craft-Rosenberg, M., & Denehy, J. (2001). *Nursing interventions for infants, children, and families.* Thousand Oaks, CA: Sage.

Kennedy, H. P., Beck, C. T., & Driscoll, J. W. (2002). A light in the fog: Caring for women with postpartum depression. *Journal of Midwifery and Women's Health, 47,* 318–330.

Martin-Arafeh, J. M., Watson, C. L., & Baird, S. M. (1999). Promoting family-centered care in high-risk pregnancy. *Journal of Perinatal and Neonatal Nursing, 13,* 27–42.

Meleis, A. I, & Trangenstein, P. A. (1994) Facilitating transitions: Redefinition of the nursing mission. *Nursing Outlook, 42,* 255–259.

Walker, L. O. (1992). *Parent-infant nursing science: Paradigms, phenomena, methods.* Philadelphia: FA Davis.

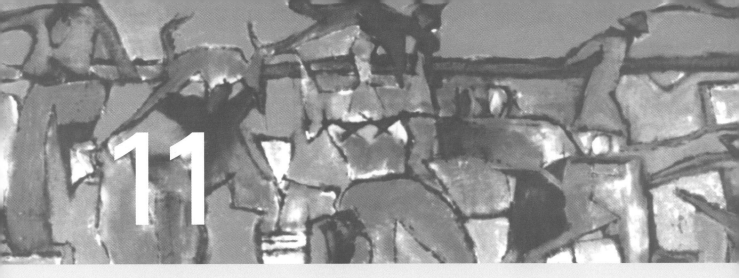

11

Family Child Health Nursing

Vivian Gedaly-Duff, DNSc, RN • Marsha L. Heims, EdD, RN
• Ann E. Nielsen, MN, RN

CRITICAL CONCEPTS

- A major task of families is to nurture children to become healthy, responsible, and creative adults.

- Most parents learn the parenting role "on the job," relying on memories of their childhood experiences in their families of origin to help them.

- Parents, as primary caretakers of their children, are charged with keeping children healthy, as well as caring for them during illness.

- Common health promotion problems of children and their families are experienced during *transition points* as individual members and the family grow and change phases.

- Because the leading causes of morbidity and mortality among youth are substance use, sexual activity, and violence (both suicidal and homicidal), there is a need for increased attention to health promotion and prevention.

- Families are the major determinant of children's well-being.

- The difference between discipline and abuse may be uncertain because of different cultural traditions, but nurses must be alert to helping families learn appropriate discipline measures.

- Families with children will experience problems specific to a disease or condition, but some have problems with *illness transitions* through acute, chronic, and end-of-life phases.

- The *family interaction model* can be used by family child health nurses to facilitate and teach healthful activities for growth in families, prevent injury and disease, and treat disease and illness conditions.

- The aim of the nurse is to help families develop appropriate ways to carry out family tasks necessary to prevent or handle illness and disease, and to promote health. During the family life cycle, the basic *family tasks* are (1) to secure shelter, food, and clothing; (2) to develop emotionally healthy individuals who can manage crisis and experience nonmonetary achievement; (3) to ensure each individual's socialization in school, work, spiritual, and community life; (4) to contribute to the next generation, by giving birth, adopting a child, or foster-caring for a child; and (5) to promote the health of family members and care for them during illness.

- Although most child-rearing families experience acute illnesses and become familiar with managing these crises, families do not anticipate that their children may have chronic illness.

- With their knowledge of family and child development, nurses can collaborate with families with chronically ill children to help them achieve developmental landmarks.

- Family child health nursing practice is affected by health policy decisions relating to legal relationships of stepfamilies and single parents, financing of health care, and services to children.

- Family child health nursing must be practiced in collaboration and cooperation with families as well as with other health professionals. In family-centered care, nurses work with families to promote health, prevent disease, and cope with acute, chronic, and life-threatening illnesses.

INTRODUCTION

A major task of families is to nurture children to become healthy, responsible, and creative adults. Parents, as primary caretakers of their children, are charged with keeping them healthy, as well as caring for them during illness. Yet most mothers and fathers have little formal education for parenting. In fact, most parents learn the role "on the job," relying on memories of their childhood experiences in their families of origin to help them.

Family nurses help families promote health, prevent disease, and cope with illness. The importance of family life for children's health and illness is often invisible, because families' everyday routines are commonplace and lie below the level of conscious awareness. However, family life influences the promotion of health and the experience of illness in children.

Families are groups with unique characteristics, including specific family memories and intergenerational relationships, family rules and routines, family aspirations and achievements, and ethnic or cultural patterns (Burr, Herrin, Beutler, & Leigh, 1988). Family changes in structure and relationships interact with these family characteristics.

Healthy outcomes for children—for example, tripling their birth weight by 1 year of age, or successfully completing high school if they have juvenile diabetes—are partially attributable to the intangible, invisible daily interactions among family members. Family characteristics related to illness are often not discussed, but they are evident in daily activities. Nurses, in collaboration with families, examine how the characteristics of families influence health.

Family child health nursing is using nursing actions that consider the relationship between family tasks and health care and their effects on family well-being and children's health. Nurses care for children within the context of their family, and they care for children by treating the family as a whole or the family as client. In both approaches, families affect their children's health, while children's health affects their families.

This chapter provides a brief history of family-centered care of children and then presents a family interaction model that can be used to guide nursing practice with families with children. A case study is used to illustrate application of the model. Finally, the chapter discusses implications for practice, research, education, and policy.

FAMILY-CENTERED CARE

Family-centered care is a system-wide approach to child health care. It is based on the assumption that families are their children's primary source of strength and support (Harticker, 1998; Lewandowski & Tesler, 2003; Stein & Perrin, 1998). Family-centered care has emerged in response to increasing family responsibilities for health care. The principles of family-centered care include the following (see Box 11–1):

1. Recognizing families as "the constants" in children's lives, while the personnel in the health care system fluctuate
2. Openly sharing information about alternative treatments, ethical concerns, and uncertainties about health care treatments
3. Forming partnerships between families and health professionals to decide what is important for families
4. Respecting the racial, ethnic, cultural, and socioeconomic diversity of families and their ways of coping

Box 11–1 **ELEMENTS OF FAMILY-CENTERED CARE**

Elements	Definition
1: The family is at the center	The family is the constant in the child's life.
2: Family-professional collaboration	Collaboration includes the care of the individual child, program development, and policy formation at all levels of care—hospital, home, and community.
3: Family-professional communication	Information exchange is complete and unbiased and occurs in a supportive manner at all times.
4: Cultural diversity of families	Honors diversity (ethnic, racial, spiritual, social, economic, educational, and geographic), strengths, and individuality within and across all families.
5: Coping differences and support	Recognizes and respects family coping, supporting families with developmental, educational, emotional, spiritual, environmental, and financial resources to meet diverse needs.
6: Family-centered peer support	Families are encouraged to network and to support each other.
7: Specialized service and support systems	Support systems for children with special health and developmental needs in the hospital, home, and community are accessible, flexible, and comprehensive.
8: Holistic perspective of family-centered care	Families are viewed as families and children are viewed as children recognizing their strengths, concerns, emotions, and aspirations beyond their specific health needs.

From Lewandowski & Tesler (Eds.). (2003). *Family-centered care: Putting it into action. The SPN/ANA guide to family-centered care*. Washington, DC: Society of Pediatric Nurses/American Nurses Association.

5. Supporting and strengthening families' abilities to grow and develop (Lash & Wertlieb, 1993)

For example, families that live with the everyday routine of a child's chronic disease not only know the pattern of the disease, drugs, and other medical treatments but also know the responses of the child and family members to these factors. Many times, health professionals fail to recognize the expertise that families acquire as they care for their children (Gedaly-Duff, Stoeger, & Shelton, 2000).

In addition to illness, nurses consider families' varying values and beliefs concerning health and family dynamics in which the sick child exists.

As a result of their ongoing involvement, families learn that health professionals base decisions on theory, research, and clinical experience but do not know specifically how their child will respond until after the interventions are completed (Paget, 1982).

❝Families acknowledge the uncertainty that surrounds their child's disease, but they want to be informed partners of the health team in decision making and valued collaborators in the care of their child (Griffin, 2003).❞

In an American society that respects diversity of opinions, a health team that includes the family is preferable to a hierarchical team with physicians at the top, nurses in between, and families at the bottom. Family-centered care brings attention back to the importance of families in health care.

COMMON THEORETICAL PERSPECTIVE: FAMILY INTERACTION MODEL

Family nurses need a theoretical model to describe, explain, predict, and prescribe child nursing care and address diverse family situations. Nurses work with families when they are healthy and ill; they see families in homes, clinics, and hospitals; they know some families for a short time and with others have ongoing relationships. The *family interaction model* must be

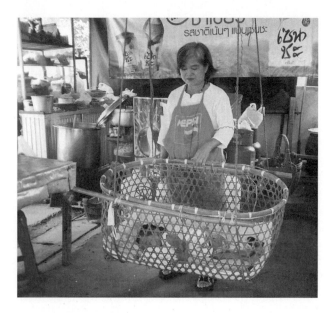

applicable to all these situations (Gedaly-Duff & Heims, 2001). By using the family interaction model, nurses help families understand and prepare for normal and situational transitions in diverse family situations.

The family interaction model is derived from *symbolic interaction theory* and *developmental theory*. (See Chapter 3 for theories on family nursing.) Based on the insights of social interactionist George Herbert Mead (1934), the model assumes that (1) meanings and responses to health, disease, and illness are created through interactions among family members and between the family and society, and (2) families' meanings and responses are influenced by family and individual development (Figure 11–1). Thus, not only do families shape their members, but also members shape their families. Much of the time, the daily nature of family activities makes meanings unspoken, and different family members may have different meanings that are not shared because each assumes that the other family member understands her/his view. When nurses understand that families and family members have unique perceptions and meanings for health or illness situations, they can help families redefine situations if necessary and create a shared family meaning. For example, a child diagnosed with sickle-cell anemia may be labeled by the family as a "son with a handicapping, painful disease." The nurse can help the family reframe the situation and create a new meaning for it by showing that children with this disease are successful in playing sports such as swimming. Reframing is a common strategy that health professionals use with patients and families. Nurses and doctors in their active management of disease demon-strate that the condition is treatable and quality of life is maintained. The family may now say, "My son is normal except for bleeding sometimes." Their boy can grow and develop but live with an episodic, painful condition.

The *developmental theory* suggests that families and individuals change over time. Families, which consist of adults and children, experience the various developmental stages of their members, and they also progress through a series of family developmental stages. Nurses, by comparing their observations of particular families to expected family and individual developmental stages, can plan appropriate care.

> ❝However, families many times do not progress through family stages as originally proposed because of divorce, blended families, or adoption; thus, the family career concept helps integrate this variability.❞

The family interaction model uses three concepts to guide nursing care: (1) family career, which includes dynamic and unique developmental and situational experiences of a family's lifetime represented by family stages and family transitions; (2) individual development, which is the expected changes in each member associated with growth and development; and (3) patterns of health, disease, and illness, which are expected behaviors in these health situations. Knowledge of these three concepts and their interactions with each other provides nurses with an understanding of the effects of health and illness on family interactions. These three concepts and their components are illustrated in Figure 11–1 and described in the next section (see Box 11–2).

Family Career

Family career is the dynamic process of change that occurs during the life span of the unique group called the family. Family career incorporates stages, tasks, and transitions. Family career is similar to family development theory in that it takes into account family tasks and raising children. However, family development theory views the family in standard sequential steps progressing from the birth of the first child to raising and launching children, to experiencing the death of a parent figure in old age (Duvall & Miller, 1985). In contrast, family career takes into account the diverse experiences of American families (Aldous, 1996). The family career includes both the expected developmental changes of the family life

Box 11–2	DEFINITIONS OF FAMILY CAREER, INDIVIDUAL DEVELOPMENT, AND PATTERNS OF HEALTH/DISEASE/ILLNESS

Term	Definition
Family career	The dynamic process of change that occurs during the life span of the unique group called the family. Whereas family development views the family in standard sequential steps or stages, family career takes into account the diverse experiences of American families that do not occur in anticipated stages.
Individual development	Physical and maturational change of the individual over time. Some theories perceive change as stages, and others describe interactional change.
Patterns of health, disease, and illness. Families and their members experience dimensions of health while managing illness among members.	*Health pattern* is behavior that promotes optimal dimensions of well-being. Family and individual health is multidimensional; therefore, a family and/or member can have a disease and be "healthy" in another dimension of health. *Disease pattern* is a set of symptoms and signs associated with pathology and treatment. *Illness pattern* is family and individual activities that manage a disease that may be acute (time-limited), chronic (live with over time), or terminal (end-of-life).

cycle and the unexpected changes of situational crises such as divorce, remarriage, adoption, and death.

The notion of family career involves the many paths that families can take during their life span. Changes do not necessarily occur in a linear fashion. For example, family development theory assumes that families raising more than one child have already experienced the stage of birthing and resulting family development tasks. Yet family career takes into account the possibility that a person may marry a partner who already has adolescent children and experience parenthood, but not the parenthood of young children. This helps explain interactions of many types of families in which the adults are married, cohabiting, single-parent, divorced, remarried, and homosexual (Gedaly-Duff & Heims, 2001). The concept of family career is thus useful because it reminds us that families are dynamic. Nurses working with child-rearing families need to be knowledgeable about family careers, which include both the stages of family development and family transition events, because these dynamics affect family health.

Family Stages

Duvall's eight stages of family development, based on the oldest child, describe expected changes in families who are raising children (Duvall & Miller, 1985). Some family careers start with marriage without children and then proceed to childbearing, preschool children, school children, adolescents, the launching of young adults (first child gone to last child leaving home), middle age of parents (empty nest to

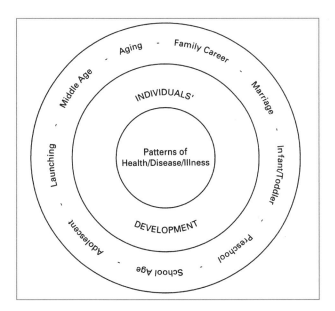

Figure 11–1 Family interaction model.

retirement), and aging of family members (retirement to death of both parents). Knowledge of *family stages* helps nurses anticipate the family reorganization necessary to accommodate the growth and development of family members. For example, families with school-age children expect children to be able to take care of their own hygiene, whereas families with infants expect to do all the hygiene care.

Family Tasks

Across all family stages, there are basic *family tasks* that are essential to survival and continuity (Duvall & Miller, 1985): (1) to secure shelter, food, and clothing; (2) to develop emotionally healthy individuals who can manage crisis and experience nonmonetary achievement; (3) to ensure each individual's socialization in school, work, spiritual, and community life; (4) to contribute to the next generation, by giving birth, adopting a child, or foster-caring for a child; and (5) to promote the health of family members and care for them during illness. The aim of the nurse is to help families develop appropriate ways to carry out the tasks necessary to prevent or handle illness and disease, and to promote health.

Family Transitions

Family transitions are events that signal a reorganization of family roles and tasks. They may be developmental or situational. Transitions are central to nursing practice because they have profound health-related effects on people (Meleis, Sawyer, Im, Hilfinger Messias, & Schumacher, 2000). *Developmental transitions* are predictable changes that occur in an expected time line congruent with movement through the eight family stages. Because they are usual, developmental transitions are also called *normative transitions*. Thus, family members expect and learn to interact differently as children grow. Sometimes families may not make the transition to an expected family stage. For example, families with children with disabilities, who are not capable of independent living, have difficulty launching their children because of lack of residential living facilities and caregivers.

Situational transitions include changes in personal relationships, roles and status, the environment, physical and mental capabilities, and the loss of possessions (Rankin, 1989; Rankin & Weekes, 2000). Situational transitions are also called *non-normative transitions*. Not all families experience each situational transition.

Further, they may occur irrespective of time or family developmental stages. For example, changes occur in personal relationships when a stepchild is integrated into the family group or when one becomes a new stepparent after divorce and remarriage. Changes in roles and status happen when an only child becomes a sibling after the family adopts a new child. Changes in the familiar environment occur when working parents move to a new job and family members adjust to a new house, school, friends, and community. Even greater changes occur when families immigrate to a new country, learn a new language and a new culture, and perhaps have to work at a lower-status job. Changes in physical and mental capabilities—for example, an illness that incapacitates a working parent—may shift caregiving activities to other members of the family and create uncertainty about skills needed (Meleis et al., 2000). A natural disaster may destroy family possessions and heirlooms, causing stress, fear, a sense of loss, and problems with family members' ways of being and interacting (Schumacher & Meleis, 1994).

Nurses should screen families for transition events because transitions (Meleis et al., 2000), both developmental and situational, are signals to nurses that families may be at risk for health problems. Families develop ways of keeping their children safe that work until the children grow. For example, an infant who is crawling may be in a playpen or swing, but when the child transitions from crawling to pulling up to standing and walking, the family needs to change the house by removing things from low tables and covering electric plugs because the child explores the floor environment by touching things with fingers and mouth (age 1 to 3 years). A situational example is a married family transitioning to a divorced family. Parents will need to think about new routines for caring for the children. In a two-parent family, one parent may have gotten breakfast ready while the other got the child dressed. Now one parent will be doing both. Nurses, by assessing families for anticipated changes related to child and family developmental transitions, as well as situational transitions, can help families plan for changes.

Individual Development

The second concept in the family interaction model is individual development. Families with children are complex groups of adults and children. Because no one perspective explains humans adequately, nurses must consider multiple dimensions of human development. Some family developmental stages are related to the growth of individual members and the differing needs of maturing human beings. A schematic overview of human development highlights the stages of individual experiences over time. Adult developmental aspects are included because adults' needs may complement or conflict with their children's.

When nurses review with families the individual family members' developmental stages that are occurring concurrently among children and adults, they assist families in their interactions. Through this review process, nurses assist families to accommodate to children's and adults' changing abilities. Table 11–1 presents three dimensions of individual development: social-emotional, cognitive, and physical. The table is meant to be a guide and is not all-inclusive. Some items may not be representative of all cultures or socioeconomic status. The table contains the following 12 columns:

- The first and second columns, *period* and *age*, are orienting time lines. The period column identifies eight stages from infancy through late adulthood, and the age column is divided into chronological years from birth through 18 years, plus the adult years beyond.
- Column 3, *social-emotional stages*, represents Erikson's perspective, which views social-emotional development across the eight stages of human life (Erikson, 1973).
- Column 4, the *radius of significant relations*, shows how the world of individuals expands as they move beyond their immediate families.
- Column 5, *stage-sensitive family developmental tasks*, provides the orientation of families as they raise and launch children (Duvall & Miller, 1985).
- Column 6, *human needs*, is a hierarchy of individual requirements ranging from basic physiological needs to the need for self-actualization (Maslow, 1970).
- Column 7, *values orientation*, reflects moral development from undifferentiated to complex stages (Bukatko & Daehler, 2004; Kohlberg, 1984). Individual family members have their own values, but their values also relate to the values of their family and community.
- Column 8 shows the *cognitive stages of development* (Bukatko & Daehler, 2004; Piaget & Inhelder, 1969).
- The *developmental landmarks* shown in column 9 are milestones that families use to measure their children's progress.

- Column 10, *physical maturation*, shows bodily changes as children grow.
- Column 11 lists the *developmental steps* that individuals experience.
- Column 12 outlines *developmental problems* associated with changes throughout the life span.

Nurses can use this table to identify expected developmental progression and potential areas of concern for families.

Patterns of Health, Disease, and Illness

The third concept that composes the family interaction model is patterns of health, disease, and illness experienced by families. Healthy behaviors promote optimal physical and social-emotional well-being. Disease is pathology. Illness represents the family activities associated with managing disease. Family interactions shape these patterns.

Health

In their daily activities, families create *health patterns*, which are the family's and family members' understandings and behaviors associated not merely with the absence of disease and incapacitation but with optimal physical, mental, and social well-being (Langford, 2004; Meister, 1991). Healthy behaviors in families include both promotional and protective actions. For example, parents may promote children's growth toward self-actualization through after-school programs that encourage school friendships and creativity. Parents prevent disease through childhood immunizations, and they avoid injuries through poison prevention efforts. Families' normative behaviors are the healthy patterns they follow as they promote and protect the health of their children and the family as a whole.

Disease

Diseases and pathological conditions are abnormal patterns of physical, social-emotional, or family processes. For example, an abnormal physical pattern is sickle-cell anemia, a genetic disease characterized by periodic pain and vaso-occlusion of cellular tissues that affects family and child life (Northington, 2000; Thomas & Westerdale, 1997). Child abuse, an abnormal family pattern, is a pattern of inappropriate and non-nurturing parenting. Families learn to recognize symptoms and signs of disease in order to treat and

Table 11–1

SOCIAL-EMOTIONAL, COGNITIVE, AND PHYSICAL DIMENSIONS OF INDIVIDUAL DEVELOPMENT

PERIOD	AGE	SOCIAL-EMOTIONAL STAGES	SIGNIFICANT RELATIONS	STAGE-SENSITIVE FAMILY DEVELOPMENT TASKS	HUMAN NEEDS	VALUES ORIENTATION
Infancy	Birth	Trust vs. mistrust (I am what I am given.)			Physiological: air, food, and shelter	
	3 mo		Primary parent	Having, adjusting to, and encouraging the development of infants		Undifferentiated
				Establishing a satisfying home for both parents and infant(s)		
	6 mo					
	9 mo					
	1 yr	Autonomy vs. shame or doubt (I am what I "will.")	Parental persons		Safety/security	
Preschool-Age	2 yr					
	3 yr	Initiative vs. guilt (I am what I imagine I can be.)	Basic family	Adapting to the critical needs and interests of preschool children in stimulating, growth-promoting ways	Belonging, rootedness, family, friends	Punishment and obedience
				Coping with energy depletion and lack of privacy as parents		
School-Age	4 yr					
	5 yr					
	6 yr	Industry vs. inferiority (I am what I learn.)	Neighborhood school	Fitting into the community of school-age families in constructive ways	Self-respect, self-esteem	

(continued on page 299)

COGNITIVE STAGES OF DEVELOPMENT	DEVELOPMENTAL LANDMARKS	PHYSICAL MATURATION	DEVELOPMENTAL STEPS	DEVELOPMENTAL PROBLEMS
Sensory-Motor Infants move from neonatal reflex level of complete self-world undifferentiation to relatively coherent organization of sensory-motor actions. They learn that certain actions have specific effects on the environment. Minimal symbolic activity is involved. Recognition of the constancy of external objects and primitive internal representation of the world begins. *Preoperational Thought (Prelogical)* Children make their first relatively unorganized and fumbling attempts to come to grips with the new and strange world of symbols. Thinking tends to be egocentric and intuitive. Conclusions are based on what they feel or what they would like to believe.	Gazes at complete patterns Social smile (2 mo) 180° visual pursuit (2 mo) Reaches for objects (4 mo) Rolls over (5 mo) Raking grasp (7 mo) Crude purposeful release (9 mo) Inferior pincer grasp Walks unassisted (10–14 mo) Words: 3–4 (13 mo) Builds tower of 2 cubes (15 mo) Scribbles with crayon (18 mo) Words: 10 (18 mo) Builds tower of 5–6 cubes (21 mo) Uses 3-word sentences (30 mo) Names 6 body parts (30 mo) Uses appropriate personal pronouns, i.e., I, you, me (30 mo) Rides tricycle (36 mo) Copies circle (36 mo) Matches 4 colors (36 mo) Talks of self and others (42 mo) Takes turns (42 mo) Tandem walks (42 mo) Uses 4-word sentences (48 mo) Copies cross (48 mo) Throws ball overhand (48 mo) Copies square (54 mo) Copies triangle (60 mo) Prints name Rides two-wheel bike Copies diamond	*Rapid (Skeletal)* Transitory reflexes present (3 mo) (i.e., Moro, sucking, grasp, tonic neck reflex) Muscle constitutes 25% of total body weight Birth weight doubles (6 mo) Eruption of deciduous central incisors (5–10 mo) Birth weight triples (1 yr) Anterior fontanel closes (10–14 mo) Transitory reflexes disappear (10 mo) Eruption of deciduous first molars (11–18 mo) Babinski reflex extinguished (18 mo) Bowel and bladder nerves myelinated (18 mo) Increase in lymphoid tissue *Slower (Skeletal)* Weight gain 2 kg per year (12–36 mo) *Rapid (Skeletal)* Weight gain 2 kg per year (4–6 yr) Eruption of permanent teeth (5.5–8 yr) Body image solidifying	Anticipation of feeding Symbiosis (4–18 mo) Stranger anxiety (6–10 mo) Separation anxiety (8–24 mo) Self-feeding Oppositional behavior Messiness Exploratory behavior Parallel play Pleasure in looking at or being looked at Beginning self-concept Orderliness Disgust Curiosity Masturbation Cooperative play Fantasy play Imaginary companions Task completion Rivalry with parents of same sex Games and rules Problem solving Achievement Voluntary hygiene	Birth defects Feeding disorders: colic, regurgitation, vomiting, failure to thrive, marasmus, feeding refusal, atopic eczema Stranger anxiety Physiologic failure to thrive Sleep disturbances, resistance or response to overstimulation Extreme separation anxiety Pica Teeth grinding Poisoning Temper tantrums, negativism Toilet training disturbances: constipation, diarrhea Excessive feeding Bedtime and toilet rituals Speech disorders: delayed, elective mutism, stuttering Physical injuries: falls Nightmares, night terrors Extreme separation anxiety Excessive thumb sucking Phobias and marked fears Developmental deviations: lags and accelerations in motor, sensory, and affective development Food rituals and fads Sleep walking School phobias Developmental deviations: lags and accelerations in cognitive functions, psychosexual, and integrative development Self-destructive behaviors Enuresis, soiling, and excessive masturbation Physical injuries: fractures

(continued on page 306)

Table 11–1 **SOCIAL-EMOTIONAL, COGNITIVE, AND PHYSICAL DIMENSIONS OF INDIVIDUAL DEVELOPMENT** *(Continued)*

Period	Age	Social-Emotional Stages	Significant Relations	Stage-Sensitive Family Development Tasks	Human Needs	Values Orientation
School-Age	7 yr			Encouraging child's educational achievement		Instrumental exchange: "If you scratch my back, I'll scratch yours."
	8 yr 9 yr 10 yr 11 yr	Identity vs. identity diffusion (I know who I am.)	Peer in-groups and out-groups Adult models of leadership	Balancing freedom with responsibility as teenagers mature and emancipate themselves Establishing post-parental interests and careers as growing parents		
Adolescence	12 yr 13 yr 14 yr 15 yr					Conventional law and order: "They mean well."
	16 yr 17 yr 18 yr					
Early Adulthood		Intimacy vs. isolation	Partners in friendship, sex, completion	Releasing young adults into work, military service, college, marriage, and so on with appropriate rituals and assistance Maintaining a supportive home base		Principled social contract
Middle Adulthood		Generativity vs. self-absorption or stagnation	Divided labor and shared household	Refocusing on the marriage relationship Maintaining kin ties with older and younger generations	Self-actualization: doing what one is capable of	
Late Adulthood		Integrity vs. despair, disgust	"Humankind" "My kind"	Coping with bereavement and living alone Closing the family home in adapting to aging Adjusting to retirement		Universal ethical principles

(continued on page 301)

COGNITIVE STAGES OF DEVELOPMENT	DEVELOPMENTAL LANDMARKS	PHYSICAL MATURATION	DEVELOPMENTAL STEPS	DEVELOPMENTAL PROBLEMS
Concrete Operational Thought Conceptual organization takes on stability and coherence. Children begin to seem rational and well-organized in their adaptation. The fairly stable and orderly conceptual framework is systematically brought to bear on the world of objects around them. Physical quantities, such as weight and volume, are now viewed as constant, despite changes in shape and size.	Simple opposite analogies Can name days of week Repeats 5 digits forward Can define "brave," "nonsense" Knows seasons of the year Able to rhyme words Repeats 4 digits in reverse Understands pity, grief, surprise Knows where sun sets Can define "nitrogen," "microscope"	_Slowest (Skeletal)_ Weight gain 2–4 kg per year (7–11 yr) Uterus begins to grow Budding of nipples in girls Increased vascularity of penis and scrotum Pubic hair appears in girls Menarche (9–16 yr) _Spurt (Skeletal)_ (Girls 1.5 yrs ahead of boys) Pubic hair appears in boys Rapid growth of testes and penis Axillary hair starts to grow Down on upper lip appears Voice changes Mature spermatozoa (11–17 yr) Acne may appear	Competes with partners Hobbies Ritualistic play Rational attitudes about food Companionship Invests in community leaders, teachers, impersonal ideals	Learning problems Psychophysiologic disorders Personality disorders: compulsive, anxious, overdependent, oppositional, overinhibited, overindependent, isolated, and mistrustful; tension discharge disorders, and sexual deviations Legal delinquency Anorexia nervosa Dysmenorrhea Sexual promiscuity Drug overdose Suicidal attempts Acute confusional state Motor vehicle accidents Schizophrenic disorders (adult type) Affective disorders; manic-depressive psychoses Involutional reactions: depression, suicide Senile disorders: chronic brain syndromes
Formal Operational Thought People can now deal effectively not only with the reality before them, but also with the world of the abstract and the world of possibility ("as if"). Cognition is of the adult type. Adolescents use deductive reasoning and have the ability to evaluate the logic and quality of their own thinking. Their increased abstract power provides them with the capacity to deal with laws and principles. Although egocentrism is still evident at times, important idealistic attitudes are developing in the late adolescent and young adult.	Knows why oil floats on water Can divide 72 by 4 without pencil or paper Understands "belfry" and "espionage" Can repeat 6 digits forward and 5 digits in reverse	Cessation of skeletal growth Involution of lymphoid tissue Muscle constitutes 43% total body weight Permanent teeth calcified Eruption of permanent third molars (17–30 yr)	"Revolt" Loosens tie to family Cliques Responsible independence Work habits solidifying Heterosexual interests Recreational activities Preparation for occupational choice Occupational commitment Elaboration of recreational outlets Marriage readiness Parenthood readiness	

Adapted from D. Prugh (1983) in _The Psychological Aspects of Pediatrics_, Philadelphia: Lea & Febiger; R. Murray Thomas (1992) in _Comparing Theories of Child Development_ (pp. 166–167, 501), Belmont, CA: Wadsworth; E.M. Duvall and B.C. Miller (1985) in _Marriage and Family Development_ (6th ed.) (p. 62), New York: Harper and Collins.

care for their children's health. For example, parents will bring their child with a fever to the physician's office or clinic. Disease is culturally defined and families are influenced by the opinions of health professionals (Kleinman, 1988). This is evident to nurses who observe families of other cultures with their own health beliefs treat their members' health problems using a mix of conventional and folk medicine (Banks & Benchot, 2001; Robledo, Wilson, & Gray, 1999; van Dyk, 2001).

Illness

In contrast to disease, which is a pathological condition, *illness patterns* are the behaviors and processes families go through to manage a condition or disease and the medical treatments that become a part of their daily lives (Corbin & Strauss, 1988). Diseases may be classified as *acute, chronic, life-threatening,* and *end-of-life* (Rolland, 2005). Families reorganize themselves and have different illness tasks for each disease. They temporarily alter daily routines to deal with the crisis of acute diseases and injuries such as communicable diseases, bone fractures, and appendicitis. After disease treatment for acute illness, however, families usually return to the family routines that were in place before the disease.

In contrast, families permanently reorganize their daily routines to accommodate ongoing, incurable diseases such as juvenile arthritis, diabetes, and asthma, as well as abnormal conditions such as cerebral palsy, seizures, or mental retardation. Family careers continue to unfold, and family tasks still need to be performed as siblings and affected children grow and develop. For example, siblings may be jealous of the attention that a chronically ill child receives from parents, and chronically ill adolescents often ignore treatments and aggravate their disease as they search for identity and try to avoid appearing different from their peers.

Families reorganize at each phase of illness, including end-of-life. They may experience the unexpectedly shortened life span of children due to sudden infant death syndrome, fatal ingestion of household poisons or medications by a toddler, cystic fibrosis, or childhood cancer. When death is inevitable, families grieve and mourn for their child. Rituals such as funerals help families remember and make the transition to ongoing life as they heal (McGoldrick & Walsh, 2005). All family members are affected and need to be included in the dying, mourning, and healing process.

As caretakers, families promote health and cope with acute, chronic, life-threatening, and end-of-life illnesses in their children. Health issues for families with children are influenced by the interacting dynamics of (1) family career, (2) individuals' development, and (3) patterns of health, disease, and illness. The family interaction model allows nurses to analyze the intersecting points of these three processes and develop interventions that assist families to care for their children's health.

FAMILY CHILD HEALTH PRACTICE AND INTERVENTIONS

This next section addresses practice and interventions for family child health nurses in four areas: health promotion, acute illness, chronic illness, and life-threatening illness. A case study follows, to illustrate use of the family interaction model.

Health Promotion

Daily routines influence the physical, mental, and social health of children, as well as the health of the family itself (Denham, 2002). Patterns of *family well-being* are facilitated by balancing the needs of individuals and the family with the resources and options available to meet these needs (Martinez, Mehesy, & Seeley, 2003; Wertlieb, 2003). Nurses help families integrate physical, social-emotional, and cognitive health promotion into family routines; in doing so, they also affirm positive patterns of health or provide alternative ones (Markson & Fiese, 2000). Because of the relationship between health behaviors and illness or death, increased attention to health promotion and prevention of unhealthy social-emotional behaviors among children and their families is needed. Nurses reduce the risk of illness and injury by shaping the family routines, rituals, and environment to encourage optimally healthy behaviors. Moreover, nurses assess for, identify, and provide interventions to reduce risk factors associated with morbidity and mortality.

The leading cause of death among children and youth, ages 1 to 24 years, is unintentional injuries. In 2001, the number of deaths from unintentional injuries for children ages 1 to 14 was 4503 (17.9/100,000) (Arias & Smith, 2003). An additional 13,871 (34.7/100,000) young people, ages 15 to 24, died from accidents, of which 10,259 (25.7/100,000) were motor vehicle crashes (Arias & Smith, 2003). Family child health care nurses can teach and support families in accident prevention. For example, teaching appropriate childproofing of the home protects toddlers from poisoning and electrical burns from uncovered electrical outlets. Furthermore, nurses minimize head trauma from bicycle accidents by teaching the importance of bicycle helmet use and locating resources for families with limited financial means for purchasing helmets.

Nurses also intervene to recognize harm from common health problems. In 2000, 15 percent of children and adolescents in the United States were overweight, an increase of 4 percent from 1994 (Federal Interagency Forum on Child and Family Statistics, 2003). Because childhood obesity is associated with significant health conditions, prevention and treatment are crucial to the child's well-being. Although genetics is a factor in development of obesity, the environment and family behaviors are also significant influences on child eating behaviors and exercise patterns. For example, family beliefs, mediated by cultural background, influence maternal feeding behaviors (Baughcum, Burklow, Deeks, Powers, & Whitaker, 1998; Bruss, Morris, & Dannison, 2003). Family interventions to prevent childhood obesity include helping caregivers to identify values concerning weight and food, educating parents to trust that children will eat the amount of food that they need, teaching parents to limit use of food as rewards to control behaviors, and emphasizing the importance of physical activity to the child's health (Baughcum et al., 1998; Hodges, 2003).

Because of developmental characteristics at this age, adolescents as a group are especially vulnerable to high-risk behaviors that can lead to illness and death. Data on the prevalence of risk behaviors among adolescents is collected by the Youth Risk Behavior Surveillance System (YRBS), using a national probability sample of 9th to 12th graders, state and local school-based surveys, and a national household-based survey (Grunbaum et al., 2002). In the United States, 71 percent of deaths for youth ages 15 to 24 in 2001 resulted from four causes—motor vehicle crashes (32 percent), other unintentional injuries (11 percent), homicide (16 percent), and suicide (12 percent) (Arias & Smith, 2003). Health behaviors that contribute to unintentional injury or to violence include use of alcohol and other substances and nonuse of seat belts. Availability of weapons in the home is also a significant risk factor for unintentional injury. Other health behaviors that contribute to mortality and morbidity include tobacco use, poor nutrition, sedentary lifestyle, and sexual behaviors that lead to pregnancies and sexually transmitted infections (Grunbaum et al., 2002).

The 2001 YRBS report showed that youth engaged in behaviors associated with significant morbidity and mortality. During the 30 days preceding the survey, 47 percent had drunk alcohol, 31 percent had ridden with a driver who had been drinking alcohol, 14.1 percent had rarely worn or had never worn a seat belt, and 24 percent had used marijuana. About one-third of all adolescents in school currently used tobacco. Forty-five percent of high-school students had sexual intercourse, and 42 percent of those surveyed reported not using a condom at last intercourse (Grunbaum et al., 2002).

Youth violence represents a significant risk for morbidity and mortality. In the United States in 1998, more than 20,000 children were killed or injured by firearms (Fingerhut & Christoffel, 2002). Adolescent aggression may not be more violent than in previous generations, but violent behaviors are now more lethal (Murray, Guerre, & Williams, 1997). Over 6 percent had carried a weapon on school property. The survey further revealed that close to 9 percent of students had been threatened or injured on school property at least once in the past year (Grunbaum et al., 2002). Black males are disproportionately affected by fatalities, with fatality rates four times those of white males ages 1 to 19 (Cook & Ludwig, 2002). Child and youth access to firearms is part of the problem. One author estimated that 50 percent of parents who own guns keep them unlocked and loaded in the home (Hardy, 2002). The American Academy of Pediatrics asserts that the most effective measure to prevent firearm injuries is to remove guns from children's homes and communities (American Academy of Pediatrics, 2004). Although interventions to prevent gun violence need to be broad-based and include legislative and community strategies, nurses can assess for presence of guns in the home and provide parental gun safety counseling, clearly identifying for parents that children are at risk for injury if a loaded gun is kept in the house (Hardy, 2002).

The mental health of children and adolescents is a growing concern because of the increasing incidence of mental illness. The 2001 YRBS report revealed that 19 percent of high-school students had felt so sad or hopeless for more than 2 weeks that they stopped doing usual activities, 14.8 percent had a suicide plan, and 8.8 percent actually attempted suicide (Grunbaum et al., 2002). Youth susceptible to drug use, unhealthy sexual behaviors, violence/aggression, and suicide often experience depression (Elliott & Smiga, 2003;

Houck, Darnell, & Lussman, 2002; Parsons, 2003). In light of these statistics, it is especially important for nurses to screen for depression and other mental illnesses, to use interventions that promote mental health in all family members, and to refer as needed. Family nurses in school-based health clinics are especially well-placed to participate in prevention programs directed at high-risk behaviors leading to sexually transmitted disease and early pregnancy, depression, injuries, substance use, suicide, and violence (Hootman, Houck, & King, 2002).

Poor school performance is correlated with increased health risk behaviors. The YRBS did not include questions about school performance, but another longitudinal study tracked eighth graders since 1988 and found that one in five students were not proficient at basic math, and 14 percent could not read adequately (Hawkins, 1997). By 10th grade, many low-performing students had dropped out (Hawkins, 1997). Family predictors of children at high risk for poor school performance include single-parent homes, family incomes of less than $15,000, older siblings who have dropped out, parents who did not finish high school, limited proficiency in English, and being at home for 2 hours a day or more without supervision (Dryfoos, 1997).

Socioeconomic factors such as poverty, lack of education, little or no health insurance, and immigrant status are strongly related to poor health (Hardy, 2002). There is evidence that behavioral symptoms of child psychiatric disorders are associated with poverty, and further that those symptoms can be reduced as the family moves out of poverty (Costello, Compton, Keeler, & Angold, 2003). Programs that provide families with employment, adequate income, day care, and health insurance have been shown to have positive effects on academic achievement, classroom behavior, and aspirations (Huston et al., 2001). Children from families from ethnic minority backgrounds are more likely to live below the poverty line and live with parents who have limited educational and/or English proficiency levels, and thus they are at risk for health problems (Kirby, Berends, & Naftel, 1999).

Families with limited financial resources and those who do not have health insurance have more difficulty with health promotion than families with insurance or other methods of payment. In the United States in 2001, 7.5 million children, 10 percent of all children, were uninsured. Eighteen percent of children whose families had incomes of less than $34,000 were uninsured (Bloom, Cohen, Vickerie, & Wondimu, 2003).

Lack of insurance tends to be correlated with lower income, but between 1994 and 2000, uninsurance rose among children from higher income groups (Holahan, Dubay, & Kenney, 2003). A recent report on access to health care in the United States indicated that Hispanic children were three times more likely than white children to have no insurance and nearly two times more likely than black children to be uninsured (Holahan, Dubay, & Kenney, 2003, p. 62). Black children were most likely to have public health care coverage (31.7 percent), followed by Hispanics (29.4 percent) and whites (11.2 percent) (Holahan et al., 2003). Furthermore, among children with special health care needs and disabilities, offspring from minority groups were more likely to be uninsured and to report being unable to get needed medical care (Newacheck, Hung, & Wright, 2002). Children who have experienced inconsistent parenting—for example, children whose mothers suffer from chronic depression or have substance abuse problems, foster children, or children whose parents are incarcerated—are at particular risk for poor health outcomes (Dube et al., 2001; Kools & Kennedy, 2003; Kotch, Browne, Dufort, & Winsor, 1999). Identification of these high-risk situations, careful assessment of needs, and knowledge of referral resources are integral to good nursing care.

Families sometimes experience conflict between family tasks and the needs of individual family members, and they must try to balance these. Often, balancing these tasks in a successful way is critical to better family and child health. For example, working parents of an infant must decide if and when they should place their child in child care. Working parents of school-age children and adolescents must decide if the children can be at home without adult supervision during the after-school period before parents return home from work. In both situations, the family task is to provide economic resources for shelter and food, and the children's need is for a trusted caretaker and safe environment. Families settle these conflicts differently. Nurses can help families resolve the issues through anticipatory guidance, which involves providing information about what to expect in various situations and how to deal with unwanted developmental problems and life changes (Limbo, Petersen, & Pridham, 2003; Pridham, 1993). Families are the major determinant of children's well-being. Nurses and other health professionals should collaborate with parents, not view parents as secondary to nurses (Bruns & McCollum, 2002). Too often in the past, professionals decided what was best for children (Darbyshire, 1993). Today, nurses are exploring parents' perceptions and definitions of health to develop more relevant health care plans. Health promotion for children occurs during parenting activities, and many American families are assisted in parenting by other child caretakers, including grandparents, and child care and after-school facilities.

Parenting and Health Promotion

Families with children promote health by practicing behaviors that advance their own physical, mental, and social well-being and that of their children. Everyday parenting activities nurture and socialize children to be healthy, responsible adults. However, parents sometimes are not aware of or do not use developmental principles. For example, one study found that parents whose socioeconomic status (SES) was higher explained their children's behavior with developmental understanding and were flexible in their parenting, but parents of lower SES used fewer explanations of development and expected their children to conform (Sameroff & Feil, 1985). Nurses might conclude that the parents with developmental understanding who are flexible in parenting are "better" parents; however, these parents are also often overanxious and worry about everything. Parents who expect conformity of their children often have themselves experienced an environment with few choices. Researchers speculated that such parents may be preparing their children to survive in a harsh environment (Pinderhughes, Dodge, Bates, Pettit, & Zelli, 2000; Sameroff & Feil, 1985). Because of the association of these factors with health, nurses need to learn more about the effects of poverty and class on family life (Hines, 1999; Nelson, 2002). Because parents' understandings of their roles and child development vary, it is important for nurses to explore parents' beliefs in order to tailor health promotion activities to families.

Discipline of children is an important part of family life. It involves establishing rules and guidelines so that children know what is expected of them. Parents may punish their children for disregarding the rules. Appropriate types of punishment include time-outs and restrictions on privileges. In American culture, physical harm resulting from punishment is considered abuse. In 2001, nearly 903,000 cases of child abuse and neglect occurred (12.4 cases per 1000 children) (U.S. Department of Health and Human Services, 2003; National Clearinghouse on Child Abuse and Neglect Information: National Adoption Information Clearinghouse, 2003). An estimated 14 percent of the children had one or more disabilities (American Academy of Pediatrics, 2001). At the same time, maltreatment can contribute to disabilities (Sullivan & Knutson, 1998). Extreme forms of inappropriate parenting are termed *child abuse* or *neglect*. "Neglect" is not providing for a child's basic physical, educational, or emotional needs (U.S. Department of Health and Human Services, 2002). "Abuse" is a comprehensive term that includes physical, emotional, and sexual harm. Hitting a child hard enough to cause bruising is considered physical abuse and is an inappropriate way to socialize a toddler to control his or her temper. The abuse may arise from parental misunderstanding of the child's expected development. For example, a 2-year-old child is physically abused for a temper tantrum because the temper tantrum is perceived as disrespect of the parent rather than as the toddler's struggle for autonomy. An appropriate way to discipline the child is to use a "time-out," or 2 minutes in a quiet place immediately after the tantrum (Bright Futures, 2002; Howard, 1991). A teenager may be verbally and physically abused at home because the assertive behavior of the adolescent is perceived by the parent as disrespectful of social values. The parent does not comprehend that the adolescent is struggling for a self-identity separate from family. The difference between discipline and abuse may be uncertain because of different cultural traditions, but nurses must be alert to helping families learn appropriate discipline measures (Stein & Perrin, 1998).

Nurses often assist families with health promotion by promoting healthy parenting strategies. They may teach parenting classes for parents and caregivers of children in various age groups. Nurses may develop and provide programs aimed at preventing the injuries associated with various ages, such as physical safety classes for school-age children with attention deficit hyperactivity disorder (ADHD) (Bentson-Royal, 1999). In addition, nurses can screen families for potentially harmful parenting situations such as child abuse and family violence by asking the questions contained in Box 11–3, Questions of Family Violence (American Academy of Pediatrics, 2001; Gedaly-Duff & Heims, 2001; Gedaly-Duff et al., 2000). Families that are stressed frequently will seek help if given the opportunity to tell about their situations. Using these screening questions, a nurse can assess the family and child for dangerous situations, teach safety, and make a referral as necessary.

> Box 11–3   **QUESTIONS OF FAMILY VIOLENCE ASSESSMENT**
>
> - Right now, who is living at home with you and your child?
> - Is everyone getting along well at home or is there a lot of stress, arguing, or fighting?
> - Has anybody ever been hit or hurt, pushed, or shoved in a fight or argument at your house?
> - Is anybody in the family in trouble with the police or in jail?
> - Is anybody worried that your children have been disciplined too harshly?
> - Is anybody worried that your children have been touched inappropriately or sexually abused?
> - Does anybody living with you or close to you drink a lot or use drugs?
> - Are there guns, knives, or other weapons at your house?
> - Has anything major (e.g., people dying, losing jobs, disasters, or accidents) happened recently?
> - What are the best part and the worst part of life for you right now?

Grandparenting and Health Promotion

Grandparents influence health promotion in child-rearing families, although grandparenting is not fully acknowledged as a way to promote health in children. Grandparents influence the values that parents bring to their parenting, because parenting values are derived in part from families of origin. In addition, grandparents provide continuity both for the nuclear family and for the extended family of aunts, uncles,

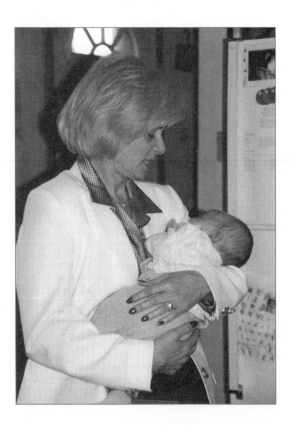

and cousins. During illness, a grandparent can serve as a valued backup, watchdog, safety valve, and stabilizing force for children and their families. Nurses who understand the influence of grandparenting on child-rearing families' health include them in their interventions. Grandparents may serve as child care providers for working families (Burton, Dilworth-Anderson, & Merriwether-deVries, 1995). Grandparents can also promote health during situational transitions such as divorce and blended families when they can provide emotional and physical support to divorced parents and children or to parents who bring children to their new marriage (Smith & Drew, 2002; Thomas, Sperry, & Yarbrough, 2000).

Grandparents may become major influences if, for instance, they raise a grandchild while a teenaged parent finishes high school or serve as primary parents to their grandchildren—for example, in the case of drug-addicted babies born to addicted parents. In 1997, 3.9 million children (5.5 percent of children under 18) were living in homes maintained by their grandparents (Bryson & Casper, 1999). In these situations, nurses must teach grandparents health promotion strategies for their grandchildren and also discuss strategies for reducing caregiver stress (Smith & Drew, 2002; Thomas et al., 2000).

Child Care, After-School Activities, and Health Promotion

One task of families is to nurture children. Families raise children without expectation of monetary reward, as a "gift" to society. Today, however, many families can no longer "give" all the work of child raising without turning to child care and after-school facilities for assistance. In 1970, 29 percent of women with children under age 6 were in the labor force; by 1990, that figure was 52 percent (Bianchi, 1995). In 1999, according to the U.S. Department of Labor Statistics, 69 percent of mothers of children under the age of 18 years were in the labor force. Approximately 50 percent worked full-time and 20 percent part-time. In 2000, 80 percent of divorced mothers of children under 18 were employed either full- or part-time (Staff of Committee on Ways and Means, 2000).

Furthermore, the number of mothers with children under 6 who work outside the home is growing. In 2000, mothers of 65 percent of children under 6 years, 61 percent of children under 3 years, and 56 percent of children under 1 year were in the workforce (Phillips & Adams, 2001). Day care arrangements for these children vary. Among preschool-age children, 14 percent are cared for in the child's own home by family members, primarily grandparents and non-relatives; 37 percent are cared for in other homes by relatives or nonrelatives; 26 percent are in child care facilities; and 22 percent are cared for by the other parent or by the mother herself at work (Staff of Committee on Ways and Means, 2000). The number of children under 18 living in single-parent households has raised concerns about loneliness, injuries, and violence (Kerrebrock & Lewit, 1999). Nurses, parents, and teachers must develop before- and after-school programs at schools, homework telephone services with teachers and teachers' aides during the school year, and community center programs during the summer months when school is not in session and single parents continue to work. Nurses can help families review the types of child care and after-school options available, select compatible philosophies for health promotion, and examine the site for health protection features. They can also participate on community boards that regulate these facilities.

In selecting day care and after-school options, protection against injuries and infections is a key issue. Nurses can provide families with a series of questions to help them check safety precautions and see how a facility will handle their children's illnesses. For example, are indoor and outdoor activity areas safe for active children? Are there functioning toilets and wash sinks that children can reach? What is the policy for children who arrive ill or develop an illness during their stay at the center? Families composed of minority groups and families with children with disabilities require special consideration when choosing child care and after-school options.

Symbolic interaction theory (White & Klein, 2002) suggests that children learn meanings of, responses to, and values about health through their interactions with their families and communities. Nurses can refer families to community resources such as federally funded Head Start programs that serve both children from economically disadvantaged families and children with disabilities (American Academy of Pediatrics, 1973). Head Start has been shown to increase high-school graduation rates and lower juvenile arrest rates, violent arrest rates, and school dropout rates (Reynolds, Temple, Robertson, & Mann, 2001). Nurses can support families in child rearing done by parents, grandparents, and day care and after-school caretakers, which is important in health promotion.

Acute Illness

Acute illness, chronic illness, and life-threatening illness present overlapping though distinct challenges for family nurses. Although members of American families experience health during 85 percent of their lifetimes, they will experience illness for 15 percent of the time (National Center for Health Statistics, 1993).

> ❝Among diseases commonly experienced in American families, asthma is significant. It is the leading cause of hospitalizations in children, as well as the leading cause of chronic illness in children less than 15 years old (Gallagher, 2002).❞

Families with children frequently experience acute illness and injury. Acute illness in children is characterized by the sudden onset of signs and symptoms; treatment can usually restore the children to the predisease state. Some examples include chickenpox, conditions such as appendicitis, and injuries such as bone fractures. Some 49 percent of ambulatory visits (71,550 visits total) by children under 15 years were for acute problems, whereas 15 percent were for care of chronic conditions and 30 percent were for preventative care (Cherry, Burt, & Woodwell, 2003).

The American health care system is encouraging more home care of acute and chronic conditions as well as more day procedures; thus families are managing their children's diseases and illnesses more than health professionals are (Liben & Goldman, 1998). Typically, families whose children undergo a day procedure such as an adenoidectomy or a tonsillectomy will care for their children at home after the first 4 to 8 hours following surgery. This presents caregiving challenges for families in managing the illness, caring for the rest of their family, and working.

Gedaly-Duff and Ziebarth (1994) studied mothers' experiences in identifying and managing their children's acute pain associated with surgery. They found that mothers learned to manage the pain through trial and error. One mother was fearful of both overdosing and under-medicating for the pain. She said:

I was concerned about giving him too much . . . and I went too long, he was extremely uncomfortable. After that I said, "It's not worth it," it took longer for the medication to get back into his system, so then I gave it every three hours, like the label said. (p. 297)

The families also altered their daily routines. Parent work schedules were rearranged and most mothers took time off to care for their children. Mothers described apprehension about the lack of sleep in the household because of their acutely ill child's irritability. Siblings were attentive, anxious, or misbehaving at the extra attention given their ill sister or brother. Most families endured the misbehavior. In such situations, parents want to protect siblings by not involving them and trying to keep life as usual; however, siblings know things have changed and do not know what to do. Nurses using anticipatory guidance can teach families to explain what is happening to the sick child and how the siblings can help.

To help families experiencing acute illness, nurses must first become aware of families' past experiences with and knowledge about acute illness. Second, nurses must alert families to potential disruptions among parents and siblings because of conflicts between family members' needs. Nurses can plan with families how to alter family routines to accommodate the temporary changes required by the acute illness and teach families how to assess the developmentally related reactions children have to acute illness, for example, how to use age-appropriate methods to assess pain. Nurses can also teach families to recognize the patterns and potential complications of acute illness. At the time of discharge, families may not hear some discharge teaching because they are concerned about their child's recovery and arrangements for going home. Nurses can facilitate follow-up care to assess the children's status and reteach what families need to learn when their child is at home.

FAMILY-CENTERED CARE

Family-centered care is a system-wide approach to child health care. It is based on the assumption that families are their children's primary source of strength and support (Harticker, 1998; Lewandowski & Tesler, 2003; Stein & Perrin, 1998). Family-centered care has emerged in response to increasing family responsibilities for health care. The principles of family-centered care include the following (see Box 11–1):

1. Recognizing families as "the constants" in children's lives, while the personnel in the health care system fluctuate
2. Openly sharing information about alternative treatments, ethical concerns, and uncertainties about health care treatments
3. Forming partnerships between families and health professionals to decide what is important for families
4. Respecting the racial, ethnic, cultural, and socioeconomic diversity of families and their ways of coping
5. Supporting and strengthening families' abilities to grow and develop (Lash & Wertlieb, 1993)

For example, families that live with the everyday routine of a child's chronic disease not only know the pattern of the disease, drugs, and other medical treatments but also know the responses of the child and family members to these factors. Many times, health professionals fail to recognize the expertise that families acquire as they care for their children (Gedaly-Duff et al., 2000).

Chronic Illness

Health conditions that (1) limit children's daily activities such as playing and going to school, (2) are long-term, and (3) are not curable or require special assistance in function are considered chronic. Depending on the definition of "chronic illness," which may include or exclude cancer and mental illness, the proportion of families with children experiencing chronic illness is estimated to be between 20 percent and 31 percent (Newacheck, Fox, & McManus, 1988; Newacheck et al., 1998). African-American and Hispanic children have less access to health care and experience more severe illness (Newacheck, Stein, Bauman, & Hung, 2003; Newacheck et al., 2002). Fifteen percent of all primary care providers' office visits are for chronic problems (Cherry et al., 2003). Although most child-rearing families experience acute illnesses and become familiar with managing these crises, families do not anticipate that their children may have chronic illness, and they are unprepared for the unknowns and uncertainties of the course of the disease, the effects on their child's development, and the effects on each family member and family life.

Chronic illnesses such as juvenile arthritis, diabetes, and asthma, as well as physical and behavioral conditions such as cerebral palsy, mental retardation, learning disability, and behavioral problems, require daily management (Federal Interagency Forum on Child and Family Statistics, 2003). Families accommodate to the effects of chronic illness on their child. The meaning of an illness can change for a family over time (Patterson & Garwick, 1994). The family's response to the illness evolves with the developmental progression of the child (Meleski, 2002). Initially, families may experience disbelief because they have assumed that children are healthy and will grow up to be independent. Families hope the disease will resolve. Sometimes families have to experience the continuing signs and symptoms before they believe the disease is not going away. For example, juvenile rheumatoid arthritis (JRA) has a pattern of inflammation and remission. Parents experiencing the remission of the disease may believe the disease is gone and stop the medication and exercise treatments. When the inflammation in the joints recurs, they begin to believe that the disease is long-term. Similarly, families may treat asthma only when the child is experiencing symptoms, rather than managing and treating the chronic inflammation of the airways that accompanies asthma. This practice can lead to acute asthma that may be life threatening (Velsor-Friedrich & Foley, 2001). Families then find ways of consistently giving medications and doing exercise treatments for their child. Nurses who recognize this process can support families as they develop new understandings of their child's illness and adjust to the chronic illness. For example, the nurse can implement a teaching program about asthma that increases parents' management of disease and conduct family workshops on issues such as sibling responses and the burden of taking care of the chronically ill child at home (Gedaly-Duff & Heims, 2001). Box 11–4 is a research study that examined the outcomes of empowering parents through asthma education.

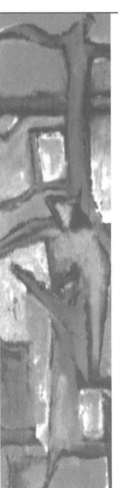

Box 11–4

RESEARCH BRIEF

Empowering Parents through Asthma Education (McCarthy et al., 2002)

Purpose of Study

Asthma is the most common chronic illness in children. Effective family management of the disease is important to child health outcomes. This study examined the effects of an empowering versus a traditional approach to asthma education. Outcome measures: (a) knowledge, (b) sense of control, (c) ability to make decisions, and (d) ability to provide care.

Methodology

In this quasi-experimental design, 57 parents whose children (ages 3 to 16 years) had asthma participated in a multi-session educational intervention (28 families in traditional approach, 29 families in empowering approach). The traditional educational approach consisted of mostly didactic format with the teacher as expert. The empowering approach recognized parental expertise, contained teaching about parent-professional partnerships, and included monthly telephone calls from a nurse to assess progress and reinforce parents' decision-making ability.

Results

The empowering teaching approach significantly increased parents' sense of control, ability to make decisions, and ability to provide care.

Nursing Implications

Using an empowering approach to family education may be more effective than information giving in supporting management of a childhood chronic illness like asthma.

Source: McCarthy, M., Herbert, R., Brimacombe, M., Hansen, J., Wong, D., & Zelman, M. (2002). Empowering parents through asthma education. *Pediatric Nursing, 28*(5), 465–473, 504.

Families use a variety of strategies to normalize the disease experience and cope with chronic illness (Deatrick, Knafl, & Murphy-Moore, 1999). Initially, families may be very watchful as they make sure that disease management and child behavior for maintaining wellness are achieved (Sullivan-Bolyai, Deatrick, Gruppuso, Tamborlane, & Grey, 2003). For example, a father may insist that he be present for all medicine giving when his child is hospitalized. This is a normal response of a family. Rather than thinking that the parent does not trust the nurse to do his job, the nurse collaborates with the parent in his role as caregiver of a child by continuing to give the medicine that he gave at home. Families spend hours at the bedside "watching over their children" (Hurst, 2001b). This is called *parent vigilance.* As they do daily care, they may not be aware that they have made changes in daily routines to accommodate to their child's chronic disease (Gedaly-Duff & Heims, 2001). When asked, however, these families describe new routines for giving medicines and new rituals such as stopping for a special hamburger after the monthly clinic visit. The nurse, by asking a family to describe how family routines have changed, helps family members recognize their flexibility. The intervention is health promoting because the family discovers its resilience and strength.

Parents generally are flexible in their approach to the health care of their children and hope that their children develop to their fullest potential in spite of disease. For example, the mother of a 5-year-old girl with juvenile rheumatoid arthritis (JRA) said:

> *Sometimes I'll see her knee seems to be swollen, but I won't say anything. I won't ask her because I figure that if it's really bad, she'll let me know. I mean, she knows she can tell me that, and then we'll figure out what it is we should do. But I'm not going to plant the seed in her mind. . . . She might always have a little bit of pain. She's not going to be very productive as a human being if she props it up on a pillow.*

Nurses and families together can create new routines to accommodate disease and continue with the family's life. For example, a 5-year-old's kindergarten class can be scheduled for the afternoon so that he can treat his JRA with a warm bath before he gets dressed in the morning. A motorized tricycle can be taken to Fourth of July picnics so that the 4-year-old with JRA can ride alongside his playmates. Grandparents can help organize a softball team to enable their grandson with JRA to play ball. A person from the community fireman squad can run for the boy with JRA (Gedaly-Duff, 1990). Researchers suggest that chronically ill adolescent children have better self-esteem when their families emphasize independence and participation in recreational activities (Weiss, Diamond, Demark, & Lovald, 2003). With their knowledge of family and child development, nurses can collaborate with families with chronically ill children to help them achieve development landmarks. Nurses should be familiar with community resources in order to facilitate family health.

A chronic illness or condition affects all members of the family. Nurses can help families look at how each member (e.g., father, mother, sibling, grandparent, family friend, neighbor, or school) is affected and discuss how to help each member of the family and the people in the community adjust to the child with a disability or chronic condition. For example, siblings may have the dilemma of telling their friends or keeping it a secret that their sister or brother has mental retardation (Faux, 1993; Sharpe & Rossiter, 2002). Sharing a book with a sibling that tells the story of a similar situation can be a useful intervention (Ahmann, 1997). Other challenges to families whose children have disabilities and chronic conditions are listed in Table 11–2.

Hospitalization

The effect of hospitalization on children and their families is a concern for nurses. In the past, parents and family had restricted visiting hours. Yet early studies of hospitalized children indicated that they suffered from a lack of family nurturance during long isolation periods. During and after World War II, Burlingham and Freud's work (1942) and Spitz's study (1945) demonstrated the negative effects of separating infants and children from their families. After reviewing this work on hospitalization, Goslin (1978) concluded that young children separated from families (particularly infants older than 6 months and children under 4 years) exhibited depression. Today, nurses know that infants and toddlers show protest, despair, and detachment behaviors when separated from their families. Young children are profoundly affected by the health care environment and the people in it. Hospitalization also causes stress and anxiety in the parents of sick children (Hurst, 2001a; Miles, Carter, Riddle, Hennessey, & Eberly, 1989; Tiedeman, 1997) and in their siblings (Morrison, 1997). Nurses who have cared for hospitalized children have found that the parents often needed care particularly when their children were undergoing unpleasant procedures (Callery, 1997a). Expert nurses now routinely include parents in their care of acutely or critically ill children

Table 11–2 STAGES, TASKS, AND SITUATIONAL NEEDS OF FAMILIES OF CHILDREN WITH DISABILITIES AND CHRONIC CONDITIONS

FAMILY STAGE	DEVELOPMENTAL TASKS	SITUATIONAL NEEDS THAT ALTER TRANSITIONS
1. Beginning family: Married couple without children.	a. Establish mutually satisfying relationship. b. Relate to kin network. c. Plan family.	a. Unprepared for birth of children with disabilities; prenatal testing or visible anomalies at birth begin the process. b. In the United States, parents usually want to know their infant's diagnosis as early as possible.
2. Early childbearing: First birth, up to developmental age of 30 mo.	a. Integrate new baby into family. b. Reconcile conflicting needs of various family members. c. Develop parental role. d. Accommodate to changes in marital couple. e. Expand relationships with extended family; add grandparent, aunt, and uncle roles.	a. Learn meaning of infant's behavior, symptoms, and treatments. b. Hampered parent role if children not able to respond to parents' efforts to interact with them (e.g., not smiling or returning sounds in response to parental cooing). c. Search for adequate health care. d. Establish early intervention programs (e.g., speech and physical therapy, special education).
3. Family with preschool children: First child at developmental age of 2 1/2–5 yr.	a. Foster development of children. b. Create parental privacy. c. Increase competence of child. d. Socialize children. e. Maintain couple relationship.	a. Formal education of disabled children begins at birth. Families may not find adequate programs until preschool years. b. Failure to achieve developmental milestones (e.g., toilet training, self-feeding, language) lead to chronic sorrow. c. Families try to establish routines for themselves and their children.
4. Family with school-age children: Oldest child at developmental age of 6–13 yr.	a. Let children go. b. Balance parental needs with children's needs. c. Promote school achievement.	a. Moving from family to community requires creating new routines and relationships. b. "Going public," explaining to others. c. Negotiating appropriate school services and curriculum. d. Behavioral problems may isolate families.
5. Family with adolescents: Oldest child at developmental age of 13 to age of leaving home.	a. Loosen family ties. b. Strengthen couple relationship. c. Emphasize parent-teen communication. d. Maintain family moral and ethical standards.	a. Continued dependency may mean children never leave home. b. Family examines how to continue family life with increasing physical growth but ongoing dependence of children.

(continued on page 312)

Table 11–2 **STAGES, TASKS, AND SITUATIONAL NEEDS OF FAMILIES OF CHILDREN WITH DISABILITIES AND CHRONIC CONDITIONS** *(Continued)*

FAMILY STAGE	DEVELOPMENTAL TASKS	SITUATIONAL NEEDS THAT ALTER TRANSITIONS
6. Launching center family: First through last child to leave home.	a. Promote independence of children while maintaining relationship. b. Build new life together. c. Deal with midlife developmental crisis.	a. Financial costs do not decrease because child still must depend on care.
7. Families in middle years: Empty nest to retirement.	a. Redefine activities and goals. b. Provide healthy environment. c. Develop meaningful relationships with aging parents. d. Strengthen couple relationship.	a. Relationships with grown children and child with special health care needs are redefined.
8. Retirement to old age: Retirement to death of both parents.	a. Deal with losses. b. Find living place. c. Adapt to role changes. d. Adjust to less income. e. Control chronic illness. f. Adjust to mate loss. g. Become aware of death. h. Review life.	a. "Living trust" is created for children with special health care needs. Planning begins for care of child after elderly parents and siblings become unable to care for adult member with special health care needs.

Gedaly-Duff, V., Stoeger, S., & Shelton, K. (2000). Working with families. In R. Nickel & L. W. Desch (Eds.), *The Physician's Guide to Caring for Children with Disabilities and Chronic Conditions*, Baltimore, MD: Paul Brooke.

(Bruns & McCollum, 2002; Gedaly-Duff & Heims, 2001). Nurses can reduce the stress for sick children, demystify the experience for their siblings, educate parents and grandparents about the children's disease, provide anticipatory guidance, and support the family as a whole during hospitalization. Nursing research that began in the 1960s has now led to open visiting hours for all family members, parent rooming-in, family preparation for procedures, and hospital play (Griffin, 2003). Box 11–5 describes preparing children and families for surgery using hospital play.

Infants and children may be hospitalized for hours, as in day surgery; for months, as in neonatal intensive care units; or repeatedly, as for chronic disease. During hospitalization families desire to participate but do not know what to do, and they often feel left out of the decision making about their children's health (Callery, 1997b). In addition, fathers and siblings are unprepared for the emotional, physical, and financial burdens of home care (Lehna, 2001).

Families are put in a difficult situation when their chronically ill children are hospitalized (Robinson, 1985). The families have been the primary caregivers at home, but now they are placed in a dependent role, as if they did not understand their child's illness pattern. Nurses who have worked with families of chronically ill children know that the families are knowledgeable about how their children respond to disease and about their developmental capabilities. To help families care for their chronically ill children, the nurse can do the following:

- Learn how the family's past experiences and expectations of disease and illness are affecting the current illness situation
- Determine whether the family is responding to a diagnosis of a new condition or is experienced in caring for their child's chronic illness
- Help families promote health in spite of illness by meeting the continually evolving needs of family members

Box 11–5 **PREPARING CHILDREN AND FAMILIES FOR SURGERY USING HOSPITAL PLAY**

Children learn by doing and playing. Using dolls and real equipment helps children know what to expect and act out their fears. Having parents observe helps them learn how to help their child using play.

Before starting, consult with the physician and parent to learn what information the child has been given. Decide the appropriate explanation for age and emotional maturity. For young children, use neutral words like "opening," "drainage," and "oozing" instead of "cut" and "bleed." Gather the visual aids (pictures, doll) and equipment to be used. Do not present too much information because the child may be overwhelmed. Plan for three sessions—why she needs surgery, what the operating room is like, and what she will feel and do after surgery.

If a child has never been in the hospital, have toys familiar to the child such as blocks, dollhouses, and stuffed animals available along with "real" equipment such as a doll with bandages similar to what the child will have, operating room masks, scrubs that nurses and doctors wear, and IV poles. The child may play with the familiar toys. As the child observes the nurse tell the story of what will happen to the doll using the "real" equipment on the doll, the child learns that it is safe to play with this equipment also.

Session 1—How will the surgery make you better?
 a. Give the child a simple explanation reinforcing what she knows.
 b. Reassure the child that no one is to blame for his condition; make it clear that nothing he did is responsible.
 c. On the doll, show where the surgery will take place and what the surgery will do to make him better.

Session 2—What will the surgery be like?
 a. Review why surgery will make her better.
 b. Talk about the steps of getting ready for surgery, such as not eating or drinking the night before, and what the operation room will smell like (alcohol), feel like (cold), and look like (big lights, a clock, people in special clothes).
 c. Child will wear special clothes (hospital gown). Note: Toddlers' body image includes keeping on their underwear since they have just finished toilet training.
 d. Put a mask on the face that has a "funny smell." Use a real anesthesia mask on the doll. Have the child do this too. This gives the child some control.
 e. Play with the thermometer, blood pressure cuff, and stethoscope for taking temperatures and listening to heartbeats and breathing on the doll, nurse, and parent.
 f. Show pictures of an operating room. Point out the "big lights," the clock, and the nurses and doctors dressed in blue (or whatever color your hospital personnel wear in the operating room suites) clothes and wearing "masks." Talk about the ride on a bed with wheels and doors that open like grocery store doors. These are things the child is familiar with and will notice.
 g. Reaffirm that parents will walk with them to the operating room and will be with them when they wake up from the surgery. Play with a mommy doll walking with the toy doll going to the operating room. Children need to know that their parents know where they are and will be there for them.

Session 3—Postoperative expectations
 Using the dolls, act out what will happen after surgery:
 a. Soreness at site of surgery
 b. Pain and medication
 c. Positioning
 d. Bandages (the word "dressing" may be a child's image of "turkey dressing" at Thanksgiving)
 e. No eating and drinking right away

INTERVENTIONS THAT PROMOTE FAMILY-CENTERED CARE

Heath care centers have a philosophy and policies that include family members as participants in decision making about child care and not as visitors (Board & Ryan-Wenger, 2000):

1. In neonatal intensive care units (NICU), nurses welcome parents as partners in the infant's care, rather than projecting the feeling that the nurse "knows best." Family attachment is facilitated by feeding infants their mothers' breast milk and helping parents touch their infant while he or she is being monitored by various machines for heart rate, respiratory rate, oxygen saturation, and so on (Bruns & McCollum, 2002).
2. In pediatric intensive care units (PICU), nurses attend to parent stress and ways of facilitating parent participation during their child's stay in the unit (Miles, Carter, Eberly, Hennessey, & Riddle, 1989) and at end of life (Burns, Mitchell, Griffith, & Truog, 2001).
3. Health care centers build a place for parents—for example, a "window seat" that converts into a bed for the parent in the intensive care unit.
4. Family and patient resource centers jointly developed by families and health care providers create a collaborative process within the health care organization.
5. Nursing assessment and actions for caring for siblings with a sister or brother with an illness (Ahmann, 1997).

- Help families accommodate to the child's developmental limitations related to the disease or condition

In carrying out these tasks, the nurse must consider the specific characteristics and manifestations of the illness, the stage of family development, and the resulting demands on relationships (Rolland, 2005). Asthma is a challenging illness that often involves acute, chronic, and life-threatening phases. The following case study involves children with asthma and their Native American families.

Life-Threatening Illness and End of Life

Families know that chronic illness, like acute injuries and diseases, may be life threatening; however, the death of a child is a rare and shocking experience for families. Even though children's deaths are often reported in television and newspaper media, the death is a distant event. Daily life in America focuses on a happy childhood and does not prepare families for the unlikely event of their children's death. Of children in the United States ages 1 year to 15 years, 12,249 (50.7 in 100,000) died from all causes in 2001. In the same year, 1415 (9.9 per 100,000) ages 1 year to 15 years died from cancer (Arias & Smith, 2003). A serious illness is characterized by hospitalization, life-threatening circumstances, and uncertainty. Much of the time, a child's disease state can be cured as in acute illness, or the child can be restored to a previous functional level. At other times, a child's bodily functions

continue to fail, and the child and family come to an end-of-life phase. Nurses can support and guide families through this traumatic experience.

Waechter's classic study (Waechter, 1971) demonstrated that children knew and worried about their illness. When children did not know exactly what was wrong, they speculated, and they sometimes thought they had done something wrong and were being punished by having the disease. Nurses can teach families how to talk to their children about their life-threatening illness. Children are aware of the seriousness of the illness from external cues such as relatives visiting from long distances and conversations that cease when they enter a room. Internal cues come from their own pain and weakness. When they are hospitalized or come to the clinic, they realize what types of patients are being treated. Families need guidance on how to answer children's questions about what is wrong, how it will affect them, and what can be done. Doka (1995) provided the following guidelines for answering children's questions about illness:

- Begin on the children's level, starting with their past experiences, such as when Grandmother was ill.
- Let the children's questions guide the conversation because sometimes adults give too much overwhelming information.
- Listen for the underlying feelings behind a comment, such as "Do you think I've gotten worse since my last visit?"

CASE STUDY ➤

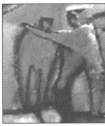

Carl Comantan is a 9-year-old boy who lives with his family in their frame house in a rural area of the northwest region of the United States. His ethnicity is Alaskan Native. His family consists of his mother Carine, his father Big Frank, and his two brothers, Sam, age 7 years, and little Frankie, age 2½ years. Carine is 4 months pregnant. Carine works at a local gas station/convenience store, and Big Frank is a part-time professional truck driver. The store where Carine works is 3 miles from their home. When Big Frank is driving, he is often gone from home for 2 to 3 days at a time. Big Frank is a partially disabled U.S. Army veteran of the Gulf War. Big Frank and Carine have been married for approximately 10 years and are common biological parents of all four of their children. Carl suffers from frequent episodes of colds (upper respiratory infections), which turn to lengthy bouts of coughing and wheezing. He frequently wheezes in the morning and when he plays outside. He goes to his aunt's house near his mother's work every day after school and often into the evening. His aunt cares for all three children while Carine works. The nearest town with a clinic or health care facility is approximately 75 miles away. The family has one vehicle, a small, one-bench-seat 1980 pickup truck with a closed canopy cover over the back. The family members travel to school, work, or a neighbor's house on foot, by bicycle, or with a neighbor who has a vehicle. Carine and Big Frank often consult with extended family members, particularly the elders, in the area concerning treatments for Carl's wheezing, coughing, and frequent infections. However, in their own household, Big Frank and Carine consider themselves equal decision makers with regard to Carl's and the other children's health and activities. Sometimes Carl improves and sometimes he does not. Carl's aunt, who is Big Frank's younger sister, has a car and has taken Carl to the distant hospital emergency room several times over the last year when he was wheezing severely. One of the Comantan family's neighbors is a registered nurse who lives 4 miles away. The nurse works in an ambulatory clinic associated with the one hospital in the town that is 75 miles away.

Consider these questions:

1. What are the features of the Comantan family's career?
2. Using the family interaction model, what patterns of health, illness, and disease do you derive from this description of the Comantan family?
3. Considering Carl's context/situation, what are potential barriers to his health and his health care? State why you included each barrier.
4. List health and health care risks and vulnerabilities for the Comantan family. State your basis for each risk or vulnerability.
5. Using information on this family's health career, construct three chronic and individual development outcomes for Carl.
6. Using concepts of family-centered nursing care and data on their family career, propose at least three health care interventions appropriate to this family. Consider two for the family and one for Carl (Liu et al., 2000; Red Horse, 1997; Rose & Garwick, 2003; Werk, Steinbach, Adams, & Bauchner, 2000).

- Allow for honest expression of anger, sadness, guilt, and ambivalence, and validate these feelings by sharing your own feelings and ways to cope with them.
- Share your own faith or philosophy, not by pronouncements that end talking, such as "We must trust in God's will," but by showing the struggle to find answers by commenting that "it is so hard to understand why this is happening."
- Ask children to tell you what they think they heard to clarify misunderstandings.
- Use other resources, such as books and films, to help with the conversation.
- Give children opportunities to express themselves in stories, games, art, and music, because play is the natural form of children's expression.

Besides teaching families home care, including adequate pain management (Ferrell, Borneman, & Juarez, 1998; Sirkia, Hovi, Pouttu, & Saarinen-Pihkala, 1998), nurses often find themselves helping parents, siblings, and grandparents work through life-and-death issues in the hospital and intensive care as well as in the home (Garros, Rosychuk, & Cox, 2003; Liben & Goldman, 1998). During the intense time of grieving over the child's shortened life span, finding ways to complete things in life that are important to the child and family can promote opportunities for family growth (Stajduhar & Davies, 1998). Guidance may also be needed to bring closure. Examples include recognizing the child's life through a journal kept in the room for all visitors to sign and write in or collecting a handprint, drawings, or favorite stories.

Nurses can use the family interaction model to support families during life-threatening illnesses and end of life. First, nurses should assess families' past experiences with a child's death. Generally families have few models for learning how to cope with this situation. Second, nurses should help families learn how children understand and cope with life-threatening illnesses. Nurses can teach them strategies for comfort care (Wolfe, Friebert, & Hilden, 2002), help them anticipate the signs and symptoms of body failure they will experience, and plan support for these families at the point of death of their child. Finally, nurses can facilitate families' grieving and mourning of the child's death through discussions about each person's needs and interpretations of the behaviors of family members (Solari-Twadell, Bunkers, Wang, & Snyder, 1995).

NURSING IMPLICATIONS

Family nurses interact with families and other health professionals and use a family perspective to guide (1) health care delivery and practice; (2) education, both for families and for other health care providers; (3) research, to systematically explore family child health nursing; and (4) health policy proposals and evaluation.

The family interaction model, which incorporates relevant components of family life, family development and transitions, and family health issues, promotes a comprehensive and holistic approach to the nursing of families. Using this model, nurses are able to collaborate with families who are in the processes of health promotion, disease prevention, and illness management.

Practice

Family child health nursing must be practiced in collaboration and cooperation with families as well as with other health professionals. In family-centered care, nurses work with families to promote health, prevent disease, and cope with acute, chronic, and life-threatening illnesses. Cooperation means talking "with" rather than "to" families about solving problems and attaining health goals, such as acquiring immunizations for family members.

❝Collaboration with families requires an even more involved relationship wherein ideas, expertise, resources, values, and ways of doing are considered by both nurse and family.❞

Both the nurse and the family initiate actions and solutions, and they work together with this information to address the health needs of the family and its members. The family interaction model provides a framework through which nurses can construct and evaluate their approaches and interactions with families with children and a framework for a collaborative approach that acknowledges and respects the individual family.

Families in America are diverse in background and lifestyle, and therefore health care systems and nurses need to understand these differences in order to be effective in problem solving and health promotion. Rather than have children and families come to hospital clinics, creating school-based and school-linked health clinics in the local schools and communities would decrease transportation barriers and help families access health care. For example, families could receive care for their school-enrolled child as well as other members of the family at school-based health clinics.

It is well known that anticipating health problems can prevent their occurrence or minimize their effects. With their close and often frequent contacts with families and their children, nurses are in a position to form a partnership with families for wellness promotion. Nurses can work collaboratively with clients to assist them in taking on self-care responsibilities appropriate to their abilities and developmental levels. For example, a school-age child is expected to dress, prepare breakfast, and get ready for school. A nurse may find that a parent is giving a child with diabetes her morning insulin injection. In this situation, the nurse would recommend that the parent begin preparing the child to do this herself in order to help her achieve her independence in self-care.

Recent reports indicate that morbidity and mortality rates in children and adolescents are often due to behavior and lifestyle and are therefore preventable. Nurses who are aware of these risk factors can intervene with children and families to help prevent or at least minimize situational and developmentally related problems. For example, nurses can discuss immunizations for vaccine-preventable diseases and safety restraints in automobiles at every health visit or encounter, regardless of the primary reason for the health care encounter. Nurses can identify health issues or risks for the family and its members by expanding assessment of children. Nurses who explore the situation of the family comprehensively will detect those individual members who are at risk. For example, in a family whose child has been newly diagnosed with a severe disease such as leukemia, a sibling may begin to fail at school due to the family situation. The nurse who assesses the whole family can identify the new behavior and facilitate a family conference so that each child understands what is happening and has an opportunity to discuss the meanings of the events, thereby keeping the focus on the family. The family can then see that other family members need attention. The family child health nurse assists the family to construct its career toward healthier outcomes for all members.

Research

Family nurses need to explore ways in which the family interactional approach can be implemented and evaluated. For example, a collaborative approach to anticipatory guidance, a commonly used yet under-explored interventional strategy, could be tested, as could long-term interventions for achieving positive health outcomes for children living in poverty. Research could also identify risk factors for families, to assist nurses and other health care providers to focus their interactions with clients. One question might be, What is the impact of a child's developmental delay on a family with impaired parents? Family nurses could identify patterns that are cues for future problems and explore the efficacy of interventions. Using an interactional approach, family child health nurses could identify factors in family and child health that are not apparent when the individual is the focus. A comprehensive family-centered approach could facilitate early screening and interventions, which could produce efficient and cost-saving strategies. For instance, the 9-year longitudinal study of children in a rural village found that family environment was a more important predictor than socioeconomic conditions in association with glucocorticoid stress and illness, suggesting that family processes may mediate links between poverty and health (Flinn & England, 1997; Wertlieb, 2003).

Education

Use of the family interaction model must be based on thorough knowledge of family development and patterns of health, disease, and illness. Family-focused care that balances health promotion, disease prevention, and illness management needs to be emphasized in formal and informal settings, as well as in academic and community programs. Educational curricula need to include opportunities for discussion and case analyses as nurses learn and/or reformulate their perspectives toward family-centered child health. Family child health nursing involves many areas of knowledge and expertise. Therefore, many educational interactions may be needed in order for changes in practice to develop. Practicing nurses, as well as those receiving their initial nursing education, need interactions in which to explore a comprehensive framework for constructing effective approaches to family child health.

Policy

Policies made at agency, institutional, regional, state, and national levels influence family health in multiple and diverse ways. For example, public policies often place single-parent families in conflicting circumstances. A parent may find a job but make too much money to qualify for state-assisted health insurance and not have enough to pay for other types of health insurance. Family nurses can influence the development of public policies through their professional organizations as well as through their individual efforts. A professional organization such as the American Nurses Association develops standards of practice and provides position papers to public servants developing health policies and laws. Policy analysis is therefore the job of every nurse.

Family child health nurses practice in many settings; therefore they need to be aware of policies that apply in and between these settings. Safe and health-promoting options are needed for families with children from infancy to adolescence. At a public policy level, family nurses must advocate for not only "adequate" but also "growth-promoting" child care facilities for the American working family. Another area in need of attention at the policy level is nutrition. Although Americans are slowly changing eating practices toward healthier diets, many gaps exist between the recommendations and actual practices. For example, iron deficiency among infants and young children is decreasing but still needs attention, and the two subgroups who are at greatest risk for nutrition-related problems are people of color and those with low income. Family child health nurses are challenged to implement policies to protect and promote nutritional health for these and other populations of children and families.

Family child health nurses can use the goals of current health care leaders and national recommendations on child health issues to guide their own policy evaluations and efforts for change. *Healthy People 2010: Understanding and Improving Health* (U.S. Department of Health and Human Services, 2000) is an example of a national guideline for family child health nurses to establish priorities of action.

SUMMARY

- Family health nurses focus on the relationship of family life to children's health and illness, and they assist families and family members to achieve well-being.
- Through family-centered care, family child health nurses enhance family life and the development of family members to their fullest potential.
- The *family interaction model* incorporates relevant components of family life and interaction, family development and transitions, and family health and illness and helps nurses take a comprehensive and collaborative approach to families.
- The family interaction model enables nurses to screen for potentially harmful situations, instruct families about health issues, and help families cope with acute illness, chronic illness, and life-threatening conditions.

STUDY QUESTIONS

1. Why is it important for family child health nurses to explore a family's developmental tasks when analyzing the family's response to an illness event?

2. What principles of family-centered care would family child health nurses use with a hospitalized infant and family?

3. Discuss with your classmates your experiences with families. Compare your expectations as you think about the behaviors of the various types of children and families with whom you are familiar and those with whom you are less familiar.

4. Compare how you, a family child health nurse, would discuss health outcomes with a family in the following situations: a family with a chronically ill child, a family with an acutely ill child, and a family with a child with a life-threatening illness. Consider families with multiple children in which one has an illness or disease and the others do not.

5. Obtain a child and/or family health policy in your city, state, country, etc. Discuss the implications of that policy for families with a chronically ill child and for a family who has few or limited financial resources or has no health insurance.

References

Ahmann, E. (1997). Family matters. Books for siblings of children having illness or disability. *Pediatric Nursing, 23*(55), 500–502.

Aldous, J. (1996). *Family careers: Rethinking the developmental perspective.* Thousand Oaks, CA: Sage.

American Academy of Pediatrics. (1973). Day care for handicapped children. *Pediatrics, 51*, 948.

American Academy of Pediatrics. (2001). Committee on Child Abuse and Neglect and Committee on Children With Disabilities. Assessment of maltreatment of children with disabilities. *Pediatrics, 108*(2), 508–512.

American Academy of Pediatrics. (2004). *Writer bytes. . .Childhood injury: It's no accident.* [Web Page]. Retrieved February 1, 2004, from http://www.aap.org/mrt/ciaccidents.htm

Arias, E., & Smith, B. L. (2003). *Deaths: Preliminary data for 2001.* Washington, DC: Department of Health and Human Services, National Center for Health Statistics, Centers for Disease Control and Prevention, National Vital Statistics System.

Banks, M. J., & Benchot, R. J. (2001). Unique aspects of nursing care for Amish children. *MCN, American Journal of Maternal Child Nursing, 26*(4), 192–196.

Baughcum, A. E., Burklow, K. A., Deeks, C., Powers, S. W., & Whitaker, R. C. (1998). Maternal feeding practices and childhood obesity: A focus group study of low-income mothers. *Archives of Pediatrics & Adolescent Medicine, 152*(10), 1010–1014.

Bentson-Royal, R. (1999). *Injury prevention in children with attention deficit hyperactivity disorder (ADHD). Presentation for Nursing 545: Health promotion in families with children* [Presentation and unpublished paper]. Portland, OR: Oregon Health & Sciences University.

Bianchi, S. M. (1995). The changing demographic and socioeconomic character of single-parent families. *Marriage and Family Review, 20*, 71–98.

Bloom, B., Cohen, R. A., Vickerie, J. L., & Wondimu, E. A. (2003). *Summary health statistics for U.S. children: National Health Interview Survey, 2001.* Washington, DC: National Center for Health Statistics.

Board, R., & Ryan-Wenger, N. (2000). State of the science on parental stress and family functioning in pediatric intensive care units. *American Journal of Critical Care, 9*(2), 106–122; quiz 123–124.

Bright Futures. (2002). *Bright Futures: Guidelines for health supervision of infants, children, and adolescents (1994; 2000; 2002)* (2nd ed., rev. ed.). National Center for Education in Maternal and Child Health/Georgetown University.

Bruns, D. A., & McCollum, J. A. (2002). Partnerships between mothers and professionals in the NICU: Caregiving, information exchange, and relationships [comment]. *Neonatal Network—Journal of Neonatal Nursing, 21*(7), 15–23.

Bruss, M. B., Morris, J., & Dannison, L. (2003). Prevention of childhood obesity: Sociocultural and familial factors. *Journal of the American Dietetic Association, 103*(8), 1042–1045.

Bryson, K., & Casper, L. M. (1999). *Coresident grandparents and grandchildren.* Washington, DC: U.S. Department of Commerce, Economics and Statistics Administration.

Bukatko, D., & Daehler, M. W. (2004). *Child development: A thematic approach* (5th ed.). Boston: Houghton Mifflin.

Burlingham, D., & Freud, A. (1942). *Young children in war time.* London: Allen & Unwin.

Burns, J. P., Mitchell, C., Griffith, J. L., & Truog, R. D. (2001). End-of-life care in the pediatric intensive care unit: Attitudes and practices of pediatric critical care physicians and nurses. *Critical Care Medicine, 29*(3), 658–664.

Burr, W. R., Herrin, D. A., Beutler, I. F., & Leigh, G. K. (1988). Epistomologies that lead to primary explanations in family science. *Family Science Review, 1*(3), 185–210.

Burton, L. M., Dilworth-Anderson, P., & Merriwether-deVries, C. (1995). Context and surrogate parenting among contemporary grandparents. In S. M. H. Hansen, M. Heims, D. J. Julian, & M. B. Sussman (Eds.), *Single parent families: Diversity, myths, and realities: Part two* (Vol. 20 [3/4], pp. 349–366). New York: The Hawthorn Press.

Callery, P. (1997a). Caring for parents of hospitalized children: A hidden area of nursing work. *Journal of Advanced Nursing, 26*(5), 992–998.

Callery, P. (1997b). Paying to participate: Financial, social and personal costs to parents of involvement in their children's care in hospital. *Journal of Advanced Nursing, 25*(4), 746–752.

Cherry, D. K., Burt, C. W., & Woodwell, D. A. (2003). National Ambulatory Medical Care Survey: 2001 summary. *Advance Data, 337*, 1–44.

Cook, P. J., & Ludwig, J. (2002). The costs of gun violence against children. *Future Child, 12*(2), 86–99.

Corbin, J. M., & Strauss, A. (1988). Illness trajectories. In J. M. Corbin & A. Strauss (Eds.), *Unending work and care: Managing chronic illness at home* (pp. 33–48). San Francisco: Jossey-Bass.

Costello, E. J., Compton, S. N., Keeler, G., & Angold, A. (2003). Relationships between poverty and psychopathology: A natural experiment [comment]. *JAMA, 290*(15), 2023–2029.

Darbyshire, P. (1993). Parents, nurses and pediatric nursing: A critical review. *Journal of Advanced Nursing, 18*, 1670–1680.

Deatrick, J. A., Knafl, K. A., & Murphy-Moore, C. (1999). Clarifying the concept of normalization. *Image—The Journal of Nursing Scholarship, 31*(3), 209–214.

Denham, S. A. (2002). Family routines: A structural perspective for viewing family health. *Advances in Nursing Science, 24*(4), 60–74.

Doka, K. J. (1995). Talking to children about illness. In K. J. Doka (Ed.), *Children mourning, mourning children* (pp. 31–39). Washington, DC: Hospice Foundation of America.

Dryfoos, J. (1997). The prevalence of problem behaviors: Implications for programs. In R. Weissberg, T. P. Gullotta, R. L. Hampton, B. A. Ryan, & G. R. Adam (Eds.), *Healthy Children 2010: Enhancing children's wellness* (pp. 17–46). Thousand Oaks, CA: Sage.

Dube, S. R., Anda, R. F., Felitti, V. J., Croft, J. B., Edwards, V. J., & Giles, W. H. (2001). Growing up with parental alcohol abuse: Exposure to childhood abuse, neglect, and household dysfunction. *Child Abuse & Neglect, 25*, 1627–1640.

Duvall, E. M., & Miller, B. C. (1985). Developmental tasks: Individual and family. In E. M. Duvall & B. C. Miller (Eds.), *Marriage and family development.* New York: Harper & Row.

Elliott, G. R., & Smiga, S. (2003). Depression in the child and adolescent. *Pediatric Clinics of North America, 50*(5), 1093–1106.

Erikson, E. H. (1973). *Childhood and society.* New York: Norton.

Faux, S. (1993). Siblings of children with chronic physical and cognitive disabilities. *Journal of Pediatric Nursing, 8*(5), 305–317.

Faville, K. (1925). The nurse as counselor in troubled homes. *The Red Cross Courier, 4,* 14–15, 22.

Federal Interagency Forum on Child and Family Statistics. (2003). *America's children: Key national indicators of well-being, 2003.* Washington, DC.

Ferrell, B. R., Borneman, T., & Juarez, G. (1998). Integration of pain education in home care. *Journal of Palliative Care, 14*(3), 62–68.

Fingerhut, L. A., & Christoffel, K. K. (2002). Firearm-related death and injury among children and adolescents. In K. Reich (Ed.), *Children, youth, and gun violence* (Vol. 12, pp. 25–37). Los Altos, CA: From *The Future of Children,* a publication of The David and Lucile Packard Foundation.

Flinn, M., & England, B. (1997). Social economics of childhood glucocorticoid stress response and health. *American Journal of Physical Anthropology, 1,* 33–53.

Gallagher, C. (2002). Childhood asthma: Tools that help parents manage it. *American Journal of Nursing, 102*(8), 71–83.

Garros, D., Rosychuk, R. J., & Cox, P. N. (2003). Circumstances surrounding end of life in a pediatric intensive care unit. *Pediatrics, 112*(5), e371.

Gedaly-Duff, V. (1990). *Family management of childhood pain: Families' experiences in care of their children's repeated pain episodes associated with chronic illness such as juvenile rheumatoid arthritis. Final report for Robert Wood Johnson Nurse Scholars Program (1988–1990).* Philadelphia: University of Pennsylvania School of Nursing.

Gedaly-Duff, V., & Heims, M. (2001). Family health care nursing. In S. M. H. Hanson (Ed.), *Family health care nursing: Theory, practice, and research* (2nd ed., pp. 243–271). Philadelphia: FA Davis.

Gedaly-Duff, V., Stoeger, S., & Shelton, K. (2000). Working with families. In R. E. Nickel & L. W. Desch (Eds.), *The physician's guide to caring for children with disabilities and chronic conditions* (1st ed., pp. 31–76). Baltimore: Paul H. Brookes.

Gedaly-Duff, V., & Ziebarth, D. (1994). Mothers' management of adenoid-tonsillectomy pain in 4- to 8-year-olds: A preliminary study. *Pain, 57*(3), 293–299.

Goslin, E. R. (1978). Hospitalization as a life crisis for the preschool child: A critical review. *Journal of Community Health, 3*(4), 321–346.

Griffin, T. (2003). Facing challenges to family-centered care. II: Anger in the clinical setting. *Pediatric Nursing, 29*(3), 212–214.

Grunbaum, J. A., Kann, L., Kinchen, S. A., Williams, B., Ross, J. G., Lowry, R., & Kolbe, L. (2002). Youth risk behavior surveillance—United States, 2001. *Journal of School Health, 72*(8), 313–328.

Hardy, M. S. (2002). Behavior-oriented approaches to reducing youth gun violence. In K. Reich (Ed.), *Children, youth, and gun violence* (Vol. 12, pp. 100–117). Los Altos, CA: From *The Future of Children,* a publication of The David and Lucile Packard Foundation.

Harticker, L. E. (1998). Core principles of family-centered health care. Advances in family centered health care. *Institute for Family-Centered Care, 4*(1), 1–20.

Hawkins, J. (1997). Academic performance and school success: Sources and consequences. In R. Weissberg, T. P. Gullotta, R. L. Hampton, B. A. Ryan, & G. R. Adams (Eds.), *Healthy children 2010: Enhancing children's wellness* (pp. 278–305). Thousand Oaks, CA: Sage.

Hines, P. M. (1999). The family life cycle of African American families living in poverty. In B. Carter & M. McGoldrick (Eds.), *The expanded family life cycle: Individual, family and social perspectives* (3rd ed., pp. 327–345). Boston: Allyn & Bacon.

Hodges, E. A. (2003). A primer on early childhood obesity and parental influence. *Pediatric Nursing, 29*(1), 13.

Holahan, J., Dubay, L., & Kenney, G. M. (2003). Which children are still uninsured and why. In C. Bennett (Ed.), *Health insurance for children* (Vol. 13, pp. 55–79). Los Altos, CA: From *The Future of Children*, a publication of The David and Lucile Packard Foundation.

Hootman, J., Houck, G. M., & King, M. C. (2002). A program to educate school nurses about mental health interventions. *The Journal of School Nursing, 18*(4), 191–195.

Houck, G. M., Darnell, S., & Lussman, S. (2002). A support group intervention for at-risk female high school students. *The Journal of School Nursing, 18*(4), 212–218.

Howard, B. (1991). Discipline in early childhood. *Pediatric Clinics of North America, 38*(6), 1351–1369.

Hurst, I. (2001a). Mothers' strategies to meet their needs in the newborn intensive care nursery. *Journal of Perinatal & Neonatal Nursing, 15*(2), 65–82.

Hurst, I. (2001b). Vigilant watching over: Mothers' actions to safeguard their premature babies in the newborn intensive care nursery. *Journal of Perinatal & Neonatal Nursing, 15*(3), 39–57.

Huston, A. C., Duncan, G. J., Granger, R., Bos, J., McLoyd, V., Mistry, R., Crosby, D., Gibson, C., Magnuson, K., Romich, J., & Ventura, A. (2001). Work-based antipoverty programs for parents can enhance the school performance and social behavior of children. *Child Development, 72*(1), 318–336.

Kerrebrock, N., & Lewit, E. M. (1999). Children in self-care. *Future Child, 9*(2), 151–160.

Kirby, S. N., Berends, M., & Naftel, S. (1999). Supply and demand of minority teachers in Texas: Problems and prospects. *Educational Evaluation and Policy Analysis, 21*(1), 47–66.

Kleinman, A. (1988). The meaning of symptoms and disorders. In *The illness narratives.* New York: Basic Books.

Kohlberg, L. (1984). *The psychology of moral development.* San Francisco: Harper & Row.

Kools, S., & Kennedy, C. (2003). Foster child health and development: Implications for primary care. *Pediatric Nursing, 29*(1), 39–49.

Kotch, J. B., Browne, D. C., Dufort, V., & Winsor, J. (1999). Predicting child maltreatment in the first 4 years of life from characteristics assessed in the neonatal period. *Child Abuse & Neglect, 23*(4), 305–319.

Langford, D. R. (2004). Family health protection. In P. J. Bomar (Ed.), *Promoting health in families: Applying family research and theory to nursing practice* (3rd ed., pp. 304–338). Philadelphia: Saunders.

Lash, M., & Wertlieb, D. (1993). A model for family-centered service coordination for children who are disabled by traumatic injuries. *The ACCH Advocate, 1,* 19–27, 39–41.

Lehna, C. (2001). Fathers' and siblings' roles in families with children in home hospice care. *Journal of Hospice & Palliative Nursing, 3*(1), 17–23.

Lewandowski, L., & Tesler, M. (Eds.). (2003). *Family-centered care: Putting it into action. The SPN/ANA guide to family-centered care.* Washington, DC: Society of Pediatric Nurses/American Nurses Association.

Liben, S., & Goldman, A. (1998). Home care for children with life-threatening illness. *Journal of Palliative Care, 14*(3), 33–38.

Limbo, R., Petersen, W., & Pridham, K. (2003). Promoting safety of young children with guided participation processes. *Journal of Pediatric Health Care, 17*(5), 245–251.

Liu, L. L., Stout, J. W., Sullivan, M., Solet, D., Shay, D. K., & Grossman, D. C. (2000). Asthma and bronchiolitis hospitalizations among American Indian children. *Archives of Pediatrics & Adolescent Medicine, 154*(10), 991–996.

Markson, S., & Fiese, B. H. (2000). Family rituals as a protective factor for children with asthma. *Journal of Pediatric Psychology, 25*(7), 471–480.

Martinez, C., Mehesy, C., & Seeley, K. (2003). *What counts: Measuring indicators of family well-being reported by The Colorado Foundation for Families and Children* (www.coloradofoundation.org). Denver, Co: The Child and Family Policy Center.

Maslow, A. H. (1970). *Motivation and personality* (2nd ed.). New York: Harper & Row.

McCarthy, M. J., Herbert, R., Brimacombe, M., Hansen, J., Wong, D., & Zelman, M. (2002). Empowering parents through asthma education. *Pediatric Nursing, 28*(5), 465–473, 504.

McGoldrick, M., & Walsh, F. (2005). Death and the family life cycle. In B. Carter & M. McGoldrick (Eds.), *The expanded family life cycle: Individual, family, and social perspectives* (3rd ed., pp. 185–201). Boston: Allyn & Bacon.

Mead, G. H. (1934). *Mind, self, and society.* Chicago: University of Chicago Press.

Meister, S. B. (1991). Family well-being. In A. L. Whall & N. Fawcett (Eds.), *Family theory development in nursing: State of the science and art* (pp. 209–231). Philadelphia: FA Davis.

Meleis, A. I., Sawyer, L. M., Im, E. O., Hilfinger Messias, D. K., & Schumacher, K. (2000). Experiencing transitions: An emerging middle-range theory. *Advances in Nursing Science, 23*(1), 12–28.

Meleski, D. (2002). Families with chronically ill children: A literature review examines approaches to help them cope. *American Journal of Nursing, 102*(5), 47–54.

Miles, M. S., Carter, M. C., Eberly, T. W., Hennessey, J., & Riddle, I. (1989). Toward an understanding of parent stress in the pediatric intensive care unit: Overview of the program of research. *Maternal Child Nursing Journal, 18*(3), 181–185.

Miles, M. S., Carter, M. C., Riddle, I., Hennessey, J., & Eberly, T. W. (1989). The pediatric intensive care unit environment as a source of stress for parents. *Maternal Child Nursing Journal, 18*(3), 199–206.

Miles, M. S., Funk, S. G., & Kasper, M. A. (1992). The stress response of mothers and fathers of preterm infants. *Research in Nursing and Health, 15*(4), 261–269.

Morrison, L. (1997). Stress and siblings. *Paediatric Nursing, 9*(4), 26–27.

Murray, M., Guerre, N., & Williams, K. (1997). Violence prevention for the 21st century. In R. Weissberg, T. P. Gullotta, R. L. Hampton, B. A. Ryan, & G. R. Adams (Eds.), *Healthy children 2010: Enhancing children's wellness* (pp. 105–128). Thousand Oaks, CA: Sage.

National Center for Health Statistics. (1993). *Health, United States, 1992 with chartbook on trends in the health of Americans* (DHHS Pub. No. PHS 93–1232). Hyattsville, MD: U.S. Government Printing Office.

National Clearinghouse on Child Abuse and Neglect Information: National Adoption Information Clearinghouse. (2003). *Child maltreatment 2001: Summary of key findings.* Washington, DC.

Nelson, A. (2002). Unequal treatment: Confronting racial and ethnic disparities in health care. *Journal of the National Medical Association, 94*(8), 666–668.

Newacheck, P. W., Fox, H. B., & McManus, M. A. (1988). Home care needs of chronically ill children. *Caring, 7*(6), 4–6, 8–10.

Newacheck, P. W., Hung, Y. Y., & Wright, K. K. (2002). Racial and ethnic disparities in access to care for children with special health care needs. *Ambulatory Pediatrics, 2*(4), 247–254.

Newacheck, P. W., Stein, R. E., Bauman, L., & Hung, Y. Y. (2003). Disparities in the prevalence of disability between black and white children. *Archives of Pediatrics & Adolescent Medicine, 157*(3), 244–248.

Newacheck, P. W., Strickland, B., Shonkoff, J. P., Perrin, J. M., McPherson, M., McManus, M., Lauver, C., Fox, H., & Arango, P. (1998). An epidemiologic profile of children with special health care needs. *Pediatrics, 102*(1, Pt. 1), 117–123.

Northington, L. (2000). Chronic sorrow in caregivers of school age children with sickle cell disease: A grounded theory approach. *Issues in Comprehensive Pediatric Nursing, 23*(3), 141–154.

Paget, M. (1982). Your son is cured now; you may take him home. *Culture, Medicine, and Psychiatry, 6,* 237–259.

Parsons, C. (2003). Caring for adolescents and families in crisis. *Nursing Clinics of North America, 38*(1), 111–122.

Patterson, J. M., & Garwick, A. W. (1994). Levels of meaning in family stress theory. *Family Process, 33,* 287–304.

Phillips, D., & Adams, G. (2001). Child care and our youngest children. In M. Larner (Ed.), *Caring for infants and toddlers* (Vol. 11, pp. 34–51). Los Altos, CA: From *The Future of Children*, a publication of The David and Lucile Packard Foundation.

Piaget, J., & Inhelder, B. (1969). *Psychology of the child.* New York: Basic Books.

Pinderhughes, E. E., Dodge, K. A., Bates, J. E., Pettit, G. S., & Zelli, A. (2000). Discipline responses: Influences of parents' socioeconomic status, ethnicity, beliefs about parenting, stress, and cognitive-emotional processes. *Journal of Family Psychology, 14*(3), 380–400.

Pridham, K. F. (1993). Anticipatory guidance of parents of new infants: Potential contribution of the internal working model construct. *Image—The Journal of Nursing Scholarship, 25*(1), 49–56.

Rankin, S. H. (1989). Family transitions. In C. L. Gilliss, B. L. Highley, B. M. Roberts, & I. M. Martinson (Eds.), *Toward a science of family nursing* (pp. 173–186). Menlo Park: Addison-Wesley.

Rankin, S. H., & Weekes, D. P. (2000). Life-span development: A review of theory and practice for families with chronically ill members. *Scholarly Inquiry for Nursing Practice, 14*(4), 355–373; discussion 375–378.

Red Horse, J. (1997). Traditional American Indian family system. *Families, Systems & Health* (formerly *Family Systems Medicine*), *15*(3), 243–250.

Reynolds, A. J., Temple, J. A., Robertson, D. L., & Mann, E. A. (2001). Long-term effects of an early childhood intervention on educational achievement and juvenile arrest: A 15-year follow-up of low-income children in public schools [comment][erratum appears in Sep. 5, 2001, *JAMA, 286*(9), 1026]. *JAMA, 285*(18), 2339–2346.

Robinson, C. A. (1985). Double bind: A dilemma for parents of chronically ill children. *Pediatric Nursing, 11,* 112–115.

Robledo, L., Wilson, A. H., & Gray, P. (1999). Hispanic mothers' knowledge and care of their children with respiratory illnesses: A pilot study. *Journal of Pediatric Nursing, 14*(4), 239–247.

Rolland, J. S. (2005). Chronic illness and the family life cycle. In B. Carter & M. McGoldrick (Eds.), *The expanded family life cycle: Individual, family and social perspectives* (3rd ed., pp. 492–511). Boston: Allyn & Bacon.

Rose, D., & Garwick, A. (2003). Urban American Indian family caregivers' perceptions of barriers to management of childhood asthma. *Journal of Pediatric Nursing, 18*(1), 2–11.

Sameroff, A. J., & Feil, L. A. (1985). Parental concepts of development. In I. E. Sigel (Ed.), *Parental belief systems* (pp. 83–105). Hillsdale, NJ: Lawrence Erlbaum.

Schumacher, K. L., & Meleis, A. I. (1994). Transitions: A central concept in nursing. *Image—The Journal of Nursing Scholarship, 26*(2), 119–127.

Sharpe, D., & Rossiter, L. (2002). Siblings of children with a chronic illness: A meta-analysis. *Journal of Pediatric Psychology, 27*(8), 699–710.

Sirkia, K., Hovi, L., Pouttu, J., & Saarinen-Pihkala, U. M. (1998). Pain medication during terminal care of children with cancer. *Journal of Pain & Symptom Management, 15*(4), 220–226.

Smith, P., & Drew, L. (2002). *Grandparenthood* (2nd ed., Vol. 3). Mahwah, NJ, & London: Lawrence Erlbaum.

Solari-Twadell, P. A., Bunkers, S. S., Wang, C. E., & Snyder, D. (1995). The pinwheel model of bereavement. *Image—The Journal of Nursing Scholarship, 27*(4), 323–326.

Spitz, R. (1945). Hospitalism. *Psychoanalytic Study of the Child, 1,* 53–74.

Staff of Committee on Ways and Means. (2000). *The 2000 "Green Book"—Background data on programs within the jurisdiction of the Committee on Ways and Means* (pdf 61–710 CC). Washington, DC: Government Printing Office, U.S. House of Representatives.

Stajduhar, K. I., & Davies, B. (1998). Death at home: Challenges for families and directions for the future. *Journal of Palliative Care, 14*(3), 8–14.

Stein, M. T., & Perrin, E. L. (1998). Guidance for effective discipline. American Academy of Pediatrics. Committee on Psychosocial Aspects of Child and Family Health. *Pediatrics, 101*(4, Pt. 1), 723–728.

Sullivan, P. M., & Knutson, J. F. (1998). The association between child maltreatment and disabilities in a hospital-based epidemiological study. *Child Abuse & Neglect, 22*(4), 271–288.

Sullivan-Bolyai, S., Deatrick, J., Gruppuso, P., Tamborlane, W., & Grey, M. (2003). Constant vigilance: Mothers' work parenting young children with type 1 diabetes. *Journal of Pediatric Nursing, 18*(1), 21–29.

Thomas, J. L., Sperry, L., & Yarbrough, M. S. (2000). Grandparents as parents: Research findings and policy recommendations. *Child Psychiatry & Human Development, 31*(1), 3–22.

Thomas, V. N., & Westerdale, N. (1997). Sickle cell disease. *Nursing Standard, 11*(25), 40–45; quiz 46–47.

Tiedeman, M. E. (1997). Anxiety responses of parents during and after the hospitalization of their 5- to 11-year-old children. *Journal of Pediatric Nursing, 12*(2), 110–119.

Tomlinson, P. S., Thomlinson, E., Peden-McAlpine, C., & Kirschbaum, M. (2002). Clinical innovation for promoting family care in paediatric intensive care: Demonstration, role modelling and reflective practice. *Journal of Advanced Nursing, 38*(2), 161–170.

U.S. Department of Health and Human Services. (2000, November). *Healthy People 2010: Understanding and improving health* (U.S. Government Printing Office, Superintendent of Documents, Washington, DC 20402–9382, Stock Number 017-001-001-00-550-9). Washington, DC: U.S. Government Printing Office.

U.S. Department of Health and Human Services. (2002). *What is child maltreatment?* Retrieved February 1, 2004, from http://nccanch.acf.hhs.gov/pubs/factsheets/whatiscan.cfm

U.S. Department of Health and Human Services, & Administration on Children, Youth, and Families. (2003). *Child maltreatment 2001* (Report No. 29–10058). Washington, DC: U.S. Government Printing Office.

van Dyk, A. C. (2001). Why me and not my neighbour? HIV/AIDS care and counselling in a traditional African context. *Curationis, 24*(3), 4–12.

Velsor-Friedrich, B., & Foley, M. K. (2001). School-based management of the child with an acute asthma episode. *AACN Clinical Issues, 12*(2), 282–292.

Waechter, E. (1971). Children's awareness of fatal illness. *American Journal of Nursing, 71,* 1168–1172.

Wald, L. D. (1904). The treatment of families in which there is sickness. *American Journal of Nursing, 4,* 427–431, 515–519, 602–606.

Weiss, J., Diamond, T., Demark, J., & Lovald, B. (2003). Involvement in Special Olympics and its relations to self-concept and actual competency in participants with developmental disabilities. *Research in Developmental Disabilities, 24*(4), 281–305.

Werk, L. N., Steinbach, S., Adams, W. G., & Bauchner, H. (2000). Beliefs about diagnosing asthma in young children. *Pediatrics, 105*(3, Pt. 1), 585–590.

Wertlieb, D. (2003). Converging trends in family research and pediatrics: Recent findings for the American Academy of Pediatrics Task Force on the Family. *Pediatrics, 111*(6, Pt. 2), 1572–1587.

White, J., & Klein, D. (2002). *Family theories.* Thousand Oaks, CA: Sage.

Wolfe, J., Friebert, S., & Hilden, J. (2002). Caring for children with advanced cancer integrating palliative care. *Pediatric Clinics of North America, 49*(5), 1043–1062.

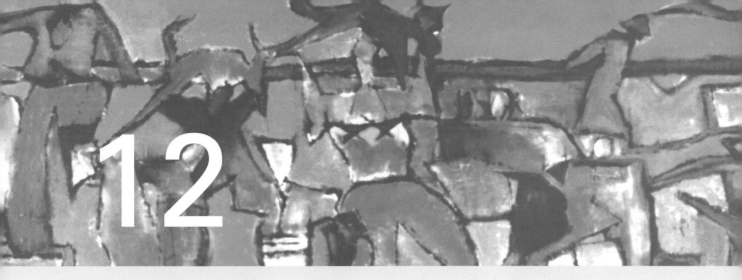

12

Family-Focused Medical-Surgical Nursing

Nancy Trygar Artinian, PhD, RN, BC, FAHA

CRITICAL CONCEPTS

- Family members who receive care in medical-surgical settings are more likely to be empowered to deal with the stressors of foreign hospital environments and thus better prepared to provide support to patients and aid in their recovery or facilitate a comfortable death.

- When planning interventions, nurses caring for families need to consider the nature of the illness, family characteristics including cultural background, the health care team's philosophy about family care, and the characteristics of the patient.

- Family theoretical models—including the structural-functional model, family systems model, and family resilience model—can provide a basis for family assessment and intervention.

- Before illness, medical-surgical nurses should direct interventions at health promotion.

- During the acute illness phase, nursing interventions should focus on providing assurance, enhancing the proximity of patient and family, managing information, facilitating comfort, and reinforcing support.

- Families in the chronic phase have been dealing with illness for a long time; thus acknowledging their experiences with illness management is important. Common family concerns in chronic illness—such as guilt, fear, uncertainty, anger, and lack of knowledge about the illness, care requirements, or resources—may require interventions.

- At end of life, interventions are directed toward helping families move through the phases of adaptation in response to the fatal illness of a family member. Families may also need help dealing with other end-of-life issues such as making decisions regarding withdrawal of life support or organ donation and witnessing cardiopulmonary resuscitation efforts.

- Nurses should assess the availability of social support, use of coping strategies, availability of personal resources, and whether the family knows what to expect once at home, as these factors positively influence their perception of readiness for discharge.

- Only when medical-surgical nurses include families in plans for care can they hope to provide unfragmented, holistic, humane, and sensitively delivered health care.

INTRODUCTION

Hospitalization is a stressful experience for patients and their families as well. Once considered the domain of only community health, mental health, or maternal-child nursing, family nursing is now recognized as an important part of care by most nurses in medical-surgical settings. Providing care to the entire family unit, as well as caring for patients in the context of their families, is crucial regardless of the setting for nursing care delivery.

The purpose of this chapter is to describe the evolution of family nursing in medical-surgical settings and to describe issues for nurses to consider as they plan care for families. Included are a review of the stressors that families often face during hospitalization and a discussion of the impact of patient hospitalization on families. This chapter examines caring for families before illness, during acute and chronic illness, and at end of life and reviews broad categories of family nursing interventions to use during any of the phases of illness. A discussion of the application of theoretical models to family medical-surgical nursing highlights the connection between theory and practice. The chapter closes with a discussion of the implications of developments in family nursing on medical-surgical practice, education, research, and health care policy.

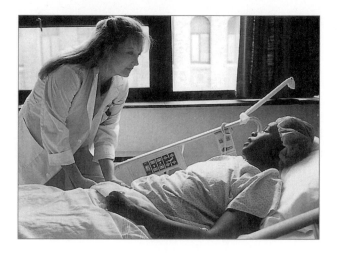

Illness or injury requiring hospitalization of a loved one has been termed a nonnormative stressor event for families; that is, it is unexpected and unpredictable. Experiencing such an event may help some families grow but may cause conflicts in others. In the case of illness or injury, home routines are disrupted and some family members may need to assume responsibilities they have never had before. In addition, parents may struggle with how much to tell their children, or children may fear that they are going to lose a parent.

IMPACT OF PATIENT HOSPITALIZATION FOR ILLNESS OR INJURY ON FAMILIES

Illness and trauma requiring admission to a hospital and/or a critical care unit is stressful for families (Lange, 2001). Not only are hospital environments foreign, but also nurses and doctors are strangers who speak another language. To add to the stress, families are often separated from their ill member soon after entering the hospital doors and are asked to go to a small, sometimes crowded, waiting room. There, they wait endlessly for someone to give them information as they deal with emotions such as fear, anger, and guilt. Some families are better prepared to deal with these stressors than others are. Researchers have found that, among 51 family members of patients who had motor vehicle accidents or gunshot wounds, increases in prior stressors, strains, and transitions were negatively related to family adaptation outcomes and that family hardiness, resources, coping, and problem-solving communication were positively related to family adaptation outcomes (Leske & Jiricka, 1998).

COMMON THEORETICAL PERSPECTIVES: ASSESSING IMPACT OF ILLNESS ON FAMILIES

Chapter 3 describes several theoretical frameworks for nursing of families. Models from the social science genre of theories—structural-functional theory, family systems theory, family stress theory, and family resilience theory—may be more helpful to medical-surgical nurses because they are concise and easy to use and do not depend on long-term relationships with families. In medical-surgical settings, the short hospital stays involved, the sometimes overwhelming needs of patients, and the many other demands on nurses' time influence their abilities to plan and deliver care to families. For the family, the first priority is to help them cope with the immediacy of the hospitalization. Thus, theories must help nurses assess and provide care for families within a short period of time. Personal philosophy, hospital unit philosophy, the nature of the nurse's clinical practice, and patient and family needs will influence the selection of the appropriate model to guide clinical practice.

Therapeutic Quadrangle

In addition to the social science theories, assessment of each component of the therapeutic quadrangle may also provide insight into the impact of the illness or injury on the family and aid in the determination of associated family care needs. The therapeutic quadrangle contains four parts: the illness, the family, the health care team, and the patient (Rolland, 1988). Caring for families in medical-surgical settings requires analyzing each of these components and designing and implementing tailor-made plans for family care accordingly.

Illness

CHARACTERISTICS OF ILLNESS

Illness is the first element of the therapeutic quadrangle. There is a great deal of variability associated with illness, and this variability is characterized by differences in the onset, course, outcome, and degree of incapacitation of the illness (Rolland, 1988). Strokes and myocardial infarctions have sudden onsets; arthritis and emphysema have gradual onsets. The type of onset may explain the amount and speed of family readjustment needed. The course of the disease may be progressive, constant, or relapsing. Cancers, rheumatoid arthritis, and emphysema are progressive; a spinal cord injury is constant; and multiple sclerosis and asthma are relapsing. Relapsing illnesses require a different kind of family adaptability from that needed with a progressive or constant course (Rolland, 1988). Moreover, the likelihood of death resulting from an illness also affects the family. Metastatic cancer and AIDS are progressive and usually fatal, whereas hypertension and arthritis are not likely to end in death if

Onset of illness—sudden or gradual

Course of illness—progressive, constant, or relapsing

Outcome of illness—recovery, chronic, or death

Degree of incapacitation of illness—physical, cognitive, or emotional dysfunction

Type and amount of treatment required by illness—medications, home care, wound care, respiratory, physical, or occupational therapy, etc.

Amount of hospital time required by illness

treated properly. Illness outcome influences the degree to which the family experiences anticipatory grief (Rolland, 1988). Thus, the expectation of future loss can alter family perceptions and problem-solving abilities. "The tendency to see the family member as practically 'in the coffin' can set in motion maladaptive responses that divest the ill member of important responsibilities" (Rolland, 1988). The degree of illness incapacitation also determines the specific adjustments required of a family. Incapacitation can result from impairment of cognition (e.g., Alzheimer's disease), sensation (e.g., blindness), movement (e.g., stroke with paralysis), or energy production (e.g., cardiovascular and pulmonary diseases). Illness incapacitation can also result from social stigma (e.g., AIDS).

The complexity, frequency, and efficiency of treatment; the amount of home care and hospital-based care required; and the frequency and intensity of symptoms vary widely across illnesses and have important implications for family adaptation (Rolland, 1988).

Family

The family is the second element in the therapeutic quadrangle. The following factors influence the family's relationships with the other elements in the therapeutic quadrangle: family flexibility, the amount of time the family has had to prepare for the illness event, the family's previous experience with illness or injury, the availability of resources to deal with the event, problem-solving ability, coping skills to assist the family in managing the illness or injury, the amount of family disruption or number of family changes caused by the event, family cohesion, structure, cultural background, and family perceptions. All of these characteristics vary dramatically from family to family, and all affect the extent and manner by which each family can handle illness of a family member.

There are a number of family tasks to consider in relation to illness (Moos, 1984). These illness-related tasks include (1) learning to deal with pain, incapacitation, or other illness-related symptoms of their ill member; (2) learning caregiving procedures; and (3) establishing workable relationships with the health care team.

Health Care Team

The third element in the therapeutic quadrangle is the health care team. Health team members vary in the priority they assign to family care, in their sensitivity to family needs, and in their knowledge and ability to assess and intervene with families. Several strategies may be used by nurses to foster positive relationships with families as shown in the following box. Strategies that inhibit relationships with families include depersonalizing the family, maintaining an efficient attitude, and displaying lack of trust in the family (Hupcey, 1998).

Fostering Positive Relationships with Families

Patient

The final element in the therapeutic quadrangle is the patient. The identity of the sick person (e.g., mother, father, grandmother, spouse, sister) and the way the patient handles illness affect family adjustment. The point in the individual's life span at which the illness occurs also influences the family's adjustment. Often illness in the prime of life is unexpected, whereas illness in old age may be anticipated. In general, the more emotionally significant the sick family member, the more disruptive the illness will be. For example, if the ill person is the one everyone in the family depended on or turned to when they needed advice or other types of help, it is more likely that the loss of their contributions to the family will be acutely missed.

FAMILY MEDICAL-SURGICAL NURSING AT VARIOUS PHASES OF ILLNESS

Medical-surgical nurses may care for families before illness, during periods of acute illness and chronic illness, and at the end of life.

Demonstrate commitment—Respond to family members as persons, spend time with the family, anticipate family needs

Persevere—Get to know a lot about the family, spend time with more difficult families

Be involved—Advocate for the family, bend or break rules when possible

Adapted from Hupcey, J. E. (1998). Establishing the nurse-family relationship in the intensive care unit. *Western Journal of Nursing Research, 20*(2), 180–194.

Health Promotion

Caring for families before illness has two aims. The first is to help all family members develop healthy lifestyles. The second is to prevent a hospitalization from affecting the family's health. Studies have shown that families play a key role in determining the health-promoting behaviors of their members (Franks, Pienta, & Wray, 2002; Denham, 2003) and that family support is important in changing both health attitudes and behaviors (Bovbjerg et al., 1995). Nurses play a critical role in facilitating health promotion within the family (Loveland-Cherry & Bomar, 2004). Before illness develops, nurses caring for patients at high risk for familial diseases such as heart disease, stroke, or cancer can suggest to the whole family ways to lower the risk of developing these diseases. Not only can this be done in the same amount of time that it takes to teach the patient alone, but also the family benefits as a whole and, at the same time, can help the patient make necessary changes in lifestyle.

The Human Genome Project

A second aim of family nursing during the health promotion period is to prevent a stress-filled hospitalization from negatively affecting the family's health. When under stress, healthy family members are at risk of numerous physical, mental, emotional, social, and financial problems of their own (Bengston, Karlsson, Wahrborg, Hjalmarson, & Herlitz, 1996; Holicky, 1996; Lenz & Perkins, 2000; Stolarik, Lindsay, Sherrard, & Woodend, 2000; Swoboda & Lipsett, 2002). Unfortunately, health care providers do not get reimbursed for providing care to family members. Consequently, the health of family members often receives little time and attention. Only a few researchers have designed studies to determine how the health-related activities and health of significant others are altered by patients' hospitalizations (Hathaway, Boswell, Stanford, Schneider, & Moncrief, 1987; Wicks, Milstead, Hathaway, & Cetingok, 1998; Leung, Chien, & Mackenzie, 2000; O'Farrell, Murray, & Hotz, 2000). Findings suggest that family members do not have a lot of concern about their personal and physical needs, that self-rated health does not improve during the illness experience, and that health practices and health deteriorate over the course of the illness.

Despite short hospital stays, there are several ways that nurses can systematically structure care to

The consequences of genetic research add another dimension to family care before illness. The Human Genome Project began in 1990 and was a 13-year effort coordinated by the Department of Energy and the National Institutes of Health. The project completed ahead of schedule in 2003 with the completion of the human genetic sequence (U.S. Department of Energy, 2004). Scientists obtained the sequence of the 3 billion base pairs making up the human genome. The order of the bases A, T, C, and G spells out the exact instructions needed to maintain and reproduce a living organism (U.S. Department of Energy, 2004). As the availability of tests to identify hereditary predisposition to chronic illnesses grows, family nurses in medical-surgical settings will need to grapple with ethical issues associated with human genetics. Family nurses will need to counsel and advise families about accessing their genetic information and responding to the knowledge that they are at higher risk for illness (Driscoll, 1998). A six-step communication skills–building intervention was designed to provide information and skills to individuals undergoing genetic testing in order to communicate effectively the results to their families (Daly et al., 2001). The six steps include the following:

1. Getting started, which entails identifying relatives who may benefit from the results and choosing the appropriate setting to communicate the results
2. Determining how much family members know about their loved one's participation in genetic testing
3. Determining how much family members want to know about their health risk
4. Sharing the genetic testing information by explaining the meaning of the test results and describing personal risk for developing the illness
5. Responding to feelings and showing support
6. Planning and follow-through, including referring family members to a local genetic counselor and sharing educational resources

promote family health. During hospitalization of a family member, nurses can facilitate family health promotion by including families in assessments at the same time the patient admission assessment is conducted; by determining the effects of patient hospitalization on the family and providing an opportunity to discuss potential coping strategies; and by intervening to address family needs such as by contacting the hospital chaplain or by arranging a family conference with the health care team.

Acute Illness

The acute phase of illness refers to the period immediately following the onset of an acute illness event, such as an acute myocardial infarction, a stroke, or coronary artery bypass surgery. Families with members who are acutely or critically ill are often seen in ICUs, cardiac care units, or emergency rooms under conditions in which they are greatly stressed because a member of their family is experiencing a life-threatening illness or injury.

Family members experience an emotional burden as a result of their relative's stay in ICU. This burden often results in anxiety and depression. One study reported that more than two-thirds of family members visiting patients in the ICU suffer from symptoms of anxiety and depression (Pochard et al., 2001). Communication among family members may become distorted because the fear, anger, and guilt that members experience may be too intense for them to handle. In some families, conflicts may be blocked or submerged during the initial period of a critical illness, but as time goes on and the family resources become depleted, conflict between members may become more obvious (McClowery, 1992, p. 561).

There are five tasks that families must accomplish during the crisis phase of illness: (1) creating a meaning for the illness event that preserves a sense of mastery over their lives, (2) grieving for the loss of the family identity before illness, (3) moving toward a position of accepting permanent change while maintaining a sense of continuity between the past and the future, (4) pulling together to undergo short-term crisis reorganization, and (5) developing family flexibility about future goals (Rolland, 1988). Understanding the work of families during the crisis phase of illness should serve to remind nurses to maintain open and caring relationships with them, as well as caution nurses to respond in a positive and sympathetic way to potential manifestations of erratic or angry family behavior.

Nurses around the world have investigated the needs of families facing acute or life-threatening illness (Molter, 1979; Leske, 1986; McLennan, Anderson, & Pain, 1996; Wagner, 1996; Lindsay et al., 1997; Kosco & Warren, 2000; Leung, Chien, & Mackenzie, 2000; Lee & Lau, 2003). The following needs were found to be most important:

- To have questions answered honestly
- To know the facts about what is wrong with the patient
- To be informed about the patient's progress, outcome, and chance for recovery
- To be called at home about changes in the patient's condition
- To receive understandable explanations
- To receive information once a day
- To have hope
- To believe that hospital personnel care about the patient
- To have reassurance that the patient is receiving the best possible care
- To see the patient frequently

The following box summarizes these family needs (Leske, 1992). In general, families' needs in a critical care unit or during the acute illness period are similar, regardless of their age, gender, relationship to the patient, and patient diagnosis (Leske, 1991). A nurse supports the family by showing compassion, concern, and sensitivity to all family needs (Leske, 1992; Wesson, 1997).

Family Needs in Acute Care

Families who receive attentive nursing care will be able to provide better comfort to their ill relative, foster improvements in care, and augment the assessment skills of health care providers. Leske's five family need categories can be used to direct nursing interventions, which should begin on initial contact with family members (Titler, Bombei, & Schutte, 1995). Providing assurance entails establishing a calm and relaxed atmosphere that will support a trusting and

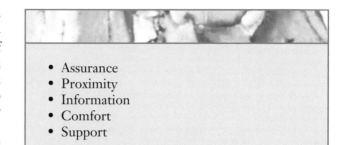

- Assurance
- Proximity
- Information
- Comfort
- Support

empathetic relationship (Leske, 1992). Enhancement of proximity means allowing family members to be near the patient by exercising flexible family visitation policies.

Information and Family Needs Studied

The need for information about the patient has been shown to be the number one identified need of families of critically ill patients, regardless of diagnosis or length of stay (Jastremski & Harvery, 1998). A study initiated to determine the level of satisfaction of family members with the care that they and their critically ill relative received found completeness of information to be associated with overall satisfaction (Heyland et al., 2002). Families require information not only upon admission and discharge but also throughout the course of the patient's stay in the hospital.

There are several ways to provide family information: educational orientation programs, classes that provide social support and information about illness management and recovery, informational packets, or unit tours. Learning the balance between too little and too much information and how to deliver it is an important skill for acute care nurses to learn (Goodell & Hanson, 1999). Additionally, nurses should consider the nature of the information to be conveyed to the family when deciding the best way to provide the information. In a study of 390 families of patients who died in an ICU, researchers found that the majority of the respondents (82.6 percent) expressed no criticism of the patient's hospital stay, 17 percent felt the information received concerning diagnosis was insufficient or unclear, and 30 percent expressed dissatisfaction regarding the information received on the cause of death (particularly among family members who were informed of the death by telephone and not in person) (Malacrida et al., 1998). A face-to-face meeting may best convey information about patient progress or prognosis, and perhaps information about self-management activities or visiting hours can be best addressed in a classroom setting or in a booklet. Investigators have tested the effectiveness of interventions to meet information needs. For example, Medland and Ferrans (1998) tested a structured communications program for family members to determine whether the program would increase family members' satisfaction with care, meet their needs for information better, and decrease disruption for the ICU nursing staff caused by incoming calls from family members. The intervention consisted of three components: (1) a discussion with a nurse approximately 24 hours after admission of the patient, (2) an informational pamphlet given at the time of the discussion, and (3) a daily telephone call from the nurse who was caring for the patient that day. The number of incoming calls from family members was significantly lower in the experimental group than in the control group. In the experimental group, satisfaction with care increased significantly from before to after the test, as did the members' perception of how well their information needs were being met (Medland & Ferrans, 1998).

Another group of investigators examined the effects of a communication team intervention on length of stay and costs for patients near the end of life in the intensive care unit (Ahrens, Yancey, & Kollef, 2003). The communication team—a physician and a clinical nurse specialist—provided daily medical updates, shared medical advice regarding treatment, and provided other information to families as needed. Compared with the control group, patients in the communication intervention group had significantly shorter stays in both the intensive care unit and the hospital and had lower fixed and variable costs. The researchers suggested that the provision of clear and direct information led to early discussion of options and support. As a result, more families elected to withhold life-prolonging treatments, resulting in decreased lengths of stays and costs.

Other findings suggest videotapes, nurse-coached volunteers, visual pamphlets, or individual counseling sessions as useful ways to impart information (Appleyard et al., 2000; Lenz & Perkins, 2000; Petterson, 2000; Oermann, Webb, & Ashare, 2003). Increasing numbers of nurses are evaluating technological methods to provide information to families. Technologies that are being explored to enhance communication with families, and to meet their information needs, include the Internet, pagers, e-mail, and telephone help lines (Carlsson, Strang, & Lindblad, 1996; Olson, 1997; Topp, Walsh, & Sanford, 1998; Brennan et al.,

2001; Jones & Brennan, 2002; Artinian et al., 2003). Before providing any information, however, it is important to use relevant cues to assess for illiteracy and modify methods of providing health information when appropriate (Artinian, Lange, Templin, Stallwood, & Hermann, 2003).

Culture and Expression of Family Needs

Family Need for Visitation during Hospitalization

Families of patients in hospitals, particularly in critical care units and emergency departments, spend a great deal of time waiting for news about their loved one. Waiting has been linked with dissatisfaction with health care services (Bruce, Bowman, & Brown, 1998). In a qualitative study designed to describe the experience of waiting, researchers found families were diligently watchful—not wanting to go far for fear of missing information (Bournes & Mitchell, 2002). Families reported the experience of waiting as "distressful," "horrible," "brutal," and "terrible."

Unfortunately, restrictive visiting policies exacerbate families' feelings of distress. During the period of acute illness, families usually encounter restrictive hospital visiting policies. They may not be able to visit their loved one in the hospital when it is convenient for them or when their work schedule permits, and frequently, they must rearrange their plans and routines to fit the policies set by the hospital. Originally, hospital visiting periods were limited so that the patient could rest and recover. However, a sound scientific basis for restricting visiting hours does not exist (Slota, Shearn, Potersnak, & Haas, 2003). In fact, one study found that "restricting visits to short time periods and terminating visits prematurely contribute to adverse hemodynamic responses in critically ill patients" (Titler & Walsh, 1992, p. 625). Another study found that patient control of family visiting in a coronary care unit (CCU) had positive effects (Lazure & Baun, 1995). Results showed that, over time, perceived control of visits and rests between visits were greater, and heart rate and diastolic blood pressure were lower, for subjects who used a visitor control device. Thus, a combination of patient and family factors may influence the nature of family visits in a CCU.

Research has uncovered several factors that should be considered when planning visiting periods with families (Clark, 1995; Gurley, 1995). Age, patients' personality characteristics, and patients' perceptions

Cultural affiliation may moderate the expression of family needs. One investigator compared African-American, Hispanic, and white family members' perceptions of the professional support they expect from critical care nurses during a family member's critical illness (Waters, 1999). In a sample of 90 family members, 30 from each cultural group, she found significant differences between the groups and suggested that critical care nurses develop interventions that respect the cultural uniqueness of family members. Interestingly, most of the white family members were wives of critically ill husbands with cardiac-related problems. African-American family members represented a variety of relatives, and responsibility for managing the physiological crisis was a collaborative effort, suggesting that critical care nurses be flexible and willing to communicate and interact with a variety of family members. In comparison to white family members, both African-American and Hispanic family members had significantly higher expectations for the critical care nurse to visit the waiting room at least once a shift to check out their concerns. In contrast to white and Hispanic family members, African-American family members had significantly lower expectations for critical care nurses to reassure them that their family member is stable enough that they could leave the waiting room or hospital for a while. Consistent with other findings in the literature, there was similarity across cultural groups. All wanted to be called at home about major changes, to have their questions answered honestly, or to be assured that their family member is receiving the best care. In sum, equitable care, dignity, and respect are universal values, but delivery of culturally effective family-centered care requires an appreciation and understanding of cultural diversity.

of the illness have been found to influence patients' visiting preferences (Simpson, 1991). For instance, older patients preferred longer visits, and extroverted patients preferred more frequent visits. Surprisingly, the more severely ill patients perceived themselves to be, the more visitors they preferred.

The diversity of patient responses to visiting policies suggests that policies should be tailored to patient and family preferences. Visiting preferences should be included in patient-family assessments (Hamner, 1990). One way to do this is to ascertain the answers to questions such as: How would you like visiting times to be handled while you are here? Who would you like to be allowed/disallowed to visit? When do you want to see visitors? How often? For how long? The answers to these questions help tailor visiting policies to meet patient-family needs.

Chronic Illness

Chronic illness imposes another set of concerns for families. A chronic illness refers to any physical or mental condition that requires long-term (more than 6 months) monitoring and/or management to control symptoms and to shape the course of the disease (Corbin, 2001). Many factors influence the effect of

chronic illness on families: the type of illness, the stage of illness, the structure of the family, the role of the patient, the life-cycle stage of the patient, and the life-cycle stage of the family (Biegel, Sales, & Schulz, 1991; Young, 1995).

The entire family system is affected when chronic illness strikes. "Normal patterns of interaction are disrupted, and there are often reassignments in tasks and roles assumed by particular family members" (Biegel, Sales, & Schulz, 1991). The family must reorganize itself around the chronic illness or disability (Steinglass, 1992). Families may make changes related to work schedules, household tasks, or provision of family income or in interpersonal areas, such as solidarity and belonging, sexuality, and love (Leventhal, Leventhal, & Nguyen, 1985).

Families and patients face both social and psychological challenges during the course of chronic illness (Hanson, 1988; Biegel, Sales, & Schulz, 1991). These include the following:

- Preventing medical crises and managing them once they occur
- Controlling symptoms
- Carrying out prescribed regimens
- Preventing or living with the sense of isolation caused by lessened contact with others

- Adjusting to changes in the course of the disease
- Normalizing interactions with others and finding the necessary money to pay for treatments or to survive, despite partial or complete loss of employment
- Confronting attendant psychosocial, marital, and familial problems

Families in the chronic phase may have to deal with a member's illness for a long time—an illness that may be constant, progressive, or episodic in nature. A key family task is to maintain normal life in the "abnormal" presence of this chronic illness and the resulting heightened uncertainty (Rolland, 1988).

As they manage their family member's illness on a day-to-day basis, families become expert caregivers. Exacerbation of a chronic illness, when it leads to hospitalization, brings expert family caregivers in contact with the health care team. Researchers have analyzed relationships between the family and the health care team from the perspective of the family members and found that these relationships moved through three stages (Thorne & Robinson, 1988). These stages reflected shifts in family trust of health care professionals.

Family members who had not had much experience with chronic illness described the first stage, naive trusting. These family members trust that health care professionals have the same perspective about caring for their ill member that they did. Families believe that their involvement on a day-to-day basis as the primary health care providers will be acknowledged and respected and that professionals will be cooperative and collaborative. Family members naively trust that health care professionals will act in their ill member's best interests. Over time, however, family members learn that their long experience is often disregarded, as is their involvement and expertise in illness management.

The second stage, the disenchantment phase, is characterized by dissatisfaction with care, frustration, and fear. Families find that it is difficult to be effectively involved in care because they have difficulty obtaining information. As trust diminishes, family relationships with health care professionals become adversarial, and families see their ill member as vulnerable and needing protection.

During the last stage, the guarded alliance phase, families renegotiate trust with health care professionals. They actively seek information and understand the differences in their perspective and that of health care professionals. Families are able to state clearly their own expectations and perceptions, an ability that leads to more satisfying care. Families and health care professionals develop a partnership in care. Nevertheless, families still experience the frustration of waiting, fear that they will not know the right questions to ask, and anger at the recognition that their own expertise is devalued.

Interventions for families experiencing chronic illness may focus on the family's cognitive, affective, and behavioral levels of functioning (Boise, Heagerty, & Eskenazi, 1996; Wright & Leahey, 2000). Cognitive interventions include giving information about the chronic illness and its treatment, giving advice about potential family responses to the illness (e.g., need for respite, possible strain on family relationships), giving information about community resources, and helping with family decision making.

Affective interventions are designed to modify intense emotions, such as guilt or anger, which may block a family's problem-solving efforts (Wright & Leahey, 2000). They include validating family members' emotional responses and helping them understand that those responses are normal, discussing with families ways to reduce their isolation, referring families to an appropriate support group, helping families open channels of communication, and helping families identify and mobilize their strengths and resources. A family's response of denial or lack of hope in the future has been identified as a major obstacle to successful patient adaptation. The hopeless family may be unable to make the necessary changes at home or learn the important aspects of the patient's care. Nurses should devise hope-facilitating strategies.

Interventions targeted at behavioral functioning are designed to help family members interact more effectively (Wright & Leahey, 2000). This goal can be accomplished by assigning specific behavioral tasks to some or all family members (Leahey & Wright, 1987; Wright & Leahey, 2000). In a recent study of 40 family members of patients 65 years or older who had been hospitalized for more than 2 days, the investigator found that 95 percent of family members preferred to participate in care and daily care activities (Li, 2002). Families may need help to coordinate responsibilities for particular caregiving activities (Gilliss, Rose, Hallburg, & Martinson, 1989). They may also need caregiving training to feel comfortable with the tasks at hand.

Other nursing interventions may be directed toward helping health care personnel work with families who are coping with chronic illness. Nurses need first to recognize the stage of their relationship (naive trust, disenchantment, or guarded alliance) with these families. Activities to promote cooperative caring must be negotiated between the nurse and the family. Being sensitive to what caregivers have experienced before hospitalization and recognizing their experience are essential to this process. Helping families access the information they need is also important; in fact, it is a prerequisite to developing a shared understanding that will help in the development of agreed-upon goals (Thorne & Robinson, 1988).

Caring for families with chronic illness presents many challenges for medical-surgical nurses. The problems and concerns that families experience differ from those in the acute illness stage. Nurses need to keep these differences in mind as they plan care.

End-of-Life Care

Sometimes nurses in medical-surgical settings encounter families who are coping with patients at the end of life. Knowledge about the process of dying can help nurses work effectively with families during this very difficult time. Family members have reported the experiences of a family member's death as including a downward spiral of prognoses, difficult decisions, feelings of inadequacy, eventual loss despite the members' best efforts, and perhaps no good-byes (Kirchhoff et al., 2002). The more the nurse knows about the family, the better, because the way a family deals with death is affected by cultural background, stage in the life cycle, values and beliefs, the nature of the illness, whether the loss is sudden or expected, the role played by the dying person in the family, and the emotional functioning of the family before the illness (Rosen, 1990; Leonard, Enzle, McTavish, Cumming, & Cumming, 1995). This knowledge of families will help nurses provide more-sensitive care as they move through the phases of end-of-life adaptation.

Phases of Adaptation

Families move through three phases of adaptation in response to the news that a family member has a fatal illness (Rosen, 1990). Various emotional responses may emerge during these phases, including disorganization, anxiety, emotional lability, or turning inward. The first phase is the preparatory phase. This phase begins when symptoms first appear and it continues through the initial diagnosis. During the preparatory phase, families experience fear and denial and may refuse to accept the prospect of death. Some family members decide to withhold all information from those whom they consider vulnerable, such as children or elderly parents (Rosen, 1990). During the period of initial symptoms, diagnosis, and treatment plan, the family may be highly disorganized and display emotional instability.

Once the family accepts the prospect of loss and begins to live with the reality of the fatal illness and the caretaking tasks of the illness, it moves into the middle phase. Families live the day-to-day challenge of dealing with physical symptoms, treatment, and care (Rosen, 1990). The family becomes less disorganized; indeed, it reorganizes to assume new roles. On the other hand, the tedium of daily care may tax the physical and financial resources of the family. If hospitalizations are lengthy or frequent, the logistics of visitation may create discord among family members (Rosen, 1990)—some members of the family may feel that others are visiting too little or too much—and unresolved family issues from the past may emerge.

The final stage, acceptance, arrives when the family accepts the imminent death and concludes the process of saying farewell. Family emotions that surfaced during the first phase but subsided during the middle phase may resurface. Family members may draw together in anticipation of their loved one's death (Rosen, 1990).

Nurses can help families with a dying relative by informing them that it is natural to pass through phases of adaptation and that they can expect to address complex issues in each phase of a fatal illness. Helping families accept their feelings and directing them to appropriate resources, such as a hospice, family support groups, social workers, and family conferences, may be useful.

Meeting Family Needs Before Death

Meeting family needs is also important. Needs of families of dying patients include the following:

1. To be with the dying person and to provide help to the dying person
2. To be informed of the dying person's changing condition and to understand what is being done to the patient and why
3. To be assured of the patient's comfort and to be comforted
4. To ventilate emotions and to be assured that their decisions were right
5. To find meaning in the dying of their loved one

6. To be fed, hydrated, and rested (Truog et al., 2001)

Although not always possible, a private room is most conducive to family emotional and physical intimacy. Usual restrictions on visitation should be relaxed as much as possible. Providing the family with an electronic pager or cellular phone may allow family members to take a break for a while without feeling out of contact (Truog et al., 2001). Attention to family well-being by providing tissues, blankets, coffee, and water is also important (Truog et al., 2001).

It is important to provide explanation about how the patient will die and what it may look like. In a descriptive study, intensive care unit nurses were asked how they prepared families for the death of their patient following withdrawal of mechanical ventilation (Kirchhoff, Conradt, & Anumandia, 2003). Forty-three descriptors were identified, of which 67.5 percent were physical sensations and symptoms. In describing dying, nurses reported telling family members about breathing patterns, sound during breathing, effort associated with breathing, skin color and temperature (e.g., pale, moist, clammy), sleepiness or decreased responsiveness, spastic movements, loss of bowel control/incontinence, and altered pupillary responses to light. The possibility of transferring the patient to another room was mentioned, and removal of unnecessary equipment was also identified.

Meeting Family Needs Following Death

Following the death, it is important to allow enough time for questions, allow the family the opportunity to view the body, and describe the events at the time of death, while conveying sensitivity and caring (Swanson, 1993; Leash, 1996). Buchanan, Geubtner, and Snyder (1996) demonstrated the importance of specialized follow-up care for surviving family members and loved ones during the year after death. Sudden, traumatic death leaves the survivors in shocked disbelief and intense emotional pain. Appropriate support and intervention can make a significant contribution to the family's eventual recovery by assisting in the normal grieving process and thus avoiding prolonged pathologic grieving (Buchanan, Geubtner, & Snyder, 1996).

Specific End-of-Life Issues

Caring for families when a member is dying is not easy. It is challenging for nurses to help families cope (Leonard, Enzle, McTavish, Cumming, & Cumming, 1995). Rarely do nurses feel comfortable and confident discussing death with patients or families. Several issues are especially difficult for nurses: discussion of use of life-saving or life-extending measures, discussion of withdrawal of life support, conveying news of sudden death, family presence during cardiopulmonary resuscitative efforts, and offering families the option of organ donation.

LIFE-SAVING OR LIFE-EXTENDING MEASURES

Frequently, illness occurs unexpectedly, and sometimes unprepared families must deal with illnesses or injuries where there is no hope for recovery. Families may have to abruptly make decisions regarding the use of life-saving or life-extending measures during the acute illness period. Patients and families may find themselves in a crisis situation with little time to discuss the options regarding life-saving measures or for making decisions about "do-not-resuscitate" (DNR) orders.

It would be ideal if health care professionals routinely discussed resuscitation preferences with patients while patients are competent to make such decisions. In reality, however, such discussions often do not take place, so health care professionals and families must make end-of-life decisions without the guidance of the patient. Families must decide between the uncertain outcomes of resuscitation and the certainty of death without resuscitation. Researchers have found that 86 percent of decisions regarding resuscitation measures involved the family, whereas only 22 percent of the patients were included in the decision making (Bedell, Pelle, Maher, & Cleary, 1986).

Several issues should be kept in mind with regard to DNR orders. First, physicians may discuss many variations of DNR orders with families. Sometimes it is appropriate, for example, to withhold chest compressions and intubation but still administer antiarrhythmic and vasopressor drugs. At other times, no life-saving measures may be administered. Nurses can help families by clarifying the various options presented to them and offering opportunities for discussion. Needless to say, decisions about DNR status are difficult to make.

The appropriate timing of discussion of DNR orders is also difficult for physicians to determine. Because nurses develop special insights as a result of the time they spend at the bedside getting to know the patient and family, they can help physicians schedule these important discussions.

Research findings suggest that four factors assisted families to make decisions about DNR status (Bedell, Pelle, Maher, & Cleary, 1986). First, an explanation of brain death criteria by the physician eased the family's ability to make a decision, as did the second factor, physician and nurse support for the family. Third, families wanted assurance that comfort measures would continue. Fourth, families found that any previous discussion they had had with the patient about life decisions was helpful in the decision-making process.

Withholding cardiopulmonary resuscitation is not the only difficult decision families are faced with. It is not uncommon during the course of stay in an ICU that hope for patient recovery fades and further treatment is considered futile. At this time, the focus of decision making changes from the pursuit of cure or recovery to the pursuit of comfort and freedom from pain until death. Decisions are needed about withdrawing treatments such as vasopressors and inotropic medication, intra-aortic balloon counterpulsation, mechanical ventilation, hemodialysis, total parenteral nutrition, and others. One study that examined deaths in an ICU over the course of a year found that 90 percent of the deaths involved withholding or withdrawing at least one life-support measure (Prendergast & Luce, 1997).

Studies have shown that less than 5 percent of ICU patients are able to communicate with health care providers at the time decisions are made about withholding or withdrawing life-sustaining therapies (Curtis et al., 2001). Health care providers must discuss these issues with family members at a time when they are under stress and struggling with making what may seem like an abrupt transition from having hope for recovery to dealing with impending death. Communication skills of nurses and physicians are critical during this time because withholding or withdrawing medical interventions involves detailed and complex conversations with patients' families (Curtis et al., 2001). Suboptimal communication can erode family trust and fuel disputes about futility of care (Fins & Solomon, 2001).

Family conferences have been suggested as one way to carry out these complex conversations with patients' families. Family conferences are attended by several members of the family and several members of the health care team (e.g., nurses, doctors, social workers, chaplain). Before these conferences, it is important for nurses to facilitate and coordinate conference planning by contacting family members and preparing them for discussion (Curtis et al., 2001).

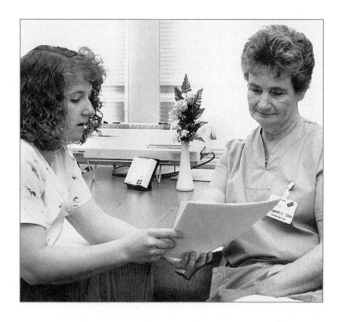

Following the conference, nurses assume responsibility for reinforcing the information given during the conference (Curtis et al., 2001). Other postconference activities include talking with family about how the conference went, asking family members whether they have questions, talking with the family members about changes in the patient's plan of care as a result of the conference or about their feelings, supporting decisions the family made at the conference, assuring the family that the patient will be kept comfortable, and locating a private room for family members to talk among themselves.

FAMILY PRESENCE DURING CARDIOPULMONARY RESUSCITATION (CPR)

During the acute illness period, the patient may suffer a sudden arrest of heartbeat and respiration, requiring cardiopulmonary resuscitation (CPR). When a patient has an arrest, the CPR team is called to the bedside. Physicians, nurses, and other health team members crowd around the patient to administer chest compressions, manually ventilate the patient, perform defibrillation, give drugs, or carry out other life-restoring activities. Until the patient's heart rhythm and respiration are restored, this is a tension-filled situation.

There is a growing acceptance that allowing families to witness resuscitation efforts is good practice (Meyers et al., 2000; Boudreaux, Francis, & Loyacano, 2002; Ardley, 2003). In 1994, the Emergency Nurses

Association (ENA) passed a resolution supporting family members at the bedside during invasive procedures and resuscitation (Boudreaux, Francis, & Loyacano, 2002). This resolution resulted in a 2001 position statement designed to assist the implementation of family presence into the practice (Emergency Nurses Association, 2001). There are advantages to having families present to watch nurses and physicians carry out resuscitative efforts. The advantages for families include the following:

- Recognizing that the patient is dying
- Feeling helpful and supportive to the patient and the staff
- Knowing that everything possible is being done
- Being able to touch the patient while he or she is still warm
- Saying whatever they need to say while there is still a chance that the patient can hear
- Recognizing the futility of further resuscitation efforts
- Facilitating the grieving process
- Accepting the reality of death (Emergency Nurses Association, 2001)

Family presence may eliminate the terrible fear of being left alone in a waiting room without knowing what is happening (Eichhorn, Meyers, Mitchell, & Guzzetta, 1996). Meyers and colleagues (2000) reported that of the 39 family members who were present for an invasive procedure or resuscitation, 95 percent said that the visitation helped them to comprehend the seriousness of the condition and to know that every possible intervention had been performed. Ninety-five percent also believed that their visit helped the patient.

On the other hand, some health care providers believe that there may be disadvantages to having families observe CPR (Boudreaux, Francis, & Loyacano, 2002; Ardley, 2003). Some clinicians believe that (1) the experience is traumatic and frightening to watch, (2) families may interfere with protocols and procedures, (3) there is not enough space at the patient's bedside for the CPR team as well as the family, (4) staff may become too stressed with family present, (5) there is an increased risk of liability, and (6) staff is not available to provide family information and support during the resuscitation (Emergency Nurses Association, 2001). However, data do not exist to support these fears. Investigators reported that there were no adverse psychological effects among family members and that the activities of health care providers were not disrupted when families were present (Belanger & Reed, 1997; Meyers et al., 2000).

Guidelines for nurses deciding when families are to be permitted in the patient's room during CPR include the following:

- Discussing the option with the family and giving them a description of what will be going on in the room
- Checking the code status with the doctor and the nurse in charge
- Assessing the room from the point of view of the family
- Accompanying the family member into the room to ensure that the family member gets an accurate explanation and has an appropriate perception of what is being done
- Not permitting family members to enter the code area while intravenous lines are being placed or while the patient is being intubated
- Letting family members in once the code is under way
- If a family member cannot handle the visit, escorting him or her from the room

Hopefully nurses will be sensitive to family needs during this stress-filled time and will consider the benefits and risks of witnessing CPR. Some families will not be able to cope with the experience, whereas others will not want to be involved. It is important to assess the family to determine whether their presence might be appropriate (Martin, 1991; Eichhorn, Meyers, Mitchell, & Guzzetta, 1996).

CULTURAL CONSIDERATIONS

Respecting the family's cultural background and use of rituals, customs, or styles to deal with death is important. For instance, in Western countries, enteral feeding is considered part of treatment. As many as 89 percent of American, 65 percent of British, and 56 percent of Belgian physicians have reported that withdrawal of feeding is acceptable; in a Japanese study, however, only 17 percent reported that they would withdraw artificial feeding (Vincent, 2001). Another example is that some Pacific Islanders may ask that a window remain open when a family member is dying, to allow the soul to leave (Mazanec & Tyler, 2003). A Muslim family might request that immediately after death, the patient's body be turned east to face Mecca, their holiest city (Mazanec & Tyler, 2003). Nurses cannot assume that families will respond to issues

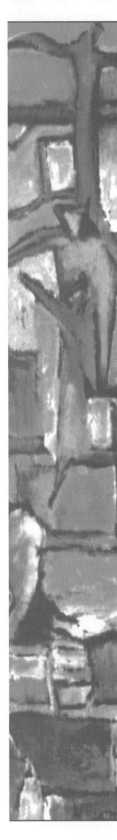

RESEARCH BRIEF

Purpose

The purpose of this study was to describe behavioral responses of family members of patients and the interactions of the family members with nurses and the patient in the trauma room.

Methods

A secondary analysis was done of 193 videotapes of trauma room care. Of these, 88 tapes showed the presence of patients' family members, for a total of 42 hours. A model of suffering served as a framework to assess behavioral and emotional states. Qualitative ethology, a method of identifying complex behaviors within the natural setting through observation and description, was used to analyze verbal and nonverbal interactions between nurses, patients' family members, and patients. Behaviors and verbal interactions of patients and their families were coded as to persons who were enduring and persons who were emotionally suffering.

Results

Whether a patient's family members entered the trauma room depended on the patient's condition, the patient's behavioral state, and the nature of the treatments. Categories of interactions included the following:

1. Learning to endure (i.e., the patient was unconscious and families stood distant from the stretcher, were trying to make sense of the situation, and looked to nurses for direction and guidance)
2. Patients failing to endure (i.e., family members were not usually admitted into the trauma room when patients were out of control; family members were admitted when patients were in pain or emotionally suffering, and family manifested enduring behaviors and tried to help patients endure)
3. Family emotionally suffering and patient enduring (i.e., family members were releasing emotion, and other family members, the patient, or the nurse attempted to ease their distress)
4. Patient and family enduring (i.e., patients and family members behaved stoically; interactions between the patient, family, and nurse were minimal; empathetic nurse responses led family member to transition to tears, withdrawal, and focus on self)
5. Resolution of enduring (i.e., when family members received news that the patient was no longer critical, an obvious release of tension occurred; family members moved into the waiting mode as they waited for the patient's transfer or discharge from the emergency department; nurses became attentive to family member needs)

Implications

These findings provide insight on which to base care of family members in an emergency department. The researchers recommended that the use of empathy is inappropriate with persons who are emotionally suppressing and are functioning in a stoic or enduring mode. These findings are also critical to the current debate on permitting family members to be present during emergency procedures.

Source: Morse, J. M., & Pooler, C. (2002) Patient-family-nurse interactions in the trauma-resuscitation room. *American Journal of Critical Care, 11*(3), 240–249.

surrounding death as they would. Cultural competence demands that nurses look at dying both through their own eyes and through the eyes of patients and their family members (Mazanec & Tyler, 2003).

CONVEYING NEWS OF DEATH

Family grief reactions manifest themselves as guilt, self-reproach, anxiety, loneliness, fatigue, shock, numbness, sleep and appetite disturbances, crying, overactivity, or confusion (Swanson, 1993). Informing the family of the death of a loved one is a challenging task. A health care professional's initial contact with the family about a death or about dying has a significant impact on the family's grief reaction. "Bad news, conveyed in an inappropriate, incomplete, or uncaring manner, may have long-lasting psychological effects on the family" (Swanson, 1993). In a survey of 54 family members of 48 patients who died in either an ICU or an emergency department, a caring attitude of the health care provider delivering the bad news was considered the most significant feature of giving bad news successfully (Jurkovich, Pierce, Pananen, & Rivara, 2000). Clarity of the message, privacy, and a news-giver who was knowledgeable and able to answer questions were also ranked as important. Touching was unwanted by 30 percent of the respondents but was encouraged or acceptable in 24 percent. Rank and attire of the news-giver were considered of little importance.

Communicating news about the death to a family should be done in person whenever possible (Truog et al., 2001). Ideally the news should be delivered in a private room that has seating available for everyone. It is important for health care providers to be attentive to their appearance, especially if they appear disheveled following resuscitative or other invasive procedures (Truog et al., 2001). Demonstrating compassion and empathy, avoiding clichés such as "He is at peace now," and avoiding unfamiliar jargon such as "code" or "vent" are important communication skills to remember.

Using the telephone to convey news of death must be considered carefully. A Gallup poll of a sample of adults living in the United States reported that when death of a family member was unexpected, 64 percent preferred to be told instead that the patient was critically ill and to come to the hospital immediately. Only 26 percent preferred to be given the news of death over the telephone (Truog et al., 2001). In a companion survey of physician practices, findings were very

similar. However, when death of the patient was expected, delivering the news of the death by telephone was more acceptable (Truog et al., 2001).

OFFERING THE OPTION OF ORGAN DONATION

Discussing organ donation with a family whose loved one has suddenly died is difficult. "Often the deceased is a young, previously healthy person who died suddenly in a tragic accident" (Hoffman & Malecki, 1990). The discussion about organ donation should take place separately from notification of the patient's death, and it should be done by someone specially trained in asking for organ and tissue donation (Truog et al., 2001). Federal regulations now stipulate that institutions are required to contact their local organ procurement organization (OPO) concerning any death or impending death (Truog et al., 2001). Once contacted, the OPO sends a representative to the hospital to ensure that the family will be approached at the appropriate time by a professional skilled in providing information about the option of organ donation and in accurately answering questions (Truog et al., 2001).

If organ donation is viewed as a consoling act, rather than as an imposition on a grieving family, offering the option of organ donation becomes easier. Organ donation benefits the family of the donor as well as the organ recipient. Hoffman and Malecki (1990) have noted that donation of organs can help families cope with their loss. Perceiving that organ donation can help someone else live, that functioning organs are not wasted, that something positive can come out of death, or that a family member can live on in someone else through donation can help families cope with their loss.

Common courtesy and sensitivity to the family's grief are important (Siminoff, 1997). The following have been found to facilitate offering of the option of organ donation:

- Using a private area
- Clearly communicating about the loved one's death
- Allowing family time to absorb the news regarding their loved one's death before asking about donation
- Assuring the family that the decision is theirs to make
- Informing the family of the possible benefits of donation

- Providing information that will assuage the family's fears regarding donation (Siminoff, 1997)
- Providing time for families to be with their loved ones and to decide about their options (Exley, White, & Martin, 2002).

Many families worry that donation is disfiguring or delays the funeral—neither is true (Siminoff, 1997). Finally, families may be confused about the costs of donation and need to be informed that the organ procurement agencies pay for all costs pertaining to the maintenance or removal of the donor organs once the family has agreed to donation (Siminoff, 1997).

PREPARING FOR PATIENT DISCHARGE

Although hospitalization is stressful for families, leaving the hospital is also stressful. Because of the prospective payment system and other efforts to control health care costs, patients are discharged quickly from the hospital (Feigin, Cohen, & Gilad, 1998). Consequently, patients and families must manage most of the patient's recovery at home. Families are even being prepared to handle very technical aspects of care, such as home mechanical ventilation for chronic respiratory failure (Glass, Grap, & Battle, 1999). Early discharge requires careful attention to discharge planning to help patients and families anticipate problems after discharge.

Numerous investigators have described the preparation of patients for discharge. Feigin and colleagues (1998) described the use of one-session group meetings to help families reduce anxieties over discharge and increase their capabilities to organize and cope with discharge. Another option is to implement an education-intensive unit incorporating a live-in family member or friend acting as a care partner, who assumes responsibility for administering all medications as a way of reducing medication error rates (Phelan, Kramer, Grieco, & Glassman, 1996). Active family participation in hospital care delivery has been found to result in fewer depressive symptoms among patients during hospitalization and at 2 weeks and 2 months posthospitalization than among a comparison group of patients (Li et al., 2003). Family caregivers also reported significantly more role rewards than comparison caregivers did at 2 weeks after hospital discharge.

Four Factors Needed for Discharge

Four factors reported by spouses as helpful in readying them for their partner's hospital discharge include (1) availability of social support, (2) use of coping strategies, (3) personal resources, and (4) knowledge of what to expect (Artinian, 1993). Consideration of these four factors suggests ways to prepare other types of families for discharge.

Social Support

Available social support can include persons who are available to give necessary information about recovery at home before discharge. Such information should include the trajectory of an uncomplicated recovery, how to distinguish between normal and unusual symptoms during recovery, signs and symptoms of complications, and activities family members can do to make the patient comfortable. Giving a phone number of someone the family can call if they have concerns is also helpful. Supplying bandages, canes, medicines, or other materials to families before they go home may be of assistance, because families do not want to have to run to the store and leave the patient alone. Post-discharge contact also may support family management of recovery at home. Telephone contact and Internet-based strategies may be useful for doing this (Darkins & Cary, 2000).

Coping Skills

Families need coping skills to manage recovery at home. These skills include problem-solving ability, ability to seek help if needed, ability to manage worry and anxiety, and ability to acquire needed information. Nurses need to assess family coping strategies to devise interventions that will fit the individual family's needs.

Personal Resources

Four categories of personal resources can help family members feel ready to take a patient home from the hospital. These categories—health and energy, time, self-confidence, and positive beliefs (Artinian, 1993)—need to be assessed by the nurse. For example, if the family member taking the patient home has numerous chronic health problems leaving him with feelings of fatigue, discharge activities and recovery at home may seem overwhelming. Assessing family members' perceptions of their own health may indicate whether the family needs additional help to manage care at home. Families who lack time to prepare for discharge because of multiple responsibilities may need encouragement to arrange for help or to plan ahead. Assessing family confidence about recovery and managing caregiving activities at home may be beneficial. Or, if a family member does not have positive beliefs about the patient's recovery and does not believe the patient is physically ready to go home, he also will not feel ready. Because optimistic beliefs can help families feel ready for discharge, it is useful to point out to families the positive signs of recovery.

Knowledge of What to Expect

The goal of preparing families for discharge is to help them know what to expect and how to assist in the patient's recovery. Inadequate preparation for discharge can contribute to hospital readmission (Martens & Mellor, 1997). Making the necessary arrangements for home care visits may complement discharge preparation.

NURSING IMPLICATIONS

The body of knowledge about medical-surgical nursing is growing, and there are many opportunities for nurses to apply this knowledge to practice, further research, education, and health policy.

Practice

In practice, medical-surgical nurses must intervene with families during all phases of an illness. "Nursing interventions for families are nursing treatments that assist families and their members to promote, attain, or maintain optimal health and functioning or to experience a peaceful death" (Craft & Willadsen, 1992). Craft and Willadsen have identified nine categories of family nursing interventions: family support, family process maintenance, promotion of family integrity, family involvement, family mobilization, caregiver support, family therapy, sibling support, and parent education. Only the first six apply to nurses in medical-surgical settings and are described in more detail in the following sections. Given the growing number of elderly Americans and the associated growth of hospitalizations due to chronic illnesses (Centers for Disease Control and Prevention, 2003; Hajjar & Kotchen, 2003), these interventions require age-specific considerations to meet the needs of aged family members.

Support

Families in medical-surgical settings are experiencing life changes and stressors and are frequently in need of support. Nurses can support the family in several ways:

- Use effective, open, and honest communication, by listening to family concerns, feelings, and questions and answering all questions or assisting the family to get answers
- Help the family acquire information
- Respect and support family coping mechanisms
- Foster realistic hope
- Assist families to make decisions through providing information about options
- Provide opportunities to visit
- Arrange family conferences to allow ventilation of family feelings
- Permit the family to make some decisions about patient care
- Clarify information

Flexible visiting hours, information booklets or flyers, and a caring attitude are practical and specific ways to support families (Henneman & Cardin, 2002). Family support groups may provide the opportunity for participants to share common experiences, build mutual support, express common concerns, foster a sense of hope, reduce anxiety, and obtain information common to the group's needs (Leske & Heidrich, 1996). Some older family members, however, may feel that sharing feelings, personal issues, and private family matters is unacceptable; thus, a support group may not be a beneficial intervention for an aged family member (Leske & Heidrich, 1996). Support groups may be more acceptable if the content focuses on information and tasks rather than on sharing feelings and concerns (Leske & Heidrich, 1996).

Process Maintenance

The illness and hospitalization of a family member upsets family routines and activities. Identifying how the acute illness episode has altered family roles and consequently disrupted typical family processes is a necessary part of maintaining family process. Offering flexible opportunities for visiting will help to meet the needs of family members and patients and can also promote maintenance of typical family processes. Family members may want to discuss with the nurse other strategies for normalizing family life.

Promotion of Integrity

Stressful hospitalizations may adversely affect the emotional bonding that family members have with one another. Nurses can promote family cohesion and unity by allowing for family visitation and facilitating open communication among family members. Scheduling a family conference to encourage all family members to voice their concerns about care management to one another and to the health care team is a way to facilitate open communication. Telling family members that it is safe and acceptable to use typical expressions of affection may also be appreciated. For example, a wife may appreciate knowing that she will not disrupt the technological equipment at her husband's bedside or disrupt equipment attached to his body if she kisses his cheek or holds his hand. Providing opportunities for private family visits can make the visits more satisfying.

Involvement

Providing physical care to their loved one during hospitalization may comfort family members, especially if the family members routinely provided physical care for the patient at home. Before encouraging family members to become involved in patient care, however, it is important to identify the family's preferences, the patient's preferences, and family members' capabilities. Family members can be involved with care in a number of ways, such as helping during mealtimes, assisting with brushing teeth, and assisting with patient positioning or range of motion.

Mobilization

Family caregivers may be experts in caring for the patient because of their many years of experience with a chronic illness. Nurses should acknowledge this family expertise and use the family's strengths through family mobilization techniques. For example, two ways to mobilize families include discussing how family strengths and resources can be used to enhance the health of the patient and establishing realistic goals with the patient and family. Collaborating with family members in planning and implementing patient therapies and lifestyle changes is another. Families may want to share information about the patient's favorite position when lying in bed, preferences in music, bedtime habits, or preferred comfort measures. Determining family cultural practices and incorporating them into plans for care is yet another way to mobilize the strengths of the family.

Caregiver Support

Frequently illnesses or injuries require patients to have an extensive period of recovery or time for adaptation to end-of-life at home. This period may be taxing on family members who are providing care as well as trying to fulfill other responsibilities of their daily life. Attentiveness to caregiver support is an important part of medical-surgical nursing. Caregiver support may include provision of the necessary information for providing care, supporting the caregiver through the grieving process, providing for follow-up health caregiver assistance through telephone calls and/or community nurse care, teaching caregiver strategies to access and maximize health care and community resources, or encouraging caregiver participation in support groups.

Education

It is no longer appropriate to study medical-surgical nursing only from the perspective of individual patient care. Faculty need to clearly define family health care practice in medical-surgical settings (Hanson & Heims, 1992) and incorporate family care into medical-surgical nursing courses and appropriate practice settings. Family assessment frameworks that lead to specific strategies for intervention also need attention in medical-surgical nursing curriculums (Hanson & Heims, 1992). Relegating the bulk of family content to specialty courses, such as community health nursing or childbearing family nursing, misleads students about the practice of family nursing. Nursing staff on medical-surgical units also need to be educated about family nursing, especially because many staff members were educated at a period when family nursing was not considered important in medical-surgical settings.

Research

Identifying family practice problems (e.g., difficulties associated with delivering care to families) and investigating the validity, relevance, cost, and benefits of potential solutions to those problems will help promote research-based practice (McCaughan, Thompson, Cullum, Sheldon, & Thompson, 2002). Designing, implementing, and testing family nursing interventions will foster the growth of medical-surgical family nursing knowledge. However, research findings about families become valuable to families only after they pass through the research utilization process. The goal of research utilization is to improve nursing care, which results in optimal family outcomes. Through research utilization, knowledge about families that is obtained from research is transferred into clinical practice. Nurses who seek to improve family care through research utilization engage in critically analyzing research literature about families, select from the literature interventions that are appropriate for their practice setting, implement the interventions, and then evaluate the family outcomes.

Health/Social Policy

Health care policies clearly influence nursing practice. Family nursing practice in medical-surgical settings can be enhanced through hospital and unit-based philosophy statements that include the family. Programs related to meeting the needs of family members should include every member of the health care team, including unit secretaries, security guards, volunteers, housekeepers, and aides (Henneman & Cardin, 2002). Policies about family visitation, family participation in care, family presence during CPR, families staying overnight in patient rooms, and families bringing in favorite foods should be evaluated in light of a family care philosophy.

In addition to advocating for families within hospitals, medical-surgical nurses should strive to assume leadership responsibilities as legislative advocates. Medical-surgical nurses are capable of providing leadership in solving the problems of our health care system that affect families requiring hospitalization and home care. Changes in public policy are needed to address issues such as the growing disparities in health care, difficulty accessing health care, lack of insurance to cover the costs of expensive medications, safe workplace environments, and others. There are several ways that medical-surgical nurses can be involved, such as by joining the American Nurses Association, keeping informed about legislative activities, or communicating with legislators by writing letters, making telephone calls, or sending e-mails.

SUMMARY

- Family members who receive care are more likely to be empowered to deal with the stressors associated with hospitalization of a family member and are therefore better prepared to provide support to patients and aid in their recovery.

- Interventions tailored for specific families need to consider the nature of the illness, characteristics of the family, the health care team's philosophy about family care, and the characteristics of the patient.
- Promoting the health of family members by focusing on the prevention of illness related to the stress of hospitalization is an important part of medical-surgical nursing.
- Family care during acute illness includes providing assurance, enhancing proximity of the patient and family, providing clear and understandable information, answering questions, facilitating comfort, and reinforcing support.
- During chronic illness episodes, it is important to acknowledge family experiences with illness management, address family concerns, and enhance knowledge and resources relative to care requirements.
- Care at the end of life includes helping family move through the phases of adaptation to death, facilitating family presence during cardiopulmonary resuscitation, assisting families to make decisions about end-of-life issues such as withdrawal of life support, conveying news of death, and assisting in a request for organ donation.
- Availability of social support, use of coping strategies, availability of personal resources, and knowing what to expect once at home positively influence a family's perception of readiness for hospital discharge.
- Excellent communication skills and positive nurse-family relationships are essential during all phases of care.
- Family support, family process maintenance, promotion of family integrity, family involvement, family mobilization, and caregiver support are nursing interventions to consider in any illness stage.
- Family-centered care in medical-surgical settings is dependent on hospital policies and procedures that consider the needs of families.
- Growing disparities in health care, difficulty accessing health care, lack of insurance to cover the costs of expensive medications, safe workplace environments, and other concerns of our health care system demand that nurses become legislative advocates on behalf of patients and their families requiring care in medical-surgical settings.

CASE STUDY ➤

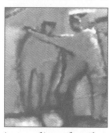

Robert Johnson, a 26-year-old single African-American teacher, received a diagnosis of AIDS a year ago. He has been HIV-positive for 4 years. His only known risk factor for AIDS is promiscuous homosexual activity when he was younger. Robert's immediate family consists of his mother Deborah and his sister Tomika. Robert's family members were deeply saddened when they learned he had AIDS. They believed he would die before he could accomplish what he wanted to do with his life. Soon after Robert's diagnosis, Tomika noticed frequent mood swings in her mother, and they began to have constant arguments over small things.

Robert regularly experiences night sweats, fatigue, and weakness, and he has ongoing weight loss, diarrhea, and malaise. Yesterday, he was admitted to the hospital for a diagnostic bronchoscopy to determine the cause of his persistent nonproductive cough, dyspnea, tachypnea, fever, chills, and chest pain. He had had one episode of Pneumocystis carinii pneumonia (PCP) in the past and was at that time diagnosed with AIDS. For the last year, Robert has feared that the next opportunistic infection would bring about his death.

Before his diagnosis, Robert was a healthy, active man. He became debilitated and has been unable to work because of extreme fatigue. He recently moved back to his mother's home and is dependent on his mother and sister for help with activities of daily living. Deborah left her job as a grocery store cashier, in part to care for Robert's care and in part because she found it difficult to deal with her coworkers' concerns that she was handling food. Tomika is single and a student. She is angered by the fact that her friends distanced themselves from her after she told them about her brother's illness. Her anger is compounded by guilt and fear: guilt because she once rejected her homosexual brother and fear because she is concerned that she may get AIDS from spending so much time caring for Robert.

Robert underwent bronchoscopy without complications. The bronchial biopsy confirmed PCP. To treat the causative organism, Robert was placed on intravenous pentamidine isethionate (Pentam), an antiprotozoal drug used to fight PCP infections. After a brief stay in the ICU, Robert was transferred to one of the hospital's medical units. Because his arterial oxygen levels continued to be low, he was given oxygen supplementation. Other care included liquid nutritional supplements, positioning in semi-Fowler's to high Fowler's position, and frequent nose and mouth care to prevent candidiasis, and his activities were clustered so that there would be periods of time to designate as rest periods.

Throughout his hospital stay, Robert's mother and sister felt that no one listened to them. They wanted to talk to the doctor and nurse every day about Robert's condition, but this never seemed possible. At times, the family felt that the staff was afraid of Robert because staff members rarely came into the room and stood at the door of the room to talk to them. Sometimes the family waited 20 minutes for Robert's light to be answered. Robert's mother was bothered by the fact that bedclothes and linens were moist from Robert's fever and sweats. She wondered why the staff did not change his gown and sheets more often.

Robert was discharged from the hospital 3 weeks after his admission. Six months later, he contracted PCP again. He was readmitted to the hospital, where he died 3 days later of respiratory failure. Deborah, Tomika, and their minister were at his bedside when he died. Nurses noted that the family appeared to accept the reality of Robert's death and mobilized themselves to participate in Robert's funeral and other tasks that would ensure their ultimate adjustment.

Discussion This case study describes how one African-American family, the Johnsons, experienced the various phases of a chronic illness and death. Describe family-focused care for the Johnsons.

STUDY QUESTIONS

1. Compare and contrast the impact of illness in the following two family situations:
   a. School teacher, married and the mother of two teenage daughters, who was hospitalized due to numbness in her lower extremities and subsequently diagnosed with multiple sclerosis
   b. Forty-five-year-old male, married and the father of a 6-year-old boy, who was diagnosed with an acute myocardial infarction and hospitalized suddenly for a percutaneous transluminal coronary angioplasty (PTCA) and stent insertion

2. Mrs. L is a 29-year-old woman who, 7 weeks ago, fell from a fourth-floor balcony while attempting to retrieve her cat and was admitted to the neurosurgical unit with severe head injuries that have resulted in a sustained coma. Twice in the first 2 weeks of her admission, and once in the sixth week, she suffered cardiorespiratory arrest and was successfully resuscitated. The neurosurgical team believes that her coma is irreversible and wants to recommend no further resuscitations. How can nurses prepare and assist Mrs. L's husband and parents with discussions about do-not-resuscitate orders?

TEACHING STRATEGIES

Assign students to carry out one of the following activities as a basis for writing a paper or for discussion in class.

1. Interview medical-surgical nurses about the experiences they have had with families on the patient care units where they work.

2. Assign students to ask nurses for copies of family-centered care policies and procedures from their medical-surgical patient care units and hospital where they work. Compare and contrast the policies and procedures.

3. Write a family-centered care philosophy statement for a medical-surgical patient care unit.

4. Interview a family member about their experience during a visit to an emergency department or hospital with another adult member of their family. What are their positive memories about the experience? Negative memories? What advice do they have for health care providers?

5. Assemble a panel of family members to give short presentations about their acute, chronic, and/or end-of-life illness experiences relative to the hospitalization of a family member.

References

Ahrens, T., Yancey, V., & Kollef, M. (2003). Improving family communications at the end of life: Implications for length of stay in the intensive care unit and resource use. *American Journal of Critical Care, 12*(4), 317–324.

Appleyard, M. E., Gavaghan, S. R., Gonzalez, C., Ananian, L., Tyrell, R., & Carroll, D. L. (2000). Nurse-coached interventions for families of patients in critical care units. *Critical Care Nurse, 20*(3), 40–48.

Ardley, C. (2003). Should relatives be denied access to the resuscitation room? *Intensive & Critical Care Nursing, 19*, 1–10.

Artinian, N. T. (1993). Spouses' perceptions of readiness for discharge after cardiac surgery. *Applied Nursing Research, 6*, 80–88.

Artinian, N. T., Harden, J. K., Kronenberg, M. W., Vander Wal, J. S., Daher, E., Stephens, Q., et al. (2003). Pilot study of a Web-based compliance monitoring device for patients with congestive heart failure. *Heart & Lung, 32*(4), 226–233.

Artinian, N. T., Lange, M. P., Templin, T. N., Stallwood, L. G., & Hermann, C. E. (2003). Functional health literacy in an urban primary care clinic. *The Internet Journal of Advanced Nursing Practice, 5*(3).

Bedell, S., Pelle, D., Maher, P., & Cleary, P. (1986). Do-not-resuscitate orders for critically ill patients in the hospital. *Journal of the American Medical Association, 256*, 233–237.

Belanger, M., & Reed, S. (1997). A rural community hospital's experience with family-witnessed resuscitation. *Journal of Emergency Nursing, 23*(3), 238–239.

Bengston, A., Karlsson, T., Wahrborg, P., Hjalmarson, A., & Herlitz, J. (1996). Cardiovascular and psychosomatic symptoms among relatives of patients waiting for possible coronary revascularization. *Heart & Lung, 25*(6), 438–443.

Biegel, D. E., Sales, E., & Schulz, R. (1991). *Family caregiving in chronic illness.* Newbury Park, CA: Sage.

Boise, L., Heagerty, B., & Eskenazi, L. (1996). Facing chronic illness: The family support model and its benefits. *Patient Education & Counseling, 27*(1), 75–84.

Boudreaux, E. D., Francis, J. L., & Loyacano, T. (2002). Family presence during invasive procedures and resuscitations in the emergency department: A critical review and suggestions for future research. *Annals of Emergency Medicine, 40*(2), 193–205.

Bournes, D. A., & Mitchell, G. J. (2002). Waiting: The experience of persons in a critical care waiting room. *Research in Nursing & Health, 25*, 58–67.

Bovbjerg, V. E., McCann, B. S., Brief, D. J., Follette, W. C., Retzlaff, B. M., Dowdy, A. A., et al. (1995). Spouse support and long-term adherence to lipid-lowering diets. *American Journal of Epidemiology, 141*(5), 451–460.

Brennan, P. F., Moore, S. M., Bjornsdottir, G., Jones, J., Visovsky, C., & Rogers, M. (2001). HeartCare: An Internet-based information and support system for patient home recovery after coronary artery bypass graft (CABG) surgery. *Journal of Advanced Nursing, 35*(5), 699–708.

Bruce, T. A., Bowman, J. M., & Brown, S. T. (1998). Factors that influence patient satisfaction in the emergency department. *Journal of Nursing Care Quality, 13*(2), 31–37.

Buchanan, H. L., Geubtner, M. D., & Snyder, C. K. (1996). Trauma bereavement program: A review of development and implementation. *Critical Care Nursing Quarterly, 19*, 35–44.

Carlsson, M. E., Strang, P. M., & Lindblad, L. (1996). Telephone help line for cancer counseling and cancer information. *Cancer Practice, 4*(6), 319–323.

Centers for Disease Control and Prevention (2003). Public health and aging: Hospitalizations for stroke among adults aged > 65 years—United States, 2000. *MMWR Weekly, 52*, 586–589.

Clark, S. P. (1995). Increasing the quality of family visits to the ICU. *Dimensions of Critical Care Nursing, 14*(4), 200–212.

Corbin, J. M. (2001). Introduction and overview: Chronic illness and nursing. In R. B. Hyman & J. M. Corbin (Eds.), *Chronic illness: Research and theory for nursing practice* (pp. 1–15). New York: Springer.

Craft, M. J., & Willadsen, J. A. (1992). Interventions related to family. *Nursing Clinics of North America, 27*, 517–540.

Curtis, J. R., Patrick, D. L., Shannon, S. E., Treece, P. D., Engelberg, R. A., & Rubenfeld, G. D. (2001). The family conference as a focus to improve communication about end-of-life care in the intensive care unit: Opportunities for improvement. *Critical Care Medicine, 29* (2 [Suppl.]), N26–N33.

Daly, M. B., Barsevick, A., Miller, S. M., Buckman, R., Costalas, J., Montgomery, S., et al. (2001). Communicating genetic test results to the family: A six-step skills-building strategy. *Family & Community Health, 24*(3), 13–26.

Darkins, A. W., & Cary, M. A. (2000). *Telemedicine and telehealth.* New York: Springer.

Denham, S. (2003). Categories of family health routines. In S. Denham (Ed.), *Family health: A framework for nursing* (pp. 178–192). Philadelphia: FA Davis.

Driscoll, K. M. (1998). The application of genetic knowledge: Ethical and policy implications. *AACN Clinical Issues, 9*(4), 588–599.

Eichhorn, D. J., Meyers, T. A., Mitchell, T. G., & Guzzetta, C. (1996). Opening the doors: Family presence during resuscitation. *Journal of Cardiovascular Nursing, 10*(4), 59–70.

Emergency Nurses Association (2001). *Family presence at the bedside during invasive procedures and resuscitation.* Des Plaines, IL: Emergency Nurses Association.

Exley, M., White, N., & Martin, J. H. (2002). Why families say no to organ donation. *Critical Care Nurse, 22*(6), 44–51.

Feigin, R., Cohen, I., & Gilad, M. (1998). The use of single-group sessions in discharge planning. *Social Work in Health Care, 26*(3), 19–38.

Fins, J. J., & Solomon, M. Z. (2001). Communication in intensive care settings: The challenge of futility disputes. *Critical Care Medicine, 29*(2 [Suppl.]), N10–N15.

Franks, M. M., Pienta, A. M., & Wray, L. A. (2002). It takes two: Marriage and smoking cessation in the middle years. *Journal of Aging & Health, 14*(3), 336–354.

Gilliss, C. L., Rose, D., Hallburg, J. C., & Martinson, I. M. (1989). The family and chronic illness. In C. L. Gilliss, B. L. Highley, B. M. Roberts, & I. M. Martinson (Eds.), *Toward a science of family nursing* (pp. 287–299). Menlo Park, CA: Addison-Wesley Publishing.

Glass, C., Grap, M. J., & Battle, G. (1999). Preparing the patient and family for home mechanical ventilation. *MEDSURG Nursing, 8*(2), 99–101, 104–107.

Goodell, T. T., & Hanson, S. M. H. (1999). Nurse-family interactions in adult critical care: A Bowen family systems perspective. *Journal of Family Nursing, 5*(1), 72–91.

Gurley, M. J. (1995). Determining ICU visiting hours. *MEDSURG Nursing, 4*(1), 40–43.

Hajjar, I., & Kotchen, T. A. (2003). Trends in prevalence, awareness, treatment, and control of hypertension in the United States, 1998–2000. *JAMA, 290*(2), 199–206.

Hamner, J. B. (1990). Visiting policies in the ICU: A time for change. *Critical Care Nurse, 10*, 48–53.

Hanson, S. M. H. (1988). Family nursing and chronic illness. In L. M. Wright & M. Leahey (Eds.), *Families and chronic illness* (pp. 2–32). Springhouse, PA: Springhouse.

Hanson, S. M. H., & Heims, M. L. (1992). Family nursing curricula in U.S. schools of nursing. *Journal of Nursing Education, 31*, 303–308.

Hathaway, D., Boswell, B., Stanford, D., Schneider, S., & Moncrief, A. (1987). Health promotion and disease prevention for the hospitalized patient's family. *Nursing Administration Quarterly, 11*(3), 1–7.

Henneman, E. A., & Cardin, S. (2002). Family-centered critical care. *Critical Care Nurse, 22*(6), 12–19.

Heyland, D. K., Rocker, G. M., Dodek, P. M., Kustsogiannis, D. J., Konopad, E., Cook, D. J., et al. (2002). Family satisfaction with care in the intensive care unit: Results of a multiple center study. *Critical Care Medicine, 30*(7), 1413–1418.

Hoffman, M., & Malecki, M. (1990). Organ procurement and preservation. In K. M. Sigardson-Poor & L. M. Haggerty (Eds.), *Nursing care of the transplant recipient* (pp. 13–34). Philadelphia: WB Saunders.

Holicky, R. (1996). Caring for the caregivers: The hidden victims of illness and disability. *Rehabilitation Nursing, 21*(5), 247–252.

Hupcey, J. E. (1998). Establishing the nurse-family relationship in the intensive care unit. *Western Journal of Nursing Research, 20*(2), 180–194.

Jastremski, C. A., & Harvery, M. (1998). Making changes to improve the intensive care unit experience for patients and their families. *New Horizons, 6*(1), 99–109.

Jones, J. F., & Brennan, P. F. (2002). Telehealth interventions to improve clinical nursing of elders. *Annual Review of Nursing Research, 20*, 293–322.

Jurkovich, G. J., Pierce, B., Pananen, L., & Rivara, F. P. (2000). Giving bad news: The family perspective. *The Journal of Trauma, Injury, Infection, and Critical Care, 48*(5), 865–873.

Kirchhoff, K. T., Conradt, K. L., & Anumandia, R. (2003). ICU nurses' preparation of families for death of patients following withdrawal of ventilator support. *Applied Nursing Research, 16*(2), 85–92.

Kirchhoff, K. T., Walker, L., Hutton, A., Spuhler, V., Cole, B. V., & Clemmer, T. (2002). The vortex: Families' experiences with death in the intensive care unit. *American Journal of Critical Care, 11*(3), 200–209.

Kosco, M., & Warren, N. A. (2000). Critical care nurses' perceptions of family needs as met. *Critical Care Nursing Quarterly, 23*(2), 60–72.

Lange, M. P. (2001). Family stress in the intensive care unit. *Critical Care Medicine, 29*(10), 2025–2026.

Lazure, L. L., & Baun, M. M. (1995). Increasing patient control of family visiting in the coronary care unit. *American Journal of Critical Care, 4*(2), 157–164.

Leahey, M., & Wright, L. M. (1987). Families and chronic illness: Assumptions, assessment and intervention. In L. M. Wright & M. Leahey (Eds.), *Families and chronic illness* (pp. 55–76). Springhouse, PA: Springhouse.

Leash, R. M. (1996). Death notification: Practical guidelines for health professionals. *Critical Care Nursing Quarterly, 19*(1), 21–34.

Lee, L. Y. K., & Lau, Y. L. (2003). Immediate needs of adult family members of adult intensive care patients in Hong Kong. *Journal of Clinical Nursing, 12*, 490–500.

Lenz, E. R., & Perkins, S. (2000). Coronary artery bypass graft surgery patients and their family member caregivers: Outcomes of a family-focused staged psychoeducational intervention. *Applied Nursing Research, 13*(3), 142–150.

Leonard, K. M., Enzle, S. S., McTavish, J., Cumming, C. E., & Cumming, D. C. (1995). Prolonged cancer death: A family affair. *Cancer Nursing, 18*(3), 222–227.

Leske, J. S. (1986). Needs of relatives of critically ill patients: A follow-up. *Heart & Lung, 15,* 189–193.

Leske, J. S. (1991). Internal psychometric properties of the Critical Care Family Needs Inventory. *Heart & Lung, 20,* 236–244.

Leske, J. S. (1992). Needs of adult family members after critical illness. *Critical Care Nursing Clinics of North America, 4,* 587–596.

Leske, J. S., & Heidrich, S. M. (1996). Interventions for aged family members. *Critical Care Clinics of North America, 8*(1), 91–102.

Leske, J. S., & Jiricka, M. K. (1998). Impact of family demands and strengths and capabilities on family well-being and adaptation after critical injury. *American Journal of Critical Care, 7*(5), 383–392.

Leung, K., Chien, W., & Mackenzie, A. E. (2000). Needs of Chinese families of critically ill patients. *Western Journal of Nursing Research, 22*(7), 826–840.

Leventhal, H., Leventhal, E. A., & Nguyen, T. V. (1985). Reactions of families to illness: Theoretical models and perspectives. In D. C. Turk & R. D. Kerns (Eds.), *Health, illness, and families* (pp. 108–145). New York: John Wiley & Sons.

Li, H. (2002). Family preferences in caring for their hospitalized elderly. *Geriatric Nursing, 23*(4), 204–207.

Li, H., Melnyk, B. M., McCann, R., Chatcheydang, J., Koulouglioti, C., Nichols, L. W., et al. (2003). Creating avenues for relative empowerment (CARE): A pilot test of an intervention to improve outcomes of hospitalized elders and family caregivers. *Research in Nursing & Health, 26,* 284–299.

Lindsay, P., Sherrard, H., Bickerton, L., Doucette, P., Harkness, C., & Morin, J. (1997). Educational and support needs of patients and their families awaiting cardiac surgery. *Heart & Lung, 26*(6), 458–465.

Loveland-Cherry, C. J., & Bomar, P. J. (2004). Family health promotion and health protection. *Promoting health in families* (pp. 61–89). Philadelphia, PA: Saunders.

Malacrida, R., Bettelini, C. M., Degrate, A., Martinez, M., Badia, F., Piazza, J., et al. (1998). Reasons for dissatisfaction: A survey of relatives of intensive care patients who died. *Critical Care Medicine, 26*(7), 1187–1193.

Martens, K. H., & Mellor, S. D. (1997). A study of the relationship between home care services and hospital readmission of patients with congestive heart failure. *Home Healthcare Nurse, 15*(2), 123–129.

Martin, J. (1991). Rethinking traditional thoughts. *Journal of Emergency Nursing, 17*(2), 67–68.

Mazanec, P., & Tyler, M. K. (2003). Cultural considerations in end-of-life care. *AJN, 103*(3), 50–58.

McCaughan, D., Thompson, C., Cullum, N., Sheldon, T., & Thompson, D. (2002). Acute care nurses' perceptions of barriers to using research information in clinical decision-making. *Journal of Advanced Nursing, 39*(1), 46–60.

McClowery, S. G. (1992). Family functioning during a critical illness: A systems theory perspective. *Critical Care Nursing Clinics of North America, 4,* 559–564.

McLennan, M., Anderson, G. S., & Pain, K. (1996). Rehabilitation learning needs: Patient and family perceptions. *Patient Education & Counseling, 27*(2), 191–199.

Medland, J. J., & Ferrans, C. E. (1998). Effectiveness of a structured communication program for family members of patients in an ICU. *American Journal of Critical Care, 7*(1), 24–29.

Meyers, T. A., Eichhorn, D. J., Guzzetta, C. E., Clark, A. P., Klein, J. D., Taliaferro, E., et al. (2000). Family presence during invasive procedures and resuscitation: The experiences of family members, nurses, and physicians. *AJN, 100*(2), 32–42.

Molter, N. (1979). Needs of relatives of critically ill patients: A descriptive study. *Heart & Lung, 8,* 332–339.

Moos, R. H. E. (1984). *Coping with physical illness, 2: New perspectives.* New York: Plenum Press.

Oermann, M. H., Webb, S. A., & Ashare, J. A. (2003). Outcomes of videotape instruction in clinic waiting area. *Orthopedic Nursing, 22*(2), 102–105.

O'Farrell, P., Murray, J., & Hotz, S. B. (2000). Psychologic distress among spouses of patients undergoing cardiac rehabilitation. *Heart & Lung, 29,* 97–194.

Olson, D. (1997). Paging the family: Using technology to enhance communication. *Critical Care Nurse, 17*(1), 39–41.

Petterson, M. (2000). Visual tools for families: A picture is worth a thousand words. *Critical Care Nurse, 20*(6), 96.

Phelan, G., Kramer, E. J., Grieco, A. J., & Glassman, K. S. (1996). Self-administration of medication by patients and family members during hospitalization. *Patient Education & Counseling, 27*(1), 103–112.

Pochard, F., Azoulay, E., Chevret, S., Lemaire, F., Hubert, P., Canoui, P., et al. (2001). Symptoms of anxiety and depression in family members of intensive care unit patients: Ethical hypothesis regarding decision-making capacity. *Critical Care Medicine, 29,* 1893–1897.

Prendergast, T. J., & Luce, J. M. (1997). Increasing incidence of withholding and withdrawal of life support from critically ill. *American Journal of Respiratory Care Medicine, 155,* 15–20.

Rolland, J. S. (1988). A conceptual model of chronic and life-threatening illness and its impact on families. In C. S. Chilman, E. W. Nunnally, & F. M. Cox (Eds.), *Chronic illness and disability. Families in trouble series* (Vol. 2, pp. 17–68). Newbury Park, CA: Sage.

Rosen, E. J. (1990). *Families facing death.* New York: Lexington Books.

Siminoff, L. A. (1997). Withdrawal of treatment and organ donation. *Critical Care Clinics of North America, 9*(1), 85–95.

Simpson, T. (1991). Critical care patients' perceptions of visits. *Heart & Lung, 20,* 681–688.

Slota, M., Shearn, D., Potersnak, K., & Haas, L. (2003). Perspectives on family-centered, flexible visitation in the intensive care setting. *Critical Care Medicine, 31*(5 [Suppl.]), S362–S366.

Steinglass, P. (1992). Family systems theory and medical illness. In R. J. Sawa (Ed.), *Family health care* (pp. 18–29). Newbury Park, CA: Sage.

Stolarik, A., Lindsay, P., Sherrard, H., & Woodend, A. K. (2000). Determination of the burden of care in families of cardiac surgery patients. *Progress in Cardiovascular Nursing, 15*(1), 4–10.

Swanson, R. W. (1993). Psychological issues in CPR. *Annals of Emergency Medicine, 22*(2; part 2), 350–353.

Swoboda, S. M., & Lipsett, P. A. (2002). Impact of a prolonged surgical critical illness on patients' families. *American Journal of Critical Care, 11,* 459–466.

Thorne, S. E., & Robinson, C. A. (1988). Health care relationships: The chronic illness perspective. *Research in Nursing & Health, 11*(293–300).

Titler, M. G., Bombei, C., & Schutte, D. L. (1995). Developing family-focused care. *Critical Care Nursing Clinics of North America, 7*(2), 375–386.

Titler, M. G., & Walsh, S. M. (1992). Visiting critically ill adults. *Critical Care Nursing Clinics of North America, 4,* 623–632.

Topp, R., Walsh, E., & Sanford, C. (1998). Can providing paging devices relieve waiting room anxiety? *AORN Journal, 67*(4), 852–854, 857–861.

Truog, R. D., Cist, A. F. M., Bracket, S. E., Burns, J. P., Curley, M. A. Q., Danis, M., et al. (2001). Recommendations for end-of-life care in the intensive care unit: The Ethics Committee of the Society of Critical Care Medicine. *Critical Care Medicine, 29*(12), 2332–2348.

U.S. Department of Energy (2004). *Human Genome Project information.* Department of Energy. Retrieved January 19, 2005, from http://www.ornl.gov/sci/techresources/Human_Genome/home.shtml

Vincent, J. (2001). Cultural differences in end-of-life care. *Critical Care Medicine, 292*(2, Suppl.), N52–N55.

Wagner, C. D. (1996). Family needs of chronic hemodialysis patients: A comparison of perceptions of nurses and families. *ANNA Journal, 23*(1), 19–26.

Waters, C. M. (1999). Professional nursing support for culturally diverse family members of critically ill adults. *Research in Nursing & Health, 22,* 107–117.

Wesson, J. S. (1997). Meeting the informational, psychosocial and emotional needs of each ICU patient and family. *Intensive & Critical Care Nursing, 13*(2), 111–118.

Wicks, M. N., Milstead, E. J., Hathaway, D. K., & Cetingok, M. (1998). Family caregivers' burden, quality of life, and health following patients' renal transplantation. *Journal of Transplant Coordination, 8*(3), 170–176.

Wright, L. M., & Leahey, M. (2000). *Nurses & families: A guide to family assessment and intervention* (pp. 155–185). Philadelphia: FA Davis.

Young, J. B. (1995). Black families with a chronically disabled family member: A framework for study. *ABNF Journal, 6*(3), 68–73.

Bibliography

Bomar, P. J. (2004). *Promoting health in families: Applying family research and theory to nursing practice.* Philadelphia: Saunders.

Denham, S. (2003). *Family health: A framework for nursing.* Philadelphia: FA Davis.

Hanson, C. L., De Guire, M. J., Schinkel, A. M., & Kolterman, O. G. (1995). Empirical validation for a family-centered model of care. *Diabetes Care, 18*(10), 1347–1356.

Vaughan-Cole, B., Johnson, M. A., Malone, J. A., & Walker, B. L. (1998). *Family nursing practice.* Philadelphia: WB Saunders.

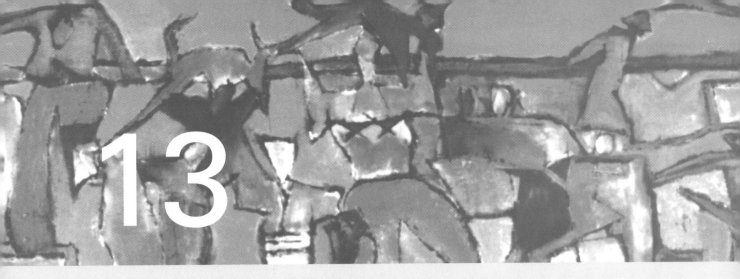

13

Family Mental Health Nursing

Helene J. Moriarty, PhD, RN, CS • Suzanne Marie Brennan, PhD, RN, CS

CRITICAL CONCEPTS

- Psychiatric mental health nurses have a long history of caring for families, but conceptualizations of the family and family interventions have evolved over the past 200 years.

- Family mental health nurses are within the subspecialty of psychiatric/mental health nursing but practice from a framework that explicitly considers the interaction between families and the mental health of individual members. The framework focuses on the mental health needs of individuals within the context of the family *and* the needs of the family as a whole.

- Common theoretical perspectives used in family

mental health nursing include Bowen's family therapy systems theory, contextual family therapy theory, structural family therapy theory, communication family therapy theory, and the biopsychosocial family systems perspective.

- Family mental health nursing interventions may focus on health promotion and management of acute illness and chronic illness.

- It is critical that family mental health nurses consider the implications of this approach for theory development, practice, education, research, and health policy.

INTRODUCTION

Psychiatric and mental health nursing is a specialized area of nursing practice that is based on the science of theories of human behavior and on the art of the therapeutic use of self (American Nurses Association [ANA], 1994; American Nurses Association [ANA], American Psychiatric Nurses Association [APNA], & International Society of Psychiatric Mental Health Nurses, 2000). The practice is directed toward both preventive and corrective efforts for mental disorders and their sequelae. We are concerned with promotion of optimum mental health for society, communities, families, and individuals. Family nursing is an integral component of psychiatric and mental health nursing, although not all nurses in this field practice family nursing. Family mental health nursing recognizes the interaction between families and the mental health of family members. It addresses the psychiatric and mental health care needs of the individual client in the context of the family, while also addressing the needs of the family as a whole.

The overall purpose of this chapter is to describe how mental health family nurses practice family-centered care in a variety of settings. The chapter begins with an overview of common theoretical perspectives in family mental health nursing to provide important background information on the ideas shaping contemporary family mental health nursing. Then, the chapter addresses family mental health nursing in health promotion, acute illness, chronic illness, and end-of-life care, using realistic case examples in inpatient and outpatient settings. The case studies also illustrate the multiple roles of the family mental health nurse. The chapter concludes with a discussion of the implications of family mental health nursing for practice, education, research, and health policy.

MENTAL ILLNESS

Mental illness is a commonly occurring and often disabling phenomenon, requiring the family mental health nurse to have expertise in the identification of risk factors and clinical symptoms, as well as the ability to provide effective pharmacological, psychological, family, and social-level interventions. Cutting across gender, racial, ethnic, socioeconomic, educational, and age parameters, mental disorders affect nearly one-quarter of the U.S. population (23.9 percent) age 18 and older and 20 percent of youth between 9 and 17 years of age (National Institute of Health [NIH] & Substance Abuse and Mental Health Services Administration [SAMHSA], 2000). Mental disorders have a negative impact on personal, social, and family system functioning. In terms of personal functioning, mental illness rivals cancer and heart disease as leading causes of disability. Depression, which affects approximately 17 million people in the United States, has been specifically identified as the leading cause of disability in developed nations (Murray & Lopez, 1996).

At a societal level, the economic consequences of mental illness are staggering, with expenditures of $74.9 billion alone on lost productivity and disability insurance payments for illness or premature death (NIH & SAMHSA, 2000). Families of persons with a mental disorder suffer as well. Stressors experienced by the family include difficulties in coping with disturbed behavior, the uncertainty and unpredictability of symptoms, and loneliness and isolation as a result of the stigma of having a mentally ill family member (Baker, 1993; Sveinbjarnardottir & Dierckx de Casterle, 1997). Additional family challenges include the need to compensate for the ill member's decline in role function and to develop strategies that effectively support the ill member in moving toward mental health. Extended care for an ill family member strains family resources and often leaves the family ill-equipped to manage the stigma, guilt, and loss that may be experienced (Baker, 1989, 1993). Across time, the burden of providing informal care places relatives in what may be a situation of risk to their own mental and physical health—predisposing them to the development of affective and anxiety disorders (Cochrane, Goering, & Rogers, 1997), as well as a variety of physiological conditions.

Unfortunately, despite the prevalence of mental illness, its many negative consequences, and the existence of effective treatment, only 25 percent of those with mental illness receive treatment in the health care system (NIH & SAMHSA, 2000). Those who do pursue treatment encounter a changing health care environment. A shift toward shortened hospital stays and increased outpatient care, along with more manageable medication protocols, have all influenced clients' treatment needs and the system of care delivery in psychiatric and mental health treatment (Baker, 1993). Increasingly, short-term psychiatric hospital admissions are designed for intensive management of acute symptoms, and early discharge places the client with continuing symptoms back in the community with the family providing the majority of care. Thus, to manage the mentally ill family member at home effectively, it is essential for families to receive support for the stressors associated with caregiving, as well as information about symptom management and community resources. Mental health nurses practicing family-centered care in a variety of settings are ideally positioned to meet the needs of the client within the context of the family and to meet the needs of the family as a whole.

Psychiatric mental health nursing focuses on the "promotion of optimal mental health, the prevention of mental illness, health maintenance, management of, and/or referral of mental and physical health problems, the diagnosis and treatment of mental disorders and their sequelae, and rehabilitation" (American Psychiatric Nurses Association, 2003b; Haber & Billings, 1993, p. 1). Thus, nurses practicing mental health and psychiatric care may be found in many settings, providing many levels of care.

The American Psychiatric Nurses Association (APNA) has delineated two practice levels of psychiatric and mental health nursing: basic and advanced (APNA, 2003a). Both are prepared to use the nursing process and theoretical frameworks to address a broad range of physical and psychosocial problems presented by clients and their families, across a variety of practice settings. In addition, both collaborate with a variety of other professions working with and on behalf of the client. Registered psychiatric mental health nurses at the basic level work with individuals, families, groups, and communities to assess mental health needs and subsequently formulate nursing diagnoses and a nursing care plan (APNA, 2003a). Advanced practice registered nurses (APRNs) in psychiatric mental health nursing have a master's degree in this specialty and are either clinical nurse specialists or nurse practitioners. Both categories of these APRNs are qualified to practice independently—diagnosing and treating mental health problems or potential mental problems in individuals, families, and larger groups. In many states, they have prescriptive authority (APNA, 2003a). Practice settings in which APRNs provide direct care include mental health centers, primary care settings, psychotherapy practices, religious organizations, hospitals, schools, health maintenance organizations (HMOs), and homes.

66 Despite the prevalence of mental illness, its many negative consequences, and the existence of effective treatment, only 25 percent of those with mental illness receive treatment in the health care system (NIH & SAMHSA, 2000). 99

HISTORICAL PERSPECTIVE

Psychiatric and mental health nurses have a long history of working with the family. However, concepts of families and family interventions have changed over the last 200 years with advances in knowledge and changes in health care delivery.

- The advent of the asylum in the 19th century began systematic care for mentally ill people. Care there was structured and routinized and stays were often indefinite.
- In the 20th century, Freud influenced care, with his theory that psychiatric symptoms were a function of the mind, rather than a brain disease. He also introduced the concept of transference, which led to one of the cornerstones of psychiatric treatment—the therapeutic relationship.
- In 1946 with the National Mental Health Act, mental illness began to receive attention through funding, research, and training. The relationship between psychiatric patients and nurses began to be studied, in an effort to identify how the nurse-patient relationship could be therapeutic for patients. The clinical specialty of psychiatric nursing emerged.
- In the mid-20th century, antipsychotic medications emerged. With the use of these medications, patients who were formerly "out of touch with reality" could better engage in therapeutic relations with staff.
- Efforts increased to provide more community-based services for the mentally ill, leading to the Community Mental Health Centers Act of 1963 and ultimately to the deinstitutionalization movement. Large numbers of chronically ill persons were released from hospitals. The focus of care shifted toward the community, a change that led to expanded roles for psychiatric nurses as individual, group, and family therapists (Peplau, 1993).

(continued on page 350)

COMMON THEORETICAL PERSPECTIVES

Psychiatric mental health nurses typically use therapeutic principles from a number of family system theories to guide their assessments and interventions with families. Psychiatric mental health advanced practice nurses, many of whom are family therapists, are more apt to base their practice on one *specific* theoretical framework; however, some advanced practice nurses use multiple frameworks. Five major theoretical frameworks are commonly employed in family mental health nursing: Bowen's family systems theory, structural family theory, contextual family theory, communication/interactional family theory, and the biopsychosocial family systems theory. There is some conceptual overlap among theories. The five theories are summarized in the following sections. Three of these theories (i.e., Bowen's, structural, and communication) are described in detail in Chapter 3.

Bowen's Family Systems Theory

One theory commonly used in family mental health nursing is Bowen's family systems theory (Bowen, 1976; Brown, 1991; Gilliss, 1973; Kerr & Bowen, 1988). This theory views the nuclear family as part of the multigenerational extended family and theorizes that patterns of relating tend to repeat themselves over generations. The theory does not "pathologize" families but, rather, encourages individuals to see their families in positive ways. Family members are guided to acknowledge that parents and relatives "did the best with what they had" (Brown, 1991).

The central assumption in this theory is that chronic anxiety is the underlying basis for dysfunction. The theory consists of eight interlocking concepts that address anxiety and emotional processes:

1. Differentiation of self
2. Triangles
3. The family projection process
4. The nuclear family emotional system
5. The multigenerational transmission process
6. Sibling position
7. Emotional cutoff
8. Societal regression

Understanding families requires understanding these concepts and the relationships among the concepts.

Differentiation of Self

The central concept is *differentiation of self*; it has two aspects. First, it refers to the capacity to be a separate yet related human being, and second, it refers to the ability to separate thought from reactive feeling. Differentiation exists on a continuum; the level of differentiation influences the ability to manage anxiety. Those at the higher end of the continuum are able to have intimate relationships, while still maintaining a sense of self. They also exhibit more thinking than reactive feeling. Because they are less reactive, they are better able to manage anxiety and to cope with stress. Those at the lower end of the continuum have more fused relationships; they are extremely close to others but are unable to maintain a basic sense of self.

They also show less thinking and more reactive feeling. Because they are more reactive, they are more anxious in times of stress and less able to cope with stress.

Triangles

A *triangle* describes a relational pattern among persons, objects, or issues. It is an emotional configuration of three members; the members may be three persons or two persons and a group, an issue, or an object. When tension mounts between two persons, one or the other moves toward the third member of the triangle to relieve the anxiety between the twosome. Triangles operate in all families but become problematic over time when they are rigid and entrenched.

Family Projection Process

The *family projection process* is the process by which parental anxiety is transmitted to children via triangles. The *nuclear family emotional system* describes how anxiety is managed: (1) through marital conflict or distance; (2) through dysfunction of a spouse; or (3) through projection onto a child or children. The *multigenerational transmission process* is the family projection process in action over several generations. *Sibling position* refers to the place and role a child assumes in the family. There is a tendency for siblings in certain positions to take on certain roles and behaviors. For example, the oldest child tends to be a responsible caretaker in the family. *Emotional cutoff* is the process of physically or emotionally separating from the family of origin as a way to handle the anxiety of fusion. *Societal regression* refers to the idea that a high level of anxiety in a society (e.g., from war or economic problems) can lead to reacting emotionally rather than in a thinking way (e.g., through riots).

Using Bowen's family systems approach, the therapist may meet with only one family member, with some members, or with all members. No matter who is present, however, the work is seen as family therapy because the therapist takes a multigenerational view of the family. The therapist and family develop a three- to four-generation genogram to examine family processes. The therapist uses this genogram to assess patterns of relationships, patterns of behavior, significant nodal events (life events), level of differentiation, level of anxiety, and triangles.

The goal of therapy is to increase the level of differentiation in the family and thus decrease anxiety within individuals and in the family. Therapy starts by helping family members learn about the family system: to see patterns of relationships and triangles over generations. It also helps individuals take responsibility for changing their position in generational patterns of relating. Family members are encouraged to develop one-to-one relationships with different family members to get to know the family system, know the triangles, and "detriangulate self." For example, a husband and wife may be encouraged to talk directly to one another about their marital problems rather than using their typical triangle (e.g., the wife complains about the husband to her mother and the husband uses work to escape from the marital tension). Family members are also assisted to take an "I position"; that is, each member is encouraged to speak for himself or herself rather than speaking for the entire family with statements such as "We feel" or "We think." In addition, therapy helps members to think instead of reacting in an impulsive, reflexive way.

Structural Family Theory

A second family systems theory is structural family theory, developed by Minuchin (1974) and his colleagues (Minuchin & Fishman, 1981; Minuchin, Rosman, & Baker, 1978). This theory emphasizes the relationship between the presenting problem and the structure of the family. Nurses and other health professionals have applied this theory to families facing problems as diverse as diabetes, asthma, eating disorders, juvenile delinquency, family violence, drug abuse, and divorce. Clinicians have also found this approach beneficial with families from varied cultural backgrounds—Jewish (Wieselberg, 1992), Italian-American (Yaccarino, 1993), Native American (Napoliello & Sweet, 1992), Asian, and Hispanic families (Navarre, 1998).

The *family structure* consists of the "invisible set of functional demands that organize the ways in which family members interact" (Minuchin, 1974, p. 51). Structure encompasses three major areas: (1) power, (2) subsystems, and (3) boundaries. The family's structure may be dysfunctional in any of these areas.

Power refers to the influence that each family member has on family processes. The theory views a hierarchy of power as necessary for effective family functioning. *Subsystems* are sets of family relationships, each with specific functions. For example, in the spousal subsystem, one function of spouses is to support each other in a relationship that fosters individual growth. The parental subsystem performs the tasks of nurturing and socializing children. In the sibling subsystem, siblings learn about peer relationships, power, and alliances. The last area, *boundaries*, includes the rules that differentiate the tasks of different subsystems. For families to function effectively, there must be clear boundaries between subsystems, with some connectedness between them. Families with boundary problems may be disengaged or enmeshed. In disengaged families with rigid boundaries, there is little communication and support among family members; only a high level of stress will evoke support from other members. In enmeshed families with diffuse boundaries, the intense togetherness hinders individuation of members; in these families, stress of one member elicits strong reactions from other members.

The goal of structural family therapy is to solve problems by altering the underlying structure of the family. The initial assessment includes these overlapping phases: (1) joining with the family to temporarily become part of the family system; (2) obtaining a description of the problem; (3) exploring the family structure by observing transactions around the problem; and (4) assessing boundary flexibility, sensitivity to members' actions, family developmental stage, family life context (sources of support and stress), and the way in which the identified patient's symptoms are related to dysfunctional family structure.

The structural therapist focuses primarily on the individual and family in the present. This approach does not negate history but acknowledges transactional patterns from the past. Nevertheless, its primary focus is on present interactions. As Minuchin (1974) noted, "Structural family therapy is a therapy of action. The tool is to modify the present, not to explore and interpret the past" (p. 14).

The therapist takes an active role in the therapy and tries to create change by transforming those aspects of the family structure that are related to the problem. Restructuring techniques result in a shift of power, subsystems, and boundaries. See Box 13–1.

Contextual Family Theory

Another major family theory is contextual family theory, which was developed by Boszormenyi-Nagy and his colleagues (Boszormenyi-Nagy & Spark, 1973; Boszormenyi-Nagy & Krasner, 1986; Cotroneo, 1982, 1986; Cotroneo & Moriarty, 1992). This is a multigenerational family theory that links concern for individuation with concern for rootedness and for significant others in one's relationship network. The relationship network includes: (1) one's legacy—the facts, events, and circumstances of the family and culture into which one is born; (2) the quality of current relationships with nuclear and extended family, peers, friends, colleagues, and the world; and (3) relational connections to the next generation (Cotroneo, Hibbs, & Moriarty, 1992). The theory has been applied to families with a wide variety of problems, such as disturbed parent-child relationships, divorce, family violence, incest, and chronic mental illness.

In contextual family theory, trust and loyalty are key multigenerational dynamics that shape a person's relationships, commitments, and expectations through the interactive process of giving and receiving care. A fundamental assumption of this theory is that living in a family requires a balance of giving and receiving care (Cotroneo, Moriarty, & Smith, 1992).

In relationships based on trust, family members are able to live as separate persons, while at the same time they are connected and available to others as resources. The contextual therapist focuses on behaviors

---

Box 13–1 RESTRUCTURING TECHNIQUES RELATED TO STRUCTURAL FAMILY THERAPY

1. Actualizing transactional patterns
2. Marking boundaries
3. Assigning tasks
4. Relabeling communication

5. Modifying mood and affect
6. Escalating stress
7. Supporting, educating, and guiding
   (Minuchin, 1974)

Source: Minuchin, S. (1974). *Families and family therapy.* Cambridge, MA: Harvard University Press.

that enhance trust and those that diminish it. The therapist assists family members to identify sources of trust and mistrust in their past and present relationships and to rebalance mistrust with resources that can be used constructively. This process of building trust requires family members to consider the merit of positions taken by other family members even when these positions oppose each other (this is termed "multidirected partiality"). The contextual therapist guides families in this process (Cotroneo, Moriarty, & Smith, 1992).

Loyalty, the other key dynamic in this theory, signifies commitments, obligations, and attachments that bind family members to each other over time. Loyalty forms the basis for family members' obligations to care for one another. In addition, whether or not one received the care one deserved and how one received care shape one's relationships with others outside the family. For example, expectations for care that were not met in the family of origin may be assigned to partners and children, tending to overburden these relationships and often distorting their reality. An assessment of at least three generations is needed to understand how loyalty expresses itself among members of a family (Cotroneo, Moriarty, & Smith, 1992).

The contextual family therapist guides family members in the following actions:

- Examining the balance of give-and-take and individuals' sense of fairness or unfairness in past and present relationships
- Inquiring into the "other side" of family members, for example, exploring one's parents' side
- Guiding family members to rebalance unfairness and helping adults make a claim on their family of origin for consideration (Cotroneo, Moriarty, & Smith, 1992)

Communication/Interactional Family Theory

Communication theorists such as Bateson (Bateson, Jackson, Haley, & Weakland, 1956), Haley (1963, 1976), Jackson (1965a, 1965b), Watzlawick (Watzlawick, Beavin, & Jackson, 1967; Watzlawick, Weakland, & Fisch, 1974), and Weakland (1976) propose that verbal and nonverbal communication among family members influences behaviors within the family. Watzlawick and colleagues (1967) presented four axioms of communication that can serve as guides for assessing communication within families:

1. All behavior, whether nonverbal or verbal, is communication and conveys a message.
2. All communication defines a relationship.
3. Persons communicate both verbally and nonverbally; the former presents more content, whereas the latter informs more about the relationship.
4. All communications are either symmetrical (equality exists and either person is free to take the lead) or complementary (one leads and the other follows).

According to this theory, dysfunctional communications, such as disconfirmation, disqualification, and incongruent messages (double-bind), are related to problematic family behaviors. *Disconfirmation* refers to the invalidation of a family member's perception of himself or herself or invalidation of his or her experience. *Disqualification* includes unclear communications such as contraindications, changes of subject, and incomplete sentences. *Incongruent messages* consist of simultaneous verbal and nonverbal messages that conflict. Strategic family therapy tries to change dysfunctional communications to clear, direct communications to change family behaviors (Haber, Hoskins, Leach, & Sideleau, 1987).

Strategic family therapists, often working with a consultation team of mental health professionals, begin by observing sequences of problematic behaviors and then identifying behaviors that maintain the problems. For example, the therapist asks the family to define a goal for treatment, stated in measurable behavioral terms. The therapist then assigns tasks to families, tries to break dysfunctional communication loops, and uses paradox. Paradoxical instruction "prescribes the symptom" or encourages the family to do more of what it has been doing (i.e., continue the status quo) rather than change. The instruction is based on the assumption that the family will instinctively resist what the therapist suggests and, therefore, will do the opposite and begin to change (Haber et al., 1987; Hare-Mustin, 1976; Stanton, 1981).

Biopsychosocial Systems View

A *biopsychosocial systems view* incorporates the consideration of many levels in work with families—biological, psychological, familial, cultural, developmental, environmental, and spiritual—and explores the interactions of these different levels (Engel, 1977, 1996; McDaniel, Hepworth, & Doherty, 1992; Wood, 1993; Wright and Leahey, 1994; Rolland, 1994). Treatment modalities may be offered at these different levels of systems. Use of a specific treatment modality does not necessarily imply an intervention directed toward the cause of the problem. Rather, treatment modalities may address issues and concerns that are present in individuals and families regardless of the possible causes of the problem.

The choice of which systems to work with and the relative importance of each system depends on the problem. Current research indicates that many mental illnesses have a biologic basis that interacts with other factors to influence the course of the illness (National Institute of Mental Health, 2002; Laraia, 2001). This suggests the use of pharmacologic interventions complemented by psychosocial and environmental supports for patients with these illnesses. There are other individual and family problems, however, where the biologic component is less obvious or may not be present—for example, in adjustment disorders, intrafamilial abuse, incest, juvenile delinquency, problems after divorce, problems after bereavement, parent-child relationship problems, and marital problems. In these cases, working with the family and possibly other psychosocial and biologic systems is warranted.

HEALTH PROMOTION

Promotion of mental health is a nursing phenomenon that is not restricted by specialty or place of health care delivery. Whether the nurse seeks to reduce the stresses experienced by the family caring for the child with a chronic condition or the stresses experienced by the aging caregiver of a terminally ill spouse, the goal is to preserve mental health.

In family mental health nursing specifically, health promotion falls in the domain of primary mental health care. This care is defined as "continuous and comprehensive services necessary for the promotion of optimal mental health, prevention of mental illness, management and/or referral of mental and physical health problems, diagnosis and treatment of mental disorders, and their sequelae, and rehabilitation" (Burgess, 1997, pp. 19–20). To help prevent mental illness, psychiatric nurses consult with health agencies and schools, provide mental health education, develop and evaluate community programs, and offer family therapy. The family may be considered the unit of care, or the family may be seen as influencing lifestyle choices that may prevent illness for individual members of the family (Danielson, Hamel-Bissell, & Winstead-Fry, 1993).

Risk Factors and Mental Health

Many risk factors for mental illness have been identified as contributing to the vulnerability of individuals and the family as a whole. With regard to depression, for example, adults and older adults are at higher risk than youth for developing this disorder. Moreover, major depression affects approximately twice as many women as men, and women who are poor, less educated, unemployed, or on welfare are at highest risk for experiencing a major depression (NIH & SAMHSA, 2003). Older adults with comorbid medical conditions are also at risk, with 12 percent of older persons hospitalized for problems such as hip fracture or heart disease receiving a diagnosis of depression. Elderly people in nursing homes also suffer from depression with rates ranging from 15 to 25 percent (NIH & SAMHSA, 2003).

For mental illness overall, the two most consistently identified risk factors are low socioeconomic status and female gender (Institute of Medicine, 1989; Lavigne et al., 1998; U.S. Department of Health and Human Services Office of Public Health and Science, 1998). Poverty is the most tenacious threat to mental health of individuals, families, and communities; it has consistently been associated with higher rates of both individual dysfunction (Raine, Brennan, Mednick, & Mednick, 1996) and family dysfunction (Costello, Farmer, Angold, Burns, & Erkanli, 1997; Lavigne et al., 1998). Moreover, poverty is complex and encompasses additional factors, such as unemployment, lack of education, and poor housing.

The higher rates of mental illness among women are also extremely complex and may be related to higher rates of poverty and sexual abuse, as well as gender-specific genetic, hormonal, and other biological differences (NIMH, 1995). Additionally, women may be predisposed to mental disorders because of role overload accompanying greater responsibilities in juggling work, family, and domestic demands (Lavigne et al., 1998). Women are also more likely to be single parents. Such gender-related risk factors may be amenable to family-level nursing preventive measures, such as identifying health and economic resources for families and assisting partners to negotiate domestic responsibilities equitably.

Beyond the compelling issue of women's unique mental health needs and risk factors, a recent NIMH-sponsored study documented a startling association between untreated maternal mental illness and a child's presentation to a mental health clinic. Specifically, this study found that 70 percent of mothers who brought their child to a child mental health clinic suffered from untreated depressive and anxiety disorders themselves (NIMH, 2001). The role of maternal mental illness as an environmental risk factor for the development of childhood emotional disturbance has been well studied. Less is known, however, about the role of paternal mental illness and the development of these disorders.

Clearly, childhood emotional disturbances, like adult mental disorders, result from an interplay of environmental and biological influences. Environmental contributors include exposure to toxins or violence; stress related to chronic poverty or discrimination; and the loss of important people through death, divorce, or broken relationships (SAMHSA, 2003). Examples of biological risk factors for mental illness in children include genetics and trauma to the central nervous system (SAMHSA, 2003).

Risk factors for both adults and children may also vary according to sociocultural contexts. For example, in a comparative study of psychiatric disorders among Native American and white youth in Appalachia, Costello and colleagues (1997) identified higher family risk factors (including poverty, violence, and substance abuse) but a lower incidence of mental illness in the Native American children. White children in this study were more likely than Native children to seek and use mental health services to deal with problems related to poverty and family deviance. The authors concluded that the relative influence of risk factors varied by the cultural context, but they also acknowledged the influence of culture on symptom expression and health-seeking behavior (Canino & Spurlock, 1997).

Interventions for Promotion

Health promotion, by definition, means early intervention targeted at specifically identified risk factors. Successful mental health promotion must be acceptable to the communities and families for whom it is intended. To that end, collaboration among community members, mental health care providers, and consumers is essential. School-based clinics that bridge the gaps between isolated individuals, families, and needed mental health care services are examples of effective community-based health promotion programs (Armbruster, Gerstein, & Fallon, 1997). Promotion of family cohesion and resilience has been found to diminish the influence of risk factors among low-income school-age children (Reynolds, 1998; Thienemann, Shaw, & Steiner, 1998). The family is

likely to serve protective functions in relation to risk factors, although further research is necessary to identify other family variables that may mediate against the pervasive influence of major risks for common mental illnesses. The following sections illustrate ways that nurses can intervene to promote mental health in the face of recognized risk factors.

Example: Divorce

In the United States, 20 percent of all first marriages end in separation or divorce within 5 years; 33 percent have dissolved after 10 years. Second marriages fare no better: 23 percent disrupt after 5 years and 39 percent after 10 years (Centers for Disease Control and Prevention, 1998). Divorce and custody disputes are life stressors that place many families at risk. In situations of intense parental conflict, children are at high risk for emotional and behavioral disturbances such as depression, low self-esteem, school problems, and antisocial behavior (Emery, 1982; Hetherington, Cox, & Cox, 1978; Hetherington, 1981; Wallerstein & Kelley, 1980). The contextual approach to custody decisions, which is derived from contextual family systems theory, can be used to minimize or prevent mental health problems in families by helping families negotiate a custody and visitation agreement (Cotroneo, Hibbs, & Moriarty, 1992; Cotroneo, Moriarty, & Smith, 1992). This approach is based on the view that the best interests of children cannot be separated from the welfare of their parents. Furthermore, examining the interests of children in an intergenerational context reflects the full reality of their relationship network and family loyalties.

Using this approach, family meetings are held that include both parents and all siblings; they may also include grandparents, aunts, uncles, and other significant persons. Each family member is asked to identify his or her own needs and commitments regarding parenting. The therapist helps the family examine the full relational context of the parents as well as the children, particularly the kind of parenting that the parents themselves received. The therapist also helps family members explore family loyalty issues and unfinished family business that may undermine trust. Cotroneo and colleagues speculate that parents who struggled with loyalty conflicts in their families of origin may use marriage and parenting of their children to reenact that struggle. Thus parents' perception of what is at stake in a custody dispute may be distorted, and their capacity for giving and sharing may be impaired (Cotroneo, Hibbs, & Moriarty, 1992).

Topical guidelines for structuring these meetings are outlined in Box 13–2. These meetings redirect the focus from blame to trust-building, so that parents can see themselves less as adversaries and more as collaborators in the care of their children. Parents learn to differentiate between issues that belong to the marriage and issues of parenting, and they also address issues from their families of origin. In this context of trust, parents are encouraged to negotiate an arrangement that they can live with and that protects the child's access to both parents (Cotroneo, Hibbs, & Moriarty, 1992).

Cotroneo and colleagues (1992) have illustrated the use of the approach with a small sample of families and through a case study. The findings suggest that the approach can help families create alternatives to continued disputation. The authors suggest using the approach as soon as a parent files for custody or visitation to promote mental health in all parties and to minimize damage to the child.

Box 13–2 GUIDELINES FOR FAMILY MEETINGS ABOUT CHILD CUSTODY DISPUTES

I. Current family situation
    a. Response of family members to separation or divorce
    b. Effects on family members
        1. What has been done to help the children deal with the situation?
        2. Contact made with significant legal, religious, psychological, social, and health care resources
II. Family genogram information
    a. Ways in which parents define and validate themselves in relation to significant others, particularly their own families of origin
        1. Patterns of expectations and commitments across three generations
        2. Gender-related issues
        3. Intergenerational history of losses, relational injuries, and injustices
III. An exploration of parenting of children (past, present, and future) and the developmental burdens and demands that are placed on children
    a. Acknowledgment of children for their contributions to the family that may have been taken for granted
    b. Exploration of the worries that children may be experiencing and how they get help when it is needed
    c. Acknowledgment of the parents for the losses, relational injuries, and injustices experienced in their families of origin
    d. Exploration of ways in which family members can work to correct injustices and exploitation in past and present relationships and repair injuries that have already been sustained
    e. Consideration of the consequences of any imbalances in giving and receiving care and fairness that exist in the family
IV. Family task (conjoint session)
    a. Describe the family situation as you see it. What are the conflicts for you?
    b. In thinking about what to do, what are you considering and why?
    c. If you could have things your way (according to your preferences), what would you do now?
    d. If you were to put your plan into action, what would happen? Do you think your plan would be successful? Why? Why not?
    e. What would be the consequences of your plan for you, your spouse or partner, and each individual child?

Source: Cotroneo, M., Hibbs, B. J., & Moriarty, H. (1992). Uses and implications of the contextual approach to child custody decisions. *Journal of Child and Adolescent Psychiatric and Mental Health Nursing,* 5(3), 17. Copyright 1992 by Nursecom, Inc. Reprinted with permission.

Example: Family Violence

The problem of family violence is another area for family health promotion. It is a sad fact that relatedness increases the likelihood of physical or sexual abuse. One out of every five American families experiences family violence. One out of four American women report that they have been physically abused by a husband or boyfriend at some time in their lives (Lieberman Research Institute, 1996). Each year, an estimated 3.3 million children in the United States witness their mother or female caretaker being abused (American Psychological Association, 1996). Approximately 1.5 million women and 834,700 men are raped and/or physically assaulted by an intimate partner (spouse, boyfriend, girlfriend, date) in the United States each year (Tjaden & Thoennes, 2000). During 2001, about 903,000 U.S. children were victims of abuse and neglect. Eighty-four percent of these child victims were maltreated by one or both parents (U.S. Department of Health and Human Services, 2003). As Dobash and Dobash (1979) stated, "Despite fears to the contrary, it is not a stranger but a so-called loved one who is most likely to assault, rape, or murder us" (cited in Strong & DeVault, 1992).

Family violence may be viewed as a severe stressor that is a symptom of family dysfunction and that leads to adverse sequelae for individual family members and the family as a whole. The term encompasses child abuse and neglect, spouse abuse, sibling abuse, teenage violence toward parents, and elder abuse. Child abuse and spouse abuse often exist together in a family.

Four forms of abuse are described in the literature—physical, emotional, neglectful, and sexual. Physical abuse is a nonaccidental injury inflicted by someone whose intent is to cause physical harm. Emotional abuse is a means of controlling through fear and degradation. It may include threats of harm, extreme and constant criticism, physical and social isolation, and false accusations. Neglect is a deliberate failure to provide for the basic human needs (e.g., food, shelter, hygiene, safety, and health care). Sexual abuse is assaultive and nonassaultive sexual exploitation; it refers to any form of sexual interaction. Incest is sexual abuse among family members; it occurs most commonly between a parent and child within a family, but it may also involve siblings. Sexual activity between a parent and a child or between an adult and a child always constitutes abuse. It does not matter whether it involves physical force or whether the child is perceived by the adult as freely engaging in sexual activity. Because of a child's age, the child cannot give informed consent. Therefore, this sexual activity always involves exploitation of the child by the adult.

Research indicates that there are three sets of factors that place families at risk for child abuse and neglect: parental characteristics, child characteristics, and family ecosystem characteristics. Parental factors include the following: (1) the parent was abused or neglected by his or her parents, (2) the parent believes in physical punishment, (3) the parent has unrealistic expectations of the child, (4) the parent is under great stress (e.g., unemployment), (5) the parent is a loner with few friends, (6) the parent sees the child as willful and purposely "bad," and (7) the parent is a substance abuser. Child characteristics include the following: (1) the child is different as a result of illness, prematurity, or disability; and (2) the child is difficult (e.g., fussy, hyperactive, demanding). Familial factors include the following: (1) the family is under great stress (e.g., poor, single-parent family, unemployed, or with other health problems), (2) the family is socially isolated, (3) the family is a patriarchal (male-dominated) household, and (4) the family has a history of abuse in the nuclear or extended family (Strong & DeVault, 1992). Identification of these risk factors is critical for family assessment and early intervention with families at risk or with families with abuse.

Prevention of child abuse is critical, given the potential for intergenerational patterns of abuse. Children who are abused and neglected in their families of origin are at higher risk for tolerating and using violence in their adult relationships (Finkelhor, 1988; Oliver, 1993).

Domestic violence is "a pattern of assaultive and coercive behaviors, including physical, sexual, and psychological attacks as well as economic coercion, that adults or adolescents use against their intimate partners" (Family Violence Prevention Fund, 1998, p. 1). It is present in all racial, ethnic, religious, educational, and socioeconomic groups. Most abuse escalates in both frequency and severity over time (AMA, 1994; Crowell & Burgess, 1996). Studies show that both men and women engage in violence toward partners, but women are most often victims of chronic battering resulting in injury (Cascardi, Langhinrichsen, & Vivian, 1992). In addition to physical injury, abused women suffer psychological sequelae, such as posttraumatic stress disorder, depression, suicidal risk, and substance abuse (Plichta, 1992).

In clinical settings, the prevalence of domestic violence is high in female patients. According to a

U.S. Department of Justice report (Rand, 1997), 37 percent of all women who sought treatment in hospital emergency departments for violence-related injuries were hurt by a current or former spouse, boyfriend, or girlfriend. Twelve to twenty-three percent of women in family practice settings reported that they were physically abused or threatened by their partners over the previous year (Hamberger, Saunders, & Hovey, 1992; Elliott & Johnson, 1995). Pregnancy is also a risk factor for domestic violence. In several studies, 7 to 18 percent of pregnant women reported physical abuse during the pregnancy (Amaro, Fried, Cabral, & Zuckerman, 1990; Berenson, Wiemann, Wilkinson, Jones, & Anderson, 1994; Norton, Peipert, Ziegler, Lima, & Hume, 1995; Parker, McFarlane, & Soeken, 1991).

Family violence causes great physical and psychological harm to adults and children, yet it is often not detected by clinicians. Nurses and health professionals in all clinical settings must look for the physical, emotional, and behavioral signs of abuse and neglect as they conduct the physical exam and patient interview and through direct questioning, such as "Have you ever been hurt by a family member?" Most victims do not spontaneously report abuse to health providers. Health professionals must consistently use screening questions in order to improve the identification of victims and the treatment of victims and families. Health professionals must also be knowledgeable of the risk factors for abuse and the reporting system for their states. In the United States, the Child Abuse Prevention and Treatment Act (1974) was amended in 1996 to mandate that specific persons, including nurses, physicians, and health care professionals, report any suspicion of child abuse (AMA, 1996).

Primary prevention of abuse involves strengthening individuals and families to enable them to better cope with multiple life stressors. For example, nurses can conduct community classes to teach parents about normal developmental challenges, such as toilet training, ways to discipline without physical punishment, and methods of conflict resolution. Secondary prevention involves identification of families at risk for violence and those who are beginning to use violence, followed by early intervention to prevent or stop the violence.

Advanced practice family mental health nurses and other mental health professionals may provide treatment to victims, perpetrators, and families. The aim is to protect the victim, stop the violence, and prevent further violence by changing family processes. Most treatment approaches over the last 10 years have focused on the victim as the primary context for treatment. However, family system approaches that consider the whole family as the unit of assessment and treatment have evolved in the United States and Europe (Cirillo & DiBlasio, 1992; Colgan-McCarthy & O'Reilly-Byrne, 1988; Cotroneo, 1986; Cotroneo & Moriarty, 1992; Gelinas, 1986).

> 66 A basic goal for mental health promotion is to assist healthy, functioning families to maintain and enhance the health of both the family and family members. 99

Families who are not experiencing severe stressors such as poverty, divorce, or violence may choose to work on issues such as stress reduction and strengthening relationships among family members. There is no such thing as a perfect family. All families have issues and concerns even if they are not experiencing severe distress. A basic goal for mental health promotion is to assist healthy, functioning families to maintain and enhance the health of both the family and family members. Health promotion for these families may take place in community educational programs or through counseling. A nurse working with the family can use a variety of approaches to enhance the family's communication and relationships.

FAMILY MENTAL HEALTH NURSING IN ACUTE ILLNESS

Some clients and families experience acute symptoms, such as suicidal ideation associated with major depression. In the year 2000, the total number of suicides in the United States was 29,350, or 1.2 percent of all deaths (Miniño, Arias, Kochanek, Murphy, & Smith, 2002; Moscicki, 2001). On an even more alarming note, it is estimated that for every suicide death there may be from 8 to 25 suicide attempts (Miniño, Arias, Kochanek, Murphy, & Smith, 2002; Moscicki, 2001). Thus, recognition and treatment of acute suicidal phenomena are a compelling clinical concern for mental health practitioners in the United States. Clients and families may also present with an acute exacerbation of a chronic illness; for example, a client with chronic schizophrenia may experience a resurgence of psychotic symptoms. Acute distress may also be associated with a severe stressor that triggers psychiatric symptoms, such as a panic attack (American Psychiatric Association [APA], 2000). Acute symptoms require early diagnosis and treatment and prompt referral for additional consultation as necessary.

When the nurse is caring for the family as client, acute individual distress is often associated with a familial crisis. For example, 15-year-old Angela attempted suicide by swallowing "a handful" of her grandmother's medication for hypertension. During the assessment, the advanced practice nurse learned that Angela thought she was pregnant. She was afraid to tell her parents because she thought it would hurt and disappoint them. When the nurse cares for the client within the context of the family, the nurse considers the relationship between the individual's symptoms and the family response to the symptoms. In either case, the meaning the family attaches to the symptom can influence the family's decision to seek care (Danielson et al., 1993).

Acute psychiatric and mental health disturbances often compel families to seek immediate care. They may seek care from the general family practitioner or go directly to an emergency department or community mental health center. In many cases, the initial screening is done by a nurse who has not been prepared as a psychiatric mental health nurse. The nurse assesses the presenting problem and then makes appropriate referrals. In the case of Angela, the nurse would first determine whether Angela had ingested a potentially lethal dose of medication, which would require immediate medical intervention. If Angela needed to be stabilized in an intensive care unit, she and her family might be seen by the psychiatric consultation liaison nurse. The role of this nurse in a medical treatment setting is to help the client and the family begin to understand the implications of the crisis that has occurred and the options for family treatment.

Once Angela's physiological safety had been established, she might be referred to a psychiatric mental health advanced practice nurse for a comprehensive assessment. Using a biopsychosocial systems perspective, the nurse would assess (1) Angela's physiological condition, (2) her mental status, including any persistent suicidal ideation, (3) the availability of family resources and support to keep the client safe, (4) the meaning the crisis had for the family, and (5) the need for psychiatric hospitalization.

In acute situations, the nurse collaborates with the family and other mental health professionals in planning for the client's care. Initial treatment may focus on assisting the client and family to open lines of communication. After resolution of the crisis, the family may be referred for family therapy to help them develop more effective coping strategies.

Inpatient Treatment

Care of the client experiencing acute distress may involve a brief admission to an inpatient psychiatric unit. Traditionally, hospitalization reinforces an individualistic view of care, in which one member is seen in the sick role and the other members of the family are seen as peripheral to the illness. Merely adding family therapy to the treatment program does not make the inpatient experience a family experience. Family-focused care can be more fully integrated into inpatient treatment programs through use of the following time-honored strategies identified by Bowers and McNally (1983):

- Plan intake conferences at the time of admission. An intake conference with the family makes it possible to assess the family as a unit and the needs of each of its members. It also serves to inform the family that care will be family-centered and indicates how they may be involved in treatment.
- Structure intensive family therapy into the treatment program. Family therapy may help the family view the presenting problem as a family problem rather than as solely the problem of the hospitalized client.
- Make family conferences a regularly scheduled activity. In inpatient settings, interdisciplinary treatment teams typically meet frequently to evaluate the client's progress toward the goals of treatment, but families are not usually included in these meetings. Family conferences involve the family in setting treatment goals and evaluating progress for the individual and family.
- Plan therapeutic leaves of absence for the individual so that family members may work

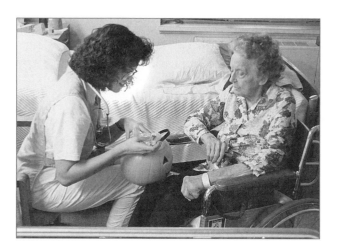

together outside the hospital setting on family treatment goals.

- Use psychiatric mental health advanced practice nurses to supervise family treatment. These specialists, who have education and experience in working with families, can both conduct family sessions and supervise others involved in family meetings and conferences.

A family-centered approach alters the traditional concept of milieu therapy (Bowers & McNally, 1983).

CASE STUDY ➤

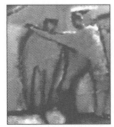

FAMILY TREATMENT ON AN INPATIENT UNIT

The following case example depicts family-focused inpatient treatment. The therapeutic goals and treatment strategies reflect a multiple systems view in addressing many levels of systems. Interventions at the family level are derived from Bowen's (1978) multigenerational family systems theory.

Jeremy G., an 18-year-old high school senior, was experiencing severe mood swings along with escalating angry, defiant behavior, school failure, and suicidal ideation. At times, Jeremy felt "on top of the world." During these periods, he felt he could accomplish almost anything. At other times, Jeremy reported "sub-zero" self-esteem. An intensive outpatient evaluation indicated that Jeremy was a gifted student and an artistic young man. His long-standing pattern of mood swings supported a diagnosis of a bipolar mood disorder called cyclothymia (American Psychiatric Association, 1994).

The family evaluation revealed that his parents had a long history of marital problems. The parents maintained emotional distance from one another, and Jeremy was distant from his father. Jeremy felt that he had tried, for many years, to get along with his father but that his father was "cold and impossible to please." Mr. G. reported having a very distant relationship with his own father. Jeremy and his mother had an unusually close, fused relationship. Jeremy's two sisters, aged 13 and 15 years, were relatively free of the triangular emotional system that occurred between Jeremy and his parents.

Jeremy and his family agreed to a 2-week hospitalization for Jeremy. He was referred for a neurological evaluation and magnetic resonance imaging (MRI) to rule out any biologic causes for his mood swings, and he began a trial of antidepressant medication for manage-

Traditionally, the family members were seen as "intruders" or visitors to the inpatient milieu and not as a part of the treatment process. Integrating the family into the inpatient setting may involve restructuring the traditional components of the milieu; for example, families need to be included in community meetings, medication groups, and discharge groups. New components may also need to be added to milieu treatment—for example, family intake conferences, multifamily therapeutic groups, and joint meetings of client, family, and staff.

ment of cyclothymia. The family agreed to participate in family therapy sessions. The therapeutic goal was to decrease emotional reactivity among family members and increase the family's level of differentiation.

In therapy, family members were encouraged to take an "I position" and to become more thoughtful in their responses to one another, rather than emotionally reactive. In addition, Jeremy was encouraged to participate in age-appropriate peer relationships. This helped Jeremy remove himself from the three-person triangular emotional system and begin to improve his self-esteem. Treatment staff helped Jeremy identify his strengths and encouraged him to pursue his dream of going to art school. In addition to attending family sessions and treatment conferences, Jeremy's parents attended a medication group to learn about the medication prescribed for Jeremy. They also attended a parenting group that focused on learning from and sharing with other parents about child-rearing issues. In separate sessions, the parents began to focus on their own marital issues. The G. family had managed their problems by submerging them and projecting their marital anxiety onto Jeremy. When the couple began to address their problems in therapy, less anxiety was projected onto Jeremy.

Mr. G.'s parents also attended several family therapy sessions. Mr. G. was encouraged to be less reactive with his own father and to work on developing a one-to-one relationship with him. As he did so, Mr. G. became more open to developing a relationship with his son. As Jeremy began to assume an "I position" in his family, he was able to express his desire for a rewarding relationship with his father. This goal was incorporated into the plans for therapeutic leaves of absence. Jeremy and his father went on several outings together to work on their relationship. Following the 2-week hospitalization, Jeremy was discharged and the family began monthly family therapy sessions to build on the successes in the hospital.

Special Considerations: When a Child Is Hospitalized

When a child with acute psychiatric symptoms requires hospitalization, the staff need to keep in mind how radical and strange hospitalization may seem to the family, which is used to having responsibility for the child (Goren, 1992). Parents may also experience doubt about their caregiving abilities and anticipate blame from the staff (DeSocio, Bowllan, & Staschak, 1997). Because the family's participation is essential to successful treatment, the staff must create an environment that is supportive to family members and must work in partnership with families (DeSocio, Bowllan, & Staschak, 1997; Goren, 1992). Given the shorter lengths of stay for children, child psychiatric nurses need to provide more individualized education to parents within less time, to prepare families for the child's quick return home (Scharer, 1999). Goren (1992) presents the following guidelines for engaging families in inpatient treatment of a child:

- Recognize the family's competencies. Given that "all families have competencies" (p. 45), staff should point out parents' strengths and emphasize the importance of using these strengths in the child's treatment.
- Replace therapeutic relationships with therapeutic systems. That is, rather than relying heavily on the traditional one-to-one therapeutic relationship, rely on the therapeutic system of child, family, and staff.
- Involve the child, family, and staff as partners in treatment planning conferences and in developing the treatment contract.

- Work through the family rather than in its place. Given that the family is the natural caregiver for the child, staff should assist the family to intervene with the child.
- Consider family-support alternatives to out-of-family placement. Rather than removing the child from the family, try to build up the family's strengths and bring in supports from the extended family and community.
- Decrease the barriers between the hospital and the community and minimize the hospital's interference with parenting. Encourage parents to take part in activities such as meals, classes, and bedtime preparation.

When these guidelines are followed, treatment becomes a process between the staff system and the family system, with the involvement of community services as well. As Goren said, "The child belongs, in the sense of what is ordinary and usual, to the family and community. The responsibility of the staff is to intervene in ways that support the child's belongingness and that increase the likelihood of rapid return to normal life" (1992, p. 46).

Outpatient Care

For some acute problems, outpatient treatment may be appropriate if there is no danger to family members or others. The following case study illustrates outpatient family treatment when a mother reported feeling overwhelmed by raising her children and questioned her ability to continue. Treatment was based on structural family theory.

CASE STUDY ➤

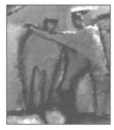

FAMILY TREATMENT IN AN OUTPATIENT SETTING

Caroline M., the mother, was a 30-year-old, single African-American woman, who was referred to the community mental health center by a female friend. Caroline lived in a three-bedroom row home with her five children: Paul, age 12; Tametrice, age 10; Sam, age 8; Nina, age 6; and Vera, age 4. Caroline had held various jobs over

the last 10 years as kitchen helper, typist, and factory worker. She had been unemployed for several months, since she quit her job because of her boss's verbal abusiveness. Presently, the family was subsisting on welfare. Caroline came to the clinic because she was very "edgy and nervous." She reported difficulty in expressing her anger toward family and friends and felt physically explosive. She was raising five children with little outside support and felt overwhelmed by this. She cared deeply about her children but questioned her ability to raise them. She had had two previous contacts at the clinic for the same reasons but reported withdrawing from therapy because she "did

(continued on page 362)

CASE STUDY ➤ *(Continued)*

not like" the therapists. During the present contact, she began work with two nurse co-therapists. Nine sessions were conducted: six sessions with the entire family, two sessions with Caroline, and one session with the children.

During the sessions, the therapists joined with the family to attempt to understand the family system and assess the family structure. The mother and Paul made up the parental subsystem. As the oldest son, Paul was a "parentified child," who was assuming many parental functions in the family; when Caroline felt overwhelmed by her parental functions, she delegated these to Paul. He attempted to meet his mother's expectations of him to receive her love and approval, but she did not acknowledge his contributions. Figure 13–1 depicts some aspects of the family's structure and the therapeutic goals for transforming these aspects. Box 13–3 outlines therapeutic goals for strengthening the parental subsystem, strengthening the sibling subsystem, and supporting the mother's personal needs.

Box 13–3   **THERAPEUTIC GOALS FOR THE M. FAMILY BASED ON STRUCTURAL FAMILY THEORY**

I. Strengthening the parental subsystem
   a. Acknowledge Caroline's stressors as a single parent.
   b. Teach Caroline about age-appropriate expectations for the children.
   c. Teach her new ways to enforce limits (e.g., through rewards or through withholding privileges).
   d. Assign tasks both inside and outside the therapy session that reinforce the parental subsystem (e.g., designation of assigned days for dishwashing).
   e. Help Caroline identify her double-bind messages and her inconsistent expectations for the children.
   f. Facilitate mobilization of supports (e.g., family, friends, church, community groups).

II. Strengthening the sibling subsystem
   a. Emphasize individual differences to mark boundaries between the children and between mother and children.
   b. Role-play or assign tasks to teach siblings ways to resolve conflicts without calling for mother.
   c. Decrease the children's competition for mother's attention by encouraging mother to designate one "special time" for each child to spend with her alone.
   d. Modify Paul's position as parentified child.
      1. Support Paul in his efforts to increase his autonomy outside the family.
      2. Acknowledge Paul's contributions to the family.
   e. Encourage activities involving only the sibling subsystem by assigning tasks requiring cooperation among siblings (e.g., Paul could teach his siblings about history or all siblings could make a present for their mother).

III. Supporting Caroline's personal needs
   a. Explore Caroline's needs for intimacy and social contact (e.g., through her relationships and social activities). Have some individual sessions with Caroline to discuss sexual issues or other issues she wishes to address without the children present.
   b. Explore the impact of Caroline's present conflict with her partner on her ability to cope with her children.
   c. Discuss possible job opportunities and completion of her general equivalency diploma.

Present Map

M and PC (executive subsystem)
....
Children (sibling subsystem)

Therapeutic Goal

M

PC : Other siblings

KEY

M = Mother
PC = Parentified child
... = Diffuse boundary
--- = Clear boundary

Figure 13–1 The map under "Therapeutic Goal" represents a clear boundary between mother and children, with Paul, the parentified child, returning to the sibling subsystem but maintaining a position of leadership among his siblings.

FAMILY MENTAL HEALTH NURSING IN CHRONIC ILLNESS

Chronic mental illness is characterized by diagnosis, duration, and disability (Bachrach, 1991). A mental illness that persists for 2 years or more is considered chronic. A lingering disability such as one that precludes the ability to return to work full-time also characterizes a disorder as chronic. Health care providers are now also using the term "severe and persistent illness" to denote chronic mental illness. For example, schizophrenia, chemical dependence, and eating disorders are considered severe and persistent mental illnesses. Prevalence rates for chronic mental illness in the United States range from 1.9 million to 2.4 million (CDC, 1999). Further, it has been estimated that about one-third of the homeless population is chronically mentally ill (Burgess, 1997). Given the prevalence of chronic mental illness, nurses and other health care professionals in many settings are likely to encounter mental illness and its related problems. For example, medical management of a client with diabetes may be complicated by severe and persistent schizophrenia. A woman's pregnancy may be complicated by a 10-year history of bulimia. Treatment of a client's alcohol abuse may need to include consideration for the client's depression.

❝The goal of wraparound services is to create an individualized package for intensive care in the home, school, and community settings.❞

Because of the encompassing nature of the label "chronic mental illness," it is difficult to generalize about treatment needs for this population. One client may lack family support and require supportive services for housing, management of medications, and a daily routine. Another client may receive family and community support, but the family may require assistance in managing the burdens associated with caring for a chronically ill family member. Wraparound services may be required for a family caring for a child with complex needs (Handron, Dosser, McCammon, & Powell, 1998). The goal of wraparound services is to create an individualized package for intensive care in the home, school, and community settings. It encompasses a strength-based, family-driven orientation that focuses on the unique needs of each child and family. In addition to improving behavioral outcomes for children engaged in wraparound services, the intensive program has been found to be a cost-effective means of maintaining children in the context of their own family, school, and community.

Cultural Perspectives on Chronicity

The family's cultural beliefs influence their perceptions and management of the client's chronic mental illness. Indeed, cultural psychiatrists (Lefley, 1990; Lefley, 1998a) have suggested that the concept of chronicity in mental illness is an artifact of cultural belief systems and expectations regarding the nature of illness. In Westernized cultures, such as the mainstream culture in the United States, chronicity may be a by-product of the treatment community's belief that serious mental illness is inherently chronic. Moreover, the bureaucratic treatment system tends to reinforce dependence and the "sick role" behavior associated with chronicity. It has also been suggested that the incidence of mental illness is greater in cultures that produce high levels of stress and offer low levels of social support. The incidence of chronicity may also be higher in cultures that provide few work opportunities for chronic patients and few supports to caregivers of chronically mentally ill persons.

In some non-Western cultures, mental illness is perceived as external to the patient and is thought to be caused by supernatural forces or possession (Skultans, 1991). In such cultures, patients and families may experience less blame and stigmatization for the illness. In addition, the family and community are likely to be more supportive, and family support is perceived as an integral component of treatment. It is also interesting that in these non-Western cultures, where mental illness is believed to be brief and temporary, the incidence of chronicity is lower (Lin & Kleinman, 1988). The differing rates of chronic mental illnesses in Western and non-Western cultures tend to support the view of cultural psychiatrists that chronicity in mental illness is a cultural artifact.

Within this Westernized multicultural society, differences in culturally determined values and belief systems abound. These differences may influence family relationships with professional, legal, and consumer communities. A family's cultural system may influence its perception of the family burden related to caring for a member with severe and persistent mental illness (Hines-Martin, 1998; Lefley,

1998b; Nahulu et al., 1996). Knowledge of culturally determined family beliefs about mental illness and perceptions of care will enhance family-provider relationships and affect treatment outcomes (Solomon, 1998; Vandiver & Keopraseuth, 1998). For example, in their work with Native American families, Johnson and Johnson (1998) found that respectful approaches to family education contributed greatly to diagnostic accuracy, treatment, and rehabilitation efficacy. When the nurse conveyed respect and interest in family cultural beliefs, it enhanced joining with the family and engagement in the treatment program.

Chronic mental illnesses that demonstrate great cultural variations include the eating disorders—anorexia and bulimia. Both disorders are found almost exclusively among women in Westernized cultures ("Eating Disorders," 1997). Family systems theories (Minuchin et al., 1978) suggest that certain types of family organization are closely related to the development and maintenance of symptoms of eating disorders. The following case example demonstrates a family mental health nursing approach to assessing eating disorders on an inpatient unit.

CASE STUDY ➤

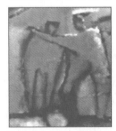

ASSESSMENT ON AN INPATIENT UNIT

Carmella was a 19-year-old woman admitted to an inpatient psychiatric unit for bulimia. She was a first generation Italian-American; her parents came from Italy to the United States. She was a freshman at an Ivy League university in the United States and had always been a hard-working student who strove for excellence in her academic work. Her physical appearance was striking; many patients on the unit referred to her as the "beautiful" patient who "could be a model." The other patients could not understand why Carmella was in the hospital because she looked so "perfect." On the unit, Carmella tried to be a peacekeeper; she avoided any expression of dissatisfaction or conflict with others and tried to please everyone—patients and staff. Carmella came from a very close and religious Italian family in which three generations lived together. In this family, there was a great emphasis on togetherness; expressions of disagreement and conflict were discouraged. On the third night of

her hospitalization, Carmella's mother visited her. Carmella's primary nurse wanted to assess Carmella's responses after the visit, based on her awareness that family factors are often related to eating disorders. Five minutes after the visit, Carmella entered the kitchen, removed two gallons of ice cream from the refrigerator, and began binge eating. The nurse followed Carmella into the kitchen and asked her what she was feeling as she began binge eating. Carmella said that she had felt "ready to explode" with anger at her mother during the visit but could not express it. This represented a breakthrough in Carmella's treatment because it was the *first time* Carmella made a connection between her feelings and her binge-eating behaviors. The primary nurse, psychiatrist, and patient continued to explore this connection in treatment. A major goal was to help Carmella develop new ways to express her anger, conflict, and disappointment in others. Family therapy, group therapy, and milieu therapy were used to address this goal. Carmella was also treated with fluoxitene, a selective serotonin reuptake inhibitor (SSRI), to address the obsessive-compulsive features of her binge-eating pattern.

Family Support: Psychoeducational Models

Family involvement in the care of clients with chronic mental illness results in better outcomes for the client. For example, family support of the patient has been shown to improve medication compliance (Mulaik, 1992) and to raise levels of satisfaction with family relations and housing (Dixon et al., 1998) in schizophrenic clients with severe and persistent mental illness. Enhanced family interaction has been related to a better quality of life (Sullivan, Wells, & Leake, 1992) and higher individual functioning (Thienemann et al., 1998) in families with a schizophrenic member. However, the burden of caring for a mentally ill family member is often overwhelming (Friedmann et al., 1997; Rose, 1996). Without adequate support, caregivers may become exhausted and relinquish their responsibilities. One of the most promising interventions to emerge since the deinstitutionalization movement is psychoeducation (McFarlane, 1997). Psychoeducational programs target the family as a unit; the benefits may be experienced by both the chronically mentally ill member and the family caregivers.

The content of psychoeducational interventions varies with the treatment philosophy as well as with the needs of the specific client and family. For example, one psychoeducational model called behavioral family management (Falloon, Boyd, & McGill, 1984) involves training families in family communication and problem solving. Another approach, called supportive family management (Zastowny, Lehman, Cole, & Kane, 1992), provides clients and families with detailed information about the illness, treatment plan, and services. Supportive family management may also include information on the availability of community services, advice on daily living, and management of client symptoms and family issues. A study (Zastowny et al., 1992) comparing these two psychoeducational interventions found similar clinical improvements with both approaches. Both interventions prevented frequent relapses and rehospitalization, decreased psychiatric symptoms, allowed a reduction in drug dosage, and improved the quality of life for patients and their families. The following case example illustrates the use of the supportive family management approach for a client with chronic schizophrenia.

CASE STUDY ➤

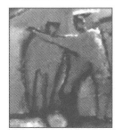

SUPPORTIVE FAMILY MANAGEMENT MODEL

Michael K., age 38, a man of Irish-American ethnicity, was first diagnosed with schizophrenia (undifferentiated type) when he was 19 years old. He had not been able to work gainfully since his initial diagnosis, and he remained at home with his mother Kathleen K., age 68, and her sister Grace W., age 63. Michael's father died when Michael was 7 years old. Thus, Michael's mother had been his only caregiver for most of his life. Michael had had more than 20 hospitalizations over the course of his illness. Hospitalization was usually precipitated by Michael's refusal to take his medications regularly. During his brief hospitalizations, Michael was stabilized on his medication and then discharged back to the care of his mother. The only follow-up care that Michael received was monthly meetings with his psychiatrist for medication management. Michael rarely kept those appointments because, in his delusional thinking, he was convinced that his medications had caused him to have cancer.

Michael's mother was afraid to push him too hard to take the medications because she feared it would cause his symptoms to worsen and Michael would become violent, as he had several times in the past.

During his most recent hospitalization for exacerbation of delusional thought patterns and disorganized speech and behavior, Michael was stabilized with an atypical antipsychotic agent and then was evaluated with magnetic resonance imaging scan (MRI) and neuropsychological testing. Consistent with findings from a number of patients with schizophrenia, Michaels's MRI showed evidence of increased lateral ventricles and decreased frontal and temporal lobe volume (Laraia, 2001). His neuropsychological testing identified a number of areas of functional impairment, including deficits in verbal memory and attention. Michael was referred to the psychoeducational treatment planning team to begin supportive family management that focused on the following:

- Education for Michael and the family about Michael's medications
- Education for Michael and the family about neuropsychological findings and their relevance for Michael's daily functioning—including compensa-

(continued on page 366)

CASE STUDY ➤ *(Continued)*

tory strategies for impaired memory and attention

- Instruction for Michael and the family on the signs and symptoms of acute exacerbations of schizophrenia
- Instruction for Michael and the family on behavior modification strategies to reinforce Michael's successful attendance in outpatient treatment and to reinforce compliance with medications
- Information for Michael and the family about the availability of public services to transport Michael to and from his outpatient appointments
- Information for Mrs. K. about the local chapter of the National Alliance for the Mentally Ill (NAMI), a family support group designed to help families understand and cope with the serious mental illness of a member
- Hotline phone numbers and local resources to help Mrs. K. if Michael became violent

A psychiatric mental health advanced practice nurse visited the family's home weekly to determine how the family was managing, to offer advice and information as needed, and to provide Mrs. K. with support. Weekly visits continued for the first 3 months after discharge from the hospital. Eventually the visits were tapered to an as-needed basis. Michael was able to stay out of the hospital for 16 months following the implementation of supportive family management. This was a dramatic change for the K. family, given Michael's history of frequent admissions to the hospital.

Although psychoeducational programs do not offer a cure for serious and persistent mental illness, they do assist clients to remain relatively free of the debilitating symptoms associated with the illness and they also provide support for family caregivers to allow them to continue in that role. Minimally, family intervention programs for the chronically mentally ill should include the following: (1) reduction of the stressful impact of the illness on the family; (2) information about the illness, patient abilities, and prognosis; (3) methods of stress reduction and problem solving; and (4) linkages to supplementary services to support the efforts of family members to maintain their patient in the community (Walsh & Anderson, 1987).

Psychiatric Home Care

Psychiatric home care services provided by advanced practice nurses are growing. Psychiatric advanced practice nurses can be reimbursed by Medicare, Medicaid, HMOs, and PPOs for home visits when the patient has a psychiatric diagnosis. Mental health services are given in the home on an intermittent basis to persons who are homebound because of their psychiatric or medical conditions. Home visits are beneficial for patients with major psychiatric illness discharged from inpatient settings, patients with increased acuity levels, and elderly patients experiencing psychosocial crises (Mohit, 2000). The beauty of home visits is that the psychiatric advanced practice nurse can observe the patient and family in their natural home environment, identify major family dynamics, and intervene quickly with the family to help the family address its problems. The nurse also functions as a case manager who coordinates all services, communicates with providers, educates the individual and family about the illness and symptom management, and provides individual and family therapy. The goal of home services is to stabilize the illness and maximize the patient's potential to remain home (Ward-Miller, 1996).

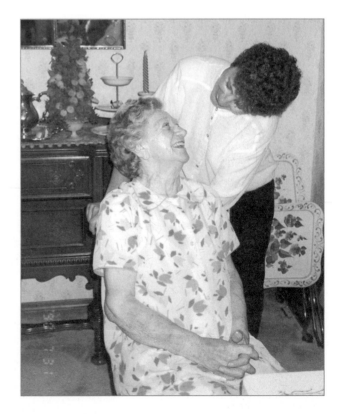

End of Life

When the family is faced with impending loss of a member, unresolved conflicts and relational patterns may become intensified. This could be an opportunity for the family to address these issues, thereby enhancing communication, trust, and intimacy. In assisting the family toward these goals, the family mental health nurse may intervene by (1) eliciting the family's multigenerational history of loss to understand better the meaning of the impending loss to the family, (2) guiding the family in constructively addressing unresolved conflicts and issues between family members and the dying individual, (3) helping the family to convey its feelings to the dying person and to say goodbye, and (4) supporting family members through the bereavement process, while remaining alert to symptoms that suggest complicated bereavement and the need for additional intervention.

> ❝When the family is faced with impending loss of a member, unresolved conflicts and relational patterns may become intensified.❞

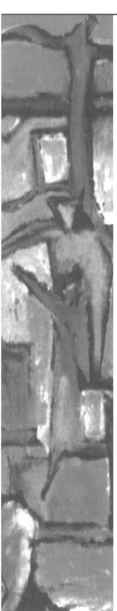

RESEARCH BRIEF: FAMILIES AND SCHIZOPHRENIA

Families caring for a member with schizophrenia face many stressors common to families caring for a member with a chronic illness. In addition, they may have experiences that are unique to living with this mental disorder.

Purpose of Study

The goal of this study was to identify themes that emerged in families living with a member who has schizophrenia. A previous study explored the influence of three family variables (family coping behaviors, family psychological distress, and family social support) and one patient variable (behavioral problems) on family functioning in families caring for a member with schizophrenia.

Methods

A qualitative approach—thematic analysis—was used to analyze written material provided by family members of individuals with schizophrenia. Data consisted of unsolicited comments by family members written on the instruments used in the previous quantitative study. Two researchers independently analyzed the material, generating separate lists of thematic categories. Through a process of abstraction and clarification, a mutually agreed-upon list of themes was generated. As a final measure of validation of the coherence and credibility of these findings, they were further evaluated by a participant of the original study.

Results

Five recurrent themes were identified: overwhelming feelings, importance of medication, legal system difficulties, family and friends, and mental health professionals. *Overwhelming feelings*, according to the authors, is a similar phenomenon to the concept of "psychological distress" used by other researchers. Examples of feelings included in this category are depression, pain, bewilderment, frustration, and fear. *The importance of medication* referred both to the positive effects of the prescribed regimen and to the deleterious patient and family consequences of noncompliance. *Legal system difficulties* encompassed families' frustration both with access to the legal system and with the system's perceived unresponsiveness to their input regarding treatment. As a category, *family and friends* reflected participants' need for additional support in caring for the member with schizophrenia, their gratitude for support received, and acknowledgement of losses of some family and friends due to the illness. *Mental health professionals* emerged as individuals who both helped and disappointed family members. Specifically, participants wished for a more collaborative relationship and assistance with caregiving responsibilities.

(continued on page 368)

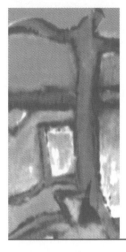

(Continued)

Nursing Implications

Findings underscore the need for family mental health nurses to (1) address the array of painful feelings experienced by family members of an individual with schizophrenia; (2) identify intervention strategies that enhance patient compliance with medications; (3) assist family members in navigating and improving the existing legal and mental health systems; (4) support family members' relationships with one another and with friends who constitute an ongoing source of needed support; and (5) acknowledge and support the family as the primary caregiving system by creating a collaborative and mutually respectful relationship throughout the course of treatment.

Source: Saunders, J. C., & Byrne, M. M. (2002). A thematic analysis of families living with schizophrenia. *Archives of Psychiatric Nursing, 16*, 217–223.

IMPLICATIONS FOR THEORY, PRACTICE, EDUCATION, RESEARCH, AND HEALTH POLICY

It is exciting that the body of knowledge about family mental health nursing is expanding. As shown in the case examples in this chapter, nurses may apply this knowledge in many different settings—in inpatient psychiatric and nonpsychiatric settings, in outpatient psychiatric and nonpsychiatric settings, in other community settings, and in the home. The expanding knowledge also has clear and compelling implications for theory development, research, education, and health policy.

Research and Theory

Concepts of families are changing. In the past, some family systems theories appeared to emphasize the relationship between family interactions and illness in a unidirectional flow from family to illness. However, clinicians and researchers now recognize the reciprocal influences between the family and illness within a sociocultural context: illness in a family member influences the family and the family may influence the course of an illness. The challenge for mental health professionals is to integrate this view into research and care of individuals and families. Family theories need to be expanded or modified to consider these reciprocal influences. It is not helpful to point a finger and blame individuals or families for illness. It is more helpful to engage the individual and family in a partnership for the benefit of both. It is also useful to draw on the patient's and family's resources in a collaborative process of goal setting and treatment. Those theories that are more resource-based need further

development and testing. No matter what the debate about the causes of problems, it is clear that both individuals and families suffer with them, and both deserve our empathy and care.

Research in the last two decades has produced major breakthroughs in genetics, immunology, and brain-behavioral relationships, increasing scientists' and mental health practitioners' understanding of biologic factors related to mental illness. For example, specific structural and functional changes in the brain have been found to be linked with schizophrenia, and DNA markers for the genetic predisposition to certain affective disorders have been identified (McBride, 1990; Laraia, 2001; NIMH, 2002). Although a familial vulnerability to schizophrenia, bipolar disorder, early-onset depression, anxiety disorders, autism, and attention deficit hyperactivity disorder has been observed, specific genetic linkages in these complex disorders have yet to be identified. Scientists now believe that these disorders are due not to a single defective gene but rather to the effects of many genes interacting with environmental factors (NIMH, 2002; Laraia, 2001).

Growing recognition of the biopsychosocial correlates of mental illness, shorter hospital stays, and the necessity for families to take primary responsibility for their member's care have led nurses and other mental health professionals to enter into a relationship with families as "partners in care." Professionals now acknowledge the benefits of basing family interventions on respect for the needs of family members and the family's collaborative role in improving patient functioning. Mental health professionals are thus combining information about the biological correlates of mental illness with a consideration of the psychological, social, cultural, and familial factors that also influence human behavior (McBride, 1990). This integrated approach (McKeon, 1990) has prompted nurses and other mental health professionals to identify and study the most effective strategies for mental health promotion in the family (O'Brien, 1998), the most effective ways to share information about a family member's schizophrenia with the family (Main, Gerace, & Camilleri, 1993), and the most effective ways to support families in caring for a schizophrenic family member in the community (Brooker & Butterworth, 1991; Zastowny et al., 1992).

In the current context of health care reform, increased emphasis must be placed on theory and research in the promotion of mental health in families, prevention of mental illness in families, and treatment of acute and chronic mental illness within families. Research on families is necessary to provide empirical support for funding family-based services. Most health care services in the United States are organized not around the family but rather around a health problem in the individual. Furthermore, reimbursement for health care is based on the individual; most third-party payers do not see the family as a client and do not accept family-level diagnoses. They provide coverage only for individual diagnoses included in the Diagnostic and Statistical Manual of Mental Disorders (DSM–IV-TR) (American Psychiatric Association, 2000), the diagnostic classification system for psychiatric illnesses.

Public Policy and Practice

In our cost-driven health care system, lengths of stays for psychiatric hospitalizations have dramatically decreased. As a result, there is an increasing reliance on families and communities to assume caregiving responsibilities and costs for members with mental illness. Families and communities are encountering a broad range of conditions that "require a more integrated view of wellness and illness, mind and body, and the biomedical and the behavioral" (Cotroneo, Kurlowicz, Outlaw, Burgess, & Evans, 2001, p. 551). Families are also shouldering much responsibility in trying to coordinate care across settings and providers in our very complex delivery system. Calls for an enhanced delivery system for mental health care are increasing (Cotroneo et al., 2001).

In our health care system, lip service is often paid to prevention services, and funding for mental health services lags behind funding for other conditions. Yet, mental health needs are often first identified in

primary care settings. Fifty percent of patients who seek treatment for mental disorders go to primary care providers for their care. Primary care providers will manage 30 percent of patients with mental disorders (Peek & Heinrich, 2000). Data showing that mental disorders contribute greatly to the overall disease burden in the United States is now receiving attention. The major impact of depression and anxiety (frequently seen in primary care) on quality of life, use of health services, and health outcomes has been recently acknowledged (Cotroneo et al., 2001; U.S. Department of Health and Human Services, 1999). Calls for collaborative practice models that integrate the biomedical and behavioral are increasing. In a landmark article in 2001 on directions for psychiatric mental health nursing, Cotroneo and colleagues stressed the need for a more integrated system of care delivery where mental health and other health professionals work together and engage patients, families, and communities as partners in health care. Psychiatric mental health nurses, who have a history of considering biopsychosocial factors and a history of collaborative relationships, can offer leadership for this delivery system (Cotroneo et al., 2001).

Education

Nursing education needs to incorporate a stronger family systems mental health focus in the curriculum, not only in mental health nursing but also in every clinical area, because all nurses encounter families that are confronting mental health issues. Undergraduate students need to learn how to assess the mental health of individuals and the family and how to intervene therapeutically with families in hospital, home, and clinic. Graduate students in psychiatric and mental health nursing need an in-depth understanding of family theories and clinical experience with family therapy in varied settings. As advanced practice nurses, they will be called on to perform comprehensive assessments and to intervene with families.

66 Nursing education needs to incorporate a stronger family systems mental health focus in the curriculum, not only in mental health nursing but also in every clinical area, because all nurses encounter families that are confronting mental health issues. 99

Access to mental health care is a serious problem for racial and ethnic nondominant people of color in the United States. Educators and clinicians are urging the development of training programs that prepare culturally competent therapists to meet the mental health needs of our diverse population (Cotroneo et al., 2001).

As stated in *Nursing: Social Policy Statement*, "the family is the necessary unit of service" (ANA, 1980, p. 5). The challenge now is for mental health nurses to embrace this idea and make it a reality in their thinking, practice, and research.

SUMMARY

- Mental health nurses who practice family-centered care are concerned with the mental health needs of the individual within the context of the family *and* the needs of the family as a whole.
- Family mental health nurses enter into relationships with families as "partners in care."
- Psychiatric mental health generalist nurses and advanced practice nurses have used varied family therapy theories to guide their understanding of family dynamics and their interventions with families.
- Using the biopsychosocial family systems perspective, family mental health nurses view clinical problems in a larger framework involving multiple systems.
- Family mental health nurses promote the mental health of individuals and families by helping individuals and families to cope with life stressors that make the family more vulnerable to emotional and physical problems.
- When a family member is hospitalized for an acute psychiatric illness, the family mental health nurse focuses on the needs of the individual and family by providing family-focused inpatient treatment.
- When working with a family member who has a chronic mental illness, the family mental health nurse recognizes that the individual and the family suffer, and both need respect, understanding, and support.
- Psychoeducational models for chronic mental illness offer support, education, symptom management, and community resources to individuals with severe and persistent mental illness and to their families.
- Family mental health nurses are advocates for families. They assist families to navigate the complex and often frustrating mental health delivery system when families are seeking mental health care.

References

Abbott, J., Johnson, R., Koziol-McLain, J., & Lowenstein, S. R. (1995). Domestic violence against women: Incidence and prevalence in an emergency department population. *Journal of American Medical Association, 273,* 1763–1767.

Amaro, H., Fried, L. E., Cabral, H., & Zuckerman B. (1990). Violence during pregnancy and substance use. *American Journal of Public Health, 80,* 575–579.

American Medical Association (AMA). (1994). *Diagnostic and treatment guidelines on domestic violence.* Chicago: AMA.

American Medical Association (AMA). (1996). *Facts about family violence.* Chicago: AMA.

American Nurses Association (ANA). (1980). *Nursing: Social policy statement.* Kansas City, MO: ANA.

American Nurses Association (ANA). (1994). *Statement on psychiatric mental health clinical practice and standards of psychiatric mental health clinical nursing practice.* Council on Psychiatric and Mental Health Nursing. Washington, DC: ANA.

American Nurses Association (ANA), American Psychiatric Nurses Association (APNA), & International Society of Psychiatric Mental Health Nurses (2000). *Scope and standards of psychiatric-mental health nursing practice* (Publication # PMH-20).

American Psychiatric Association (APA). (2000). *Diagnostic and statistical manual of mental disorders* (4th ed., text revision). Washington, DC: APA.

American Psychiatric Nurses Association (APNA). (2003a). *Frequently asked questions (FAQ's) about psychiatric nursing.* Retrieved from http://www.apna.org/faq/aboutnursing.html

American Psychiatric Nurses Association (APNA). (2003b). *APNA position paper on psychiatric-mental health nursing practice.* Retrieved from http://www.apna.org/resources/positionpapers.html

American Psychological Association (APA). (1996). *Violence and the family: Report of the APA Presidential Task Force on Violence and the Family* (p. 11). Washington, DC: Author.

Armbruster, P., Gerstein, S. H., & Fallon, T. (1997). Bridging the gap between need and service utilization: A school-based mental health program. *Community Mental Health Journal, 33,* 199–211.

Bachrach, L. (1991). The chronic patient: Community psychiatry's changing role. *Hospital and Community Psychiatry, 42,* 573–574.

Baker, A. F. (1989). Living with a chronic schizophrenic can place great stress on individual family members and the family unit: How families cope. *Journal of Psychosocial Nursing, 27,* 31–36.

Baker, A. F. (1993). Schizophrenia and the family. In C. S. Fawcett (Ed.), *Family psychiatric nursing* (pp. 342–355). St. Louis: Mosby Year Book.

Bateson, G., Jackson, D., Haley, J., & Weakland, J. (1956). Toward a theory of schizophrenia. *Behavioral Science, 1*(19), 251–275.

Berenson, A. B., Wiemann, C. M., Wilkinson, G. S., Jones, W. A., & Anderson, G. D. (1994). Perinatal morbidity associated with violence experienced by pregnant women. *American Journal of Obstetrics and Gynecology, 170,* 1760–1769.

Berkey, K. M., & Hanson, S. M. (1991). *Pocket guide to family assessment and intervention.* Philadelphia: Mosby Year Book.

Boszormenyi-Nagy, I., & Krasner, B. (1986). *Between give and take: A clinical guide to contextual theory.* New York: Brunner/Mazel.

Boszormenyi-Nagy, I., & Spark, G. (1973). *Invisible loyalties.* New York: Harper & Row.

Bowen, M. (1976). Theory in the practice of psychotherapy. In P. J. Guerin (Ed.), *Family therapy: Theory and practice* (pp. 42–90). New York: Gardner Press.

Bowen, M. (1978). *Family therapy in clinical practice.* New York: Jason Aronson.

Bowers, J., & McNally, K. (1983). Family-focused care in the psychiatric inpatient setting. *Image: The Journal of Nursing Scholarship, 15,* 26–31.

Brain imaging and psychiatry. Part I. (1997, February). *Harvard Mental Health Letter, 13*(8), 1–4.

Brooker, C., & Butterworth, C. (1991). Working with families caring for a relative with schizophrenia: The evolving role of the community psychiatric nurse. *International Journal of Nursing Studies, 28,* 189–200.

Brown, F. H. (Ed.). (1991). *Reweaving the family tapestry.* New York: W.W. Norton.

Burgess, A. W. (1997). Psychiatric nursing. In A. W. Burgess (Ed.), *Psychiatric nursing: Promoting mental health* (pp. 11–34). Stamford, CT: Appleton & Lange.

Canino, I. A., & Spurlock, J. (1997). Mental health issues of culturally diverse and underserved children. *Journal of the Association for Academic Minority Physicians, 8,* 63–66.

Cascardi, M., Langhinrichsen, J., & Vivian, D. (1992). Marital aggression. Impact, injury, and health correlates for husbands and wives. *Archives of Internal Medicine, 152,* 1178–1184.

Centers for Disease Control and Prevention. (1998). *Cohabitation, marriage, divorce, and remarriage in the United States* (Series Report 23, Number 22, 103 pp., Public Health Service 98-1998). Hyattsville, MD: National Center for Health Statistics.

Centers for Disease Control and Prevention. (1999). *Fastats A-Z, mental health.* Retrieved from http://www.cdc.gov/nchswww/fastats/mental.htm

Chafez, L., & Barns, L. (1989). Issues in psychiatric caregiving. *Archives of Psychiatric Nursing, 3*(2), 61–68.

Child Abuse Prevention Treatment Act. (1974). United States federal legislation (Public Law 93-247). Washington, DC: U.S. Government.

Cirillo, S., & DiBlasio, P. (1992). *Families that abuse: Diagnosis and therapy* (J. Neugroschel, Trans.). New York: Norton.

Clements, I. W., & Roberts, F. B. (Eds.). (1983). *Family health: A theoretical approach to nursing care.* New York: Wiley & Sons.

Cochrane, J. J., Goering, P. N., & Rogers, J. M. (1997). The mental health of informal caregivers in Ontario: An epidemiological study. *American Journal of Public Health, 87,* 2002–2007.

Colgan-McCarthy, I., & O'Reilly-Byrne, N. (1988). Mis-taken love: Conversations on the problem of incest in an Irish context. *Family Process, 27,* 181–199.

Costello, E. J., Farmer, E. M., Angold, A., Burns, B. J., & Erkanli, A. (1997). Psychiatric disorders among American Indian and white youth in Appalachia: The Great Smoky Mountains study. *American Journal of Public Health, 87,* 827–832.

Cotroneo, M. (1982). The role of forgiveness in family therapy. In A. Gurman (Ed.), *Questions and answers in family therapy* (Vol. 2, pp. 241–244). New York: Bruner/Mazel.

Cotroneo, M. (1986). Families and abuse: A contextual approach. In M. Karpel (Ed.), *Family resources* (pp. 413–437). New York: Guilford Press.

Cotroneo, M., Hibbs, B. J., & Moriarty, H. (1992). Uses and implications of the contextual approach to child custody decisions. *Journal of Child and Adolescent Psychiatric and Mental Health Nursing, 5*(3), 13–26.

Cotroneo, M., Kurlowicz, L. H., Outlaw, F. H., Burgess, A. W., & Evans, L. K. (2001). Psychiatric-mental health nursing at the interface: Revisioning education for the specialty. *Issues in Mental Health Nursing, 22,* 549–569.

Cotroneo, M., & Moriarty, H. (1992). Intergenerational family processes in the treatment of incest. In A. Burgess (Ed.), *Child trauma: Issues and research* (pp. 293–305). New York: Garland.

Cotroneo, M., Moriarty, H., & Smith, E. (1992). Managing family loyalty conflicts in child custody disputes. *Journal of Family Psychotherapy, 3*(2), 19–38.

Crowell, N. A., & Burgess, A. W. (1996). *Understanding violence against women.* Washington, DC: National Academy Press.

Danielson, C. B., Hamel-Bissell, B., & Winstead-Fry, P. (1993). *Families, health, and illness: Perspectives on coping and intervention.* St. Louis: Mosby Year Book.

Daro, D., & Wang, C. (1997). Current trends in child abuse reporting and fatalities: Annual fifty state survey. Chicago, IL: NCPCA.

DeSocio, J., Bowllan, N., & Staschak, S. (1997). Lessons learned in creating a safe and therapeutic milieu for children, adolescents, and families: Developmental considerations. *Journal of Child and Adolescent Psychiatric Nursing, 10,* 18–26.

Dixon, L., Stewart, B., Krauss, N., Robbins, J., Hackman, A., & Lehman, A. (1998). The participation of families of homeless persons with severe mental illness in an outreach intervention. *Community Mental Health Journal, 34,* 251–259.

Dobash, R. E., & Dobash, R. (1979). *Violence against wives: A case against the patriarchy.* New York: Free Press. Cited in B. Strong & C. DeVault (1992). *The marriage and family experience* (5th ed., p. 468). New York: West.

Eating disorders. Part II. (1997, November). *Harvard Mental Health Letter, 14*(5), 1–4.

Elliott, B. A., & Johnson, M. M. (1995). Domestic violence in a primary care setting. *Archives of Family Medicine, 4,* 113–119.

Emery, R. (1982). Interparental conflict and the children of discord and divorce. *Psychological Bulletin, 92,* 310–330.

Engel, G. L. (1977). The need for a new medical model: A challenge for biomedicine. *Science, 196,* 129–136.

Engel, G. L. (1996). From biomedical to biopsychosocial: I. Being scientific in the human domain. *Families, Systems & Health, 14,* 425–433.

Falloon, I. R. H., Boyd, J. L., & McGill, W. (1984). *Family care of schizophrenia.* New York: Guilford Press.

Family Violence Prevention Fund (1998). *Health care response to domestic violence: Fact sheet.* San Francisco, CA.

Fawcett, J., & Whall, A. (1991). Family theory development. In *Nursing: State of the science and the art.* Philadelphia: FA Davis.

Finkelhor, D. (1988). *Stopping family violence.* Newbury Park, CA: Sage.

Friedmann, M. S., McDermut, W. H., Solomon, D. A., Ryan, C. E., Keitner, G. I., & Miller, I. W. (1997). Family functioning and mental illness: A comparison of psychiatric and nonclinical families. *Family Process, 36,* 357–367.

Gelinas, D. (1986). Unexpected resources in treating incest families. In M. Karpel (Ed.), *Family resources* (pp. 327–358). New York: Guilford.

Gilliss, J. M. (1973). *Family therapy in clinical practice: An abstract.* Unpublished manuscript, University of Pennsylvania School of Nursing, Philadelphia.

Goren, S. (1992). Practicing in partnership with families in the inpatient setting. *Journal of Child and Adolescent Psychiatric and Mental Health Nursing, 5*(3), 43–46.

Haber, J., Hoskins, P. P., Leach, A. M., & Sideleau, B. F. (1987). *Comprehensive psychiatric nursing* (3rd ed.). New York: McGraw-Hill.

Haber, J., & Billings, C. (1993). Primary mental health care: A vision for the future of psychiatric-mental health nursing. *ANA Council Perspectives, 2*(2), 1.

Haley, J. (1963). *Strategies of psychotherapy.* New York: Grune & Stratton.

Haley, J. (1976). *Problem-solving therapy.* San Francisco: Jossey-Bass.

Hamberger, L. K., Saunders, D. G., & Hovey, M. (1992). Prevalence of domestic violence in community practice and rate of physician inquiry. *Family Medicine, 24,* 382–387.

Handron, D. S., Dosser, D. A., McCammon, S. I., & Powell, J. Y. (1998). "Wraparound": The wave of the future: Theoretical and professional practice implications for children and families with complex needs. *Journal of Family Nursing, 4,* 65–86.

Hare-Mustin, R. (1976). Paradoxical tasks in family therapy: Who can resist? *Psychotherapy: Theory, Research and Practice, 13,* 128–130.

Herrick, C. A., & Goodkoontz, L. (1989). Neuman's systems model for nursing practice as a conceptual framework. *Journal of Child and Adolescent Psychiatric Nursing, 2*(2), 61–67.

Hetherington, E. (1981). Children and divorce. In R. Henderson (Ed.), *Parent-child interaction: Theory, research, and practice* (pp. 35–58). New York: Academic Press.

Hetherington, E., Cox, M., & Cox, R. (1978). The aftermath of divorce. In J. Stevens & M. Mathews (Eds.), *Mother/child, father/child relationships* (pp. 149–176). Washington, DC: National Association for Education of Young Children.

Hines-Martin, V. P. (1998). Environmental context of caring for severely mentally ill adults: An African American experience. *Issues in Mental Health Nursing, 19*, 433–451.

Institute of Medicine. (1989). *Research on children and adolescents with mental, behavioral and developmental disorders.* Report of a study by a committee of the Institute of Medicine (Division of Mental Health and Behavioral Medicine), National Academy of Sciences. Washington, DC: National Academy Press.

Jackson, D. D. (1965a). Family rules: Marital quid pro quo. *Archives of General Psychiatry, 12*, 589–594.

Jackson, D. D. (1965b). The study of the family. *Family Process, 4*, 1–20.

Johnson, C. A., & Johnson, D. L. (1998). Working with Native American families. *New Directions for Mental Health Services, 77*, 89–96.

Jones, S. L. (1999). NAMI: A convention worth noting. National Alliance for the Mentally Ill. *Archives of Psychiatric Nursing, 13*, 1–2.

Kerr, M. E., & Bowen, M. (1988). *Family evaluation.* New York: W. W. Norton.

Laraia, M. (2001). Biological context of psychiatric nursing care. In G. W. Stuart & M. T. Laraia (Eds.), *Principles and practice of psychiatric nursing* (7th ed., pp. 88–119). St. Louis: C.V. Mosby.

Lavigne, J. V., Arend, R., Rosenbaum, D., Binns, H. J., Christoffel, K. K., & Gibbon, R. D. (1998). Psychiatric disorders with onset in the preschool years: II. Correlates and predictors of stable case status. *Journal of the American Academy of Child and Adolescent Psychiatry, 37*, 1255–1261.

Lefley, H. (1990). Culture and chronic mental illness. *Hospital and Community Psychiatry, 41*, 277–286.

Lefley, H. P. (1998a). The family experience in cultural context: Implications for further research and practice. *New Directions for Mental Health Services, 77*, 97–106.

Lefley, H. P. (1998b). Family culture and mental illness: Constructing new realities. *Psychiatry, 61*, 335–355.

Lieberman Research Institute (1996, July–October). Tracking survey conducted for the Advertising Council and the Family Violence Prevention Fund.

Lin, K. M., & Kleinman, A. M. (1988). Psychopathology and clinical course of schizophrenia: A cross-cultural perspective. *Schizophrenia Bulletin, 14*, 555–567.

Main, M. C., Gerace, L. M., & Camilleri, D. (1993). Information sharing concerning schizophrenia in a family member: Adult siblings' perspectives. *Archives of Psychiatric Nursing, 7*(3), 147–153.

McBride, A. B. (1990). Psychiatric nursing in the 1990s. *Archives of Psychiatric Nursing, 4*, 21–28.

McDaniel, S., Hepworth, J., & Doherty, W. (1992). *Medical family therapy. A biopsychosocial approach to families with health problems.* New York: Basic Books.

McFarlane, W. R. (1997). Fact: Integrating family psychoeducation and assertive community treatment. *Administration and Policy in Mental Health, 25*, 191–198.

McKeon, K. L. (1990). Introduction: A future perspective on psychiatric mental health nursing. *Archives of Psychiatric Nursing, 4*, 19–20.

Miniño, A. M., Arias, E., Kochanek, K. D., Murphy, S. L., & Smith, B. L. (2002). Deaths: Final data for 2000. *National Vital Statistics Reports, 50*(15). Hyattsville, MD: National Center for Health Statistics.

Minuchin, S. (1974). *Families and family therapy.* Cambridge, MA: Harvard University Press.

Minuchin, S., & Fishman, H. C. (1981). *Family therapy techniques.* Cambridge, MA: Harvard University Press.

Minuchin, S., Rosman, B. L., & Baker, L. (1978). *Psychosomatic families: Anorexia nervosa in context.* Cambridge, MA: Harvard University Press.

Mohit, D. (2000). Psychiatric home care and family therapy: A window of opportunity for the psychiatric clinical nurse specialist. *Archives of Psychiatric Nursing, 14*, 127–133.

Moltz, D. A. (1993). Bipolar disorder and the family: An integrative model. *Family Process, 32*, 409–423.

Mood disorders: An overview. Part I. (1997, December). *Harvard Mental Health Letter, 14*(6), 1–4.

Moriarty, H. J., & Shepard, M. (2000). Mental health family nursing. In S. Hanson (Ed.), *Family health care nursing: Theory, practice, and research* (2nd ed., pp. 300–325). New York: Davis.

Moscicki, E. K. (2001). Epidemiology of completed and attempted suicide: Toward a framework for prevention. *Clinical Neuroscience Research, 1*, 310–323.

Mulaik, J. S. (1992). Noncompliance with medication regimens in severely and persistently mentally ill schizophrenic patients. *Issues in Mental Health Nursing, 13*, 219–237.

Murray, C. J. L., & Lopez, A. D. (Eds.). (1996). *The global burden of disease and injury series, volume 1: A comprehensive assessment of mortality and disability from diseases, injuries, and risk factors in 1990 and projected to 2020.* Cambridge, MA: Published by the Harvard School of Public Health on behalf of the World Health Organization and the World Bank, Harvard University Press. Retrieved from http://www.who.int/msa/mnh/ems/dalys/intro.htm

Nahulu, L. B., Andrade, N. N., Makini, G. K., Yuen, N. Y., McDermott, J. F., Danko, G. P., et al. (1996). Psychosocial risk and protective influences in Hawaiian adolescent psychopathology. *Cultural Diversity and Mental Health, 2*, 107–114.

Napoliello, A. L., & Sweet, E. S. (1992). Salvador Minuchin's structural family therapy and its application to Native Americans. *Family Therapy, 19*, 155–165.

National Institute of Health & Substance Abuse and Mental Health Services Administration. (2000). *Healthy People 2010.* Retrieved from http://www.healthypeople.gov/Document/HTML/Volume2/18Mental.htm#_Toc486932699

National Institute of Mental Health, D/ART Campaign. (1995). *Depression: What every woman should know* (Pub No. 95-3871). Retrieved from http://www.nimh.nih.gov/publicat/depwomenknows.cfm

National Institute of Mental Health. (1999). *Schizophrenia research at the National Institute of Mental Health.* Retrieved from http://www.nimh.nih.gov/publicat/schizresfact.htm

National Institute of Mental Health. (2001). *NIMH research on women's mental health: FY1999-FY2000.* Retrieved from http://www.nimh.nih.gov/wmhc/highlights.cfm#2a

National Institute of Mental Health. (2002). *Gene hunting* (NIH Publication No. 01-4600). Retrieved from http://www.nimh.nih.gov/publicat/huntgene.cfm

Navarre, S. E. (1998). Salvador Minuchin's structural family therapy and its application to multicultural family systems. *Issues in Mental Health Nursing, 19*, 557–570.

Norton, L. B., Peipert, J. F., Zieler, S., Lima, B., & Hume, L. (1995). Battering in pregnancy: An assessment of two screening methods. *Obstetrics and Gynecology, 85*, 321–325.

O'Brien, S. M. (1998). Health promotion and schizophrenia. Year 2000 and beyond. *Holistic Nursing Practice, 12*, 38–43.

Oliver, J. E. (1993). Intergenerational transmission of child abuse: Rates, research, and clinical implications. *American Journal of Psychiatry, 150*(9), 1315–1324.

Parker, B., McFarlane, J., & Soeken, K. (1994). Abuse during pregnancy: Effects on maternal complications and birth weight in adults and teenage women. *Obstetrics and Gynecology, 84*, 323–328.

Patel, V., Todd, C., Winston, M., Gwanzura, F., Simunyu, E., Acuda, W., & Mann, A. (1998). Outcome of common mental disorders in Harare, Zimbabwe. *British Journal of Psychiatry, 172,* 53–57.

Peek, C. J., & Heinrich, R. L. (2000). Integrating behavioral health and primary care. In M. E. Maruish (Ed.), *Handbook of psychological assessment in primary care* (pp. 43–91). Mahwah: Lawrence Erlbaum.

Peplau, H. E. (1993). Foreword. In C. S. Fawcett (Ed.), *Family psychiatric nursing* (pp. vii–ix). St. Louis: Mosby Year Book.

Plichta, S., (1992). The effects of women abuse on health care utilization and health status: A literature review. *Women's Health Issues, 2,* 1154–1173.

Raine, A., Brennan, P., Mednick, B., & Mednick, S. A. (1996). High rates of violence, crime, academic problems, and behavioral problems in males with both early neuromotor deficits and unstable family environments. *Archives of General Psychiatry, 53,* 544–549.

Rand, M. R. (1997, August). *Violence-related injuries treated in hospital emergency departments.* U.S. Department of Justice. Washington, DC: Bureau of Justice Statistics.

Reynolds, A. J. (1998). Resilience among black urban youth. Prevalence, intervention effects, and mechanisms of influence. *American Journal of Orthopsychiatry, 68,* 84–100.

Rolland, J. S. (1994). *Families, illness and disability: An integrative treatment model.* New York: Basic Books.

Rose, L. E. (1996). Families of psychiatric patients: A critical review and future research directions. *Archives of Psychiatric Nursing, 10,* 67–76.

Scharer, K. (1999). Nurse-parent relationship building in child psychiatric units. *Journal of Child and Adolescent Psychiatric Nursing, 12,* 153–167.

Shepard, M. P., & Moriarty, H. J. (1996). Family mental health nursing. In S. M. H. Hanson & S. T. Boyd (Eds.), *Family health care nursing* (pp. 303–326). Philadelphia: FA Davis.

Skultans, V. (1991). Women and affliction in Maharashtra: A hydraulic model of health and illness. *Culture, Medicine and Psychiatry, 15,* 321–359.

Solomon, P. (1998). The cultural context of interventions for family members with a seriously mentally ill relative. *New Directions for Mental Health Services, 77,* 5–16.

Stanton, M. D. (1981). Strategic approaches to family therapy. In A. Gurman & D. Kniskern (Eds.), *Handbook of family therapy.* New York: Brunner/Mazel.

Strong, B., & DeVault, C. (1992). *The marriage and family experience.* New York: West.

Substance Abuse and Mental Health Services Administration (SAMHSA) National Mental Health Information Center (2003).*Children's and adolescents' mental health.* Retrieved from http://www.mentalhealth.samhsa.gov/publications/allpubs/CA-0004/default.asp

Sullivan, G., Wells, K. B., & Leake, B. (1992). Clinical factors associated with better quality of life in a seriously mentally ill population. *Hospital and Community Psychiatry, 43,* 794–798.

Sveinbjarnardottir, E., & Dierckx de Casterle, B. (1997). Mental illness in the family: An emotional experience. *Issues in Mental Health Nursing, 18,* 45–56.

Thienemann, M., Shaw, R. J., & Steiner, H. (1998). Defense style and family environment. *Child & Human Development, 28,* 89–198.

Tjaden, P., & Thoennes, N. (2000). *Extent, nature, and consequences of intimate partner violence: Findings from the National Violence against Women Survey.* Report for grant 93-IJ-CX-0012, funded by the National Institute of Justice and the Centers for Disease Control. Washington, DC: NIJ.

U.S. Department of Health and Human Services. (1999). *Mental health: A report of the surgeon general—Executive summary.* Rockville, MD: U.S. Department of Health and Human Services, Substance Abuse and Mental Health Services Administration, Center for Mental Health Services, National Institutes of Health, National Institute of Mental Health.

U.S. Department of Health and Human Services, Children's Bureau. (2003). *Child maltreatment 2001.* Washington, DC: U.S. Government Printing Office.

U.S. Department of Health and Human Services Office of Public Health and Science. (1998). *Healthy People 2010 objectives: Draft for public comment.* Washington, DC: U.S. Government Printing Office.

Vandiver, V. L., & Keopraseuth, K. O. (1998). Family wisdom and clinical support: Culturally relevant practice strategies for working with Indochinese families who care for a relative with mental illness. *New Directions for Mental Health Services, 77,* 75–88.

Wallerstein, J., & Kelly, J. (1980). *Surviving the breakup.* New York: Basic Books.

Walsh, F. (1987). New perspectives on schizophrenia and the family. In F. Walsh & C. M. Anderson (Eds.), *Handbook of family therapy* (pp. 3–18). New York: Haworth Press.

Walsh, F., & Anderson, C. M. (1987). Chronic disorders and families: An overview. In F. Walsh & C. M. Anderson (Eds.), *Chronic disorders and the family* (pp. 3–18). New York: Haworth Press.

Ward-Miller, S. (1996). The psychiatric clinical specialist in the home care setting. *Nursing Clinics of North America, 3,* 519–525.

Watzlawick, P., Beavin, J., & Jackson, D. (1967). *The pragmatics of human communication.* New York: Norton.

Watzlawick, P., Weakland, J., & Fisch, R. (1974). *Change: Principles of problem formation and problem resolution.* New York: W. W. Norton.

Weakland, J. H. (1976). Communication theory and clinical change. In P. J. Guerin, Jr. (Ed.), *Family theory: Theory and practice.* New York: Gardner Press.

Whall, A. L. (1991). Family system theory: Relationship to nursing conceptual models. In A. L. Whall & J. Fawcett (Eds.), *Family theory development in nursing: State of the science and art* (pp. 317–341). Philadelphia: FA Davis.

Wieselberg, H. (1992). Family therapy and ultra-orthodox Jewish families: A structural approach. *Journal of Family Therapy, 14,* 305–329.

Wood, B. L. (1993). Beyond the "psychosomatic family": A bio-behavioral family model of pediatric illness. *Family Process, 32,* 261–278.

Wright, L., & Leahey, M. (1994). *Nurses and families. A guide to family assessment and intervention* (2nd ed.). Philadelphia: FA Davis.

Yaccarino, M. E. (1993). Using Minuchin's structural family therapy techniques with Italian-American families. *Contemporary Family Therapy, 15,* 459–466.

Zastowny, T. R., Lehman, A. F., Cole, R. E., & Kane, C. (1992). Family management of schizophrenia: A comparison of behavioral and supportive family treatment. *Psychiatric Quarterly, 63,* 159–186.

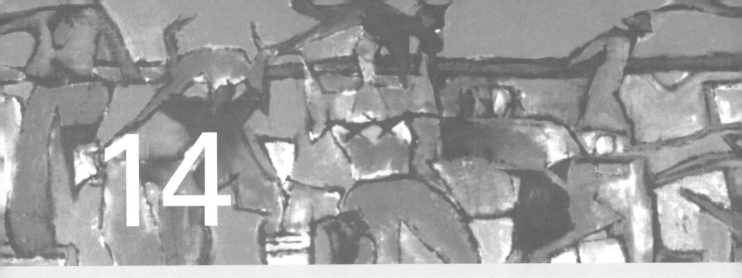

14

Gerontological Family Nursing

Mary LuAnne Lilly, PhD, RN

CRITICAL CONCEPTS

- Families are the primary providers of care and support for elderly kin.

- Multiple and competing demands are typical in contemporary families and can undermine family cohesiveness, particularly when demands exceed family resources.

- Gerontological family nurses can assist elderly individuals and their families through the application of specialized knowledge related to individual and family development, health maintenance, acute and chronic illness, family caregiving dynamics, interpersonal communication, referral resources, and evidence-based interventions.

- Theoretical models informed by family systems theory provide a useful framework for organizing and understanding data, selecting interventions, and evaluating outcomes.

- Gerontological family nurses possess a working knowledge of currently available supplemental resources (e.g., Agency on Aging, Alzheimer's Association, Meals on Wheels) for referral purposes.

- Gerontological family nurses must be aware that social, economic, and cultural forces interact to limit or expand the availability, accessibility, and affordability of supplemental services for families.

- Many older persons with chronic conditions are able to remain in the community. The family, not the formal health care system, provides 80 to 90 percent of care to its elderly members, including medical and nursing care, personal services such as transportation, and help with household tasks and shopping.

- Women have always been the traditional caregivers and they continue to provide nearly two-thirds (66 percent) of the family care given to older members. This figure remains constant, even though more women than ever are in the workforce.

INTRODUCTION

Our society is aging rapidly. Although this demographic shift is influencing every institution in our society, none are more affected than the family and health care. With increasing longevity, there is an increase in chronic, incapacitating conditions. At the same time, as efforts to contain health care costs intensify, more and more responsibility for care and assistance is being shifted into the community. Unfortunately, the current health care delivery is oriented primarily toward meeting the needs of the individual, not the family unit. Consequently, many families "go it alone," seeking professional help only during emergencies or periods of acute illness. Some family researchers have raised questions about the family's capacity to continue to assume increasing responsibility for informal care under the present system.

In our society, nearly every family is concerned with the well-being of at least one elderly member. Contemporary families balance workplace responsibility, child care/child-rearing commitments, and civic involvement. The family is where members learn about health and illness and also where most care is given and received throughout life. Consequently, the family has great potential as an ally in maintaining and restoring the health of its members, particularly the elderly.

The purpose of this chapter is to provide an overview of gerontological family nursing. Using a holistic, theory-based approach to working with families, gerontological family nurses are uniquely able to exert a positive influence in the lives of older persons and their loved ones by assisting them both physically and psychologically. To do so, however, the nurse builds an effective partnership with the family to maximize its capabilities, minimize its vulnerabilities, and serve as a bridge to the formal care system. Thoughtful, well-planned nursing interventions that recognize and use family strengths promote the health of the members and prevent or alleviate many of the negative outcomes of illness. The challenges, decisions, and transitions faced by many families as they move through later life are also examined in this chapter, as are the many facets of the nurse's role in working with families to provide care and services to their older members.

66 Thoughtful, well-planned nursing interventions that recognize and use family strengths promote the health of the members and prevent or alleviate many of the negative outcomes of illness. 99

COMMON THEORETICAL PERSPECTIVES

Families are like individuals in that each has a life cycle with predictable developmental stages and changes. The changes that families experience over time are like those in a kaleidoscope. The turn of events, whether an accumulation of small changes or the advent of a major stressor, results in the creation of a new pattern from the existing components of family life. Whereas some changes are subtle, others are more dramatic, but the changing patterns unfold progressively.

Until the occurrence of a stressor event or crisis that demands change, families maintain fairly stable patterns of interaction over time. Events that demand change take two forms: normative and nonnormative. Normative changes or transitions are those expected, somewhat predictable maturational life events, such as marriage, birth of the first child, retirement, and death of a spouse in old age. Although these are expected changes, a period of floundering or crisis may occur until the family adjusts. Nonnormative crises, on the other hand, are not predicted or expected and may occur with little warning. Examples include the diagnosis of a serious chronic illness, the accidental death of a family member, a job transfer, the unexpected unemployment of a primary breadwinner, or adult children having to move back home with parents. The suddenness of the event does not allow the family to plan or rehearse options, and there can be considerable family disequilibrium, confusion, and distress until the family establishes new patterns in roles and responsibilities.

The ways in which families work together to meet these demands and changes, maintain equilibrium, and meet the needs of members have been studied extensively from the perspective of family systems theory. Two system-based models provide a framework for understanding and working effectively with aging families. The first is the Family Life Cycle Model, which provides a view of how families change over time (Aldous, 1978; Carter & McGoldrick, 1980; Duvall & Miller, 1985). It points out places in family development where changes in status and roles are likely to occur, and it can be useful in predicting many facets of family behavior and vulnerability. The second model is the Resiliency Model of Family Stress, Adjustment, and Adaptation (McCubbin & McCubbin, 1993). This approach to the family is concerned with how families negotiate change and adapt to stressful life events over time, particularly to stressors such as illness. The approach is especially useful because it incorporates the characteristics of the individual members, the family system, and the community, all of which interact to shape the course of family behavior and adaptation. It also stresses the importance of family resilience and the natural healing qualities of family life.

Life Cycle of Older Families

The family's life cycle includes the various stages of development of the family system over time. These stages are convenient divisions that help to study a process that, in real life, flows from one stage to another without a pause or break.

Stages divide the lifetime of a family into distinctive periods that are marked by changes in status and roles. Stages are initiated by critical events that can originate either inside or outside the family system. Internal events in the older family include becoming a couple again after launching the last child, becoming grandparents, experiencing the onset of physical or cognitive incapacity in a spouse or elderly parent, or the death of the spouse. Events originating outside the family may occur in connection with education or work life and include retirement or starting a second career.

As with the development of individuals, each stage requires the completion of certain tasks to move on to the next stage. Duvall and Miller (1985, p. 318) identified eight family developmental tasks of the aging couple:

1. Making satisfying living arrangements as aging progresses
2. Adjusting to retirement income

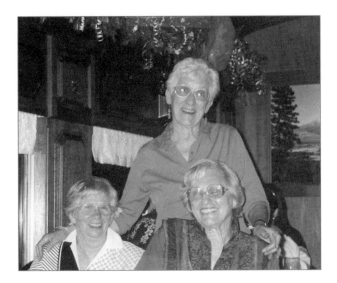

3. Establishing comfortable routines
4. Safeguarding physical and mental health
5. Maintaining love, sex, and marital relations
6. Remaining in touch with other family members
7. Keeping active and involved
8. Finding meaning in life

As families move from one stage into the next, changes in earlier interaction patterns create changes within the family system. Schumacher and Meleis (1994) identified transitions as a concept central to nursing. Client-nurse contact may occur as a result of individual or family response to situational, developmental, or health status transitions. In an earlier work, Brubaker (1983) identified four common events that initiate significant transitions in the careers of aging families. Each requires family members, either willingly or unwillingly, to participate in negotiating the change. These are the following:

- The empty nest, or launching of children into independence
- Retirement of one or both spouses from employment
- An incapacitating illness that compromises independence or requires institutionalization
- Disruption of the family through death
- Need for relocation or change in living arrangements because of declining health or functional abilities

Assessment of the Life Cycle

The Family Development Model provides a framework within which to assess both existing and potential strengths and vulnerabilities in the family. The results of the assessment can be built into the plan of care using anticipatory guidance, education, and support. In the life cycle of the family, roles, responsibilities, individual developmental tasks, career demands, and resources are rarely synchronized. Therefore, understanding the timing and intersection of internal and external events is crucial in determining family vulnerability. It is especially important to examine critical role transitions within the family— recent, current, or anticipated—because some have greater potential than others for causing stress and vulnerability.

Transitions within older families occur when roles and responsibilities start to shift across the generations. Middle-aged children often find their aging parents coming to them for emotional support, advice, and other forms of help. This may occur at a time when their own children are leaving home, the family's financial resources are stretched to pay for college tuition, and the mother is returning full-time to the workforce. For the older generation, the changes brought by retirement, possible loss of income, and physical decline may bring fear and trepidation. Reaching out to their children for help is often a disturbing and even humiliating experience. As much as they need the help, they may have great difficulty in asking for it.

As elderly members begin to develop signs of physical or cognitive decline that threaten their independence and capacity for self-care, several things are likely to happen. There may be a shift in the traditional hierarchical structure as parental authority and influence decline, which brings shifts in roles, responsibilities, and boundaries. Adult children are confronted with the filial crisis, a concept introduced by Blenkner (1965) in an attempt to explain the experience of adult children when parent care becomes necessary. The children are forced to face the fact that their belief that their parents will "be there" forever is a fantasy. Instead of continuing to be the recipient of parental nurturance, they must become the nurturing ones— both to their parents and to the younger generation. Middle-aged children's sense of loss and distress may be intensified because they must admit to their own mortality as their aging parents must acknowledge their decline, need for help, and loss of independence (King, Bonacci, & Wynne, 1990).

As the parents' need for care and assistance increases, the adult children, particularly adult daughters, may find themselves caught in the middle between the needs of the older and the younger generation. This group has been described as the sandwich generation (Brody, 1981). These family members are a vulnerable group because as the need to provide care for others increases, the caregivers often neglect their own needs (Bunting 1989).

Resiliency Model of Family Stress, Adjustment, and Adaptation

The Resiliency Model of Family Stress, Adjustment, and Adaptation developed by McCubbin and McCubbin (1993) provides a framework for understanding a family's response, adjustment, and finally, adaptation to stress over time. This framework is useful for understanding the demands and challenges that older families experience and allows for assess-

ment and intervention at many points to promote adaptation. The resiliency model evolved from Hill's (1958) earlier formulation of family vulnerability to crisis events and the subsequent development of the double ABCX family stress and adaptation model developed by McCubbin and Patterson (1983). The model is oriented toward adaptation, which is its central concept. Adaptation is the outcome of family efforts to bring a new level of balance, harmony, coherence, and functioning to a family crisis situation over time. The model includes a number of interacting components that influence successful or unsuccessful family adjustment.

The Stressor and Its Severity

"A stressor is a demand placed on the family that produces, or has the potential of producing, changes in the family system" (McCubbin & McCubbin, 1993, p. 28). The event or demand can influence many aspects of family life including health, roles and responsibilities, and boundaries. Severity is determined by the degree to which the stressor threatens the stability of the family. In many older families, the stressor event is the onset, or recognition through diagnosis, of the deterioration in health of an older member.

Family Vulnerability: Pileup and Life-Cycle Changes

Vulnerability is the degree of fragility in the interpersonal and organizational state of the family. It is influenced by the number of normative changes in the family's life cycle and by the accumulation or pileup of demands from inside or outside the family. The model outlines six categories of stresses and strains that contribute to a pileup of demands as a family attempts to adapt to a stressor such as illness.

1. The illness and related hardships over time
2. Normative transitions in individual family members and the family as a whole
3. Prior family strains accumulated over time
4. Situational demands and contextual difficulties
5. The consequences of family efforts to cope
6. Intrafamilial and social ambiguity that provides inadequate guidelines on how families should act or cope effectively (McCubbin & McCubbin, 1993, p. 37)

Specific demands might include economic stress due to poor health, heavy health care expenses, need to relocate, death of a member, or adult children leaving or returning home.

Family Types: Family-Established Patterns of Functioning

The family type is characterized by fairly stable, observable patterns of functioning. Two family attributes that are important in helping families manage chronic illness are a moderate degree of cohesion and flexibility. These facilitate a spirit of cooperation, open communication, and negotiation as change becomes necessary.

Family Resistance Resources: Capabilities and Strengths

Resistance resources are capabilities and strengths that enable the family to manage the stressor and prevent major upheaval in their functioning. The following critical family resources have been identified by McCubbin and McCubbin (1993): economic stability, cohesiveness, flexibility, hardiness, shared spiritual beliefs, open communication, traditions, celebrations, routines, and organization.

Resources outside the family are also important to adaptation. These include the family's social support network of friends and neighbors, as well as community-based agencies such as day-care centers, respite programs, and self-help groups. Social support serves to protect and insulate the family from the effects of stress and promotes recovery from crisis. The elders, especially the very old elders, or those without available family, may have a limited social support network because of poor health, restricted mobility, limited finances, deaths of friends, and lack of transportation.

Family Appraisal of the Stressor

Appraisal includes the family's perceptions and definition of the stressor and its accompanying hardships, as well as the family's perceptions of their available resources and the actions needed to meet the demands and regain family balance. If family members perceive the situation as hopeless or beyond their ability to manage, they may not be able to recognize and use available resources or seek additional resources. Therefore, they will be at high risk for maladaptation. On the other hand, if they can accept the situation and see it as a challenge that they can deal with, they are more likely to engage in constructive efforts to manage the situation.

Family Problem Solving and Coping

The model includes a consideration of the problem-solving skills and coping strategies the family uses to manage the demands created by the stressor. Steps in the problem-solving process include (1) organizing the stressor into manageable components, (2) identifying alternative management strategies, and (3) taking steps to resolve the problem. Coping includes family patterns and a wide range of efforts to maintain and strengthen the family, obtain family and community resources, and attend to the well-being and developmental needs of family members.

Family Response: Stress and Distress

When a stressor occurs that necessitates family management or change, it causes tension in the family. If this tension is not resolved or at least brought within manageable limits, it becomes stress. Stress occurs when there is a perceived imbalance between the demands on the family and its resources and capabilities. If balance is not restored, family distress may occur and the stress can even threaten the stability and integrity of the family system.

Together, the Family Life Cycle Model and the Resiliency Model of Family Stress, Adjustment, and Adaptation provide a comprehensive framework for assessing the aging family's strengths and areas of vulnerability in times of stress and change. This is a crucial aspect of assisting families to adapt positively to their changing lives.

GERONTOLOGICAL FAMILY NURSING

Family gerontological nursing occurs in the context of a health services system where care is directed toward the elderly individual. Given the limitations inherent in the current system, the goal of family gerontological nursing is to work in partnership with the family to maintain optimal functioning, restore health, and prevent or reduce the effects of illness in the older members. To accomplish this, the nurse helps families provide care to their older loved ones that promotes the optimal health and functioning of all members, regardless of age and regardless of health. The nurse uses skillful, thoughtful communication to assist family members to define and clarify problems, solve problems, set limits, and clarify boundaries and family roles. Sometimes when the demands of family caring exceed the family's resources and compromise its well-being, the nurse is called on to help the family choose other forms of care. To be successful, the nurse focuses assessment, planning, management, intervention, and evaluation of care on the family as a unit. An extensive background in the biological sciences and the physical aspects of health and illness is also important in working with older families because it allows the nurse to monitor physical symptoms and teach family members to carry out medical regimens and nursing care procedures (Box 14–1).

Practice Settings and Roles

Because the types and levels of care needed by older persons vary widely, gerontological family nurses practice in a variety of settings. For example, home health agencies, such as visiting nurse services, have special programs that provide various levels of care in the elderly person's home. Some general hospitals in urban areas provide follow-up care of older patients after hospitalization for acute illness. Gerontological family nurses also practice in long-term care facilities, mental health centers, inpatient psychiatric units, specialized clinics such as Alzheimer's centers or geriatric institutes, interdisciplinary group practices with primary care physicians, hospices, and nurse-managed clinics in the community.

By its very nature, gerontological family nursing challenges the nurse to assume a variety of roles that include advocate, health care broker, liaison, health teacher, family counselor, consultant, and case manager. Because many conditions and illnesses in the elderly are chronic, the nurse's relationship with a family may extend over time. During periods of greatest need, the nurse may even be viewed as a part of the family.

Demographic Trends

The older population—persons 65 years or older—numbered 35 million in 2000 and represented 12.4 percent of the U.S. population. The *Morbidity and Mortality Weekly Report* (*MMWR*), February 2003, estimated that by the year 2030, 19.6 percent of the U.S. population (71 million persons) will be 65 years old or over (Centers for Disease Control, 2003). The older population itself is getting older. According to the *MMWR*, the 80-year-and-older population will double by 2030, increasing from 9.3 to 19.5 million.

Advances in biomedical science have reduced early deaths from acute diseases and have prolonged life for those with chronic conditions such as cancer and heart disease. Unfortunately, living longer also brings increased possibilities for debilitating illnesses and conditions, such as Alzheimer's disease, diabetes, arthritis, and stroke. A 2003 *MMWR* revealed that 80 percent of persons age 65 and over have at least one chronic condition. Because age is commonly accompanied by one or more chronic health problems, an older person can be deprived of independence by limitations in the ability to function and carry out self-care activities. Help may be needed with at least one of the following daily activities: bathing, dressing, transfers, toileting, moving indoors, and taking medications. Assistance may also be required with household tasks, meal preparation, shopping, transportation, and management of finances (Altman & Taylor, 2001).

The "oldest old" (≥85 years) are more likely to experience multiple, interacting illnesses and circumstances that result in a condition known as "frailty." *Frailty* is a nonspecific clinical term associated with functional decline and includes anorexia, weight loss,

---

Box 14–1   UNIQUE ATTRIBUTES OF GERONTOLOGICAL FAMILY NURSING

- Demographic shifts and social trends will dramatically increase demands for the specialized knowledge and skills possessed by gerontological family nurses.
- Gerontological family nurses can expect opportunities for practice in a variety of settings and roles.
- Assessment of developmental issues and health status for individuals and families provides essential data for the gerontological family nurse.
- Skillful management of acute and chronic illness by the gerontological nurse, in collaboration with other members of the health care team, can mean the difference between recovery and rehabilitation or decompensation and frailty in an elderly individual.
- Ethical and legal discussion related to aging, genetics, resource allocation, and end-of-life care will demand the attention and input from gerontological family nurses and the entire health care team in order to ensure the well-being of our elderly citizens.

impaired mobility, falls, fatigue, muscle weakness and wasting, cognitive impairment, and coping difficulty. "Frail" individuals are at highest risk for adverse outcomes in response to minimal changes in their internal and external environments (Brody, 1985; Hammerman, 1999).

In spite of these facts, only 5 percent of the population 65 years of age and older live in long-term care facilities (Gavan, 2003). The majority of elderly persons who live in nursing homes are older, female, Caucasian, unmarried, lacking social support, and living with multiple health problems. Over 50 percent of nursing home residents have some form of dementia (Medina-Walpole & Katz, 2003). It is clear that many older persons with chronic conditions are able to remain in the community with the care and assistance of family and friends.

About 53 percent of older noninstitutionalized persons live in a family setting; the remaining 47 percent live alone or with a nonrelative (Gavan, 2003). A recent report on baby boomers and their aging parents revealed that 54 percent of boomers were providing care for children, parents, or both (AARP, 2001). Seventy percent of boomers reported that they were dealing adequately with caregiving demands; still, almost half reported guilt about not doing enough. Eighty percent of boomers engaged in social support, defined as telephone calls and visits, as a caregiving activity. Some important ethnic and racial differences were present among older boomers. For example, African-American boomers are less likely to have two living parents and tend toward a broad definition of family, including siblings and other relatives. Hispanic boomers are family focused, assume heavy caregiving responsibilities, and tend to experience significant guilt. Seventy-five percent of Asian-American boomers believe that children should take care of parents, whereas only 50 percent of other boomers agree. Older white boomers report less stress and guilt about caregiving and are the least likely to assume a caregiving role for elderly parents (AARP, 2001).

Social Trends

Over the past few decades, an immense body of research has focused on the nature of family relationships, including the informal caregiving network within the aging family. (See Given & Given, 1991, for a comprehensive review.) Reciprocal patterns of support and care have remained the norm throughout the life cycle of the family, although they tend to shift as the older generation experiences more financial and

health problems (Brody, 1985; Gaugler, Kane, & Kane, 2002). However, changing social roles and norms are reflected in public discussion, legal challenges, and legislative action around the definition of marriage and family. For example, in the relatively recent past, a discussion of heterogeneity in family constellation might have referred to single-parent, divorced, or blended families. More recently, gay and lesbian couples have established families, adding to the heterogeneity in family makeup. Research is needed to understand the similarities and differences in nontraditional family development, which often takes place in a nonfacilitative or openly hostile environment. The long-term impact of these nontraditional families for the care and support of aging kin is unknown (Fredriksen, 1999). Changing marriage and family-related norms, combined with smaller families, a mobile workforce, and a dual-earner standard of living, may loosen family ties and increase dependency on non-kin support for elderly family members. On the other hand, innovative approaches to "distance caregiving" could facilitate, nurture, and maintain family involvement in the lives of elderly kin (Antonucci & Schulz, 2003; Rosenblatt & Steenberg, 2003). Undoubtedly, social, economic, and legal forces will exert significant impact on all families, traditional and nontraditional. For a thorough presentation of sociocultural influences on family health, see Chapter 7 of this text.

Caregiving in Older Families

The family, not the formal health care system, provides 80 to 90 percent of care to its elderly members, including medical and nursing care, personal services such as transportation, and help with household tasks and shopping (Dilworth-Anderson & Gibson, 1999; Faison, Faria, & Frank, 1999; Hanley, Wiener, & Harris, 1991; Brody, 1985). The family responds to emergencies, provides acute care and assistance, and initiates and maintains links with the formal care system as necessary. The frailer an elderly member becomes, the more responsibility for care the family assumes (Biegel & Blum, 1990; Hanley et al., 1991). Despite this evidence, there is a lingering myth among many nurses that family members, especially adult children, do not provide care for elderly family members when they need it but instead rely on formal services such as nursing homes. In truth, adult children are providing more assistance and more difficult care to their elderly parents than in the past (Gavan, 2003; O'Neill & Sorenson, 1991; Brody, 1985).

Further, the prospective payment system has shortened hospital stays, sending people home "quicker and sicker" and creating more pressure on the family to provide care that they may be unprepared to provide. Unfortunately, help in the form of community-based support services is sparse, poorly funded, uncoordinated, or absent altogether (Faison, Faria, & Frank, 1999). This is especially true for families in rural areas (Henderson, 1992; Lee, 1993).

Who Provides Care?

The support and care given by all family members are usually lumped together under the term "family caregiving." Closer examination reveals, however, that one individual assumes primary responsibility of caregiver, and care usually is given by one member at a time (Tennstedt, Crawford, & McKinlay, 1993). When the elderly person is married, the spouse is first in line. Adult children are usually less involved in the care of a married parent, relying instead on the other parent to provide the majority of care. This approach may work satisfactorily unless the caregiving parent's health is also declining. Many elderly couples do not receive the assistance they need because they hide the seriousness of the difficulties from the rest of the family until a crisis occurs.

When there is no spouse available, the children, usually a daughter or daughter-in-law, assume the caregiving role. If there are no children, another family member, such as a sibling, niece, or nephew, may step in to help provide care. These more-distant relatives generally do not provide the intensity of care that spouses or children provide; instead, they serve more as intermediaries to obtain care from formal sources.

Women have always been the traditional caregivers, and they continue to provide nearly two-thirds (66 percent) of the family care given to older members. This figure remains constant, even though more women than ever are in the workforce (the percentage of working women rose from 48 percent in 1980 to 58 percent in 2000) (Chao, 2001). Daughters outnumber sons as caregivers by four to one (Brody, 1990). In addition, women provide more hours of care and are more likely to give assistance with personal hygiene, household tasks, and meal preparation. Men, on the other hand, more typically help with financial management, transportation, and home repairs (Dwyer & Coward, 1991; Stone, Cafferata, & Sangl, 1987). Although women provide the bulk of care, the contributions of men should not be overlooked. They frequently provide support and affection to the

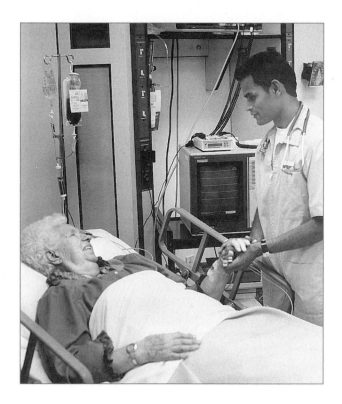

primary caregiver. Moreover, many elderly husbands assume the role of primary caregiver if their wives become ill or disabled, meeting their personal care needs and taking over household tasks.

At What Price Family Caregiving?

Research findings over the past several decades consistently point to the key role that family relationships play in helping older members maintain their independence and health (Field, Minkler, Falk, & Leino, 1993; Fletcher & Winslow, 1991; Shanas, 1979; Stone et al., 1987), and indeed, the term "family caregiving" has become so common that its meaning is taken for granted. Providing informal assistance to family members is a normative and usual activity throughout life. When does it cross the bounds of what is expected and ordinary and become extraordinary care? Biegel, Sales, and Schulz (1991) pointed out that "caring for a family member who has a chronic illness involves a significant expenditure of time and energy over potentially long periods of time, involves tasks that may be unpleasant and uncomfortable, is likely to be nonsymmetrical, and is often a role that had not been anticipated" (p. 17). Depending on the type and stage of the illness, the tasks and responsibilities can vary greatly over time.

Although family caregiving of elderly members will no doubt continue, researchers have raised questions about the capacity of family caregivers to provide the bulk of long-term care to the elderly (Baille, Norbeck, & Barnes, 1988; Brody, 1981, 1985; Brody, Litvin, Hoffman, & Kleban, 1992). Brody (1985) noted that "parent care has become a normative but stressful experience for individuals and families and its nature, scope, and consequences are not yet fully understood" (p. 19).

Fortunately, since Brody's 1985 observation, research on caregiving, stress, and health-related outcomes has provided valuable, though still incomplete, information for assessment, intervention, and further research in the family caregiving domain. Some of the negative consequences of caring for older loved ones, especially those with dementing illnesses such as Alzheimer's disease, have been well documented over time and include physical and emotional illness, social isolation, financial burdens, and mortality (Cattanach & Tebes, 1991; Pinquart & Sorensen, 2003; Schulz & Beach, 1999; United Hospital Fund, 1997).

Significant "downstream" negative effects of emotional distress, including depressive symptoms and clinical depression, are in part due to the production of proinflammatory cytokines, which, in turn, promote inflammatory processes. Rozanski, Blumenthal, and Kaplan (1999) identified three pathophysiological effects of depression: hypercortisolemia, impaired platelet function, and arrhythmogenic changes in heart rate and vagal control. Alterations in physiological processes are linked to a number of conditions including diabetes, cancer, arthritis, and cardiovascular disease (Harris et al., 1999; Kiecolt-Glaser, McGuire, Robles, & Glaser, 2002; Kronfol, & Remick, 2000; Schulz et al., 2000).

Long-term family care during chronic illness may increase the potential for abuse and neglect among family members, including mistreatment of an elderly ill member and mistreatment of other family members by the ill person (Paveza et al., 1992; Pillemer & Finkelhor, 1988, 1989; Semple, 1992; Williams-Burgess & Kimball, 1990). Risk may increase when the elderly person has a dementing illness such as Alzheimer's disease, with reports of 57 to 65 percent of those persons becoming aggressive toward family members at some time (Hamel et al., 1990; Ryden, 1988). In 2002 the American Medical Association, in collaboration with experts in medicine, nursing, social work, public health, and law, published *Diagnostic and Treatment Guidelines on Elder Abuse and Neglect*. These guidelines provide valuable up-to-date information on elder abuse facts, interviewing, assessment, intervention, and treatment and prevention. State-by-state contact information for Adult Protective Services and Ombudsman Program Directors is also included; the guideline is free and available to the public (Box 14–2).

Other Pressures Facing Families

Conflicts between caregiving and other responsibilities can produce tremendous role strain and overload. These conflicts can strain the adult child's relationship with the elderly parent (Sherrell & Newton, 1996). Competing demands have been found to contribute to the most pervasive consequence of caregiving: emotional stress (George & Gwyther, 1986). Two important sources of caregiver stress are competing familial obligations and conflict with work (Stone et al., 1987). One large study found that many women either quit their jobs or cut their hours to care for their elderly relative (Brody, 1985).

Societal trends influence the structure of contemporary families and thus affect their caregiving capacity. The increasing divorce rate has brought about more single-parent families, most of them headed by working women. In addition, the steadily decreasing birth rate since World War II means that as the need for caregivers increases there will be fewer family caregivers available. Many couples are postponing childbearing, which means that in the future they will be providing care to their elderly parents while they are still responsible for dependent children.

The demands on family caregivers are intensified as hospital stays are shorter and care shifts to the family in the community. At the same time, more elders are going to need more long-term care, which is rarely covered by insurance. These trends have created a dilemma for many older families. Faced with the need for expensive long-term care, many elderly couples are forced to "spend down" their assets to qualify for medical coverage, which may leave the healthier spouse with seriously reduced resources.

The fierce pride that many older people take in their independence and lifelong self-sufficiency means that they try to avoid accepting government assistance at any cost. To protect hard-earned assets, these older persons may attempt to get by and deny their need for formal care until a medical crisis occurs. These strategies can place added stress on the entire family because it may be unaware of the seriousness of an elderly member's health problems until the crisis occurs. This situation can also place unanticipated demands on family members for immediate care and

Box 14–2 REPORTING ELDER ABUSE

Who Do I Call If I Suspect Elder Abuse?

Each one of us has a responsibility to keep vulnerable elders safe from harm. The laws in most states require helping professionals in the front lines—such as doctors and home health providers—to report suspected abuse or neglect. These professionals are called mandated reporters. Under the laws of eight states, "any person" is required to report a suspicion of mistreatment.

Call the Police or 9-1-1 Immediately If Someone You Know Is in Immediate, Life-Threatening Danger.

If the danger is not immediate, but you suspect that abuse has occurred or is occurring, please tell someone. Relay your concerns to the local adult protective services, long-term care ombudsman, or police. For a list of reporting numbers, go to this important link: Where to Report Abuse.

If you have been the victim of abuse, exploitation, or neglect, you are not alone. Many people care and can help. Please tell your doctor, a friend, or a family member you trust, or call the Eldercare Locator help line immediately.

You can reach the Eldercare Locator by telephone at 1-800-677-1116. Specially trained operators will refer you to a local agency that can help. The Eldercare Locator is open Monday through Friday, 9 A.M. to 8 P.M. Eastern Time.

Source: National Center on Elder Abuse. (2003). *FAQ's about elder abuse.* Retrieved April 27, 2004, from http://www.elderabusecenter.org

---

assistance for which they are unprepared. This is the context in which gerontological family nurses must work to optimize the health of elderly clients and their families.

Health Promotion

The 20th century has seen an impressive increase in life expectancy for elders because of advances in health care (e.g., improved control of hypertension) and alterations in health behaviors (e.g., smoking cessation, dietary modification). Currently, the leading causes of death among the elderly include cardiovascular disease, cancer, stroke, respiratory disease, falls and other accidents, diabetes, renal disease, and hepatic disease. Major chronic conditions include arthritis, dental disease, high blood pressure, cardiac disease, vision problems, osteoporosis, hearing problems, depressive disorders, diseases of the vascular system, and activities of daily living (ADL) and instrumental activities of daily living (IADL) dependencies (American Association for World Health, 1999; Rubenstein, 1996–1997).

Elders in the 21st century will have even greater opportunities to benefit from research-based informa-

tion on maintaining health and avoiding illness and disability (Rubenstein, 1996–1997). *Healthy People 2010* recognizes the increasing physical and mental health needs of an aging population and identifies a number of health promotion and disease prevention objectives (U.S. Department of Health and Human Services, 2000). The gerontological family nurse is in a key position to inform and influence the health-related interactions and behaviors of elders and family members.

Most causes of mortality and morbidity are amenable to primary or secondary preventive interventions. Primary interventions aim to prevent the onset of illness; secondary interventions aim to detect disease before the appearance of symptoms (Rubenstein, 1996–1997). Examples of primary interventions include influenza immunizations, regular dental exams, regular physical activity, avoidance of tobacco and excessive alcohol use, avoidance of excessive sun exposure, elimination of environmental hazards, maintenance of a nutritionally adequate diet, and maintenance of prosthetic devices (e.g., hearing aids, glasses, dentures). Examples of secondary interventions include screening and early intervention for cancer, elevated blood pressure, cholesterol, and blood sugar. Secondary preventive interventions also include screening, treatment, and referral for depression, dementia, and functional loss in elderly individuals (American Association for World Health, 1999; Rubenstein, 1996–1997).

Primary and secondary preventive practices can greatly improve the health status of elderly individuals and add to the quality of life for elders and involved family members. Recommendations, interventions, referrals, and follow-ups should be research-based and systematic and should proceed from a thorough history and physical, hopefully with the participation of elders, family, and the interdisciplinary treatment team. To increase elder participation in and compliance with health promotion and illness prevention strategies, it is imperative that gerontological family nurses be up-to-date and proactive in providing information, education, intervention, and referral to elders and their families.

Acute and Chronic Illness: The Family Conference

The initial contact with the older person frequently occurs when help is sought for an acute or worsening health problem. Following the medical evaluation, the family nurse should set up a conference that includes the elder and all other family members who may be involved in providing care and assistance. The physician and other members of the health care team, such as the social worker, visiting nurse, and physical therapist, are to be included as needed.

Step 1

The first step is to establish a working partnership with the family so that they are comfortable in expressing their feelings, ideas, and concerns. The goal of the conference is to provide support and information and to help them set realistic goals by clarifying what needs to be done, establishing a plan of action, and determining the best way to carry it out.

Start by obtaining the family story by using the concepts from the assessment and interventions in Chapter 8. Explore each member's perceptions of the current stressor: the elderly member's illness or condition. Do they understand the diagnosis? What do they believe that it will mean in terms of changes or demands on the family? How are they defining the situation in relation to themselves, to a spouse, or to a parent? What resources are available to them personally, within the family, and in the community? How do they perceive those resources? What other stressful events and transitions are occurring, for example, health problems, job stress, or other family disruptions? How have they coped with other stressful events or periods in the past? Did they pull together (cohesion) and make adjustments (flexibility) or did they freeze and pull apart?

Step 2

The family's priorities, both as individuals and as a group, should be brought into the open and discussed. Priorities include what they hope to accomplish in their elderly member's care as well as their individual personal goals. Financial concerns, time constraints, and generational responsibilities should be discussed openly. The elderly member's wishes, priorities, and expectations must be included for a plan to be successful.

Step 3

Step 3 is to help the family establish caregiving goals that are realistic and acceptable (Kashner, Magaziner, & Pruitt, 1990). Some elderly members' desire to remain in their own home may be so strong that rather than leave, they would accept mediocre care or no care at all. They may also have an unspoken expectation that the adult children will "pitch in" and help. This belief may create increasing tension and stress in the family because the adult children, while wanting their loved one to have the best care possible, may be unaware of this expectation or be unable to deliver the assistance needed because of other demands.

It may be helpful to inquire whether any family members have ever promised the elderly member, "I will never put you in a nursing home. I will always take care of you, no matter what happens." Many family members, especially wives and daughters, make this well-meaning but unrealistic commitment either under duress, as a result of guilt or denial, or as a form of reassurance to an aging relative. It can, however, have a profoundly negative effect on the family when they face difficult caregiving decisions. Through open, guided discussion, nurses help families view the situation realistically so that they can face appropriate alternatives when necessary.

Step 4

All family members should have an opportunity to express the0ir priorities and goals for caregiving. The effects of the illness require inevitable role and structural changes in the family. The next focus of the family conference is helping the family evaluate how they plan to work together to meet not only the needs of the elderly member but also those of the other members. The day-to-day care expectations should be made explicit, including the responsibilities of individual members and the plan for emergencies and other contingencies, such as illness or vacations.

Whatever their role in caregiving, all family members should be taught about the illness or condition, including the actual caregiving activities and the resources required. The designated caregiver and those less directly involved in day-to-day care will know the actual requirements for care and the resources necessary. Proactive education and clear role expectations can prevent conflict and misunderstanding between family members at a later time.

In facilitating the family conference, the nurse must ensure that decisions are made with the full participation of the elderly person whenever possible, even if the person has an early dementing disorder. It is also necessary to help the family coordinate its caregiving activities over time. The nurse can lay the groundwork for formal assistance by connecting the family with appropriate community resources, such as adult day care, respite care, in-home health services, support groups, and family workshops or classes.

It is highly desirable, whenever possible, to visit the elderly person at home with family caregivers present. Visiting on the family's "turf" tends to strengthen the nurse's therapeutic alliance with the family; at the same time, it is possible to see the family's usual patterns of interaction and evaluate the home in terms of safety and available resources.

End-of-Life Care

Sensitive and skilled end-of-life care for patients and family members is a critical domain for gerontological family nurses. Steinhauser and associates (2000) identified six common concerns for patients and family experiencing the end of life. These include the following:

- Management of symptoms
- Communication about treatment
- Making preparations for death
- Completing and contributing
- Maintaining personal identity
- Trusting relationship with nurse and doctor

In order to address these concerns, nurses and other health care providers must be willing and able to assist the patient and family in the clarification of goals and in the articulation of expectations and fears related to mortality and the process of dying. Patients and family members should be approached with patience, recognizing that information may need to be repeated and repeatedly processed to be understood and integrated. As the elder and the family live through the end-of-life experience, conflicts and misunderstandings may occur, goals may change, and new priorities may surface. In the midst of this dynamic process, the gerontological family nurse must maintain a steady, reliable, open stance providing assistance, guidance, and referral as needed and requested. As much as possible, the nurse should strive for an environment conducive to intra- and interpersonal growth for the patient and family up to, including, and following the moment of death (Lorenz & Lynn, 2003).

Legal Concerns

Legal counsel is an important aspect of caregiving that is often overlooked until a health crisis. Planning for short- and long-term care, including incapacity, ensures that elderly persons' wishes are known and honored and prevents family guesswork, hassles, misunderstanding, and conflicts. Planning proceeds from a frank sharing of information about supplementary health and long-term care benefits, pensions, Social Security income, property, and other assets. In addition, families need accurate and timely information about Medicare benefits and limitations along with state-specific Medicaid rules to make informed decisions about planning for short- and long-term care.

Sometimes elderly individuals and family members neglect discussions of legal, financial, and end-of-life issues. Broaching these issues may trigger defensiveness, embarrassment, anxiety, and uncertainty for adult children and their elderly kin. Gerontological family nurses can initiate exploration and discussion of legal, financial, and end-of-life issues during the psychosocial component of a comprehensive assessment. In addition, the nurse has an ideal opportunity to normalize a broad range of thoughts, feelings, and reactions to this process and to provide support and encouragement.

Finally, the nurse can offer general information and referrals to specialists in elder law. Elder-law specialists advise elders and family members about estate planning, living wills, advance directives, health care representatives, power of attorney, and guardianship, in addition to answering questions related to complex rules and regulations. Although general legal and financial planning information can be accessed via online resources (e.g., Alzheimer's Association Website), this information cannot replace legal counsel.

Spiritual Concerns

Elders' spiritual needs must not be overlooked or minimized (Fahey, 2003; Reed, 1991). Religious affiliation and spiritual beliefs have an important place in many older persons' lives, influencing perspectives on suffering, loss, and death. Indeed, some elderly individuals may experience an intense need to address troubled relationships, to ask for forgiveness, and to make amends. Seeking consultation from or making a referral to a specialist in pastoral care may provide an opportunity for spiritual and emotional healing and a more peaceful death (Fahey, 2003). In addition, churches, parishes, synagogues, or temples are great sources of formal and informal support for the elderly (Dilworth-Andersen & Gibson, 1999).

NURSING IMPLICATIONS

Many factors demand that gerontological family nursing be an essential component of nursing practice, nursing curricula, and nursing research. The driving forces for the prominent agenda of elderly and their families are the increase in aging populations, increase in longevity, and the shift of health care to the family in the community.

Practice

One of the challenges of gerontological family nursing is incorporating both health promotion and disease prevention strategies along with participating in the monitoring and management of acute and chronic illness. The role of the gerontological family nurse includes teaching, giving advice, providing encouragement and support, and advocating for the family within the health care delivery system. Establishing a therapeutic alliance with the elderly members and the rest of their family is crucial for health promotion, prevention, and management. To do this successfully, it is necessary to view the family as a system, not as individual victims who need to be rescued. It is important to recognize that adult children often experience powerful feelings of abandonment, anger, and guilt when their parents' health fails. These emotions may alternate with denial of the seriousness of their parents' health problems. Older spouses may also experience these feelings, especially when the healthier spouse has always been dependent on the person

who is declining; frequently, it is the nurse in the home, hospital, or clinic who first notices the frustration and tension in family caregivers. The family's negative or angry feelings may be temporarily displaced onto the nurse or other professional caregivers and mistakenly interpreted as hostility or treatment resistance. In reality, these feelings are a natural response to a tragic, sad, irreversible situation (King et al., 1990). It is often helpful at this point to explain to the family that these are normal reactions and help them explore their perceptions of the situation and its meaning for them. In situations that involve long-term caregiving, it may be useful to refer family members to support groups or to teach them stress management techniques (Dellasega, 1990).

Policy

Given current social and demographic trends, it is certain that the future will bring increasing demands for family caregiving of elderly members. At a time when biomedical breakthroughs are succeeding in slowing or halting chronic conditions, managed care is shifting more care into the community and placing even greater responsibility for care on family members. Creation of the National Family Caregiver Support Program (NFCSP) is tangible evidence of a move toward policy-level recognition and valuing of the contribution made by families to the care of elderly citizens. The NFCSP, developed by the Administration on Aging (AoA) in 2000, was designed to promote state and local partnerships in offering five basic family caregiver services. These services include respite, counseling and support, information, service access assistance, and limited supplementary care (Cuellar, 2002).

Clearly, state and federal legislation will not remedy all issues and needs related to family caregiving for elderly individuals. For example, the Family and Medical Leave Act will not solve the dilemma of caregivers who cannot afford to take leaves without pay. For such families, a tax credit similar to the Child and Dependent Care Tax Credit should be explored (Stone et al., 1987). However, passed, pending, and proposed legislation can simplify access to services by reducing or eliminating financial, geographic, and information-related barriers to services.

The vulnerability of the growing group of caregivers must be addressed. Failure to do so will result in increased mental and physical health problems for overburdened family members and, ultimately, increased costs to society. The informal family caring system is a national resource that must be protected and supported, not overwhelmed. No institution can replace the support and care given by family members; rather, elderly persons' needs for care are best served by a combination of formal and informal services. The development of affordable support services in the community is increasingly important to supplement family caregiving, such as respite care, homemaker services, adult day-care centers, and neighborhood wellness clinics. The challenge is to provide appropriate, accessible forms of tangible assistance with caregiving and not simply view family members as unpaid workers who need to be "cheered on" in their caregiving work (Brody, 1985; United Hospital Fund, 1997).

Research

The challenges facing the aging family are complex. To meet the needs of our noninstitutionalized elderly, we need answers to many questions. For example, what functions do formal and informal care systems perform best? What balance of formal and informal services is needed to meet the care needs of the elderly? How can caregivers balance competing family and work demands, and what interventions are effective in reducing caregiver distress (Knight, Lutzky, & Macofsky-Urban, 1993)? Only recently has it been recognized that abuse and violence are serious problems in older caregiving families. What are the factors that contribute to the aggression and violence, and under what conditions do they occur?

> **"**No institution can replace the support and care given by family members; rather, elderly persons' needs for care are best served by a combination of formal and informal services.**"**

Studies of interventions for elders with various illnesses and chronic conditions need to be conducted with family caregivers in the home, to test the effectiveness of approaches to specific care situations. Finally, further research is needed to determine the best ways to reach older families of various ethnic and racial backgrounds and develop care options that they will accept (Connell & Gibson, 1997).

Education

Gerontological nursing is a recognized speciality, grounded in a body of knowledge and guided by

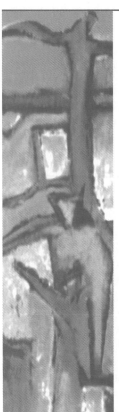

RESEARCH BRIEF

Purpose
To examine the effects of a psychoeducational intervention for family caregivers of persons with Alzheimer's disease or a related disorder.

Methodology
This was a 4-year, longitudinal, quasi-experimental design, aimed at testing a theory-based, psychoeducational intervention. The sample consisted of 245 community-based dementia caregivers in four states: Iowa, Minnesota, Indiana, and Arizona. Caregivers in the treatment group received an individualized treatment plan based on the Progressively Lowered Stress Threshold Model. Caregivers in the comparison group received "usual care," including information on Alzheimer's disease, support group referral, and case management.

Results
Caregivers in the treatment group experienced improved outcomes in mood, decreased distress over care recipient's problem behaviors, decreased burden related to caregiving, and increased satisfaction and mastery related to caregiving compared with controls.

Implications for Nursing
Nurses can have a positive impact on caregiving outcomes using a theory-based, psychoeducational intervention in the community setting.

Source: Buckwalter et al. (2000). Family caregiver home training based on the progressively lowered stress threshold model. *Sigma Theta Tau Monograph on Aging.*

standards of care. Unfortunately, preparation of nurses for practice in this speciality is inadequate for both current and future care demands. In a 2000 report titled *Older Adults: Recommended Baccalaureate Competencies and Curricular Guidelines for Geriatric Nursing*, the American Association of Colleges of Nursing and the John A. Hartford Foundation Institute for Geriatric Nursing identified limited undergraduate preparation in geriatric nursing as an important cause for the shortage of nurses in this practice area. This report specified competencies and curriculum guidelines for professional nursing education in the care of frail and healthy older adults. In 2003, Congress funded the Nurse Reinvestment Act, providing needed support for implementing suggestions contained in the 2000 report.

In February 2003, Congress, in recognition of the national nursing shortage, appropriated funding for the Nurse Reinvestment Act of 2002. Funding mechanisms in the act include scholarships for individual students of nursing, loan repayment grants for faculty in schools of nursing, and importantly, geriatric nurse training grants for schools of nursing. Geriatric nurse training grants aim to

(1) provide training to individuals who will provide geriatric care for the elderly; (2) develop and disseminate curricula relating to the treatment of the health problems of elderly individuals; (3) train faculty

members in geriatrics; or (4) provide continuing education to individuals who provide geriatric care (Nurse Reinvestment Act, 2002).

The Nurse Reinvestment Act, and specifically the geriatric nurse training grant, serves as a policy-level statement on the importance of course work, clinical experience, faculty expertise, and lifelong learning to ensure "accessible, quality nursing care for the growing geriatric population" (American Association of Colleges of Nursing & John A. Hartford Foundation, 2000; Reinhard, Barber, Mezey, Mitty, & Peed, 2002).

SUMMARY

- In our society, families are the providers of care for the elderly.
- Families are faced with multiple competing demands and limited resources.
- Gerontological nurses can apply their specialized knowledge and skills to assist families in the care of elderly kin.
- Theory provides useful frameworks for organizing and interpreting data and for selecting appropriate interventions.
- Knowledge of local, state, and federal resources related to aging, families, caregiving, and chronic illness will enhance the nurse's ability to make appropriate referrals.

CASE STUDY WITH STUDY QUESTIONS ➤

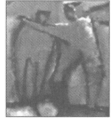

THE JOHNSONS

Mary Johnson lives in the family home, where she and her husband James raised their three children. Mary is a 72-year-old woman and has been living alone since the death of James, 10 years earlier. Thanks to a small pension from James's retirement, along with Mary's Social Security pension, Mary has been able to live comfortably but not extravagantly through careful management of her resources. Mary has led an active life, walking daily, babysitting for grandchildren, teaching in Sunday school, participating in the church Ladies' Club, and volunteering at the neighborhood senior center. Mary has a close relationship with her three daughters and their families and enjoys regular, if not daily, contact. In the past few years, Mary's daughters have expressed concerns about

the changing character of the neighborhood. Many of Mary's friends and neighbors have either died or moved away.

Recently Mary was taken to the hospital emergency room after a fall at church. Mary became dizzy and then "blacked out"; she sustained a broken wrist and an evulsion wound to her right shin. Mary's condition was stabilized and she was transferred to a transitional care unit for rehabilitation. Mary made good progress in her recovery; discharge is anticipated within the week.

Mary is adamant about returning to the family home when discharged. She recognizes that she will need continued assistance and is concerned about burdening her daughters and their families with her care. Discharge planning is complicated by the following factors: (1) Mary will need some assistance with activities of daily living (ADLs) and instrumental activities of daily living (IADLs) for at least 6 weeks, (2) special wound care is necessary because of Mary's

(continued on page 390)

CASE STUDY ➤ *(Continued)*

diabetes and impaired circulation, (3) Mary's bedroom and bath are on the second floor (there is a half bath on the first floor), and (4) although Mary's daughters live within a 10-minute drive, they work full-time and have teenage children involved in numerous school and extracurricular activities. A family conference is scheduled by Mary's primary nurse to plan for her care after discharge.

1. Present this case to your classmates or colleagues using the Resiliency Model of Family Stress, Adjustment, and Adaptation. Include the concepts of stressors, vulnerabilities, typology, resources, and appraisal in your discussion.
2. Discuss the importance of comprehensive and appropriate discharge planning in optimizing Mary's return to previous status and reducing the risk of Mary's increasing disability or frailty.
3. A change in health status can disrupt important activities and relationships. For example, prior to her accident, Mary engaged in a physically and socially stimulating routine. Identify possible physical and mental health outcomes for Mary related to decreased activity and social contact.
4. The gerontological family nurse is aware of the increased stress experienced by family caregivers. What resources, referrals, or anticipatory counseling would be appropriate for Mary's daughters?
5. Conducting a family meeting is a complex task, requiring the ability to process information from multiple sources (family members) and from multiple levels (verbal, nonverbal). As this process occurs, the nurse is also responding based on his or her prior history, nursing experience, family experiences, immediate environmental demands, fatigue, and mood. Review the four-step plan included in the text. Based on your knowledge and awareness of yourself, assess your probable areas of strength and limitation in conducting a family meeting.
6. List and describe three common normative events that can trigger significant transitions in families.
7. Review the legal issues included on the Alzheimer's Association and National Center on Family Caregiving Websites. After reviewing this information and considering Mary's situation, what action(s) would you recommend for Mary Johnson and her daughters?

References

AARP. (2001). *In the middle: A report on multicultural boomers coping with family and aging issues.* Washington, DC: AARP.

Aldous, J. (1978). *Family careers. Developmental change in families.* New York: John Wiley & Sons.

Altman, B., & Taylor, A. (2001). *Women in the health care system: Health status, insurance, and access to care.* Rockville, MD: Agency for Healthcare Research and Quality.

American Association of Colleges of Nursing & John A. Hartford Foundation. (2000). *Older adults: Recommended baccalaureate competencies and curricular guidelines for geriatric nursing care.* Washington, DC, & New York, NY: Authors.

American Association for World Health. (1999). *Healthy aging, healthy living: Start now!* Washington, DC: Author.

American Medical Association. (2002). *Diagnostic and treatment guidelines on elder abuse and neglect.* Retrieved from http://www.ama-assn.org

Antonucci, T., & Schulz, R. (2003). Families, social support, and caregiving. In W. Hazzard, J. Blass, J. Halter, J. Ouslander, & M. Tinetti (Eds.), *Principles of geriatric medicine and gerontology* (5th ed., pp. 255–263). Chicago: McGraw-Hill.

Baille, V., Norbeck, J., & Barnes, L. (1988). Stress, social support, and psychological distress of family caregivers of the elderly. *Nursing Research, 37*(4), 217–222.

Biegel, D. E., & Blum, A. (1990). *Aging and caregiving: Theory, research, and policy.* Newbury Park, CA: Sage.

Biegel, D., Sales, E., & Schulz, R. (1991). *Family caregiving in chronic illness.* Newbury Park, CA: Sage.

Blenkner, M. (1965). Social work and family relationships in later life with some thoughts on filial maturity. In E. Shanas & G. J.

Streib (Eds.), *Social structure and the family: Generational relations.* Englewood Cliffs, NJ: Prentice-Hall.

Brody, E. M. (1981).Women in the middle and family help to older people. *Gerontologist, 25,* 19–29.

Brody, E. M. (1985). Parent care as a normative family stress. *Gerontologist, 25,* 19–29.

Brody, E. M. (1990). *Women in the middle: Their parent care years.* New York: Springer.

Brody, E. M., Litvin, S., Hoffman, L., & Kleban, M. (1992). Differential effects of daughters' marital status on their parent care experiences. *Gerontologist, 32,* 58–67.

Brubaker, T. H. (Ed.). (1983). *Family relationships in later life.* Newbury Park, CA: Sage.

Buckwalter, K. C., Gerdner, L. A., Hall, G. R., Kelly, A., Kohont, F., Richards, B. S., & Sime, M. (2000). Family caregiver home training based on the progressively lowered stress threshold model. In *Gerontological nursing issues for the 21st century.* Indianapolis, IN: Center Nursing Press: A Division of Sigma Theta Tau International.

Bunting, S. (1989). Stress on caregivers of the elderly. *Advances in Nursing Science, 11,* 63–73.

Carter, G. A., & McGoldrick, M. (1980). *The family lifecycle: A framework for family therapy.* New York: Family Press.

Cattanach, L., & Tebes, J. K. (1991). The nature of elder impairment and its impact on family caregivers' health and psychosocial functioning. *Gerontologist, 31,* 246–255.

Centers for Disease Control. (2003). Public health and aging: Trends in aging—United States and worldwide. *Morbidity and Mortality Weekly Report, 52,* 101–106.

Chao, E. (2001). *Report on the American workforce.* Washington, DC: U.S. Bureau of Labor Statistics.

Connell, C., & Gibson, G. (1997). Racial, ethnic and cultural differences in dementia caregiving: Review and analysis. *Gerontologist*, *37*, 355–364.

Cuellar, N. (2002). The impact of health policy on family caregiving. *Geriatric Nursing*, *23*, 284–285.

Dellasega, C. (1990). Coping with caregiving: Stress management for caregivers of the elderly. *Journal of Psychosocial Nursing*, *28*, 15–22.

Dilworth-Andersen, P., & Gibson, B. (1999, Fall). Ethnic minority perspectives on dementia, family caregiving, and interventions. *Generations*, 40–45.

Duvall, E. M., & Miller, B. C. (1985). *Marriage and family development* (6th ed.). New York: Harper & Row.

Dwyer, J. W., & Coward, R. T. (1991). A multivariate comparison of the involvement of adult sons versus daughters in the care of impaired parents. *Journal of Gerontology*, *46*, S259–S269.

Fahey, C. (2003). Spirituality and the elderly. In W. Hazzard, J. Blass, J. Halter, J. Ouslander, & M. Tinetti (Eds.), *Principles of geriatric medicine and gerontology* (5th ed., pp. 347–351). Chicago: McGraw-Hill.

Faison, K., Faria, S., & Frank, D. (1999). Caregivers of the chronically ill elderly: Perceived burden. *Journal of Community Health Nursing*, *16*, 243–253.

Field, D., Minkler, M., Falk, R., & Leino, E. (1993). The influence of health on family contacts and family feelings in advanced old age: A longitudinal study journal of gerontology. *Psychosocial Sciences*, *48*, 8–28.

Fletcher, K. R., & Winslow, S. A. (1991). Informal caregivers: A composite and review of needs and community resources. *Family Community Health*, *14*(2), 59–67.

Fredriksen, K. (1999). Family caregiving responsibilities among lesbians and gay men. *Social Work*, *44*, 142–155.

Gaugler, J., Kane, R., & Kane, R. (2002). Family care for older adults with disabilities: Toward more targeted and interpretable research. *International Journal on Aging and Human Development*, *54*, 205–231.

Gavan, C. (2003). Successful aging families. *Holistic Nursing Practice*, *17*, 11–18.

George, L. K., & Gwyther, L. P. (1986). Caregiver well-being: A multidimensional examination of family caregivers of demented adults. *Gerontologist*, *26*, 253–259.

Given, B. A., & Given, C. W. (1991). Family caregivers for the elderly. *Annual Review of Nursing Research*, *9*, 77–101.

Hamel, M., Gold, D., Andres, D., Reis, M., Dastoor, D., Grauer, H., & Bergman, H. (1990). Predictors and consequences of aggressive behavior by community-based dementia patients. *Gerontologist*, *30*, 206–211.

Hammerman, D. (1999). Toward an understanding of frailty. *Annals of Internal Medicine*, *130*, 945–950.

Hanley, R., Wiener, J., & Harris, K. (1991). Will paid home care erode informal support? *Journal of Health Politics, Policy, and Law*, *16*, 507–521.

Harris, T., Ferrucci, L., Tracy, R., Corti, C., Wacholder, S., Ettinger, W., Heimovitz, H., Cohen, H., & Wallace, R. (1999). Associations of elevated interleukin-6 and c-reactive protein levels with mortality in the elderly. *American Journal of Medicine*, *106*, 506–512.

Henderson, M. C. (1992). Families in transition: Caring for the rural elderly. *Family Community Health*, *14*(4), 61–70.

Hill, R. (1958). Generic features of families under stress. *Social Casework*, *49*, 139–150.

Kashner, T. M., Magaziner, J., & Pruitt, S. (1990). Family size and caregiving of aged patients with hip fractures. In D. E. Biegel & A. Blum (Eds.), *Aging and caregiving: Theory, research, and policy* (pp. 184–203). Newbury Park, CA: Sage.

Kiecolt-Glaser, J., McGuire, L., Robles, T., & Glaser, R. (2002). Emotions, morbidity, and mortality: New perspectives from psychoneuroimmunology. *Annual Review of Psychology*, *53*, 83–107.

King, D. A., Bonacci, B., & Wynne, L. (1990). Families of cognitively impaired elders: Helping adult children confront the filial crisis. *Clinical Gerontologist*, *10*, 3–15.

Knight, B. G., Lutzky, S., & Macofsky-Urban, F. (1993). A meta-analytic review of interventions for caregiver distress: Recommendations for future research. *Gerontologist*, *33*, 240–248.

Kronfol, Z., & Remick, D. (2000). Cytokines and the brain: Implications for clinical psychiatry. *American Journal of Psychiatry*, *157*, 683–694.

Lee, H. J. (1993). Health perceptions of middle, "new middle," and older rural adults. *Family Community Health*, *16*, 19–27.

Lorenz, K., & Lynn, J. (2003). Care of the dying patient. In W. Hazzard, J. Blass, J. Halter, J. Ouslander, & M. Tinetti (Eds.), *Principles of geriatric medicine and gerontology* (5th ed., pp. 323–334). Chicago: McGraw-Hill.

McCubbin, H. I., & McCubbin, M.A. (1993). Families coping with illness: The resiliency model of family stress, adjustment, and adaptation. In C. B. Danielson, B. Hamil-Bissel, & P. Wynstead-Fry (Eds.), *Families, health and illness: Perspectives on coping and intervention* (pp. 21–63). St. Louis: C.V. Mosby.

McCubbin, H. I., & Patterson, J. M. (1983). Family transitions: Adaptation to stress. In McCubbin & C. R. Figley (Eds.), *Stress and the family. Vol. 1: Coping with normative transitions* (pp. 5–25). New York: Brunner/Mazel.

Medina-Walpole, A., & Katz, P. (2003). Nursing home care. In W. Hazzard, J. Blass, J. Halter, J. Ouslander, & M. Tinetti (Eds.), *Principles of geriatric medicine and gerontology* (5th ed., pp. 197–209). Chicago: McGraw-Hill.

Neugarten, B. L. (1968). Adult personality: Toward a psychology of the life cycle. In B. L. Neugarten (Ed.), *Middle age and aging* (pp. 137–147). Chicago: University of Chicago Press.

Nurse Reinvestment Act. (2002). Pub. L. No. 107–205, 116 Stat. 811.

O'Neill, C., & Sorenson, E. S. (1991). Home care of the elderly: A family perspective. *Advances in Nursing Science*, *13*(4), 28–37.

Paveza, G. J., Cohen, D., Eisdorfer, C., Freels, S., Semla, T., Ashford, J., Gorelick, P., Hirschman, R., Luchins, D., & Levy, P. (1992). Severe family violence and Alzheimer's disease: Prevalence and risk factors. *Gerontologist*, *32*, 493–497.

Pillemer, K., & Finkelhor, D. (1988). The prevalence of elder abuse: A random sample survey. *Gerontologist*, *28*, 51–57.

Pillemer, K., & Finkelhor, D. (1989). Causes of elder abuse: Caregiver stress versus problem relatives. *American Journal of Orthopsychiatry*, *59*, 179–187.

Pinquart, M., & Sorensen, S. (2003). Differences between caregivers and noncaregivers in psychological health and physical health: A meta-analysis. *Psychology and Aging*, *18*, 250–267.

Reed, P. G. (1991). Self transcendence and mental health in the oldest-old adult. *Nursing Research*, *2*(1), 43–163.

Reinhard, S., Barber, P., Mezey, M., Mitty, E., & Peed, J. (2002). *Initiatives to promote the nursing workforce in geriatrics*. New Brunswick, NJ: Rutgers Center for State Health Policy.

Rosenblatt, B., & Steenberg, C. (2003). *Handbook for long-distance caregivers*. San Francisco: National Center on Caregiving.

Rozanski, A., Blumenthal, J., & Kaplan, J. (1999). Impact of psychological factors on the pathogenesis of cardiovascular disease and implications for therapy. *Circulation*, *99*(16), 2192–2217.

Rubenstein, L. (1996–1997, Winter). Update on preventative medicine for older people. *Generations*, 47–53.

Ryden, M. (1988). Aggressive behavior in persons with dementia living in the community. *Alzheimer's Disease and Associated Disorders International Journal*, *2*(4), 342–355.

Schulz, R., & Beach, S. (1999). Caregiving as a risk factor for mortality: The Caregiver Health Effects Study. *JAMA*, *282*(23), 2215–2219.

Schulz, R., Beach, S., Ives, D., Martire, L., Ariyo, A., & Kop, W. (2000). Association between depression and mortality in older adults: The Cardiovascular Health Study. *Archives of Internal Medicine*, *160*(12), 1761–1768.

Schumacher, K., & Meleis, A. (1994). Transitions: A central concept in nursing. *Image: Journal of Nursing Scholarship, 26,* 119–127.

Semple, S. H. (1992). Conflict in Alzheimer's caregiving families: Its dimensions and consequences. *Gerontologist, 32,* 648–655.

Shanas, E. (1979). The family as a social support system in old age. *Gerontologist, 19,* 3–9.

Sherrell, K., & Newton, N. (1996). Parent care as a developmental task. *Families in Society: The Journal of Contemporary Human Services, 77,* 174–181.

Steinhauser, K., Christakis, N., Clipp, E., McNeilly, M., McIntyre, L., & Tulsky, J. (2000). Factors considered important at the end of life by patients, family, physicians, and other care providers. *JAMA, 284*(19), 2476–2482.

Stone, R., Cafferata, G., & Sangl, J. (1987). Caregivers of the frail elderly: A national profile. *Gerontologist, 27,* 616–626.

Tennstedt, S., Crawford, S., & McKinlay, J. (1993). Is family care on the decline? A longitudinal investigation of the substitution of formal long-term care services for informal care. *The Millbank Quarterly, 71,* 601–624.

United Hospital Fund. (1997). *Initiatives: Facts about family caregiving.* Retrieved from http://www.uhfnyc.org/initiat/fhcpfaq.htm

U.S. Department of Health and Human Services. (2000). *Healthy people 2010.*

Williams-Burgess, C., & Kimball, M. J. (1990).The neglected elder: A family systems approach. *Journal of Psychosocial Nursing, 30*(10), 21–25.

Bibliography

Aranda, M., & Knight, B. (1997). The influence of ethnicity and culture on the caregiver stress and coping process: A sociocultural review and analysis. *Gerontologist, 37,* 355–364.

Archbold, P. G. (1983).The impact of parent-caring on women. *Family Relations, 32,* 39–45.

Buckwalter, K. C., Gerdner, L. A., Hall, G. R, Kelly, A., Kohont, F., Richards, B. S., & Sime, M. (2000). In *Gerontological nursing issues for the 21st century.* Indianapolis, IN: Center Nursing Press: A Division of Sigma Theta Tau International.

Cohen, D., & Eisdorfer, C. (1986). *The loss of self: A family resource for the care of Alzheimer's and related disorders.* New York: W.W. Norton.

Connell, C., & Gibson, G. (1997). Racial, ethnic and cultural differences in dementia caregiving: Review and analysis. *Gerontologist, 37,* 355–364.

Dillehey, R. C., & Sandys, M. R. (1990). Caregivers for Alzheimer's patients: What we are learning from research. *International Journal of Aging and Human Development, 30,* 263–285.

Given, C. W., Collins, C. E., & Given, B. A. (1988). Sources of stress among families caring for relatives with Alzheimer's disease. *Nursing Clinics of North America, 23,* 69–83.

Hogstel, M. O. (1990). *Geropsychiatric nursing.* St. Louis: C.V. Mosby.

Lachs, M. (2003). Elder mistreatment. In W. Hazzard, J. Blass, J. Halter, J. Ouslander, & M. Tinetti (Eds.), *Principles of geriatric medicine and gerontology* (5th ed., pp. 1593–1598). Chicago: McGraw-Hill.

Neundorfer, M. M. (1991a). Coping and health outcomes in spouse caregivers of persons with dementia. *Nursing Research, 40,* 261–265.

Neundorfer, M. M. (1991b). Family caregivers of the frail elderly: Impact of caregiving on their health and implications for interventions. *Family Community Health, 14,* 48–58.

Pratt, C. C., Schmall, V. L., Wright, S., & Cleland, M. (1985). Burden and coping strategies of caregivers to Alzheimer's patients. *Family Relations, 34,* 27–33.

Pruchno, R. A., & Potashnik, S. L. (1989). Caregiving spouses: Physical and mental health in perspective. *Journal of the American Geriatic Society, 37,* 697–705.

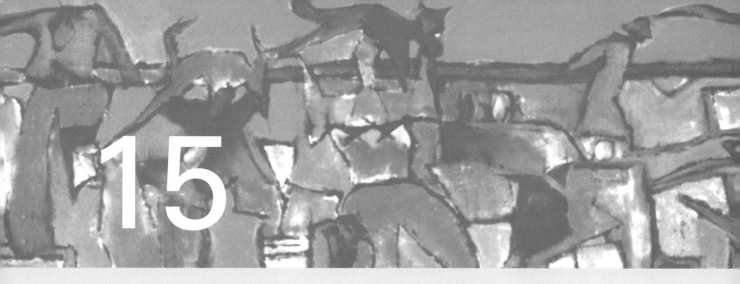

15

Families and Community/Public Health Nursing

Debra Gay Anderson, PhD, RNC • Kacy Allen-Bryant, RN, BSN

CRITICAL CONCEPTS

- Protecting the health of families is crucial for ensuring the health of the community.
- Community and public health nursing utilize theories and models to care for families in the community.
- Community and public health nurses practice in a variety of settings, which include the homes of families in the community.

- Three levels of prevention—primary, secondary, and tertiary—are used by community and public health nurses.
- Research, nursing education, and health care policy affect the care of families.

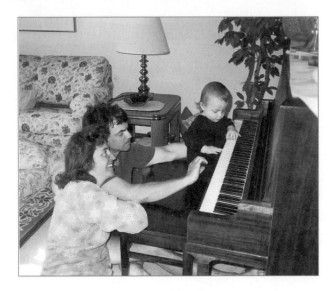

Community/public health nurses have a long history of working with families, and they recognize that the health of individuals is intertwined with the health of families and the community. Families have a major impact on the health of individuals; that impact can be positive or negative. For example, families are assumed to provide social support, which is both health-promoting and restoring for their members. However, this support may instead be negative or absent, in which case family members' health may be compromised (Anderson, 1996). The health of families is important to every community's well-being. In fact, the health of communities is measured by the collective health of its individuals and families (e.g., the rate of low-birth-weight infants born to single mothers in a community; number of uninsured children in a region). Violence, poverty, employment rates, and homelessness are indicators of the community's and family's health. The character of the community and its ability to deal with health issues influences the well-being of all who live there. This chapter describes how the principles and practice of family nursing and community health nursing are integrated to yield what might be called family-centered community/public health nursing.

WHAT IS COMMUNITY/PUBLIC HEALTH NURSING?

Community as client is inherent in community health nursing practice. The community client may be a location in space and time such as a neighborhood, a city, or a state. The community may be an *aggregate of people* with similar characteristics, such as all people infected with HIV, those diagnosed with juvenile-onset diabetes, or homeless families. The community client may describe groups who have a specific function (Shuster & Goeppinger, 1996), such as a nurse's organization that provides education on gun safety or a group of parents who work to decrease teen suicide. The use of the term "community" in this chapter reflects all of these views of community as a client.

The practice of community and public health nursing encompasses both caring for the community as a whole and caring for individuals and families within the community. According to the Association of Community Health Nursing Educators (ACHNE, 1995), the definition of community health nursing is

> *The synthesis of nursing theory and public health theory applied to promoting and preserving the health of populations. The focus of community health nursing is the community as a whole, with nursing care of individuals, families, and groups being provided within the context of promoting and preserving the health of community. (p. 2)*

For the purpose of this chapter, the definition of public health nursing from the Public Health Nursing Section of the American Public Health Association (1996) is most useful:

> *Public health nursing is the practice of promoting and protecting the health of populations using knowledge from the nursing, social, and public health sciences.*

These definitions of community/public health nursing suggest that the underlying target of care is the community; the community is either the direct or the ultimate client. Individuals, families, and groups are subunits of the community and receive either direct care in the context of being a member of the community client or indirect care as a result of being a member of the community client. Although family nursing should be evident in every clinical setting, it is particularly important in community/public health nursing where nurses seek to empower families to achieve and maintain wellness through health promotion and education (Duffy, Vehvilainen-Julkunen, Huber, & Varjoranta, 1998; Spoth, Kavanagh, & Dishion, 2002).

Traditional Community Health Nursing Roles

Working with individuals, families, and groups in the context of community involves one set of nursing roles and interventions, whereas working directly with the community as a client involves others. Clark (1996) categorizes these nursing roles as (1) client-oriented, (2) delivery-oriented, and (3) group-oriented. Client-oriented roles are directed toward providing services to clients and include the roles of caregiver, educator, counselor, referral source, role model, advocate, primary care provider, and case manager. Delivery-oriented roles are directed toward facilitating the operation of the health care delivery system and indirectly enhance the care of clients. These roles include those of coordinator, collaborator, liaison, and discharge planner. Lastly, group-oriented roles are directed toward promoting the health of the population of a community and include the roles of case finder, leader, change agent, community care agent, and researcher. Client-oriented and delivery-oriented roles are used most frequently when providing care to individuals, families, and groups in community settings, whereas group-oriented roles are used when care is directed toward the community.

Not all community health nurses perform all of these roles. Often the setting and employing agency determine which roles are utilized. In addition, the core functions of public health have changed and strengthened many community health roles. These ideas will be further explained later in this chapter.

Community/Public Health Nursing Today

Over the past 30 years, community/public health nursing has grown, partly due to societal developments beginning in the late 1960s. Nurses began to recognize that the entire community needs health services, not just the sick poor. In addition, other nursing specialists such as home health nurses began practicing outside the hospital setting, and some focused their practice on the care of the family. Furthermore, changes in the health care delivery system, such as the emergence of managed care systems and decrease in preventive services covered by Medicare and Medicaid (Institute of Medicine, 2003), began to blur the distinctions between private, public, and nonprofit services. All of these developments led community/public health nurses to reexamine their scope of practice (Spradley, 1985).

As a result, there are two branches or foci of care: (1) community as client, with the family as an important subunit, and (2) the family as the central unit of service within the community setting. Regardless of

HISTORICAL PERSPECTIVE

Visiting nurses, or nurses who provide care in patients' homes, were described as early as the pre-Christian eras in India, Egypt, Greece, and Rome (Gardner, 1928). Visiting nursing is documented from the 11th to 16th centuries in Europe, with both secular and religious orders providing care (Rue, 1944).

In the mid-1800s, the importance of health promotion and disease prevention began to be recognized. Community health nurses, or visiting nurses, then expanded their roles to include health education as well as sick care, and in order to function effectively, they directed their care not only to individuals but also to families (Gardner, 1928; Rue 1944). Recognizing that nurses were more effective when care involved all family members, Lillian Wald established a home visiting service in the homes of the sick poor over 100 years ago (Kuss, Proulx-Girouard, Lovitt, Katz, & Kennelly, 1997). Wald developed guidelines for nursing of families in the home (Rue, 1944; Whall, 1986). Furthermore, Wald went beyond caring for families during an illness to being a forceful advocate of economic and social reform to effect societal change that would improve the overall health of families and communities (Kuss et al., 1997).

In the early 1900s, subspecialties in community health nursing developed. Some nurses cared for mothers and infants, others cared for those with communicable diseases, and others worked with the mentally ill. Moreover, community health nurses began seeing individuals in other settings besides the home, including clinics, tenements, day nurseries, schools, and industries (Spradley, 1985). Despite recognizing the importance of family, community health nurses did not fully direct their practice to the family as a unit of care until the 1950s. The family as a unit of care then remained the orienting perspective for community health nurses until the 1970s (Spradley, 1985).

the differing viewpoints of community health nurses, working with families remains an important component of community/public health nursing.

In 1998, the World Health Organization's (WHO) European Region identified 21 health targets for the next century (Fawcett-Henesy, 1998). Comprehensive primary health care is the method to be used in achieving the goals. Of particular importance is the focus on families, workplaces, the local community, and other settings that include multiple generations living together. The importance of targeting families in the community to improve health is a challenge for health care providers worldwide.

COMMON THEORETICAL PERSPECTIVE

Many theoretical perspectives on the family are available to guide community health nursing practice. Not surprisingly, nursing models for families reflect two prevalent schools of thought in community/public health nursing today. Some espouse the view that the family is the unit of care and the community is context, whereas others focus on the community as client and view the family as a subunit (see Chapter 1). Zerwekh's (1991) Family Caregiving Model for Public Health Nursing outlines a framework that supports providing care to families within a community. The Core Public Health Functions Model provides guidance in the provision of nursing care for families and addresses both views of the family as the client within the community and the family as a part of the community client.

Family Caregiving Model for Public Health Nursing

Zerwekh's (1991) Family Caregiving Model for Public Health Nursing continues to be a useful framework for providing care to families in the community (Ackerman, 1994; Collins & Reinke, 1997). This model was created on the basis of descriptions by expert community health nurses of home visiting activities that made a difference in the outcomes for maternal-child clients. From these descriptions, 16 competencies were identified and a model of their relationships was developed (Figure 15–1). The focus of this model is the family and developing the ability of members to take charge of their lives and make their own choices. Nurses' actions are aimed at encouraging family self-help through believing in the family's ability to make

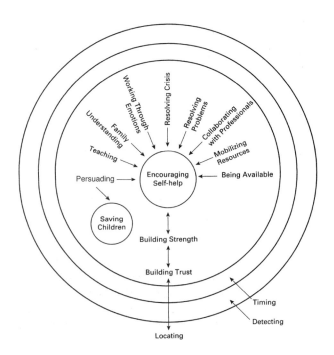

Figure 15–1   Zerwekh's Caregiving Model for Public Health Nursing.

choices and aiding them to believe in themselves. Appropriate nursing actions include listening to the family's needs, expanding the family's vision of choices, and feeding back reality so that the family sees patterns in their lives and the consequences of their decisions.

The first three competencies establish the foundation for family caregiving: (1) locating the family, (2) building trust, and (3) building strength. After this foundation is laid, eight encouraging self-help competencies are employed when working with families:

1. Being available
2. Mobilizing resources
3. Collaborating with other professionals
4. Resolving problems
5. Resolving crises
6. Working through emotions
7. Fostering family understanding
8. Teaching
9. Persuading

Three of these competencies help to foster community: being available, mobilizing resources, and collaborating with other professionals. Thus, the model acknowledges that the community is the context for family care.

If family self-help cannot be achieved and the nurse finds that a family member is still at risk, two additional forceful competencies are employed: (1) persuading, which includes the use of reasoning, confronting, and threatening action (for example, calling child protective services); and (2) saving the children. In these at-risk situations, the nurse's responsibility for children (or individuals at risk) becomes primary.

Two competencies are used simultaneously with the other competencies and are ongoing during the care of the family. These are called encompassing competencies. The first of these, timing, relates to the speed of introducing an intervention and has three dimensions: (1) detecting the right time to initiate the action, (2) persisting in implementing the intervention, and (3) futuring, whereby the nurse considers the present action based on a view of the future (e.g., the child's development). The second encompassing competency, detecting, uses comprehensive assessment to identify potential and actual health problems.

Core Public Health Function Model

The Core Public Health Function Model addresses assessment, policy development, and assurance as the three primary functions of public health (Institute of Medicine, 2003; Washington State Core Public Health Functions Task Force, 1993). Public health nurses, administrators, and educators from Washington State collaborated to develop the public health nurse's role within the Core Public Health Function Model. Each core function will be described and the role of the public health nurse for each will be discussed. Individual, family, and community levels will be included because each level affects family.

Assessment

The trust that public health nurses have earned from their clients, agencies, and private providers provides them with ready access to populations that are otherwise difficult to access and engage in health care. In addition, they have knowledge of current and emerging health issues through their daily contact with high-risk and vulnerable populations. This trust and knowledge provide the foundation for the activities shown in Table 15–1.

Policy Development

Public health nurses are uniquely qualified to influence and develop policy at the individual, family, and

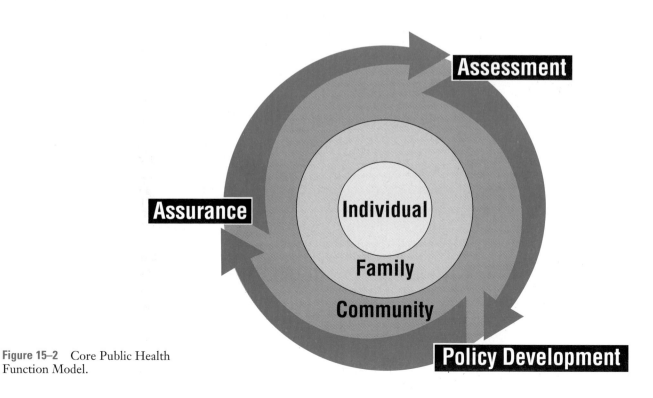

Figure 15–2 Core Public Health Function Model.

Table 15–1   PUBLIC HEALTH NURSE ASSESSMENT STRATEGIES

COMMUNITY	FAMILY	INDIVIDUAL
1. Analyze data on and needs of specific populations or geographic area. 2. Identify and interact with key community leaders, both formally and informally. 3. Identify target populations that may be at risk. These populations may include high-density low-income areas, preschools, primary and secondary schools, and elderly. 4. Participate in data collection on a target population. 5. Conduct surveys or observe targeted populations, such as preschools, jails, and detention centers, in order to gain a better understanding of needs.	1. Evaluate a specific family's strengths and areas of concern. This involves a comprehensive assessment of the physical, social, and mental health needs of the family. 2. Evaluate the family's living environment, looking specifically at support, relationships, and other factors that might have a significant impact on family health outcomes. 3. Assess the larger environment in which the family lives (the block or specific community) for safety, access, and other related issues.	1. Identify individuals within the family who are in need of services. 2. Evaluate the functional capacity of the total individual through the use of specific assessment measures, including physical, social, and mental health screening tools. 3. Develop a nursing diagnosis for the individual that describes a problem or potential problem, etiology, and contributing factors. 4. Develop a nursing care plan for the individual.

community level. Public health nurses synthesize and analyze data collected from individuals, families, and communities in making policy decisions. The information obtained at the assessment level will be used to make decisions at the organizational and community level. Activities to influence policy development include those listed in Table 15–2.

Assurance

Assurance activities are the direct individual-focused services that public health nurses have provided over the past several years. This was due, in large part, to programmatic funding and Medicaid reimbursement that focused on the individual rather than on population-focused services. Although the current shift in emphasis is toward assessment and policy development, critical assurance activities for the public health nurse remain (see Table 15–3).

The Family Caregiving Model for Public Health Nursing and the Core Public Health Function Model form the basis for nursing interventions for families in the community.

HEALTH PROMOTION AND DISEASE PREVENTION

Several concepts basic to community/public health nursing have set the direction for care provided to individuals, families, groups, and communities. *Health promotion, disease prevention, primary prevention, secondary prevention, tertiary prevention, epidemiology, risk,* and *case finding* will be defined, and examples from the *Healthy People 2000* and *Healthy People 2010* documents (U.S. Public Health Service, 1996; U.S. Department of Health and Human Services, 2000) will be used to demonstrate each concept.

Health Promotion and Disease Prevention Defined

Health promotion includes activities that improve or maintain the well-being of people (Albrecht & Swanson, 1993). Teaching families conflict resolution skills is an example of a health promotion activity. Disease prevention includes those activities that protect families from actual or potential diseases and

Table 15–2 ACTIVITIES TO INFLUENCE POLICY DEVELOPMENT

COMMUNITY	FAMILY	INDIVIDUAL
1. Provide leadership in convening and facilitating community groups to evaluate health concerns and develop a plan to address the concerns. 2. Recommend specific training and programs to meet identified health needs. 3. Raise awareness of key policy makers about health regulations, budget decisions, and other factors that may affect the health of communities negatively. 4. Recommend programs to target populations such as child care centers, retirement centers, jails, juvenile detention facilities, homeless shelters, work sites, and minority communities. 5. Act as an advocate for the community and individuals who are not willing or able to speak to policy makers about issues/programs of concern. 6. Work with business and industry to develop employee health programs.	1. Recommend new or increased services to families based on identified needs. 2. Recommend programs to meet specific families' needs within a geographic area. 3. Facilitate networking of families with similar needs/issues. Guide policy makers on specific issues affecting clusters of families. 4. Request additional data and analyze information to identify trends in a group or cluster of families. 5. Identify key families in a community who may either oppose or support specific policies or programs and develop appropriate and effective intervention strategies to use with these families.	1. Recommend or assist in the development of standards for individual client care. 2. Recommend or adopt risk classification systems to assist with prioritizing individual client care. 3. Participate in establishing criteria for opening, closing, or referring individual cases. 4. Participate in the development of job descriptions to establish roles for various team members who will provide service to individuals.

disabilities and their consequences (Albrecht & Swanson, 1993; Hassmiller, 1996); it occurs at three different levels: primary, secondary, and tertiary prevention (Leavell & Clark, 1958). Water fluoridation and accident control programs are examples of preventive activity.

Primary Prevention

Primary prevention focuses on preventing the occurrence of health problems. The four leading causes of death for adolescents and young adults aged 15 to 24 are motor vehicle accidents, other unintended injuries, homicide, and suicide. Schools can be instrumental in decreasing youth violence and injury through education, the expansion of after-school sports, and other activities for young people (U.S. Public Health

Service, 1996). In rural New Mexico, for example, tribal leaders and other members of the Jicarilla Apache Tribe have engaged in a suicide prevention effort in schools and a public education campaign to make the community aware of the problem. The number of suicide attempts has dropped and no suicides were recorded in 1995 (U.S. Public Health Service, 1996).

Secondary Prevention

Secondary prevention activities are designed to identify and treat health problems early. Secondary prevention activities are carried out during the early stage of an acute or chronic illness. The Milwaukee Women's Center initiated a public awareness campaign designed to decrease violence against women. The Center's messages about family and intimate partner violence are

Table 15–3 **CRITICAL ASSURANCE ACTIVITIES FOR THE PUBLIC HEALTH NURSE**

COMMUNITY	FAMILY	INDIVIDUAL
1. Provide service to target populations such as child care centers, preschools, work sites, minority communities, jails, juvenile detention facilities, and homeless shelters. Interventions may include health screening, education, health promotion, and injury prevention programs.	1. Provide services to a cluster of families within a geographic setting. Services may be provided in a variety of settings including homes, child care centers, preschools, and schools. Services may include physical assessment, health education and counseling, and health and developmental screening.	1. Provide nursing services based on standards of nursing practice to individuals across the age continuum. These services may encompass a variety of programs including, specifically, First Steps and Children with Special Health Care Needs and, more generally, child abuse prevention, immunizations, well-child care, and HIV/AIDS programs.
2. Improve quality assurance activities with various health care providers in the community. Examples include education on new immunization policies; educational programs for communicable disease control; and assistance in developing effective approaches and support techniques for high-risk populations.	2. Provide care in a nursing clinic to a specific group of families in a geographic location.	2. Assess and support the individual's progress toward meeting outcome goals.
3. Maintain safe levels of communicable disease surveillance and outbreak control.		3. Consult with other health care providers and team members regarding the individual's plan of care.
4. Participate in research or demonstration projects.		4. Prioritize the individual's needs on an ongoing basis.
5. Provide expert public health consultation in the community.		5. Participate on quality assurance teams to measure the quality of care provided.
6. Ensure that standards of care are met within the community.		

displayed on the local buses. Because of the visibility, the number of calls to domestic violence hotlines and agencies increased, including calls from men admitting they need help (Healthy People 2010, 2000).

Tertiary Prevention

Tertiary prevention is aimed at correcting health problems and preventing further deterioration. It is used with both acute and chronic health problems.

For example, in the school shooting incident at Columbine High School in Colorado, twelve students and one teacher were killed and the two student gunmen committed suicide. In this case, tertiary prevention focused on rebuilding the community, dealing with the grief and fears of individuals, families, and the entire community, and developing community prevention strategies to help prevent such a violent act from occurring in the future. Since the terrorist attacks on the United States on September 11, 2001, public health nurses have employed tertiary prevention activities such as mental health counseling for victims and emergency workers and development of emergency preparedness measures (Martinelli, 2003).

> 66 Community health nurses use concepts from epidemiology to promote health and prevent disease. 99

Risk

Epidemiology is a science that is concerned with health events in human populations (Valanis, 1999). An important epidemiological concept is risk, which refers to the probability that individuals in a community will be affected by a health problem. Community health nurses assist in identifying individuals, families,

and populations at risk for health problems by using case-finding methods, such as review of health statistics, screening programs, and contact tracing (Freeman & Heinrich, 1981). One example of the use of risk assessment took place in a school-based program in Dayton, Ohio. Adolescents who were identified as high risk for becoming perpetrators or victims of violence were enrolled in the Positive Adolescent Choices Training (PACT) program. Adolescents in the program showed reductions in violent confrontations and improvements in managing conflict.

All of the aforementioned strategies are useful both when the family is the focus of care and when the community is client. Although the major focus of community health nursing is on health promotion and disease prevention, these concepts are applicable during various other phases of the health–illness trajectory.

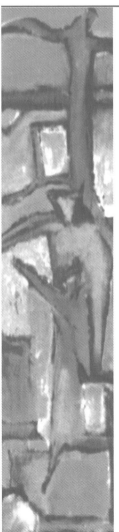

RESEARCH BRIEF

Purpose

Current literature identifies factors that are associated with women who have experienced homelessness; these factors include history of domestic violence, history of child abuse, substance abuse, poverty, and lack of social support. The purpose of this study was to examine further the link between social support, homelessness, and the families of origin of women who have a history of homelessness. The family of origin is the group that reared and socialized the woman during childhood, regardless of biological ties. The dynamics of the relationships formed within the family of origin affect adult relationships later in life (Stroufe & Fleeson, 1986). The study also evaluated the difference in the levels of intimacy and autonomy in the families of origin of homeless and never-homeless women. In addition, the levels of reciprocity and conflict in past and current social support networks were also compared.

Methodology

Researchers used a descriptive correlational design to complete the study. Subjects were recruited in the Greater Portland Area via flyers, newspaper advertisements, and informational sessions at local homeless shelters, housing complexes, and public meeting places. Three groups of women over the age of 18 were recruited: 94 homeless women, 88 never-homeless women who were victims of child abuse, and 73 never-homeless women who had never experienced child abuse. Women in the homeless group were required to have one or more periods of homelessness for 1 to 12 months at a time.

The subjects were asked to complete questionnaires with research team members present. The Interpersonal Relationship Inventory (IPRI) was used to measure current social support. Childhood social support was measured through the use of the IPRI-A, a version of IPRI. Autonomy and intimacy levels were determined using the Family-of-Origin Scale. Sociodemographic data was collected after the completion of the questionnaires.

Results

The average number of people per family was significantly higher for the women in the homeless group. Examination of the scores for current social support showed a significant

(continued on page 402)

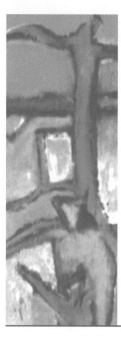

(Continued)

difference between the homeless group and the other two groups; the homeless group's score was much lower. Reciprocity and conflict scores also possessed a significant difference between the homeless group and the other two groups. A dissimilarity was also demonstrated between the conflict scores of the never-homeless/abused group and the never-homeless/not-abused group. Analysis of childhood social support, autonomy, and intimacy uncovered that the never-homeless/not-abused group had significantly higher reciprocity, lower conflict, and more autonomy and intimacy than the other two groups. The remaining two groups did not have significant differences for childhood social support, autonomy, and intimacy.

Nursing Implications

Results of this study demonstrate the need for community/public health nursing interventions that are targeted toward improving familial relationships. Moreover, community/public health nurses need to assist at-risk individuals and families in accessing and maintaining social support networks.

Anderson, D. G., & Rayens, M. K. (2004). Factors influencing homelessness in women. *Public Health Nursing,* *21*(1), 12–23.

Strategies for Health Promotion and Disease Prevention for Families in the Community

Many health promotion and disease prevention strategies are directed at both families and communities. Clark (1996) outlined five categories of health promotion and disease prevention strategies: (1) health appraisal, (2) health education, (3) lifestyle modification, (4) provision of a healthy environment, and (5) development of effective coping skills. In addition, *Promoting Health/Preventing Disease: Objectives for the Nation* (U.S. Department of Health and Human Services, 1980) suggests that (1) planning and providing health services (e.g., family planning clinics), (2) instituting health legislation and regulations, (3) offering economic incentives, and (4) developing health technology (e.g., Websites for support groups) are measures to promote health. Although community health nurses generally are not involved in technology development, they frequently use other measures in the care of the family as client in the community setting and in the care of community as client.

The Family as Client in the Community Setting

Health appraisal, education, and ensuring access to care are key activities of community/public health nurses when dealing with families in the community.

Health Appraisal

An initial health-promoting and disease-preventing strategy is to conduct a health appraisal of families and their environments for the purpose of identifying strengths and potential risks to health. Appraisal of the family's environment is a unique function of community health nursing. If possible, the community health nurses make home visits to directly observe the environment and develop appropriate interventions based on the availability of resources in that home environment. The community health nurse who works in a school or occupational setting also directly appraises the effects of these environments.

An environmental appraisal includes assessment of physical, psychological, social, and economic environments. Assessment of the physical environment of the home includes examination of safety hazards, such as condition of paint, age of housing, fire extinguishers, and dangerous playground equipment; facilities for hygiene, such as running water and indoor plumbing; items to meet basic needs, such as food, heating, cooking facilities, and refrigeration; and objects that promote social, emotional, and physical development, such as toys and books. A similar assessment can be applied to other settings. The neighborhood also should be assessed for level of violence, safety hazards, availability of transportation, access to needed goods and services, access to recreational facilities, and the presence of environmental pollutants (Clark, 1996).

The community health nurse appraises the family's psychological, social, and economic environment. In the home, family communication patterns, role relationships, family dynamics, emotional strengths, coping strategies, and child-rearing and discipline practices can be assessed directly. The effects of the social environment (e.g., religious practices, culture, social class, economic status, and social support system) on health can be assessed on a home visit. In settings other than the home, factors that promote the psychological and social growth of individual family members should be evaluated.

Education

Education is essential to the promotion of health and the prevention of disease in families. After completing the health appraisal, the community health nurse reinforces health promotion and provides health information and teaching in areas identified as at risk. The four determinants of health—environment, social/lifestyle, biology, and health care/medical—provide a useful framework for developing a health teaching plan (University of Southern Mississippi School of Nursing, 2003).

The community health nurse uses a variety of strategies to modify risky lifestyles identified in the health appraisal. Teaching and health information can be used to discuss immunizations, nutrition, rest, exercise, use of seat belts, and abuse of harmful substances such as alcohol and drugs. The community health nurse may refer the family to programs and resources that assist in lifestyle modifications (e.g., smoking cessation classes, exercise programs).

Health teaching based on appraisal of the physical environment might include information on child safety and prevention of falls. Other teaching might focus on psychological or social environmental problems, such as family communications or dealing with peer pressure. In some situations, the community health nurse promotes a healthy environment by providing information to community members outside the family. For example, community health nurses working in schools might need to inform officials about playground hazards or poor food-handling practices.

Access to Resources

A major health promotion strategy is ensuring access to health promotion and prevention services, including immunizations, family planning, prenatal care, well-child care, nutrition, exercise classes, and dental hygiene. These services may be provided directly by the community health nurse in the home or in clinics, schools, or work settings. In some cases, the community health nurse facilitates access to these services through referrals, case management, discharge planning, advocacy, coordination, and collaboration.

Community as Client and Nursing Care of Families

When nursing care focuses on the community as client with the goal of promoting health and preventing disease, nurses use strategies and interventions similar to those used with families. However, strategies are refocused toward the community. Other nursing actions are program planning and policy development.

One strategy for promoting the health of families when the community is client is to conduct a community assessment or health appraisal of a community to identify potential and actual health risks to all individuals and families living in the community. After potential health risks are identified, the community health nurse intervenes to temper these risk factors.

A community assessment involves collecting health and social data about the population, the social institutions (e.g., health and social services, economics, education, safety and transportation, recreation, politics and government, and communication), and the environment (physical, psychological, and social). Demographic information about the population provides information regarding possible health problems. For example, a community with a large population of children under 5 years of age might benefit from strategies aimed at increasing competence in parenting and increasing immunizations. Information on social institutions is helpful in assessing the adequacy of the community's resources. Such information can indicate whether there are enough pediatricians, whether municipal transportation is available to go to hospitals and clinics, or whether fire and emergency services are staffed for immediate response. Assessment of the environment includes evaluating the types and adequacy of sewage and water treatment and investigating for the presence of disease-bearing insects such as the ticks that cause Lyme disease.

Methods of gathering data for a community assessment include windshield surveys, interviews with key informants, analysis of secondary data gathered by health departments such as morbidity and mortality rates, and large population surveys. A windshield survey is the motorized equivalent of simple observation. Through an automobile windshield, many dimensions of a community's life and environment are carefully observed (Stanhope & Lancaster, 2004). Via this method, data can be collected about families in the community—for example, the proportion of single-parent families or the number of day-care facilities. A detailed description of community assessment is beyond the scope of this chapter; however, most community health nursing texts provide guidance for implementing a community assessment.

Once data has been collected, it is analyzed to identify the community's health problems, that is, to make "community diagnoses." An example of a community diagnosis is "The children are at risk for lead poisoning due to the amount of old housing stock in the community." After community diagnoses are made, researchers develop goals to correct the problems and develop program plans to intervene.

Program planning includes the following:

- Identification of potential solutions to the problem
- Analysis and comparison of alternative solutions
- Selection of one program and/or solution
- Development of program goals and objectives
- Identification of resources
- Development of the specific activities of the program
- Development of methods to evaluate the program

Usually program planning involves multidisciplinary teams of health and non-health professionals. The community and its families also should be involved in the planning and implementation to ensure that the program meets their needs. During this process, community health nurses employ the group-oriented roles of community care agent, leader, and change agent. Community families and leaders, nurses, nutritionists, weight loss experts, and physical fitness instructors convening to plan a program to prevent obesity in a community is an example of interdisciplinary program planning that involves the community and families.

Awareness of the need to design community health programs with a family-centered approach has grown over the past 20 years. For example, in 1986, Congress passed PL 99-457, the Education for All Handicapped Children Act, and mandated that services be provided to the families of children with developmental disabilities as well as to the child (Shelton, Jeppson, & Johnson, 1987). Since then, the Association for the Care of Children's Health (ACCH) has developed a definition of family-centered care that many other groups working with families have adopted (Korteland & Cornwell, 1991, p. 57). Box 15–1 lists the elements of family-centered care. Community health nurses can facilitate development of health programs that are supportive to families by using these elements to guide program planning and implementation.

Box 15–1   **ELEMENTS OF FAMILY-CENTERED CARE**

1. Recognition that the family is the constant in the child's life whereas service systems and personnel within those systems fluctuate
2. Facilitation of parent-professional collaboration at all levels of health care
3. Sharing of unbiased and complete information with parents about their child's care on an ongoing basis in an appropriate and supportive manner
4. Implementation of appropriate policies and programs that are comprehensive and provide emotional and financial support to meet the needs of families
5. Recognition of family strengths and individuality and respect for different methods of coping
6. Understanding and incorporation of the developmental and emotional needs of infants, children, and adolescents and their families in health care delivery systems
7. Encouragement and facilitation of parent-to-parent support
8. Assurance that the design of health care delivery systems is flexible, accessible, and responsive to family needs
9. Respect for the racial, ethnic, cultural, and socioeconomic diversity of families

Source: Korteland, C., & Cornwell, J.R. (1991). Evaluating family-centered programs in neonatal intensive care. *Children's Health Care, 20*(1), 56–61. With permission.

The work of David Olds and his colleagues (1997) shows the effectiveness of family-centered care and the effectiveness of community/public health nursing home visitation. Nurses visited low-income, unmarried mothers and their children. The families with home visitation had significantly improved health outcomes. The home visitation reduced the number of the mothers' subsequent pregnancies, the use of welfare, child abuse and neglect, and criminal behaviors for up to 15 years after the first child's birth (Olds, 2002).

The home-visit nursing program (Olds et al., 1998) was found to reduce serious antisocial behavior and substance use as the high-risk children in the study entered adolescence. As adolescents, they ran away less, were arrested and convicted less, were less promiscuous, and smoked and drank less than comparable adolescents. The results of this work show how home visits in the community are beneficial for high-risk families and demonstrate how intervention by community/public health nurses is essential for the effectiveness of this visitation program.

Another strategy for promoting health and preventing disease from a community-as-client perspective is policy development and implementation. Community health nurses frequently interact in local and state policy by alerting policy makers about the health problems in their communities. Nurses give direct accounts of the effects these health problems have on families in the community. They write letters, make telephone calls, testify before committees, and take part in other political activities to create awareness of the health problem. Nurses sit on advisory boards and task forces at all levels: community, city, county, state, and national. In these positions, nurses directly influence policy to promote health and prevent disease.

Once a health problem is recognized, community health nurses work with others to propose and shape policy solutions. The community health nurse's perspective on a proposed policy's effect on families is important to the development of health proposals. Community health nurses have a role in the implementation of these policies to ensure optimum results for family health.

ACUTE AND CHRONIC ILLNESS CARE

Nursing care for families in the community involves secondary and tertiary prevention, specifically for those families who have members with either an acute or a chronic illness.

Secondary Prevention in Families with Acute and Chronic Illness

Secondary prevention strategies include (1) early detection of health problems in families and communities, (2) referral for further evaluation and treatment, and (3) health teaching about the potential illness and the need for follow-up. Screening for detection of illness is a major function of community health nurses and is accomplished through health appraisals, as described previously in this chapter, and by using screening tools and methods. Many screening procedures are available for detecting health problems in family members of all ages and in the family as a whole. These procedures and instruments are discussed in other chapters in this text.

Once community health nurses detect a health problem, they initiate appropriate nursing care and/or make referrals to nurse practitioners or physicians for medical evaluation of the condition and treatment. The community health nurse is responsible for ensuring that the patient receives the needed health care.

The referral process includes identifying the need for referral, identifying appropriate health resources, preparing the client for the referral, communicating with the referral agency, and evaluating the outcome of the referral for the client (Clark, 1996). During this time, the community health nurse also provides health education and information about the significance of positive screening results and the need for follow-up treatment of the condition. Clients vary in their ability to find and use health care resources. Clemen-Stone, Eigisti, and McGuire (2002) suggest that there are three levels of nursing intervention in the referral process. Level I clients are dependent on the nurse to identify needed health care resources, coordinate referrals, and assist the patient to use the referral services. Level II clients are moderately independent. They seek information from the nurse and may need some help in identifying resources and in completing the referral process. Level III clients are independent; after they are given information about health resources, they can complete the referral process.

Tertiary Prevention in Families with Acute and Chronic Illness

Tertiary prevention focuses on (1) monitoring the health problem, (2) providing treatments, (3) providing health education, and (4) promoting adjustment to the illness. One tertiary prevention strategy is to monitor the individual's physical condition. Follow-up health appraisals provide information that can be compared with the initial health appraisal data to chart progress. For example, the nurse monitors the diabetic client's blood glucose levels to determine whether the treatment is effective. Another tertiary prevention strategy is to provide nursing treatments to correct the illness and prevent further health problems. In these instances, the community health nurse provides direct patient care such as dressing changes, medication administration, and range of motion. In some communities, home health nurses employed by private agencies provide these treatments; in other communities, community health nurses from public health departments provide this care. Home health nursing is a subspecialty of community health nursing; however, home health nurses in private agencies tend to provide more intensive technological nursing care. School nurses and occupational health nurses also provide direct nursing interventions.

A third tertiary prevention strategy is to provide health teaching to the patient and the family to help them carry out prescribed treatments. The nurse also provides information about the disease and the ways to prevent further problems. A fourth tertiary prevention strategy is to assist the patient and family in coping with the illness through counseling or to help mobilize other support resources within the family and the family's extended network or in the community.

Community assessment, program planning and implementation, case finding, community education, and health policy development can also be appropriate as secondary and tertiary prevention measures. Strategies utilizing these measures, in relation to the care of the family as client, can be carried out in a variety of community settings.

END-OF-LIFE CARE

Many of the same interventions that are used with acute and chronic illness are also used with families in the community at the time of a family member's death. Home health and hospice nurses often work with individual families to provide nursing care, education, and referrals for other services, such as legal aid and respite services for the caregivers. After the death, community/public health nurses provide grief counseling for the family. In the case of relatives who die at home, nurses often act as a liaison between the family and the hospital or funeral home to arrange the pickup of the body. They may also direct the family to the proper organizations for assistance with burial and costs associated with the funeral.

Community/public health nurses may also indirectly assist families with end-of-life care. This assistance comes in a variety of forms, which include planning programs to support families with dying loved ones and lobbying for laws that affect end-of-life issues. Nurses frequently participate in state, federal, and medical organizations' committees that make decisions concerning such matters as advanced directives and do-not-resuscitate orders (American Association of Colleges of Nursing, 2002).

IMPLICATIONS OF COMMUNITY/PUBLIC HEALTH NURSING FOR PRACTICE, EDUCATION, RESEARCH, AND HEALTH CARE POLICY

Several implications for study and change exist for community/public health nursing. These implications include the areas of nursing practice, education, research, and health care policy.

Practice

Although nurses have focused on the family unit in the community for many years, there are still many obstacles to family-centered care. First of all, nurses must have access to families in order to provide care; thus care needs to be provided in settings where families

---

NURSING INTERVENTIONS FOR ACUTE AND CHRONIC ILLNESS WHEN THE COMMUNITY IS CLIENT

Care for families with acute and chronic illnesses at the community level involves using (1) community assessment to identify significant acute and chronic health problems in the community, (2) planning and providing screening and treatment services, (3) identifying those at risk for particular acute and chronic illnesses, (4) providing community educational programs, and, in some instances, (5) developing health policy. These strategies focus on acute and chronic health problems in the community.

commonly reside. These include homes, the schools where younger family members spend a large portion of their day, the occupational settings where adult members are easily located, and sites where the elderly congregate.

In addition, barriers to care of families in the community need to be removed. Most health agencies, even those that espouse a family focus, in reality direct care to the individual. Patient records usually contain data only about the individual. Family members have separate records. Family assessment data may exist in only one family member's record or, more commonly, are not recorded at all. This fragmentation makes it difficult to view the family as a unit. In the past, there were legal constraints to recording one individual's assessment information in another's record because of confidentiality. The Health Insurance Portability and Accountability Act (HIPAA) established a privacy rule that increased the protection of individuals' health records and limited the ability to disclose health information (U.S. Department of Health and Human Services, 2003). HIPAA limits the amount of health information that can be disclosed to family members; this limitation can impede the care of families. Some agencies have not found ways to overcome these legal barriers.

Education

Nursing education needs to emphasize the interplay between the health of the community and the health of families. Undergraduate students who learn community-focused interventions can promote the health of families. Graduate students specializing in family and community health nursing study the theoretical perspectives of community-focused and family-focused interventions. Practica that include family-centered nursing provide students with opportunities to practice theoretical perspectives and are important at both the undergraduate and graduate level of nursing.

Research

Research is needed to identify common family health problems in the community, resources to meet family needs, and effective organization of services to promote family health and coping. A possible research topic includes minority and low-socioeconomic-status families and access to health care; family cultural values and the effects on nutrition, weight, and health is also a needed research area. Program evaluation is necessary to determine the effectiveness of interventions and to develop a strong base for funding of programs.

Research is also needed to determine which intervention strategies are most effective in promoting family health and preventing family illness. Research on the effects of home visiting on individual health problems needs to be broadened to include the effect on family problems.

Health Care Policy

Policy-level barriers to providing family-centered care in the community include the current organization of health services and reimbursement for health care. Health services in the community frequently are not family-focused but are arranged according to specific health problems (e.g., sexually transmitted diseases) or by age and/or life stage (e.g., prenatal care, teenage clinics). This skewed approach occurs because funding is allocated for specific services, which precludes health providers from focusing on the family as a unit and forces, instead, a focus on the specific health problem or life stage of the individual.

Reimbursement for health care is designed to promote an individual focus. Only specific health conditions or treatments are reimbursable. Reimbursement is paid for the individual presenting the problem; most insurance does not recognize the family as a client or accept family health diagnoses. Lastly, it frequently happens that not all family members are covered by health insurance and that reimbursement is thus limited to those who are covered.

Medicaid is a state program that provides health care coverage to elderly, disabled, and persons of low socioeconomic status. Recent changes in states' Medicaid programs threaten to affect not only the health care of

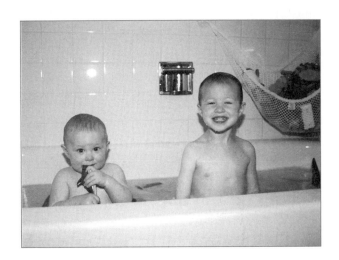

covered family members but also the financial and emotional stability of the entire family. In Kentucky, for example, Medicaid coverage for home health care, nursing homes, and outpatient care was decreased to save the state $250 million (Henry J. Kaiser Family Foundation, 2003). Such cutbacks decrease individuals'

access to care; the burden of cost then falls on individuals and families, who often must change their lifestyles to provide care. To remove the barriers created by inadequate reimbursement and lack of insurance, there need to be health policy changes. A strong nursing voice will help to effect these changes.

CASE STUDY ➤

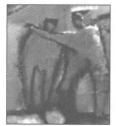

THE YORKE FAMILY

The following case study describes a typical community health nursing role. The scope of activities and breadth of responsibility described here are common to many community health nurses.

Catherine Parker, PHN, is a community health nurse for Monroe County Health District. She has a caseload of 50 families who live in the northwest section of the county. The health department sponsors 15 clinics a week, including clinics for prenatal care, well-child, family planning, immunizations, sexually transmitted diseases, and hypertension. In addition, public health nurses (PHNs) work closely with environmental health professionals. Catherine works Tuesday and Thursday mornings in the prenatal care and well-child clinics. She also works with the hospital's discharge coordinator to identify patients who need community services after leaving the hospital. Monroe County Health District's Nursing Department is responsible for providing school health services to the county's three elementary schools, two middle schools, and one high school. Catherine spends one afternoon a week at the high school. Recently, Catherine was asked to be on a task force to develop protocols for working with mothers with substance abuse; this group meets monthly. In addition, the State Health Department is planning to implement a child health information tracking system and has directed each county to conduct a feasibility study. Catherine is surveying the young families in her caseload for their views on having their children's health information available to multiple health providers.

Last week when Catherine was doing discharge planning at the County Hospital, she realized that the Yorke family could use additional services and arranged a postpartum home visit. Gina Yorke, aged 23 years, delivered her fourth child 1 week ago and is now at home. Gina's husband, Rob Yorke, aged 24 years, is an unemployed logger receiving job retraining at the

local community college. The other three children are aged 13 months, 2 years, and 3 years. Rob's parents live nearby. The Yorkes recently moved to Monroe and live in a rural part of the county. Gina received late prenatal care at the Monroe Health Clinic. The family lives in a rented, two-bedroom house 15 miles from town. Rob uses the only car for transportation to classes.

The Yorkes are just one of many families who live in the rural part of the county. There is no public transportation. Most families that live in this area rent their homes because it is less expensive than buying. The median family income of the people residing in this area is $12,120 a year. The mean age of the residents in this area is 25 years. Most houses have indoor plumbing with running water; the water comes from the county system. All houses have septic tanks. In the past year, three methamphetamine labs have been discovered in the area; adolescent substance abuse is a problem.

Catherine returns to visit the Yorke family for a 6-week postpartum follow-up. She weighs and measures the new baby and measures the infant's head circumference. The baby is gaining weight adequately and appears to be healthy. Gina Yorke also is feeling well and has had her 6-week checkup with the nurse midwife at the health department.

Gina mentions that the 2-year-old is not feeling well. He feels hot and has a rash on his chest. Catherine takes the child's temperature and it is 101°F. He has a runny nose and congestion in his chest. The rash on his trunk has vesicles; Catherine determines that he has varicella (chickenpox). None of the other children have had chickenpox, nor do they have any symptoms yet.

Catherine teaches Gina to take the child's temperature and discusses skin care and hygiene. She also emphasizes the importance of giving the child fluids and makes suggestions for diet. Catherine tells Gina that the child should be kept isolated from people outside the household until the vesicles are dried. If the child becomes more ill, Gina should call the doctor at the health clinic. Catherine asks Gina whether any

(continued on page 409)

of her family can help her with the care, and Gina indicates that Rob's mother is available. Catherine returns in a week to find that the family is coping well, although the other children now have caught varicella.

County health statistics indicate that there is a high incidence of lead poisoning in young children, particularly children in rural areas. It is possible that the source of lead is the water pipes, as older homes have plumbing that used to be soldered with lead; also, many of these older homes were painted with lead-based paints. Nearby, there also is a factory that makes lead pipe fittings; this factory has been cited by the Environmental Protection Agency for high levels of toxic waste emission.

While working in the well-child clinic, Catherine Parker screens all children for high lead blood levels. Gina Yorke brings her children to this clinic for preventive care, and when the children are tested, all are found to have lead in their blood. Follow-up care is planned and implemented. This comprehensive and interdisciplinary care is typical of a family receiving health care services from a county health department.

Case Study Discussion Questions

1. Apply Zerwekh's Family Caregiving Model for Public Health Nursing and the Core Public Health Function Model to the Yorkes' situation and planning for care.
2. How would the care given by Catherine Parker be different if she had an individual rather than a family focus?
3. How do the geography of the community and the availability of resources influence the Yorkes' health?
4. What types of prevention strategies is Catherine Parker using in caring for the Yorkes?
5. Are there other strategies that would be helpful?
6. What actions should Catherine Parker take at the community level to improve the Yorkes' health?

SUMMARY

- Community/public health nurses are concerned with the health of individuals, families, groups, and communities.
- The settings in which community/public health nurses work vary and include public and private health agencies, schools, and occupational sites.
- Community/public health nurses utilize concepts from public health including epidemiology, health promotion, and illness prevention.
- Community/public health nurses employ a large repertoire of roles. These roles vary according to whether the nurse is focusing on the family as the unit of care in the context of the community or focusing on the health of the community with families being a subunit.
- Health intervention strategies used by community/public health nurses include the following:

- Individual, family, and group health appraisals
- Community assessment
- Health education
- Referral to community resources
- Monitoring health problems
- Providing treatments
- Coordinating care and planning and providing health services
- Instituting health legislation and regulations

SQ STUDY QUESTIONS

1. Describe the target of care for community/public health nursing.

2. Identify nursing's historical roots in caring for families in community settings.

3. Analyze how the practices of family and community/public health nursing interface.

4. Define the following: epidemiology, public health nursing, community as client, aggregate of people, health promotion, disease prevention, and primary, secondary, and tertiary prevention.

5. List at least one example of a public health intervention for each level of prevention.

6. Identify a policy that affects families in your community.

References

Ackerman, P. M. (1994). *Competencies for the practice of effective public health nursing: Confirmation of Zerwekh's Family Caregiving Model.* Unpublished doctoral dissertation, University of Colorado, Denver, CO.

Albrecht, M., & Swanson, J. M. (1993). Health: A community view. In J. M. Swanson & M. Albrecht (Eds.), *Community health nursing: Promoting the health of aggregates* (pp. 3–12). Philadelphia: WB Saunders.

American Association of Colleges of Nursing. (2002). *Peaceful death: Recommended competencies and curricular guidelines for end-of-life nursing care.* Retrieved August 10, 2004, from http://www.aacn.nche.edu/publications/deathfin.htm

American Nurses Association. (1980). *A conceptual model of community health nursing.* Kansas City, MO: ANA.

American Public Health Association, Public Health Nursing Section. (1996). *The definition and role of public health nursing—A statement of the public health nursing section.* Washington, DC: Author.

Anderson, D. G. (1996). Homeless women's perceptions about their families of origin. *Western Journal of Nursing Research, 18,* 29–42.

Anderson, D. G., & Rayens, M. K. (2004). Factors influencing homelessness in women. *Public Health Nursing, 21*(1), 12–23.

Anderson, E. T., & McFarlane, J. M. (1988). *Community as client, application of the nursing process.* Philadelphia: JB Lippincott.

Association of Community Health Nursing Educators (1995). *Perspectives on theory development in community health nursing.* Louisville, KY: Author.

Butterfield, P. (1993). Thinking upstream: Conceptualizing health from a population perspective. In J. M. Swanson & M. Albrecht (Eds.), *Community health nursing: Promoting the health of aggregates* (pp. 68–80). Philadelphia: WB Saunders.

Clark, M. J. (1996). *Nursing in the community* (2nd ed.). Stamford, CT: Appleton & Lange.

Clarke, P. N. (1998). Nursing theory as a guide for inquiry in family and community health nursing. *Nursing Science Quarterly, 11*(2), 47–48.

Clemen-Stone, S., Eigisti, D. G., & McGuire, S. L. (2002). *Comprehensive family and community health nursing* (6th ed.). St. Louis, MO: CV Mosby.

Collins, A. M., & Reinke, E. (1997). Use of a family caregiving model to articulate the role of the public health nurse in infant mental health promotion. *Issues in Comprehensive Pediatric Nursing, 20*(4), 207–216.

Cookfair, J. M. (1996). *Nursing care in the community* (2nd ed.). St. Louis: Mosby.

Cooley, M. (1995). *A family perspective in community health nursing, community health nursing: Theory and practice.* Philadelphia: WB Saunders.

Coontz, S. (1992). *The way we never were.* New York, NY: Basic Books.

Cottrell, L. S. (1976). The competent community. In B. H. Kaplan, R. H. Wilson, & A. H. Leighton (Eds.), *Further explorations in social psychiatry* (pp. 195–209). New York: Basic Books.

Duffy, M. E., Vehvilainen-Julkunen, K., Huber, D., & Varjoranta, P. (1998). Family nursing practice in public health: Finland and Utah. *Public Health Nursing, 15*(4), 281–287.

Fawcett-Henesy, A. (1998). Speaking out. *Nursing Times, 94*(23), 23.

Feldman, H. R. (Ed.). (1995). *Nursing care in a violent society: Issues and research.* New York: Springer Publishing Company.

Freeman, R. B. (1970). *Community health nursing practice.* Philadelphia: WB Saunders.

Freeman, R. B., & Heinrich, J. (1981). *Community health nursing practice* (2nd ed.). Philadelphia: WB Saunders.

Gardner, M. S. (1928). *Public health nursing.* New York: Macmillan.

Henry J. Kaiser Family Foundation. (2003, January 22). Kaiser daily health policy reports round up coverage of recent state efforts to reduce Medicaid costs. Retrieved May 30, 2003, from http://www.kaisernetwork.org/daily_reports/rep_index.cfm?hint=3$DR_ID=15631

Higgs, Z. R., & Gustafson, D. D. (1985). *Community as a client: Assessment and diagnosis.* Philadelphia: FA Davis.

Institute of Medicine. (2003). *The future of the public's health.* Washington, DC: National Academy Press.

Korteland, C., & Cornwell, J. R. (1991). Evaluating family-centered programs in neonatal intensive care. *Children's Health Care, 20*(1), 56–61.

Kuss, T., Proulx-Girouard, L., Lovitt, S., Katz, C., & Kennelly, P. (1997). A public health nursing model. *Public Health Nursing, 14*(2), 81–91.

Leavell, H. R., & Clark, E. G. (1958). *Preventive medicine for the doctor in his community.* New York: McGraw-Hill.

Martinelli, A. (2003). *Solving the shortage of nurses.* Retrieved February 19, 2004, from www.modbee.com/24hour/opinions/story/994860p

McClennan Reece, S. (1998). Community analysis for health planning: Strategies for primary care practitioners. *The Nurse Practitioner, 23*(10), 46–59.

Oberg, C. N., Bryant, N. A., & Bach, M. L. (1994). *America's children: Triumph or tragedy.* Washington, DC: American Public Health Association.

Olds, D. L. (2002). Prenatal and infancy home visiting by nurses: From randomized trials to community replication. *Prevention Science, 3*(3), 153–172.

Olds, D. L., Eckerode, J., Henderson, C. R., Kitzman, H., Powers, J., Cole, R., Sidora, K., Morris, P., Pettitt, L. M., & Luckey, D. (1997). Long-term effects of home visitation on maternal life course and child abuse and neglect, Fifteen-year follow-up of a randomized trial. *Journal of the American Medical Association, 278*(8), 637–643.

Olds, D. L., Henderson, C. R., Jr., Cole, R., Eckenrode, J., Kitzman, H., Kuckey, D., Pettitt, L., Sidora, K., Morris, P., & Powers, J. (1998). Long-term effects of nurse home visitation on children's criminal and antisocial behavior. *JAMA, 280*(14), 1238–1244.

Olds, D. L., Henderson, C. R., Jr., Tatelbaum, R., & Chamberlin, R. (1986). Improving the delivery of prenatal care and outcomes of pregnancy: A randomized trial of nurse home visitation. *Pediatrics, 77*(1), 16–28.

Olds, D. L., Henderson, C. R., Jr., Tatelbaum, R., & Chamberlin, R. (1988). Improving the life-course development of socially disadvantaged mothers: A randomized trial of nurse home visitation. *American Journal of Public Health, 78*(11), 1436–1445.

Olds, D., Hill, P., & Rumsey, E. (1998). *Prenatal and early childhood nurse home visitation.* Washington, DC: U.S. Department of Justice.

Olds, D., Kitzman, H., Cole, R., & Robinson, J. (1997). Theoretical foundations of a program of home visitation for pregnant women and parents of young children. *Journal of Community Psychology, 25*(1), 9–25.

Olds, D., & Korfmacher, J. (1997). The evolution of a program of research on prenatal and early childhood home visitation: Special issue introduction. *Journal of Community Psychology, 25*(1), 1–7.

Olds, D., Pettitt, L., Robinson, J., Henderson, C., Jr., Eckenrode, J., Kitzman, H., Cole, B., & Powers, J. (1998). Reducing risks for antisocial behavior with a program of prenatal and early childhood home visitation. *Journal of Community Psychology, 26*(1), 65–83.

Public Health Nursing Directors of Washington. (1993). *Public health nursing within core public health functions.* Olympia, WA: Washington State Department of Health.

Rue, C. B. (1944). *The public health nurse in the community.* Philadelphia: WB Saunders.

Saha, A., Cole, A. F., & Linder, B. M. W. (1992). Education in family and community health: The challenge faced by a new medical school. *Medical Education, 26,* 478–481.

Shelton, R., Jeppson, E., & Johnson, B. (1987). *Family-centered care for children with special health care needs.* Washington, DC: Association for the Care of Children's Health.

Shuster, G. F., & Goeppinger, J. (1996). Community as client: Using the nursing process to promote health. In M. Stanhope &

J. Landcaster (Eds.), *Community health nursing* (pp. 289–314). St. Louis: CV Mosby.

Sidel, R. (1986). *Women and children last: The plight of poor women in affluent America*. New York: Penguin Books.

Spoth, R. L., Kavanagh, K. A., & Dishion, T. J. (2002). Family-centered preventive intervention science: Toward benefits to larger populations of children, youth, and families. *Prevention Science, 3*(3), 145–152.

Spradley, B. W. (1985). *Community health nursing: Concepts and practice* (2nd ed.). Boston: Little, Brown.

Stanhope, M., & Knollmueller, R. N. (1996). *Handbook of community and home health nursing: Tools for assessment, intervention, and education* (2nd ed.). St. Louis: Mosby.

Stanhope, M., & Lancaster, J. (2004). *Community and public health nursing* (6th ed.). St. Louis: Mosby.

Stroufe, L. A., & Fleeson, J. (1986). Attachment and the construction of relationships. In W. W. Hartup & Z. Rubin (Eds.), *Relationships and development* (pp. 51–71). Hillsdale, NJ: Lawrence Erlbaum Associates.

Swanson, J. M., & Nies, M. A. (1997). *Community health nursing: Promoting the health of aggregates* (2nd ed.). Philadelphia: WB Saunders.

University of Southern Mississippi School of Nursing. (2003). *Public health nursing: Pioneers of health care reform.* Retrieved August 12, 2004, from http://www.nursing.usm.edu/FacAccess/lundy/Powerpoints/chnursing_ch37.ppt

U.S. Department of Health and Human Services. (1980). *Promoting health/preventing disease: Objectives for the nation.* Washington, DC: Author.

U.S. Department of Health and Human Services. (2000). *Healthy People 2010: Understanding and improving health* (2nd ed.). Washington, DC: U.S. Government Printing Office.

U.S. Department of Health and Human Services. (2003). *HIPAA privacy rule and public health.* Washington, DC: U.S. Government Printing Office.

U.S. Public Health Service. (1993). *Healthy People 2000 review* (94-1232-1). National Center for Health Statistics. Hyattsville, MD: U.S. Department of Health and Human Services.

U.S. Public Health Service. (1996). *Healthy People 2000: Progress review: Violent and abusive behavior.* Department of Health & Human Services, Public Health Service. Retrieved November 26, 1996, from http://odphp.osophs.dhhs.gov/pubs/hp2000/progrvw/violprog.htm

Vahldieck, R. K., Reeves, S. R., & Schmelzer, M. (1989). A framework for planning public health nursing services to families. *Public Health Nursing, 6*(2), 102–107.

Valanis, B. (1999). *Epidemiology in health care* (3rd ed.). Stamford, CT: Appleton & Lange.

Washington State Core Public Health Functions Task Force. (1993). *Core public health functions.* Olympia, WA: Washington Department of Health.

Washington State Department of Health. (1996). *Public health improvement plan: A blueprint for action.* Olympia, WA: Author.

Whall, A. L. (1986). The family as the unit of care in nursing: A historical review. *Public Health Nursing, 3*(4), 240–249.

Williams, D. M. (1997). Vulnerable families: A study of health visitors' prioritization of their work. *Journal of Nursing Management, 5,* 19–24.

Yach, D. (1992). The use and value of qualitative methods in health research in developing countries. *Social Science & Medicine, 35*(4), 603–612.

Zerwekh, J. V. (1991). A family caregiving model for public health nursing. *Nursing Outlook, 39*(5), 213–217.

Zimmerman, S. L. (1992). *Family policies and family well-being: The role of political culture.* Newbury Park, CA: Sage Publications.

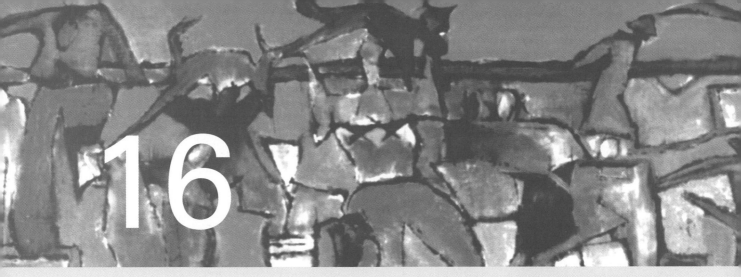

16

Families with Chronic Illness

Jane M. Kurz, PhD, RN • *Margaret P. Shepard, PhD, RN*

CRITICAL CONCEPTS

- Chronic illnesses challenge families throughout the family life span.
- Challenges are more stressful at times of transitions.
- The Rolland Family Systems and Illness Model provides a framework for nurses for family-centered care.

- Nurses should include all family members when assessing families and planning care.
- Nurses help families manage chronic illnesses, anticipatory losses, and ambiguous losses at all stages of the family life cycle by using a variety of strategies.

INTRODUCTION

Chronic illness is expected to be the major health problem of the 21st century. These illnesses typically include conditions that have existed for 3 months or longer, do not resolve spontaneously, and are rarely cured (Centers for Disease Control and Prevention, 2003). Chronic illness may affect physical, emotional, intellectual, social, or spiritual functioning. The goal of care for more than 125 million Americans currently living with chronic illnesses is to slow the disease progression and to manage symptoms (Centers for Disease Control and Prevention, 2003). Researchers suggest that 20 million (approximately 31 percent) American children under the age of 18 live with some chronic illness (Meleski, 2002). In addition, nearly half of all adults with chronic illnesses have more than one condition. Wolff, Starfield, and Anderson (2002) report that 88 percent of the population over the age of 65 years has one or more chronic conditions. More than 1.7 million Americans die of chronic illness each year, which represents 70 percent of all U.S. deaths. One-third of those deaths occur with individuals under the age of 65 years. Five chronic diseases (heart disease, cancer, stroke, chronic pulmonary diseases, and diabetes) cause more than two-thirds of all deaths annually. Regardless of deaths, the most common illnesses include cardiovascular disease, arthritis, upper respiratory diseases, and respiratory infection. Note that as of 1996, AIDS became recognized as a chronic illness as protease inhibitors became more available (Siegel & Lekas, 2002). Mental illnesses, also chronic, affect 20 million Americans (Partnership for Solutions, 2002). Sixty percent of these individuals also have additional chronic illnesses.

There are several reasons for the trend toward an increase in chronic illnesses. Advances in technology and medications have allowed individuals to live longer with illnesses that in the past would have caused early death. Life expectancy has increased dramatically over the last century. In 1900 it was 45 years and now it is over 74 years for men and women (Hammonds-Smith, 2003). The population is also aging as baby boomers born between 1950 and 1965 are reaching middle and late adulthood.

Chronic illness costs are often difficult to measure and are frequently underestimated. Actual reimbursable services, clearly identified under various insurance programs, account for 75 percent of health care costs yearly (Wolff, Starfield, & Anderson, 2002). Accounting procedures do not typically address out-of-pocket expenses related to professional care and medications or related expenses paid by families. Related expenses can include supplies, equipment, home modifications, and respite care. Lost income secondary to illness or caregiving, decreasing quality of life, and lost income due to early death all contribute to the economic implications of chronic illness. At present, annual direct costs are estimated at $200 billion for medical care (Ignatavicius & Workman, 2002). Individuals with a mental illness and other comorbidities tend to spend more for inpatient and outpatient care, using more health care providers as the number of chronic illnesses increases. Having one comorbidity tends to double expenses, and having three comorbidities triples annual expenses (Partnership for Solutions, 2002). It is expected that direct medical costs associated with chronic illness will continue to rise and double to more than $1 trillion by 2020 (Greco, 2001).

FAMILIES AND CHRONIC ILLNESS

Family responses to chronic illness vary according to many factors. These include characteristics of the ill person (e.g., age, gender, developmental stage), presence of additional stressors, coping skills, resources, beliefs, and characteristics of the illness. Some factors will contribute to adaptive responses such as family coping skills, availability of social support, and family beliefs that the illness situation is manageable. Other factors will contribute to the intensity of the stressful demands experienced by the family; these may include insufficient resources such as money, time, and emotional support. The key to successful adaptation is a balance between demands and resources. Most families manage well, but for some, a chronic illness can contribute more stressful demands than the family can reasonably meet with their usual resources.

For example, Bud and Marilyn are the parents of three young children and they are successfully managing many of the stressors common to developing families, such as mortgage payments, providing care for Marilyn's aging mother, Bud's long work hours as he strives for a promotion, and meeting all of the children's developmental needs. After Marilyn was diagnosed with chronic fatigue syndrome, the family experienced many changes. Marilyn was no longer able to work; her loss of income was financially stressful, so Bud took a part-time job. Marilyn assumed more of the child care responsibilities, although her fatigue frequently prevented her from finishing anything. As a result, the children missed things such as deadlines for homework, soccer practice, and health care appointments. Marilyn's mother was having difficulty managing her chronic health problems because Marilyn could not drive her to the pharmacy or the grocery store. Although only one family member developed a chronic illness, each member, and the family as a system, experienced changes in response to the demands presented by the illness.

Caregiving Demographics

The family of the 21st century looks different from the family of the early 20th century. In 1900, family trees were shaped like pyramids with one or two older adults followed by several children (2–15) who contributed many grandchildren (10–30). In the current century, families appear more like beanpoles with one or two adults followed by one or two children who produce one or two grandchildren and one or two great-grandchildren. The old old (individuals over the age of 85 years) are the fastest-growing segment of the population. The number of available caregivers is much fewer for older adults of this century. Some families find caregiving to be a source of stress as they juggle work and other family obligations. Older caregivers are typically spouses (predominately wives), parents, or grandparents. Long-term caregiving has negative effects on family members. Researchers have noted depressed immune functioning, higher rates of depression, higher psychotropic drug use, and more physical exhaustion than noted with the non-caregiving families (Gerdner, Buckwalter, & Reed, 2002).

A newly developing phenomenon is grandparents assuming the parental role permanently for grandchildren as a result of their own children's death secondary to trauma or infectious disease (especially AIDS). In the past, grandparents might assume parental roles for their children when the parents were incapacitated due to drug addiction, incarceration, or other medical problems. There was the understanding that this parental role was temporary and that biological parents would assume their roles in time. Parenting grandparents today take on the challenges that were part of an earlier family life cycle at a time when they are facing changes in their income, roles, and health. Not all individuals consider the caregiver role negatively, however. Winston (2003) reported that some grandmothers welcomed a second chance to raise a child and reported satisfaction with the situation and a lack of loneliness.

Conversely, it sometimes is the young adult who becomes the caregiver of the older family member in the home. Lackey and Gates (2001) surveyed adults retrospectively who provided care for family members with chronic physical illnesses when they were young children or teens. The caregiving tasks most cited were personal care and household tasks. The negative aspects included less available time for schoolwork and friends, but the positive aspects were becoming closer with the family, increased pride in being helpful and learning new skills, and becoming more caring and nurturing. Almost everyone in this study stated that they would allow their children to assume a caregiver role if needed.

Spouses

By age 65 years, 96 percent of all Americans have married at least once (Schmaling & Sher, 2000). Married or cohabiting partners are often listed as the strongest support person for the individual with chronic illness and a buffer against stress. A bidirectional effect is noted with both spouses in the presence of chronic illnesses. This means that as the patient experiences a change in adaptation to the disease process, quality of life, and well-being, the well spouse experiences similar changes. Additionally, marital quality as a source of stress or support can have both a physical and a psychosocial impact on the well and the ill partner. This has been noted with couples dealing with depression, heart disease, renal disease, and cancers (Coyne, Thompson, & Palmer, 2002; Orth-Gomér et al., 2000; Rohrbaugh, Cranford, Shoham, Nicklas, Sonnega, & Coyne, 2002; Schmaling & Sher, 2000; White & Grenyer, 1999). Coyne, Rohrbaugh, Shoham, Sonnega, Nicklas, and Cranford (2001) found that a good marriage influenced patient survival, especially wives, in the presence of severe congestive heart failure. Not only do partners share the stress and responsibility associated with chronic illness, but they also often have a risk for the same disease as the ill partner (especially depression, diabetes, hypertension, ischemic heart disease, peptic ulcer disease, asthma, and chronic obstructive pulmonary disease) because they share the same environment and health behaviors (Hippisley-Cox, Pringle, Crowne, & Hammersley, 2002).

Parents/Children

The impact of parental chronic illness on sons and daughters is often forgotten. There is a paucity of studies that focus attention on well children in the family system in the presence of chronic disease. Several researchers have examined adolescents living with a parent with a chronic illness (e.g., AIDS, cancer, depression, head injury, and renal disease) and reported conflicting results (Bonica & Daniel, 2003; Dorsey, Chance, Morse, Forehand, & Morse, 1999; Gilber & Refaeli, 2000; Perlesz, Kinsella, & Crowe, 1999; Smith & Soliday, 2001). Negative effects included depression, poor school performance, role confusion, and poor quality of life. Positive outcomes include resilience, increased self-esteem, and family cohesiveness (Mukherjee, Sloper, & Lewin, 2002). These mixed results reflect the relationships of other variables, such as coping strategies, economic resources, and support networks.

Impact of children's illness on parents falls within several general areas, including illness and treatment tasks, family's attitudes toward the illness, and caregiver burden (Meleski, 2002). This will be discussed more extensively later in this chapter. Unfortunately, the impact of chronic illness on child siblings has not been extensively researched. In the few available reported studies, researchers detail positive and negative outcomes. Snethen and Broome (2001) described how siblings' involvement in clinical trials changed the participants' family routines, increased workload for all, produced less involvement with their ill brother or sister, and resulted in their own separation from family and friends. In contrast, Gallo, Breitmayer, Knafl, and Zoeller (1992) found that children with a sibling with a chronic condition did not experience greater problems in behavior and social competence.

COMMON THEORETICAL PERSPECTIVE: FAMILY SYSTEMS AND ILLNESS MODEL

Rolland's model provides a framework for assessing, planning, and intervening with families dealing with chronic illness (Rolland, 1998). It offers a psychosocial orientation with a systems perspective, which was described in Chapter 2.

Model Dimensions

Rolland conceptualizes the framework as a three-dimensional picture composed of three intersecting lines. Each line meets at a single point to represent the relationship among the three major dimensions or components: illness types, time phases, and components of family functioning (i.e., family system variables). Picture two corner walls in a room touching each other and the floor simultaneously. These three structures represent those major dimensions for the

---

HISTORICAL PERSPECTIVE

Chronic illness is a relatively new concept that emerged along with the 20th-century advances in health care. Prior to the second half of the previous century, there were many children crippled with conditions such as polio or tuberculosis; many adults were *handicapped* or *disabled* from similar illnesses or farm and industrial accidents. When a child was born with a disease such as spina bifida, interventions were minimally effective and the child often died in infancy. Families were urged to "forget this child" that would be the source of "nothing but grief" and to relegate care and custody to large state or county institutions. Children with cerebral palsy or adults with diabetes who were cared for in the home often lived foreshortened lives.

Advances in modern medicine eradicated many illnesses and have replaced conditions that were formally considered terminal—such as diabetes, heart disease, and asthma—with the current chronic counterparts. Today, even conditions like HIV-AIDS and certain cancers, once almost certainly lethal, have been reclassified as chronic conditions. As people with chronic illnesses began living longer, concern for quality of life and civil rights of the disabled grew.

At present, shorter-length hospitalizations mean that more care is being provided in the home. Many clinicians and researchers were at first concerned about the impact of caregiver burden on quality of life for other members of the family. Mothers were found to be depressed, fathers were more absent and distant from the family system, and siblings were scarred by their own feelings of guilt, anger, and depression. More recently, however, there has been a focal change in the way families with a member with a chronic illness are perceived; there is increased recognition of the strength on which members rely in their daily coping with chronic illness. Given adequate support and resources, many families grow stronger and thrive as they master the tasks of caring for a member with a chronic illness.

family system in the presence of chronic illness. An examination of each dimension is helpful.

Illness Types

Illness types, a classification system, links biological and psychosocial components and clarifies relationships between family and illness. The two broad categories are incapacitating and non-incapacitating illnesses. It encompasses onset, course, outcome, and incapacitation. Chronic illnesses have either an acute or a gradual onset. In acute-onset illness, families must rapidly mobilize crisis management skills as they react to changes in a short amount of time. Rolland divides chronic illness into three general courses. The course can be progressive (family member's disability worsens in a stepwise or gradual manner, e.g., Alzheimer's disease), constant (initial event is followed by a stable biological course and the chronic phase is characterized by clear-cut limitations or deficits), or relapsing-episodic (alternation of stable, low symptoms with symptom flare-ups or exacerbation). Initial expectation of the outcome has a significant impact on families. The continuum ranges from fatal (e.g., metastatic cancer) to nonfatal (e.g., cerebral palsy). An intermediate category, unpredictable, includes illnesses that shorten the life span but have the possibility of sudden death (e.g., diabetes, sickle-cell disease). The extent,

kind, and timing of incapacitation or disability will affect the degree of family stress. This can involve impairments in cognition, sensation, movement, stamina, or a combination of several of these. In some constant illnesses, the disability is worse at the beginning (as in spinal cord injury). In progressive illnesses, the disability is worse in the late stages (as in multiple sclerosis).

The pictorial representations in Figures 16–1 and 16–2 might help you understand the various parts of this dimension.

Time Phases

Time phases, the second dimension, help explain some differences in chronic illness's impact on families. There are three major phases. Picture a straight line with arrows at both ends. On the extreme left side is the crisis or initial phase and on the extreme right is the terminal phase. The chronic phase is in the middle of the line. The crisis phase is the symptomatic period before diagnosis and the initial period of adjustment after diagnosis. Families often describe it as the "long haul" or "problems without end" (Rolland, 1994). In the terminal phase, issues related to death and mourning predominate. Each phase has its own developmental tasks that nurses and families need to address to maximize successful family adaptation.

Incapacitating Category

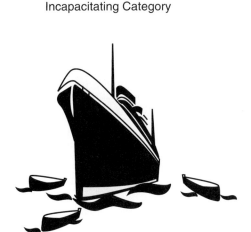

Non-Incapacitating Category

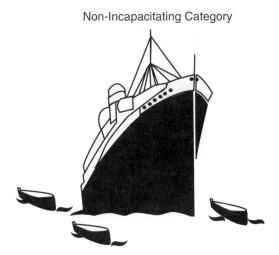

Each ship represents one broad category. Each category has three major subdivisions (fatal, shortened life span, and non-fatal) represented by the three rowboats, which are on the side of every ship.

Figure 16–1 Categories of chronic illness.

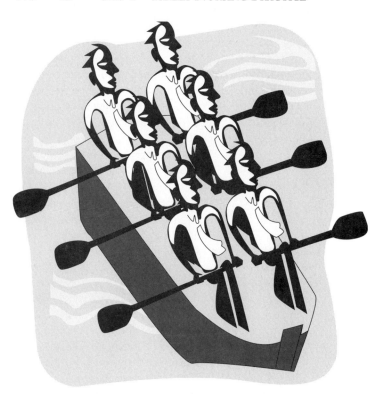

Each rowboat has two or three benches that can accommodate two rowers. The rower represents the acute or gradual onset of the illness.

Figure 16–2 Rowboats.

Each bench represents the course of the illness: progressive, relapsing or constant. Each bench contains two rowers: one who represents the acute onset of that illness group and one that represents the gradual onset of that illness group.

SAMPLE UNIVERSAL FAMILY DEVELOPMENTAL TASKS ASSOCIATED WITH EACH TIME PHASE

Crisis phase	Establish relationship with health care team.
	Learn about illness and treatments.
	Cope with interventions associated with illness.
	Develop a sense of family competence.
	Grieve loss of pre-illness family identity.
Chronic phase	Acknowledge permanency of changes.
	Maintain normal family life.
	Develop autonomy for all family members.
	Reestablish realistic expectations.
	Communicate openly.
	Maintain flexibility with family roles.
	Formulate future plans.
Terminal phase	Acknowledge impending loss.
	Discuss end-of-life issues.
	Begin process of family reorganization.

Components of Family Functioning

Key family variables include individual and family life cycles (as presented in Chapter 5), multigenerational patterns, and beliefs systems that are influenced by culture, ethnicity, and gender. This model emphasizes the fit between the illness's psychosocial demands and the family's strengths and vulnerabilities (Rolland, 1999a). Nurses can help families to address phase-related tasks in sequence to optimize outcomes. Family members and nurses should work together to set goals that reflect components of family functioning relevant to type and phase of illness. This empowers families, gives realistic hope, and offers a sense of control. Interventions focus on family tasks and coincide with the critical transition points. Transitions occur as the illness cycle progresses and the family has new illness-related demands. Alerting families at these times to the need for reevaluating their structure and coping strategies assists with health promotion, health maintenance, and disease prevention.

Beliefs—Normality

A family's belief of what is normal and what is abnormal is associated with a family's adaptation to chronic illness (Rolland, 1998). There are normative illnesses and nonnormative illnesses. *Normative illnesses* are common and predictable, but *nonnormative illnesses* tend to be unexpected and more traumatic for families. When illnesses occur at the "right time," families tend to have access to internal and external resources needed to adapt to changes associated with the illness. For the older married couple with adult children, heart disease in either spouse would not be the same challenge as it would be for the newly married couple who is just starting a career and procreation. The older couple would have more financial resources (savings, fewer general expenses, retirement plan), seniority status, sick leave, and disability benefits. The older couple typically has more experience with successfully coping with various stressors. They have also had the opportunity to watch peers successfully (and unsuccessfully) deal with heart disease. Their network of social supports tends to be wider. For the younger couple with heart disease, there are pressures to continue with the usual developmental tasks associated with life-cycle goals, such as rearing children. It might be necessary for them to revise original goals or allow a longer time to complete family goals. Having access to other young couples with similar situations (e.g., support groups) provides opportunity to create a normalizing context (Rolland, 1998).

Families usually have a general conceptualization of how the typical family deals with a chronic illness similar to what they are experiencing. They will measure themselves as individuals and as a family unit against this ideal. If the family believes that every family has some chronic health problem and seeks help from professionals, then that family would find no loss of esteem and no shame in accessing health care providers or agencies. Conversely, if a family believes that families should take care of themselves and be self-sufficient in the presence of all challenges, accessing health professionals would be a blow to family esteem and the family would perceive itself as weak and abnormal.

Families who successfully adapt to chronic illness often described themselves as "normal," or able to reconstruct life with chronic illness. In this quest for *normality*, families develop a sense of balance, empowerment, and control. This is an active process as families reshape their world and adjust their expectations. Post–lung transplant families provide a good example. Kurz (2001) interviewed well spouses of lung transplant recipients. As they progressed post-transplant at home, patients had episodes of rejection or infection that necessitated intravenous medications via a central catheter. Spouses reported that initially they felt unprepared to complete this task and would view it as a crisis. In the early months, they experienced feelings of sadness and anxiety with the news of the need for intravenous medications at home. In later months, the need and administration of intravenous medications were treated as routine events and part of normal life.

Kralik (2002) suggests that this normality as a quest for ordinariness is affected by cultural and social expectations. Women with various chronic illnesses reported that families expected them to minimize the disruption their illness caused in others' lives by continuing to fulfill their roles. Those roles included contributing to the household income or keeping the house tidy. If the women with chronic illnesses were able to maintain that aspect of their lives, then families judged their families to be "normal." However, it is clear that this normality is a nonlinear process. Families can consider themselves "normal" for a period of time until the next crisis or acute event occurs. Then, they need to work on reconstructing their life in the presence of the new situation.

Knafl and Deatrick (2002) use the term "normalization" to describe the successful management process used by many families of children with chronic conditions. This process entails the following:

- Acknowledging the condition and its potential to threaten lifestyle
- Adapting a "normalcy lens" for defining child and family
- Engaging in parenting behaviors and family routines that are consistent with the normalcy lens
- Developing a treatment regimen that is consistent with a normalcy lens
- Interacting with others based on a view of the child and the family as normal

Normalization is an ongoing process of actively accommodating the child's evolving physical, emotional, and social needs. Acknowledging the condition is essential as the foundation of normalization. There is no denial involved; rather, the family is making a statement that "this child is a part of our family, and our family is just like every other family." The child's age and the condition's severity affect the ability of the family to use the process of normalization (Knafl & Deatrick, 2002; Rehm & Franck, 2000).

TYPOLOGIES OF FAMILIES (WITH CHRONIC ILLNESS) ACROSS THE LIFE CYCLE

A life-cycle perspective provides the background for examining the interface of the individual, the illness, and the family system. Using a family life-cycle model can help nurses think proactively about potential family stresses and strategies to improve coping skills and facilitate family adaptation.

Newly Married Families

All couples at this stage of the family life cycle are focusing on the formation of the marital system and realignment of relationships with extended families and friends to include the partner or spouse. If the illness was present during the courtship, couples tend to romanticize the situation and avoid examining the long-term potential difficulties. Chronic illnesses diagnosed during this stage are untimely and challenging. Couples might have discussed a plethora of issues related to roles, work, finances, children, sex, intimacy, vacations, space, time, eating habits, and so on prior to and after becoming a couple, but chronic illness forces a reexamination and renegotiation of those issues. Attention is focused on relationship quality (i.e., satisfaction or dissatisfaction) and couple interaction. Gay and lesbian couples with chronic illness deal with the same issues as heterosexual couples, with the possible addition of social stigma (Rolland, 1998).

Researchers have linked being part of a couple with better health outcomes in the presence of chronic illnesses (Schmaling & Sher, 2000). Diseases with a mild level of severity (nonfatal, mild incapacitation, or nonprogressive) may require some life structure revisions but not radical changes. The newlywed woman who has a new onset of diabetes, for example, might need to reexamine and revise plans for future children. The couple's desire could be affected by the knowledge of medical outcomes or opportunities for adoption. However, diseases of greater severity (fatal or constant, incapacitating) require major life structure revisions. An example is a man married for 4 months who develops primary pulmonary hypertension and needs aggressive medical interventions to maintain life. Unless both partners are willing to become active participants in his care, he might be forced to return to his family of origin (his parents) for disease-related caretaking. Dreams for a stable couple relationship might be threatened temporarily or permanently.

Families with Young Children

At this stage, parents normally are adjusting the marital system to make space for children, adapting to the parental role, and realigning their relationships with extended family members. These tasks—challenging in themselves—change in the presence of chronic illness. Many families perceive the early diagnostic period and acute exacerbations of the illness as times of crisis causing family disequilibrium. All crises challenge family coping; the family must learn to adapt. Family perceptions, problem-solving strategies, coping repertoire, and usual patterns of functioning will moderate the family's ability to adapt to the new situation (McCubbin & McCubbin, 1993).

For example, the Carter family learned to manage the multiple crises inherent in the management of their son Ron's factor VIII deficiency hemophilia. When Ron was a baby, they felt that each bleeding episode was a life-threatening crisis that sent them speeding to the emergency room. Although each bleeding episode remains potentially life threatening, Ron and his parents have developed a repertoire of skills for managing them and increased confidence in their ability to manage successfully. The additional resources that the family acquired with time and experience enabled them to manage Ron's symptoms so that bleeding episodes were no longer perceived as crises.

The new experience of parenting is a developmental crisis that presents with many challenging tasks and a wide array of feelings, ranging from intense joy to paralyzing self-doubts and uncertainty. Couples experience

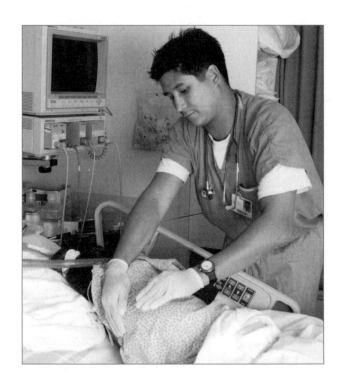

substantial role changes as they add dimensions of motherhood and/or fatherhood to the more familiar roles as partners. Even feeding and changing the new baby are challenging at first, let alone knowing how to decipher the meaning of the baby's cries and other signals of distress. When the baby is born with a congenital illness, the parents' transitions are increasingly complex. Most couples are understandably ill-prepared to meet the added challenges; they lack medical knowledge and, in their relative youth, they may not have previous experiences coping with such intense crises. The hormonal changes that mothers experience in the early days following delivery may contribute to increased emotional lability, and it may be confusing to her and her partner. They are catapulted into grief for the healthy child they only dreamt about and they may experience guilt at their ambivalent feeling for the ill child.

Parents have described the time between their initial awareness of the child's symptoms and the leveling of a diagnosis as overwhelming, characterized by uncertainty and a sense of "groping in the dark" (Sobel & Cowan, 2003). The family response may include shock, disbelief, denial, disgust, relief, guilt, despair, hate, rage, or confusion. Conversely, parents may experience great relief when a diagnosis is made just because it eliminates some of the uncertainty. Some parents, however, describe new areas of uncertainty. Parents may wonder how the condition will affect the family as a whole and each of the individual members. Some may find that their "taken-for-granted world" has been destroyed as they begin to learn to manage under very uncertain conditions. Some factors that affect the responses of parents and others include the following:

1. The visibility of the condition
2. Whether there are functional limitations (Silver, Westbrook, & Stein, 1998)
3. The presence or absence of mental retardation
4. The expectation of pain for the child
5. The uncertainty about changes in the condition
6. The parents' experience with others who have chronic conditions
7. The preconceived ideas about the condition that might engender reactions that are incongruent with the reality of the condition

Well siblings might view the chronic illness as either a significant stressor or a normal situation. Older siblings may be more aware of the family system changes that accompany the diagnosis of a chronic illness. On the other hand, siblings born after the child with the chronic illness never experienced life without an ill sibling, so they are more likely to perceive the situation as "normal." Moreover, when the family achieves "normalization" as described previously, all siblings are likely to adapt well to their situation and view it as within a range of normal life experiences. For some, having a sibling with a chronic condition engenders feelings of isolation, rejection, anxiety, helplessness, resentment, guilt, or depression. These feelings may be greater at the time of diagnosis, hospitalization, or acute exacerbations of the chronic condition. Siblings often lack current information and have decreased access to other family members. Children may perceive an imbalance between the importance of their needs and those of the affected siblings. In addition, well siblings often lack the ability to control or affect the many and perhaps serious changes within the family. They often guess (sometimes incorrectly) about the chronic condition and the resulting health status.

Effects of a condition or its treatment, such as hair loss, flatulence, or copious secretions, may be embarrassing for school-age and older siblings. Simultaneously, children also want to protect the affected sibling from derisive statements or stares of others. Many positive effects may also be borne from having a sibling with a chronic condition, including greater maturity, supportiveness, and independence (Williams et al., 2002).

Parents frequently view selected aspects of some chronic conditions as disruptive to their relationship with their children. Examples include parents of children with cystic fibrosis who must perform postural drainage, the decreased physical contact that might be required if the child has osteogenesis imperfecta, or the blood testing and insulin injections required by children with diabetes. Parenting a child with a chronic condition involves qualitatively different work than parenting a child without a chronic condition. Concurrently, parents struggle with establishing discipline and setting limits for all children that are consistent with family and individual needs. For example, some families fear punishing or setting consequences for the ill child because "their condition is punishment enough already," so they may also struggle with treating all of the children equally. Well sibling vocal complaints of unequal treatment will heighten the parents' struggle. When the presence of an ill sibling places added responsibility on well siblings, parents may perceive it as placing undue burden on the well sibling. Again, this will contribute to parents' struggle with discipline and limit setting.

Families of Adolescents with Chronic Illness

This stage marks the shifting of parent-child relationships to permit adolescents to move in and out of the system. Normally, there is increasing flexibility of family boundaries to include children's independence. Families with more than one adolescent engage in the tasks of this stage until the last child transitions to a level of maturity and the family progresses to the next stage. Adolescents will challenge parental authority and power in their quest for autonomy, creating conflict and instability. Typically adolescents are at the peak of health, and death is relatively rare.

66 Chronic illness complicates adolescent development and family task completion. 99

Because of risk-taking behaviors and violence, accidents are the leading causes of disability for adolescents. Adolescents' lifestyle factors (smoking, drug and alcohol abuse, and nutritional disorders) are common factors associated with family distress. Chronic disorders that were diagnosed either in childhood (e.g., asthma) or in adolescence (e.g., lupus) place an increasing strain on adolescents' concerns regarding body image, independence, and relationships with peers at home and at school. Specific illnesses with life-threatening capability and periods of exacerbation and remission (e.g., IDDM) amplify self-sufficiency issues with strict medical regimens and periods of poor control (Dashiff & Bartolucci, 2002). This can lead to parental overprotectiveness and modification of expected behaviors. Many chronic illnesses influence adolescents' daily self-care practices with respect to scheduled medications, diet, exercise, lab monitoring, and health care provider visits. Kyngas (2000) reported that 50 percent of adolescents with long-term conditions do not comply with care recommendations. This noncompliance could reflect adolescents' attempts to make their own decisions, anger related to having a chronic illness, or poor judgment in the presence of peers. Individual and family interventions addressing these will be discussed later.

Families with chronically ill adolescents (where the disease began in childhood) often have developed long-term relationships with health care teams. In the late part of this stage, health care for the adolescent moves from children's health care services to adult services. This transition has the potential of causing increased physical stress for the adolescent and feelings of loss for all family members. Planned transition to adult health care services should involve the collaboration of all family members and health care team members and should emphasize promoting independence for chronically ill adolescents (Fleming, Carter, & Gillibrand, 2002).

Families of Adolescents with Parental Chronic Illness

Some families deal with parental chronic illness, which affects well adolescents. Adolescence is a time of turmoil and high morbidity rates on many indicators, such as sexually transmitted disease rates, alcohol consumption, drug use, and depression. Several studies highlighted at the introduction of this chapter demonstrate conflicting outcomes with adolescents. Family outcomes in this situation can be both positive (spending time with the ill parent, being close as a family, and adolescents being more independent) and negative (role confusion, tension, repression). The impact of parental illness on well adolescents has not been examined in depth. One might postulate that some negative effects are due to ill or well parents' distraction with treatment, their own or their partner's depression, or other competing concerns (e.g., money). A strong support system is essential to individual and family well-being. Issues related to communication, roles, and care burden are important to all families with children throughout the life cycle. Common interventions need to be tailored for family members but could focus on encouraging family exchange of information and feelings and working on improved coping strategies.

Families Launching Children

During this life-cycle stage, families are usually involved in launching children and shifting roles. It is expected that children will leave home to embark on careers, pursue education, and form their own marital system. However, if chronic illness is diagnosed in a family member at this time or if a previously progressive chronic illness changes to a relapsing course, then the chronic illness interferes with this stage of the life cycle. It tends to disrupt the family members developmentally and force them to turn inward. Thus, the adult children might delay leaving for college, marrying, living independently, or assuming more adult roles. This stage of the life cycle could be prolonged indefinitely or until the illness reaches the terminal phase. Because this is also a time when the couple should be renegotiating their relationship as a dyad, marital satisfaction and cohesiveness could be negatively affected.

SANDWICH GENERATION

- Usually describes a daughter or daughter-in-law
- Characterized by competing responsibilities for aging parents, children, spouse, and career
- High risk for caregiver role strain in presence of chronic illness
- Suggested interventions:
  - Help families to reestablish realistic priorities.
  - Encourage caregiver to ask for help.
  - Assist families to find services through employers or state agencies for home-delivered meals, health care services, homemakers, and so on.
  - Explore resource networks for child care or elder care options.
  - Suggest that families consider flextime or alternative work arrangements.

Illnesses that were constant and stable (e.g., glaucoma, hypertension, irritable bowel syndrome) allow the family to continue on their developmental tasks. The life-cycle phase continues as expected where family members distance themselves from each other and assume new roles and relationships.

Other factors that must be considered when exploring this stage of the life cycle are longevity of the surviving older generation and adult children's socioeconomic factors. Children who left home sometimes return to their family of origin as a result of divorce or high unemployment rates at this time. Couples at this stage are truly the sandwich generation as they care for older- and younger-generation family members. These individuals could be stress buffers or sources of stress in the presence of chronic illnesses.

Families in Later Life

At this stage of the life cycle, older family members focus on maintaining functioning in the presence of physical or psychological decline. Chronic illnesses force older couples to recognize potential loss of independence, income, and companionship as they deal with loss of friends and other family members. Illnesses that were previously constant or progressive have evolved into the preterminal or terminal phases. At this time of life, some illnesses have led to incapac-

itation. The most prevalent conditions are arthritis, hearing impairment, heart condition and hypertension, and depression (Ebersole & Hess, 2001). In response to these changes in the chronic illnesses, transitions occur in families as some roles and responsibilities shift across generations. Family members often confront for the first time the reality of the absence of their older family member. When there is only one parent left, there is increased strain on adult children as they assume more caregiving functions. In addition, they start to confront their changing position as the oldest generation in their family.

Disequilibria might develop in couples with changes in the chronic illness phase in one partner. Families provide 80 to 90 percent of the long-term caregiving in the United States, and they frequently extend themselves beyond their limits to care for an elder with chronic illnesses (Ebersole & Hess, 2001). Informal caregiving and emotional support can be in the form of money, tasks, direct physical care, transportation, frequent telephone calls, and visits. The most typical caregiving relationship is between spouses, and women experience more burden and psychological distress in the caregiving role than men do (Marks, Lambert, & Choi, 2002).

Couples in later life will choose to modify plans for retirement, travel, and new relationships as they manage the effects and responsibilities of chronic illness. Coping with chronic illness includes learning to deal with daily challenges, retaining control over decision making, and, for some, maintaining strong religious beliefs (Davis & Magilvy, 2000). End-of-life issues are usually addressed or reexamined within the family with regard to advance directives, hospice, and care for survivors.

Coping with the stress of chronic illness continues even after an elderly family member leaves the family home for a nursing home. Family members who were "doing everything" daily are often relegated to the bedside and are less actively involved. This new role can create stress for the family and the patient. Nurses are in a key position to help families remain involved in care and decisions at an appropriate level that does not increase family or staff burden. See the Research Brief for results of the Family Involvement in Care intervention.

FAMILY TASKS AND NURSING ROLES

Nurses can help families cope with chronic illnesses by supporting their efforts with family cohesion, effective communication, flexible boundaries, and adaptability.

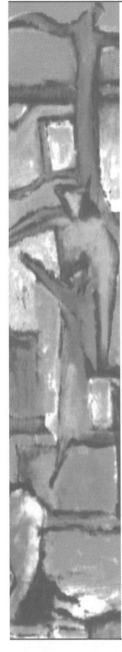

RESEARCH BRIEF

Purpose of Study

To test the effects of the Family Involvement in Care (FIC) intervention with family caregivers of individuals with dementia and staff in special care units.

Methodology

- *Design:* Quasi-experimental with nonequivalent control group with repeated pretest and posttest measures.
- *Sample:* Family members ($N = 185$) and nursing staff ($N = 845$) from 14 nursing homes in the United States. Seven homes were the experimental sites and seven were the control sites.
- *Measures:* Family members completed Family Perceptions of Caregiving Role (FPCR) and Family Perceptions of Care (FPC) at baseline and four follow-up times for 10 months. Staff completed Staff Perceptions of Caregiving Role (SPCR), Caregiver Stress Inventory (CSI), and Attitude towards Families Checklist (AFC) every 6 months for 24 months. Resident characteristics, measured with the Functional Abilities Checklist (FAC), were used in hierarchical linear modeling analyses.
- *Intervention:* This was a protocol for family and staff negotiation of a written partnership agreement. Family members had four educational sessions and staff had 8 hours of training.

Results

The intervention had a statistically significant effect on family caregiver outcomes (emotional reaction to caregiver role, perceptions of relationships with staff, and perceptions of care for relative) and staff outcome (staff perceptions of family caregiving role). Positive effects were noted when family members were of the same generation as client but not for the younger generation. It did not reduce families' perception of staff conflict or increase staff's perception of partnerships.

Nursing Implications

This nursing intervention is empirically supported for use with caregiving families of institutionalized individuals with dementia. Future researchers might want to examine effects of the timing of the protocol and longitudinal effects on staff turnover, absenteeism, or job satisfaction. Protocol might need to be adjusted according to age of caregiver.

Mass, M. et al. (2004). Outcomes of family involvement in care intervention for caregivers of individuals with dementia, *Nursing Research, 53*, 76–85.

These were the major predictors of positive adaptation (Rolland, 1994). In the next sections, we will examine characteristics of the various phases of chronic illness and sample nursing interventions that facilitate family coping.

Acute Phase

Chronic illnesses can start as acute illnesses presenting symptoms suddenly or can evolve as a disruption interrupted by episodes of crises. Results for the affected individual can be a shortened life span, decreased quality of life, or death. In this phase, the increased demands on the family are compressed into a brief time period and the family's rapid response is necessary. Family members must mobilize resources and coping strategies quickly.

Initially, families will experience a period of confusion following the stress of acute illness. Researchers have described families progressing through six phases before they return to their baseline of functioning: high anxiety, denial, anger, remorse, grief, and reconciliation (Hopkins, 1994). Families might differ in the sequence of the phases and the rate at which they progress through these phases. Regardless of the cause of illness, the main family task is to regain stability.

To assess the family in the acute phase, nurses must ask about other stressors occurring in the family and coping strategies that the family used. This can be accomplished through interviews and written questionnaires. Rolland suggests that family assessments focus on four major components of family functioning: family structure and organizational patterns, communication processes, multigenerational patterns and family life cycle, and finally, family belief system. These components are addressed in more detail under the section titled "Chronic Phase." There should be an effort to gather information from all the significant members of the family and not just the most willing or available family member (e.g., the mother or wife). Interventions should include active listening, early and frequent family contact, and frequent patient updates. Nurses should encourage families to gather accurate information about the illness and treatments. Families sometimes need guidance in establishing priorities for themselves. Providing information on family and community resources can prove helpful. Referrals to other health care professionals if there are continued problems in coping or adaptation are appropriate.

Anticipatory Loss

Anticipatory loss involves a wide range of intense emotional reactions in response to an expected or threatened loss over the course of the chronic illness. *Anticipatory loss* could be the family's potential loss of the ill family member, the loss of the intact family, or the expectation of disability or death by the ill family member. Effects of anticipatory loss vary with the multigenerational experiences of real or threatened losses, the kind of illness, its long-term psychosocial demands, and the amount of uncertainty about prognosis (Rolland, 1994). Common family responses include minimization, hypervigilance and overprotectiveness, separation anxiety, anger and resentment, exhaustion, and desperation. Family members' feelings often oscillate between pleasure that their family member is still alive with them and guilt that they want their ill relative present in spite of pain and suffering. Conversely, family members might have guilt that they are planning for their loved one's absence prior to their actual loss. Anticipatory loss does provide time for the family members to rehearse their reactions before the loss actually occurs.

Consider this example. Antoinette moved in with her son, his wife, and their three children 2 years ago, after her last hospitalization for congestive heart failure. She has become progressively more dyspneic, and her ankle edema makes walking more and more difficult. Her medications have been increased. There are times recently when she finds she is tearful as she considers what her life will be when she cannot walk to the corner store. Her grandchildren also seem to be avoiding her as they discuss their upcoming family vacation to the mountains. Her son and his wife meanwhile have been arguing more often lately over the amount of salt in their dinners. He insists that they do not need to change their dietary habits, but his wife wants to buy low-sodium foods for everyone and remove all salt from the house. During a home health visit, the nurse notices Antoinette's sadness and wonders if the sadness and other recent changes are signs of anticipatory loss.

To determine whether this is occurring, the nurse needs to assess the entire family. Planning a visit at a time when all are present would facilitate this assessment. Questions regarding previous or concurrent losses should be posed to all. Encouraging all members to share concerns is often a good opener. Assisting the family members to identify strengths and prepare them for possible grief reactions is helpful. The nurse should initiate a dialogue to explore options available and possible actions. Interventions should include health teaching regarding what to expect in the future, identifying signs of pathological responses, and highlighting possibilities for growth for the family in the presence of this chronic illness. Referrals to agencies or support groups may reduce grief responses.

There should be a feeling of trust so that direct expressions of feelings can occur. This trust is a bidirectional phenomenon between nurses and patients and families. Thorne and Robinson (1988, 1989) found in their studies that a reciprocal trust has a significant impact on patient perceptions and satisfaction with health care. They have confirmed from their research studies that trust evolves in three stages: naive trust, disenchantment, and guarded alliance. They advise nurses that trust is difficult to develop but that it involves the health care professional cultivating competence in the family and eventually viewing the family as competent. The health care professional's view stimulates the patient and family to feel more confident in their skills in managing the illness and to make valid decisions on their own behalf. To achieve this trust, there must be sharing of accurate information, flexibility in relationships, and collaboration in treatments. Finally, there needs to be recognition of individual limitations and system constraints.

In Antoinette's case, the home health care nurse was able to meet with the entire family one Thursday evening after dinner. After she completed Antoinette's routine assessment, she arranged to have the family sit in the living room. She asked each what they thought the future held for them and the family. Their responses surprised each other. Each frequently exclaimed, "I had no idea you felt that way!" and "I think about that too!" After an hour, they all agreed that they were feeling sad and responding to events that had not occurred yet. The nurse named various strengths that she had noted in the last visits. She did not offer false hope and recognized that Antoinette would continue to experience physical deterioration. She encouraged them to continue to talk to each other. Antoinette's daughter-in-law was receptive to calling the American Heart Association to get more information about support groups. The home health care nurse will continue to monitor this family during subsequent visits.

Ambiguous Loss

Ambiguous loss (i.e., an unclear loss) is the most stressful loss that families can experience (Boss, 1999). An actual death of a family member is a real loss. However, some losses are not as clear or obvious to society. Ambiguous loss disrupts families by confusing family dynamics. It forces family members to question family membership and roles. The danger is that it can result in immobilization and prolonged grief. It is like a death where there is a major loss in the family. Conversely, it is unlike death because the family member is still present on some real level and the family cannot mourn. Families dealing with ambiguous loss do not have the advantage that death offers, with rituals and formal supports that aid in adjustment and adaptation. The two following examples will clarify this concept.

In the presence of chronic illness, there are two types of ambiguous losses. In one situation, the family member is physically absent but psychologically present. Consider this construction worker who is in the rehabilitation unit with a cervical spinal cord injury at C_4 and multiple fractures complicated by infection.

Sam, age 44, was the primary wage earner in a family with two teenage children and a wife, Mary, who worked part-time as a cashier. He was a person who viewed himself as "in charge" of his family, and the family always sought his approval for all decisions. He had a stormy 2-month hospitalization prior to moving to the rehabilitation center. It is unclear as to when he actually will come home. His children continue to attend school and their part-time jobs. The oldest son had been planning to attend college, and he should have completed applications at this time. Prior to the accident, the family had planned to visit a few campuses over the next few months, but those visits never occurred. Mary has returned to work and her routine household tasks. She has written a few checks to pay bills, but the budget was always Sam's job. The hot-water heater has started to malfunction, but she has not called a repairperson because "that was Sam's specialty." She complains to everyone that she is tired of these "house problems," tired of the boys always fighting, and tired of worrying about Sam. She confides to her mother that she has experienced a 10-pound weight loss and cannot sleep at night. Mary continues to visit Sam weekly and seeks his advice on everything before committing to any action. Unfortunately, Sam frequently falls asleep during their visits and is therefore unable to make decisions. Will this family always be frozen or will they reorganize their roles and move forward?

A second type of ambiguous loss is a situation where the family member is physically present but psychologically absent. This can occur in the presence of certain chronic mental illnesses, head injury, Alzheimer's disease, and coma. Consider the example of Marie, who has been married for 32 years in a happy relationship. She and Jim raised their three children in the same house over the last 30 years. Grandchildren, children, and friends visited frequently until 9 months ago. Jim had become forgetful and had periods of confusion at the time of their 30th wedding anniversary. He had always been fastidious in his dress and work, but he slowly lost interest in grooming and activities. Eventually, he stopped playing guitar. Evidence of cognitive decline became obvious to others at work and home, and he "retired" from his job as manager. Marie started to provide more direct care. In the past, she always prepared meals and laid out his clothes. Lately, as Jim sits and stares at his food or clothes, she finds that she must help him dress or feed himself. His verbal outbursts have frightened family and friends, and they have not visited for several months. Marie telephones a friend to share that she feels so alone and does not know how much more she can take. She adds, "I am married and my husband is here, but I have no husband."

These are not dysfunctional families. There has been a real loss, but recognition and subsequent grieving are not possible. Confusion freezes the grieving process. The typical results include anxiety, depression, and somatic complaints. These are normal reactions to a complicated situation. Nurses should routinely ask questions about family events that provide evidence for ambiguous losses. Clinicians must provide information to families, explore creative ways to manage the associated stressors, and guide their reorganization of family roles. Networking with other families facing similar situations has proven helpful. One woman, who was having difficulty adjusting to her husband's progressive cognitive decline, reported that she was able to place herself as head of the family, his former role, by removing her wedding and engagement rings. Once they were in a drawer, she was able to assume those family tasks, care for him, and reduce her own sadness and distress.

Chronic Phase

Chronic illness offers challenges and opportunities for growth for all families at every stage of the life cycle. It is more of a challenge when the illness is "off-time" or occurring simultaneously with other life-cycle transitions, because the possibility of meeting individual or family goals can become very skewed (Rolland, 1999a). Families need to be flexible and maintain open family communication. Couples must discuss the illness and its impact on their roles and responsibilities and the dynamics of their relationship. Parents often question how much to share with young children. When age-appropriate information is shared, parents can address fears, explore feelings, and correct any misconceptions. Often, imagination is worse than reality.

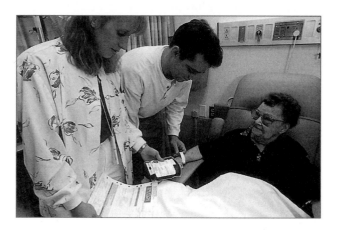

Families need to develop an "our challenge" attitude toward the illness. If it is only the patient's problem, there will be imbalances of power and control. A major risk is that families identify exclusively with the illness and the illness shapes the boundary of what is considered normal family life. One example of that would be a woman who was treated surgically for breast cancer 30 years ago but has not worked since her surgery in case she has further need for surgery and chemotherapy. Her husband resents his burden of being the sole breadwinner but feels he has no right to vocalize his concerns because of her "illness." Meanwhile, none of the adult children has ever moved more than 10 miles away, in spite of opportunities to move, because the cancer might resurface again.

Chronic illness can be used as a crutch to help the affected family member gain other positive responses. Family members can prevent this trap by working together as a unit to handle specific problems or decisions. Often, roles change as chronic illness persists over time. Families who have traditional roles, for example, might need to shift responsibilities in order to meet family goals. The 55-year-old construction worker with worsening renal failure and diabetes previously divided the household tasks with his wife so that she did the inside work and he did the outside work. Now he is on medical leave at home during his adjustment to hemodialysis, and he is more involved in monitoring their children. His wife has increased her work hours to meet expenses. The children have also become involved with his direct care and assumed more responsibility with household tasks. Conflicts will develop unless this family negotiates the new roles and responsibilities in the presence of this chronic illness.

Family members often need to develop mastery with new skills and plan for potential future crises. Parents and children will need to discuss what resources can be activated when they are needed. Kurz and Cavanaugh (2001) found that couples who were waiting for lung transplantation had developed telephone call lists for their children to alert friends and family of the surgical event. Several also had grandparents on standby to take care of children when the transplant candidate needed to leave for the hospital. Simultaneously, there needs to be a balance between individual needs and family needs.

When health care providers assess families in the chronic phase of illness, they gain a more holistic view by using a broad family assessment tool. It should encompass family form and structure, communication, resources, family patterns, and family function

FAMILY ASSESSMENT FOCUS

Family Structure and Organizational Patterns

- Who lives at home?
- Do family members consider pets part of the family? If so, seek information about each pet.
- Who are the other significant relatives (extended family)?
- Where do they live?
- Describe how child-rearing decisions are made.
- How are home maintenance tasks accomplished?
- Are there any family rules?

Communication Processes

- What are the family's financial needs?
- How does this family meet their financial needs?
- What strengths does this family have?
- Who is working and where?
- Are they satisfied with their work type (or employer)?
- How effectively do family members communicate?
- How does the family deal with conflict?

Multigenerational Patterns and the Family Life Cycle

- How does this family cope typically with stresses?
- What experiences have the family members had with chronic illness in their past?
- Have the family members described their experiences with health professionals?
- How is the health of all the family members?
- What types of supports does this family have? Who will give help?
- Where is this family in the life cycle?

Family Belief System

- What are the family's key beliefs about the specific illness?
- What are the goals that this family has identified?
- What are the options with this illness for the family?
- How does each family member think this illness will affect him or her? The family?
- How would a healthy family cope with your situation?
- Are there any family traditions or celebrations that are important?

(Potter & Perry, 2003). Using a genogram helps to conceptualize membership and structure, interaction patterns, medical history, and other important family information (see Chapter 8 for more details).

Family at the Chronic Phase

Interventions for the family at this phase need to help them master these challenges associated with chronic illness and family adaptation. Families need to understand the expected patterns of demands over the course of the disorder, develop an understanding of themselves as a functioning unit, become cognizant of the individuals and family life cycles so that they can remain aware of the fit between the illness and developmental issues, and finally, explore the beliefs and multigenerational legacies and their construction of meaning about the illness, health problems, and caregiving systems (Rolland, 1999a). Families managing a great number of stressors with limited resources may experience greater challenges than families with fewer stressors or more resources do. Sharing the genogram in multiple-family discussion groups offers members the ability to see clearly their family patterns and to stimulate discussions. Each meeting can be tailored to address family skills and coping strategies to build resources. Family members have reported that group support by peers and professionals has been helpful. Planning and implementation is with, rather than for, the family.

Another general resource to facilitate family coping is helping to provide accurate information about the condition, treatment options, and community resources (e.g., adaptive equipment and support services). A diagnosis sets some on a search for information, and this is the first step toward having some control over the situation (Hobbs, Perrin, & Ireys, 1985; Swallow & Jacoby, 2001). Nurses should support this quest for information as a coping strategy by sharing information and directing families to appropriate literature, health experts, and organizations. Nurses must encourage families to ask questions and then should take the time to answer them. Providing written information or allowing taping during information sessions is helpful. Nurses must anticipate the need for repetitive education and explanations using teaching strategies appropriate to the learner. One might also consider that in certain cultures it is considered inappropriate to ask questions of health care providers. Nurses could deal with this by initiating a statement that many families do not understand some aspects of the care or treatment (identify the specific topic for the involved family) and by volunteering to provide more in-depth information. Nurses can also evaluate the family's knowledge of essential information by asking questions or observing the patient or family member demonstrate a technique or treatment. This will provide evidence of the family's knowledge level and need for more information.

Furthermore, nurses can help the family put the diagnosis in perspective. Nurses begin by assessing what expectations and knowledge the family already has. If there are misconceptions, clarify them. Parents, especially, need timely, sufficient information to be full and active participants in the decision-making process. An insufficient understanding of the child's illness and treatment needs has been linked to poor adherence and excess risk for acute exacerbations of the condition (Dosa, Boeing, & Kanter, 2001). Children should be given developmentally appropriate

information. Nurses must gauge the level of information to meet the child's and family's needs and periodically assess how each is responding to and using the information. Information and written material that is overly simplistic, too complex, or inappropriately timed is not helpful and may ultimately alienate the family.

Use of the Internet has greatly increased the range of information to which families have access. As a result, nurses may be required to clarify information and respond to sophisticated questions posed by family members. Nurses should periodically update their knowledge of information sources available on the Internet so that they can direct families to appropriate resources and warn them about inflammatory or inaccurate Internet sites.

Ultimately, many families will also search for some level of meaning by asking the question "Why me?" Often they will identify religious, philosophical, or scientific reasons for the child's condition. Family functioning can be enhanced if families have a more positive than negative interpretation and are able to define the chronic condition and resultant situations within a previously existing personal, medical-scientific, and/or religious worldview (Copeland & Clements, 1993). Nurses can encourage family members to discuss their search for meaning with one another as well as with the nurse, other families in the same situation, or a supportive friend or spiritual advisor.

Establishing normality is important because it focuses on family and not the condition. In this process, family tasks and activities may be reorganized so that the illness regime becomes a routine part of family life. Parents who have used normalization techniques have discovered these techniques on their own. Parents may go through a series of stages as they learn to care for their child on a day-to-day basis. Nurses can facilitate this by recognizing the normalcy, the strengths, and the weaknesses of the family system, by being open and supportive concerning the condition and treatment, and by actively involving the family in all aspects of care. Reinforcing the family's successful use of these tactics can improve self-esteem and motivate further development.

Siblings

Some interventions are specific to a family life-cycle stage. To help prepare for the hospitalized child's needs, for example, nurses can accompany families on a predischarge home visit (Bakewell-Sachs et al., 2000). A thorough assessment of the home environment can facilitate parent teaching and identify unanticipated situations. For instance, sometimes siblings complain that the chronically ill child is treated more leniently. Parents may be unaware that they are treating their children with different standards or may say, "Of course I'm not as strict with him. Look at all he has to put up with." This question of discipline is crucial. Discipline supplies both limits and structure and should be consistent within families and between siblings. It is appropriate for the nurse to question families about methods and consistency of discipline.

Consider Frankie, a fourth grader who has been sent to the school nurse today with complaints of a headache and "bellyache." He has had the same complaints several times in the last 4 weeks. Today's physical exam reveals nothing abnormal. The nurse is aware that his brother, an eighth-grade student at the same school, recently started hemodialysis. She encourages him to rest in a reclining chair while she "works." During the next hour, Frankie shares that he thinks he caused his brother's illness because he brought home a stray dog that was sick. Frankie asks, "How would I know if my kidneys were not working?" and "Do you think it is fair that my brother gets to sleep all day and I have to go to school even if I have a headache? I have to do dishes every night now and he never does them."

The nurse responds to his questions and encourages him to vocalize his feelings. At the end of an hour, Frankie states that he feels better and wants to return to class. The nurse decides to call his parents for a family conference about Frankie's frequent somatic symptoms.

Siblings are usually very aware of their negative feelings, which may include anger, feelings of being neglected, fears of causality, contagion, guilt, or responsibility, and other founded and unfounded feelings. Nurses should tell children that their emotions are acceptable but should also clarify misconceptions. Nurses, in conjunction with the parents, can confirm a sibling's perception that he or she has been receiving less attention and tell the child that it is okay to feel angry about receiving less attention. Siblings' perceptions of the home environment are likely to differ from the impressions of their parents. This is another reminder that providers should speak directly with siblings, rather than relying on impressions of parents. Siblings may benefit from being involved in caregiving responsibilities if they are interested in doing so and if the tasks are within their developmental ranges. Throughout the course of the chronic condition,

information for the siblings needs to be updated for two primary reasons. First, what is known about the condition changes, both as the affected child and parents learn more about the condition and because this particular child's manifestations of the condition might change. Second, siblings' developmental levels change, thereby changing their ability to integrate information.

Spouses

Siblings are not the only group who might feel neglected. Spouses in a family with chronic illness also need attention. The presence of a chronic condition often increases the stress in a family, so some assume that the rate of family dissolution is greater. To the contrary, carefully controlled studies have indicated neither differences in marital functioning nor differences in the rates of divorced or single-parent families among families of children with chronic conditions. Although divorce is not more prevalent, tension and stress are more common than in families without a child with a chronic condition (Sullivan-Bolyai, Sadler, Knafl, & Gillis, 2003). The negative relationship between strain and distress was mediated by the frequency and duration of social and recreational activities. Nurses can facilitate family adjustment by encouraging family outings, recreation, and private time for spouses or partners.

Adolescents

Nurses' interventions for families with adolescents should focus on preventing developmental complications. Nurses need to suggest or initiate discussions addressing physical effects of medications, surgery, or treatments and ways to reduce or cope with effects. Parents of chronically ill adolescents tend to be resistant to adolescent efforts leading to independence. Nurses can help families by teaching adolescents self-care skills and encouraging them to monitor their treatment needs. If nurses find adolescents having little contact with peers, they might need to explore with the adolescent and family how to facilitate peer interactions. Adolescents have commented that they often felt marginalized by the health care community as if they were merely observers in their own care (Woodgate, 1998; Young, Dixon-Woods, Windridge, & Heney, 2003). Nurses can prevent this from occurring by routinely asking adolescents to share ideas and concerns with them and their families. If the illness becomes unstable due to noncompliance, nurses should discuss what happened and how to prevent a reoccurrence. Nurses could suggest that other family members use this strategy instead of a reprimand. Nurses and other family members might collaboratively develop problem-solving skills related to the illness by asking, "What would you do if . . . ?" or "What would you say if he said . . . ?"

NURSING IMPLICATIONS

To achieve best outcomes, nurses can no longer focus care solely on one family member. There must be an increase in collaborative efforts with all family members in the presence of chronic illness in all settings.

Practice

Family-centered care and a trusting relationship with health care providers are pivotal to successful treatment (American Academy of Pediatrics, 2001; Cohen & Wamboldt, 2000). Family-centered care includes a respectful and accepting emotional climate developed between family and all clinicians. Complementary and alternative medicines (CAM) have been increasingly integrated into mainstream treatment options (American Academy of Pediatrics, 2001). In fact, many CAM uses of herbs, acupuncture, reflexology, and guided imagery have proven efficacious. Many CAM techniques, however, have not been rigorously tested. Nurses may want to incorporate accurate knowledge of CAM in their practice plans and include them routinely in family history taking and interventions. Additionally, with the advent of new genetic information and technology, nurses will need to integrate new genetic information in their patient teaching strategies. Patients, families, and nurses have been using the Internet for the latest information. Use of advanced technology will continue to impact the way nursing care is delivered. Video conferencing will allow nurses to conduct interviews and modified assessments and communicate in real time at a distance.

Finally, there is a demand that nurses routinely implement interventions that are based on the best available empirical evidence. Nurses are very familiar with monitoring and intervening with patients' disease-specific health problems and health promotion activities. Several nursing leaders have emphasized that it is important for clinicians to identify and implement interventions based on illness types as opposed to specific illness (Knafl & Deatrick, 2003). As an example, the family with a mother who has emphysema has needs that are similar to those of the family with multiple sclerosis or scleroderma. Nurses might find it more efficient to create family interventions based on the commonalities. The families are dealing with progressive illnesses with a gradual onset that have the probability of shortening the patient's life span. Knafl and Gillis (2002), in their systematic review focusing on family research and chronic illness, report that nursing studies fell into two broad groups: descriptive studies of a family's response to illness and explanatory studies of variables that contributed to a family's response to illness. There were few studies that focused on nursing interventions. It is expected that this trend will change in the next few years because many nursing organizations and funding groups have identified the need to measure the effectiveness of nursing interventions as a top priority (Hinshaw, 2000). Nurses should continue to search for studies that support their interventions.

Over the past decade, the health care delivery system has changed dramatically. In 2000 only 60 percent of all U.S. nurses were employed within the hospital setting (McEwen, 2002). Nurses in the future will find that they typically are working with families who have a family member with a chronic illness in the home environment, extended-care facilities, community settings (e.g., schools), or ambulatory care settings (e.g., clinics, dialysis units). Changing demographics (e.g., the aging population) will also influence the types of families for which nurses care. They will find that they are often working with families that include an individual older than 65 years of age. Unfortunately, the scarcity of resources—specifically, the nursing shortage, lack of access to quality health services, and the rising costs of health care—will shape nursing interventions to focus on helping families become more self-reliant and independent. Nursing interventions will involve more teaching about specific direct-care techniques and strategies to improve family communication skills.

Education

Nursing education frequently focuses on the patient with chronic illness as a member of a family. Nursing graduates of the 21st century must be prepared to collaborate with families, communities, and other health care professionals. With family-centered care, nurses acknowledge the family's developmental needs, recognize family strengths, and support family efforts.

Nursing educators need to assess undergraduate and graduate curricula to verify that there is a family focus in every area. There must be a deliberate movement in education from the individual client as a family member (family in context) to a family-focused approach. Students at all levels must gain expertise with skills in assessing and planning interventions for families dealing with chronic illness and not solely for individual clients. Since the mid-1960s, there has been the expansion of the family nurse practitioner programs throughout the United States to deliver family-centered care. It is expected that this trend will continue in the future. However, a review of guidelines for interventions for adult and family nurse practitioners reveals that few authors direct attention to the entire family as a unit. Nursing actions are directed toward the client with the chronic illness. At the doctoral level, there are schools that list "family" as an area of concentration where nurses have the opportunity to shape their studies to examine families dealing with chronic illnesses. As increasing numbers of nurses complete doctoral work with a family focus, these individuals will be able to assume leadership roles to shape curriculum at all levels of nursing to incorporate families coping with chronic illness.

Research

Researchers, as was noted with educators, need to examine health and chronic illness from a family perspective and not just from the perspective of individuals. More research is needed to explore the interactions between biological factors, the patient's psychological well-being, and the family's adaptation. A paradigm shift in the last decade calls researchers to focus on family strengths and positive outcomes and not on family weaknesses and negative outcomes. There is a need to identify factors and interventions that contribute to family resiliency. Many descriptive studies have imparted new knowledge that has served as the basis for planning interventions. It is time to move beyond mere description and plan outcome studies of nursing interventions, educational strategies, and policy.

Additionally, researchers often design studies focusing on families with a disease-specific approach. Results cannot be generalized to broader populations. It would be fruitful to examine families with a more generic approach with the idea that chronically ill families face common challenges and develop common coping strategies regardless of diagnosis (Meleski,

2002; Stein, 1998). In addition, the increasing availability of genetic risk screening for a variety of chronic diseases will have an impact on families in the future (Rolland, 1999b). Very little is known as to how families will cope with positive and negative test results and long-term consequences across all ethnic and social groups.

Traditionally, researchers have used one family member (i.e., the mother or wife) to provide data for the entire family. The advantages of a single informant might include having the best source for information, reduced costs, and efficient use of time. However, the strategy results in a possibly biased perception, faulty information, and the inability to generalize. Triangulation of data sources would enhance the depth and breadth of findings. Multiple family members as informants used concurrently or sequentially can provide a broader perspective (Astedt-Kurki, Paavilainen, & Lehti, 2001; Shepard, Orsi, Mahon, & Carroll, 2002). Cross-sectional studies provide snapshots of the examined topics; longitudinal studies would allow researchers and clinicians to track trends in family events and outcomes.

Health Policy

There is an underutilization of research in the formation of public policy. Several had suggested that this is due to a communication gap between researchers, practitioners, and policy makers (Bogenschneider, Friese, & Balling, 2002; O'Donnell, 2003). Nurses have the ability to influence public policy at the local, state, national, and international levels in many ways. There has been increased emphasis across nursing organizations and state nursing boards to improve nurses' role in shaping public policy. Leaders from several nursing organizations served on the steering committee that created goals and work plans published in "Nursing's Agenda for the Future" (2002). Some strategies included the following:

- Moving nurses into policy-maker positions
- Collaborating with stakeholders for the development of specific policies
- Reporting reliable data for legislatures' use
- Monitoring health policy's congruency with standards of nursing education and practice

Families dealing with chronic illness face a complex health care system that is difficult to navigate. Private insurance companies and government plans typically do not deal efficiently with long-term problems. Many social and health care policies do not address the economic and social consequences of families living in the presence of a chronic illness and their desire for independence and productive lives for all family members.

Home care and community settings are preferred places of care by families and patients; however, Medicaid and Medicare rarely cover home care services. Patients and families could avoid costly hospitalizations with the use of home health care services, child and adult care programs, or assisted living arrangements. Unfortunately, these services are inaccessible due to insurance noncoverage and high costs. The estimated value of "free" family caregiving services is $257 billion (NCFR, 2003). Families often pay for some long-term costs (e.g., equipment, supplies, services) out of their personal funds. Federal and state governments have supported caregivers with the enactment of the Family and Medical Leave Act, which enables family caregivers to take unpaid leave from their jobs without threats of job loss. This might reduce psychological stress but it also increases economic stresses. As the population continues to age, policy makers will need to recognize a greater need for caregiving supports in the form of tax credits, tax deductions, and cash vouchers for families. Respite programs provide families with needed breaks from caregiving activities. They provide brief opportunities for families to regain stability and strength to maintain positive caregiving roles. Unfortunately, families presently find respite programs unaffordable. Nurses are ideal leaders in the formation of a statewide or national respite program that uses a coordinated system of accessible community-based respite care services for planned and emergency breaks. Legislatures will not formulate policies that are family-friendly until there is strong pressure from interested individuals and groups.

Grandparent caregivers are a recently emerging group as sequelae of chronically ill or dying adults who are unable to fulfill their parental role. These custodial, caregiving arrangements, even after parental death, are usually informal. If legislatures expanded the definition of family to include grandparents raising grandchildren, many would be eligible for government programs that pay for health care services and nursing care. Typically, grandparents do not receive child support, public assistance, or enough Social Security benefits to cover child-related costs. Nurses, in collaboration with consumers, could work toward health care policies that allow for subsidized child care, respite care, or training programs for children with special needs.

Nurses should also give attention to the opposite end of the family life cycle—families with young children. The health and economic benefits of breastfeeding for infants and mothers, for example, is well documented. Federal, state, and local agencies need to be strong advocates for the WIC Breastfeeding Promotion campaign. Benefits among the states vary and often do not meet families' priority needs. Some states offer economic support for education programs focusing on new fathers and new mothers. These not only teach psychomotor skills but also strengthen communications skills and partner relationships. Nurses can educate legislatures on the value of educational programs, home care visits, use of lactation consultants, and full coverage for breast pumps for working mothers. Finally, nurses need to inform nursing colleagues about public policy issues and processes. This is done initially within basic nursing curricula and continues within professional organizations. Nurses working within organizations can scan current legislatures and issue alerts when public statements from nurses are warranted. Experts have identified holding a health policy planning summit with key consumer groups to plan collaborative efforts as a primary strategy to shape public policy ("Nursing's Agenda for the Future," 2002). A single nurse can be effective to change policies.

SUMMARY

- To achieve best outcomes, nurses can no longer focus care solely on one family member. There must be an increase in collaborative efforts with all family members in the presence of chronic illness in all settings.
- A theoretical model provides a framework for family assessment, goal formation, and nursing interventions.
- Chronic illness complicates individual (but especially adolescent) development and family task completion.
- If family members consider the illness as only the patient's problem, there will be imbalances of power and control.
- Nurses are in a unique position to help families cope with chronic illness across the family life cycle.
- Nurses can affect the effects of chronic illness in educational, research, and public policy arenas.

STUDY QUESTION

1. A family with two school-age sons was involved in a motor vehicle accident, and the father is now in a permanent vegetative state. Name two possible outcomes for this family with unresolved ambiguous loss.

References

American Academy of Pediatrics Committee on Children with Disabilities. (2001). Counseling families who choose complementary and alternative medicine for their child with a chronic illness or disability. *Pediatrics, 107,* 598–601.

Astedt-Kurki, P., Paavilainen, E., & Lehti, K. (2001). Methodological issues in interviewing families in family nursing research. *Journal of Advanced Nursing, 35,* 288–293.

Bakewell-Sachs, S., Carlino, H., Ash, L., Thurber, F., Guyer, K., Deatrick, J. A., & Brooten, D. (2000). Home care considerations for chronic and vulnerable populations. *Nurse Practitioner Forum, 11,* 65–72.

Bluebond-Longer, M. (1996). *In the shadow of illness: Parents and siblings of the chronically ill child.* Camden, NJ: Rutgers University Press.

Bogenschneider, K., Friese, B., & Balling, K. (2002). Spanning the great divide: Strategies for linking research and policymaking from the policy institute for family impact seminars. *NCFR Family Focus On: Bridging Research and Practice, FF14,* 1–3.

Bonica, C., & Daniel, J. (2003). Helping adolescents cope with stress during stressful times. *Current Opinion in Pediatrics, 15,* 385–390.

Boss, P. (1999). *Ambiguous loss: Learning to live with unresolved grief.* Cambridge, MA: Harvard University Press.

Centers for Disease Control and Prevention. (2003). *Chronic disease prevention.* Retrieved October 18, 2003, from http://www.cdc.gov/nccdphp/power_prevention/pop_epidemic.htm

Cohen, S. Y., & Wamboldt, F. S. (2000). The parent-physician relationship in pediatric asthma care. *Journal of Pediatric Psychology, 25,* 69–77.

Copeland, L. G., & Clements, D. B. (1993). Parental perceptions and support strategies in caring for a child with a chronic condition. *Issues in Comprehensive Pediatric Nursing, 16,* 109–121.

Coyne, J., Rohrbaugh, M., Shoham, V., Sonnega, J., Nicklas, J., & Cranford, J. (2001). Prognostic importance of marital quality for survival of congested heart failure. *The American Journal of Cardiology, 88*(5), 526–529.

Coyne, J., Thompson, R., & Palmer, S. (2002). Marital quality, coping with conflict, marital complaints, and affection in couples with a depressed wife. *Journal of Family Psychology, 16*(1), 26–37.

Dashiff, C., & Bartolucci, A. (2002). Autonomy development in adolescents with insulin dependent diabetes mellitus. *Journal of Pediatric Nursing, 17,* 96–106.

Davis, R., & Magilvy, J. (2000). Quiet pride: The experience of chronic illness by rural older adults. *Journal of Nursing Scholarship, 32*(94), 385–390.

Dorsey, S., Chance, M., Morse, E., Forehand, R., & Morse, L. (1999). Children whose mothers are HIV infected: Who resides in the home and is there a relationship to child psychological adjustment? *Journal of Family Psychology, 13*(1), 103–117.

Dosa, N. P., Boeing, N. M., & Kanter, R. K. (2001). Excess risk of severe acute illness in children with chronic health conditions. *Pediatrics, 107,* 499–504.

Ebersole, P., & Hess, P. (2001). *Geriatric nursing & healthy aging.* St. Louis: Mosby.

Fleming, E., Carter, B., & Gillibrand, W. (2002). The transition of adolescents with diabetes from the children's health care service into the adult health care service: A review of the literature. *Journal of Clinical Nursing, 11,* 560–567.

Gallo, A. M., Breitmayer, B. J., Knafl, K. A., & Zoeller, L. H. (1992). Well siblings of children with chronic illness: Parents' reports of their psychological adjustment. *Pediatric Nursing, 18,* 23–29.

Gerdner, L., Buckwalter, K., & Reed, D. (2002). Impact of a psychoeducational intervention on caregiver response to behavioral problems. *Nursing Research, 51,* 363–374.

Gilber, O., & Refaeli, R. (2000). The relationship between adult cancer patients' adjustment to the illness and that of their parents. *Families, Systems & Health, 18,* 5–17.

Greco, J. I. (2001). Who cares: Chronic illness in America [Video]. In M. Cogswell (Producer), *PBS Programming, Fred Friendly Seminars at the Columbia University Graduate School of Journalism in association with Thirteen/WNET New York.* Princeton, NJ: Films for the Humanities and Sciences.

Hammonds-Smith, M. (2003, April). NCFR fact sheet: Helping families meet the needs of older adults. Retrieved November 1, 2003, from http://www.ncfr.org

Hinshaw, A. (2000). Nursing knowledge for the 21st century: Opportunities and challenges. *Journal of Nursing Scholarship, 32*(2), 117–123.

Hippisley-Cox, J., Pringle, M., Crowne, N., & Hammersley, V. (2002). Married couples' risk of same disease: Cross-sectional study [electronic version]. *British Medical Journal, 325,* 636.

Hobbs, N., Perrin, J. M., & Ireys, H. T. (1985). *Chronically ill children and their families.* San Francisco: Jossey-Bass.

Hopkins, A. (1994). The trauma nurse's role with families in crisis. *Critical Care Nurse, 14*(2), 35–41.

Ignatavicius, D., & Workman, M. (2002). Rehabilitation concepts for acute and chronic problems. In D. Ignatavicius & M. Workman (Eds.), *Medical-surgical nursing: Critical thinking for collaborative care* (4th ed., pp. 119–120). Philadelphia: WB Saunders.

Knafl, K., & Deatrick, J. (2002). The challenge of normalization for families of children with chronic conditions. *Pediatric Nursing, 28,* 49–56.

Knafl, K., & Deatrick, J. (2003). Further refinement of the family management style framework. *Journal of Family Nursing, 9,* 232–256.

Knafl, K., & Gillis, C. (2002). Families and chronic illness: A synthesis of current research. *Journal of Family Nursing, 8,* 178–198.

Kralik, D. (2002). The quest for ordinariness: Transition experienced by midlife women living with chronic illness. *Journal of Advanced Nursing, 39,* 146–154.

Kurz, J. (2001). The roller coaster ride of spouses of lung transplant recipients. *Journal of Advanced Nursing, 34,* 493–500.

Kurz, J., & Cavanaugh, J. (2001). Stressors and coping strategies used by well spouses of lung transplant candidates. *Families, Systems & Health, 19,* 181–197.

Kyngas, H. (2000). Compliance of adolescents with chronic diseases. *Journal of Clinical Nursing, 9,* 549–556.

Lackey, N., & Gates, M. (2001). Adults' recollection of their experiences as young caregivers of family members with chronic physical illnesses. *Journal of Advanced Nursing, 34,* 320–328.

Marks, N., Lambert, J., & Choi, H. (2002). Transitions to caregiving. Gender and psychological well-being: A prospective U.S. national study. *Journal of Marriage and Family, 64,* 657–667.

McCubbin, H., & McCubbin, M. (1993). Family coping with health crisis: The resiliency model of family stress, adjustment and adaptation. In C. Danielson, B. Hamel-Bissell, & P. Winstead-Fry (Eds.), *Families, health, and illness.* St. Louis: Mosby.

McEwen, M. (2002). *Community-based nursing: An introduction.* Philadelphia: Saunders.

Meleski, D. (2002). Families with chronically ill children. *American Journal of Nursing, 102*(5), 47–54.

Morrison, L. (1997). Stress and siblings. *Paediatric Nursing, 9,* 26–27.

Mukherjee, S., Sloper, P., & Lewin, R. (2002). The meaning of parental illness to children: The case of inflammatory bowel disease. *Child: Care, Health Development, 28,* 479–485.

Nursing's agenda for the future: A call to the nation. (2002, April). Retrieved from http://www.NursingWorld.org/paf

O'Donnell, D. (2003). The politically active nurse. In J. Catalano (Ed.), *Nursing now* (3rd ed., pp. 347–372). Philadelphia: FA Davis.

Orth-Gomér, K., Wamala, S., Horsten, M., Schenck-Gustafsson, K., Schneiderman, N., & Mittleman, M. A. (2000). Marital stress worsens prognosis in women with coronary heart disease: The Stockholm Female Coronary Risk Study. *Journal of the American Medical Association, 284*(23), 3008–3014.

Partnership for Solutions. (2002, May). Better lives for people with chronic conditions. Retrieved October 18, 2003, from http://www.partnershipforsolutions.org

Perlesz, A., Kinsella, G., & Crowe, S. (1999). Impact of traumatic brain injury on the family: A critical review. *Rehabilitation Psychology, 44,* 6–35.

Potter, P. A., & Perry, A. G. (2003). Caring in families. In *Fundamentals of nursing* (5th ed., pp. 138–153). St. Louis: Mosby.

Rehm, R., & Franck, L. (2000). Long-term goals and normalization strategies of children and families affected by HIV/AIDS. *Advanced Nursing Science, 23,* 69–82.

Rohrbaugh, M., Cranford, J., Shoham, V., Nicklas, J., Sonnega, J., & Coyne, J. (2002). Couples coping with congested heart failure: Role and gender differences in psychological distress. *Journal of Family Psychology, 16,* 3–13.

Rolland, J. (1994). *Families, illness & disability: An integrative treatment model.* New York: Basic Books.

Rolland, J. (1998). Beliefs and collaboration in illness: Evolution over time. *Family, Systems & Health, 16,* 7–25.

Rolland, J. (1999a). Parental illness and disability: A family systems framework. *Journal of Family Therapy, 21,* 242–266.

Rolland, J. (1999b). Families and genetic fate: A millennial challenge. *Family, Systems & Health, 17,* 123–132.

Schmaling, K., & Sher, T. (2000). *The psychology of couples and illness: Theory, research & practice.* Washington, DC: American Psychological Association.

Shepard, M., Orsi, A., Mahon, M., & Carroll, R. (2002). Mixed-methods research with vulnerable families. *Journal of Family Nursing, 8,* 334–352.

Siegel, K., & Lekas, H. (2002). AIDS as a chronic illness: Psychosocial implications. *AIDS, Supplement, 16,* S69–S76.

Silver, E., Westbrook, L., & Stein, R. (1998). Relationship of parental psychological distress to consequences of chronic health conditions in children. *Journal of Pediatric Psychiatry, 23,* 5–15.

Smith, S., & Soliday, E. (2001). The effects of parental chronic kidney disease on the family. *Family Relations, 50,* 171–177.

Snethen, J., & Broome, M. (2001). Children in research: The experiences of siblings in research is a family affair. *Journal of Family Nursing, 7,* 92–110.

Sobel, S., & Cowan, C. (2003). Ambiguous loss and disenfranchised grief: The impact of DNA predictive testing on the family as a system. *Family Process, 42,* 47–57.

Stein, R. E. K. (1998). Children with chronic conditions in the 21st century. *Journal of Urban Health, 75*(4), 732–738.

Stewart, M., Davidson, K., & Meade, D. (2001). Group support for couples coping with a cardiac condition. *Journal of Advanced Nursing, 33,* 190–199.

Sullivan-Bolyai, S., Sadler, L., Knafl, K., & Gillis, C. (2003). Great expectations: A position description for parents as caregivers: Part I. *Pediatric Nursing, 29,* 457–461.

Swallow, V. M., & Jacoby, A. (2001). Mothers' coping in chronic childhood illness: The effect of presymptomatic diagnosis of vesicoureteric reflux. *Journal of Advanced Nursing, 33,* 69–78.

Thorne, S., & Robinson, C. (1988). Reciprocal trust in health-care relationships. *Journal of Advanced Nursing, 13,* 782–789.

Thorne, S., & Robinson, C. (1989). Guarded alliance: Health care relationships in chronic illness. *Image: Journal of Nursing Scholarship, 21,* 153–157.

Trief, P., Orenforff, R., & Weinstock, R. (2001). The marital relationship and psychological adaptation and glycemic control of individuals with diabetes. *Diabetes Care, 24,* 1384–1389.

White, Y., & Grenyer, B. (1999). The biopsychosocial impact of end-stage renal disease: The experiences of dialysis patients and their partners. *Journal of Advanced Nursing, 30,* 1312–1320.

Williams, P. D., Williams, A. R., Graff, J. C., Hanson, S., Stanton, A., Hafeman, C., et al. (2002). Interrelationships among variables affecting well siblings and mothers in families of children with a chronic illness or disability. *Journal of Behavioral Medicine, 25*(5), 411–424.

Wilson, S., Bladin, P., & Saling, M. (2001). The burden of normality: Concepts of adjustment after surgery for seizures. *Journal of Neurology, Neurosurgery & Psychiatry, 70,* 649–656.

Winston, C. (2003). African-American grandmothers parenting AIDS orphans: Concomitant grief and loss. *American Journal of Orthopsychiatry, 73,* 91–100.

Wolff, J., Starfield, B., & Anderson, G. (2002). Prevalence, expenditures, and complications of multiple chronic conditions in the elderly. *Archives of Internal Medicine, 162,* 2269–2276.

Woodgate, R. L. (1998). Adolescents' perceptions of chronic illness: "It's hard." *Journal of Pediatric Nursing, 13*(4), 210–223.

Young, B., Dixon-Woods, M., Windridge, K., & Heney, D. (2003). Managing communication with young people who have a potentially life-threatening chronic illness: Qualitative study of patients and parents [electronic version]. *British Medical Journal, 326,* 305.

Bibliography

Allen, J. (Ed.). (2002). *Using literature to help troubled teenagers cope with end-of-life issues.* Westport, CT: Greenwood Press.

Bomar, P. (2004). *Promoting health in families: Applying family research and theory to nursing practice* (3rd ed.). Philadelphia: Saunders.

Boss, P. (Ed.). (2003). *Family stress: Classic and contemporary readings.* Thousand Oaks, CA: Sage Publications.

Clark, C. (2003). *In sickness and in play: Children coping with chronic illness.* New Brunswick, NJ: Rutgers University Press.

Josl, D. (2002). *Invisible caregivers: Older adults raising children in the wake of HIV/AIDS.* New York: Columbia University Press.

Kramer, B., & Thompson, E. (2002). *Men as caregivers: Theory, research and service implications.* New York: Springer Publications.

Rice, V. (2000). *Handbook of stress, coping and health: Implications for nursing research, theory and practice.* Thousand Oaks, CA: Sage Publications.

Vaughan-Cole, B., Johnson, M., Malone, J., & Walker, B. (1998). *Family nursing practice.* Philadelphia: Saunders.

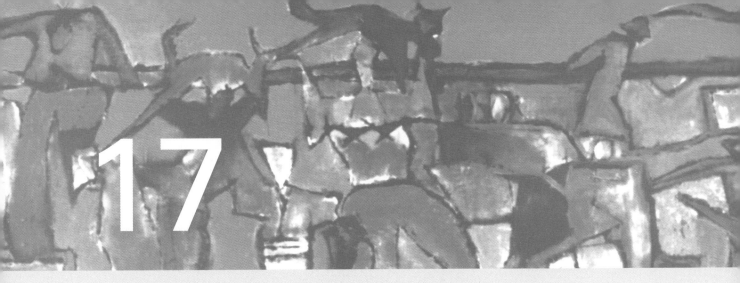

17

Genomics, Family Nursing, and Families across the Life Span

Janet Karen D. Williams, PhD, RN, CPNP, CGC, FAAN •
Dr. Heather Skirton, PhD, MSc, RGN, Dip Counselling, Registered Genetic Counsellor (UK)

CRITICAL CONCEPTS

- Genetics is the area of family nursing where family most intimately comes into play because it has not only a social and caregiving connection but also a biological one.

- Biological members of a family may share the risk of disease due to genetic factors. However, it is often difficult to ascertain the extent of shared genetic risks because family members who live together may also be exposed to risk of disease due to common environmental influences.

- The term "genetic disease" is commonly used to describe conditions that are directly attributable to a *mutation* in one *gene* or a *chromosomal* abnormality.

- A change in gene structure can be due to a range of environmental influences (such as drugs, radia-

tion, and carcinogens) but also commonly occurs sporadically.

- Gene mutations have been identified for some inherited disorders. In some cases, one mutation is found in all those who have the condition (e.g., Huntington disease), but in other cases, not all persons with the condition will have the identical gene mutation or even mutations in the same gene (e.g., tuberous sclerosis).

- Issues connected with genetic disease are relevant to nurses working in all fields of nursing, from reproductive medicine and obstetrics to the care of the elderly.

- Individuals in families have individual responses to learning about genetic aspects of health and illness. These responses are shaped by personal coping

437

styles, as well as by family values, beliefs, and patterns of communication regarding medical information.

- When peoples' beliefs about their risk of a genetic condition are informed by family experiences, the scientific information provided by the nurse may be rejected as not being applicable to that particular family.

- There are a number of specific ethical issues that arise frequently in the practice of genetic nursing.

One of these is *confidentiality*. Although genetic information is personal and private, it may also have implications for the health of other family members.

- Nurses who specialize in genetic nursing are master's prepared and focus their nursing practice on patient groups that have genetic conditions.

- Genes control all functions of the human body at the cellular level.

INTRODUCTION

Some illnesses "run in families," and people commonly wonder if they, or their children, will develop a disease that is present in their parents or grandparents. The ability to apply understanding of genetics in the care of families is a priority for nurses and for all health care providers, reflecting the rapidly expanding body of knowledge on genetic influences on health and illness emerging from genomic research (NCHPEG, 2000). This integration of genetic knowledge, attitudes, and skills is especially important for nurses who care for families. Implications of genetic discoveries on the health of families are not yet well understood and represent an important challenge for all health providers, including nurses (Feetham, 1999). Families can be defined from both a biological viewpoint and a social viewpoint. Family members who are biologically related may share genetic risk factors that they have inherited from common ancestors. Family members, regardless of their biological kinship, support each other in seeking and maintaining healthy growth and development. Much of what is known about the health care needs of persons with genetic conditions has focused on the individual, with less attention directed toward the persons' biological and socially defined family. This chapter describes nursing responsibilities for families of persons who have, or are at risk of having, genetic conditions. These responsibilities are described for families prior to conception, families seeking genetic information to promote health, management of multiple health problems during chronic illness, and families of persons with genetic conditions who are nearing the end of life. All nurses, regardless of their areas of practice, should be prepared to apply an understanding of the impact of genetic risk factors on the health of individuals and their families.

The purpose of this chapter is to describe the relevance of genetic information within families when there is a question about genetic aspects of health or disease for members of the family. Family nursing knowledge is incomplete without attention to the impact of genetic factors that influence health and disease on health and functioning of individuals as well as family units. Content in this chapter describes situations throughout the life span of family members, where nursing knowledge of genetic concerns is necessary in order for the nurse to provide comprehensive assessment, interventions, and evaluation of nursing care.

❝Issues connected with genetic disease are relevant to nurses working in all fields of nursing, from reproductive medicine and obstetrics to the care of the elderly.❞

❝Genetic nursing is not new, but the breadth and depth of genetic knowledge and its applications in nursing practice are rapidly changing.❞

COMMON THEORETICAL PERSPECTIVES

There are many theories that can support the development of nursing competence in caring for families with a genetic condition. These include the Health Belief Model (Janz, Wren, Schottenfeld, & Guire, 2003; Finney Rutten & Iannotti, 2003) and theories of behavioral coping styles (Miller, 1995; Rees & Bath, 2000). However, three theoretical models that pertain directly to nursing in this context will be described in this chapter. These are (1) lay representations of illness, (2) need for cognitive closure theory, and (3) family systems theory.

HISTORICAL PERSPECTIVES

Genetic nursing is recognized in the United States by the American Nurses Association as a specialty (ISONG, 1998). Genetic nursing is not new, but the breadth and depth of genetic knowledge and its applications in nursing practice are rapidly changing. Over 30 years ago, maternal child health nurses provided nursing care to families of newborn infants who were screened for phenylketonuria and other inherited metabolic disorders (Bowe, 1995). Communication of options for prenatal screening and diagnosis became an additional nursing responsibility when maternal serum alpha-fetoprotein (MSAFP) levels were recognized as a means to identify fetuses at risk to have *neural tube defects* (NTDs) (Grant, 2000). Prior to the 1990s, the majority of genetic health care services focused on diagnosis and management of conditions that were relatively uncommon and had specific *Mendelian* patterns of inheritance. This changed, however, with the increasing understanding of the role of familial predisposition to cancer, especially cancer of the breast, ovary, and colon (Hodgson & Maher, 1999). The discovery of mutations in genes associated with familial breast and ovarian cancer (Miki et al., 1994) and hereditary colon cancer (Cole & Sleightholme, 2000) made *predictive genetic testing* possible for families where there was a strong family history of cancer. With the completion of the comprehensive sequence of the human *genome*, scientists are identifying genetic factors that contribute to relatively common diseases (Collins, Green, Guttmacher, & Guyer, 2003). These discoveries create the expectations that all nurses will recognize genetic risk factors in families, provide accurate information about genetic tests, and integrate genetics into all nursing care activities (Jenkins & Collins, 2003). Genetics educational materials are now available for oncology nurses (Oncology Nursing Society, 2003). Nurses can now become credentialed as genetic nurse specialists or advanced practice genetic nurses through the Genetic Nursing Credentialing Commission (GNCC, 2003).

The Lay Representation of Illness

Lau and Hartmann (1983) developed an original theory of lay representation of disease that included five domains. The individual uses these to create a psychological construct of the illness. The five domains are as follows:

- Disease identity (name, signs, and symptoms)
- Timeline
- Consequences
- Causes
- Controllability

The information covered by the five domains can be acquired through personal experience, information provided by others (including health professionals), and experience of other related situations. For example, a woman who gives birth to a baby with a congenital heart defect may construct a representation of that condition based on her previous experience of a childhood friend who had surgery for a heart defect, information gathered from both fictional and nonfictional media sources, and the information provided to her by staff caring for her baby. Her reaction to the diagnosis will be congruent with her own representation but may not be entirely consistent with the actual extent of the defect and the prognosis.

The illness representation (Lau, 1997) is used as a basis to assess the extent of the threat to health (Leventhal et al., 1997). This is important when the individual is faced with a number of potential measures for dealing with the threat, and in particular if those measures require potentially life-changing decisions. In terms of a genetic condition, the decisions made by one person could significantly affect other family members. For example, one parent may decide not to continue with a pregnancy because she perceives the threat of a prenatally diagnosed condition to be very great. If the other parent does not share the illness representation, the decision may cause conflict. The impact of the decision by one family member to be tested for a breast cancer gene mutation could have an impact on other family members, who will become aware of their own increased risk if the test is positive.

The representation of illness varies over time, as the person passes from one life stage to another and as the information gathered about the condition changes (Leventhal & Crouch, 1997). This is relevant to genetic nursing, as the decision made by a patient at one point in time may subsequently alter. For this reason, it is important that patients feel able to recontact the genetic service to renew discussions and perhaps alter plans that were previously made. Richards (1993) has emphasized that professionals who provide genetic services should be aware of the lay representation of genetic disease that exists within each family, as well as within each individual. These beliefs should be addressed as part of the provision of genetic health care (Skirton & Eiser, 2004).

Need for Cognitive Closure

The psychological concept known as the "need for cognitive closure" is defined by Webster and Kruglanski (1994) as an individual preference for certainty and discomfort with ambiguity. Kruglanski (1989) developed the theory as an extension of lay epistemic theory in an attempt to create a concept that was not situation-specific but rather could be applied universally to knowledge acquisition. He proposed that knowledge acquisition occurs in two stages: construct formation (based on previously acquired knowledge) and construct testing. If the evidence obtained through testing supports the hypothesis, the construct will be reinforced. This theory is relevant to genetic counseling, as evidence indicates that clients develop a lay theory to explain the genetic condition in the family (Richards, 1993). Webster and Kruglanski (1994) proposed that the motivation to seek new information was due to the individual's need for cognitive closure.

The theory of the need for cognitive closure (Manetti, Pierro, Kruglanski, Taris, & Benzinovic, 2002) therefore describes the individual differences in a person's motivation to seek information. There are five domains in the "need for closure" model:

- Preference for order
- Discomfort with ambiguity
- Decisiveness
- Desire for predictability
- Closed-mindedness

The authors describe those who have a strong drive to obtain information to help them resolve uncertainties as having a high need for cognitive closure. Those who are more psychologically comfortable with uncertainty are described as having a low need for closure. Although a person may or may not have a tendency to strive for closure, this individual characteristic is not absolutely fixed and may alter with circumstances to some extent, particularly where there is some degree of accountability. For example, a

person may generally have a low tendency to seek certainty, but this may alter in circumstances of extreme importance to the future of themselves or their families. Skirton (2001) demonstrated that individuals who sought or accepted a genetic referral tended to seek certainty and in fact preferred bad news to uncertainty. A person with a high need for certainty will usually be more likely to pursue information about the condition as a method of coping with the diagnosis or genetic risk, whereas those with a low need for certainty may cope best by avoiding information until dealing with it is imperative. This theory partly explains differences in the approach of family members toward dealing with the genetic condition, risk information, and genetic testing. Family members with a higher need for closure will be more driven to seek information from professionals or other sources, such as the Internet, whereas those with a low need for certainty may actively avoid any discussion or reminders of the genetic condition. It is evident in clinical practice that these fundamental differences in approach can cause lack of understanding and even hostility within families, for example, when a family member requests predictive testing for an adult-onset disease such as Huntington disease or familial breast cancer while relatives refuse even to discuss the risk.

This theory can help nurses understand the stance of some patients who are not receptive to health care education, even when it may alter their health status, such as information about available screening procedures.

Family Systems Theory

Family systems theory is used by family therapists as a basis for psychotherapeutic interventions when more than one person in a family is seeking help. It is frequently used to help the family modify behavior patterns that have become problematic (Dallos & Draper, 2000). The family unit works as a system, and the theory is based on the observation that forces operate both externally and internally in any system. When a force is applied, the family adjusts to regain its former equilibrium. This is termed *homeostasis*. The ability of the system to respond to external pressure can be used therapeutically. For example, therapists can use interventions to enable the family to improve its ability to function as a unit (e.g., when one or more family members are exhibiting behaviors that are an expression of conflicts in the family).

Communication within families is vital to enable information relevant to the genetic risk to be shared by all those whose lives may be potentially affected. The family systems theory describes the types of relationships that exist within families that have an influence on the communicative styles in the family.

Relationships within a family may have several characteristics. For example, if the relationship is described as an alliance, individuals are considered to have equal status and their ability to make personal decisions is likely to be respected. Because it is considered important that a person has the right to have information that could have a personal impact, genetic information is likely to be shared, even if it is distressing. By contrast, when the family operates on a hierarchical structure, differentials in power exist between family members. This may lead to those with greater power making decisions about the dissemination of genetic information to those lower in the hierarchy. A family member may withhold relevant information when that person believes that others should be protected from information that may cause anxiety (Skirton, 2001). A coalition type of relationship exists when two or more members of the family collude against another member. In communication terms, this could result in information being shared selectively within the family. Flexibility is an aid to family survival, and within a functional family, there is fluidity in relational styles. For example, parents may operate as an alliance for the majority of the time, as a coalition when setting boundaries for an unruly child, and in a hierarchy when key financial decisions are made.

Relational boundaries also have an important influence on communication and decision making in families. Where the relationships are boundaried, family members have an understanding of their own identity in relation to that of others. This facilitates individual decision making. However, between some family members, particularly parent and offspring, boundaries may be enmeshed. The boundary between one individual and another is indistinct because the psychological separation process is incomplete. Where the boundary is enmeshed, the individual may have difficulty in making personal decisions and will rely on the input of the other family member to decide a course of action. Family members are said to be disengaged when the emotional connection between them is sparse. In this case, an individual may fail to see the relevance of genetic information to others or reason that personal information is confidential even from family members to whom it would be relevant.

Family systems therapists use a number of interventions to help the family to change communication styles. One of these is using metaphors. This can be useful when a nurse is helping families understand or communicate genetic information. For example, a family may feel frustrated at the lack of empathy for others shown by a person affected with Huntington disease. Guilt about those feelings may prevent the family from addressing the problem. Using an animal as a metaphor for the disease, such as saying that the disease is like "a wolf that is devouring their loved one," may enable the family members to express their rage at the situation without attaching blame to the affected person (Dallos & Draper, 2000). However, although the family systems theory can be an extremely useful tool in facilitating adaptation by families, it may not be suitable for use in cultures outside those in which it was developed (Rothbaum, Rosen, Ujiie, & Uchida, 2002).

HEALTH PROMOTION

Family members who are biologically related may share risks for health problems that have a major genetic component. After recognizing these risks, family members can determine whether they want more information about how to maintain their health and manage problems that may occur if they develop an inherited disorder. All nurses should be able to conduct a risk assessment that includes obtaining a genetic family history (American Association of Colleges of Nursing, 1998). A specific type of family history assessment is used when health professionals need to identify inherited risks for disease. The genetic family tree (pedigree) provides information about a potential inheritance pattern and recurrence risks for individual family members. Information on standardized pedigree symbols and the construction of a genetic family pedigree are available on the NCHPEG Website (NCHPEG, 2003). Taking a family history is a nursing skill that requires technical expertise and knowledge of what needs to be asked, as well as sensitivity to very personal or distressing topics and an awareness of the ethical issues involved. Information given by the patient may be confidential and should not be shared with other family members unless consent is sought and given.

Genetic Risk Assessment and Family Tree

Genetic risk assessment is based on the drawing of a genetic family history in the form of a three-generation pedigree, using standardized symbols (NCHPEG, 2003). The use of a genogram is not appropriate for this purpose, as it does not clearly identify health status of individuals that may put them at risk of disorders that have a genetic component. The purpose of drawing the family tree is to enable medical information to be set into the context of the family structure for interpretation by health care providers. In order to maintain privacy of medical information, health care providers should not share a genetic family pedigree with other family members without the permission of the person who provided the information.

It is best to start with the patient and the immediate family and then complete one side of the family before moving to the other. Drawing the family tree for at least three generations often provides important data on the potential inheritance pattern. Where a condition affects both males and females and is present in more than one generation, a *dominant* condition is suspected (Figure 17–1). Conditions affecting mainly males, with no evidence of male-to-male transmission, will increase suspicion of an *X-linked recessive* condition (Figure 17–2). When there is more than one child affected of only one set of parents, it may be evidence of a *recessive* condition.

Nurses should not assume that a condition is genetic merely because more than one family member has it. Family members who are subject to similar environmental influences may develop similar conditions, without a genetic basis. One such example is a family with a strong history of lung cancer. Bob was a 62-year-old man affected by lung cancer, and his two brothers and father had all died from lung cancer. Bob was very concerned about a genetic predisposition that

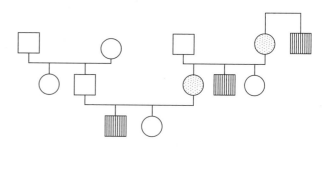

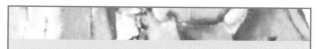

Heterozygote (carrier) of X-linked recessive disorder

Male with X-linked recessive disorder

Figure 17–2 X-linked recessive pedigree.

could be passed to his grandsons. Taking a social family history revealed that Bob's father and every male member of his family had worked underground as coal miners from the age of 14 years. In addition, they had all smoked at least 40 cigarettes a day from adolescence. The women in the family had not smoked, nor worked in the mines, and none had developed cancer. In this family, the cancer could be attributed to environmental rather than inherited causes.

A genetic nursing assessment includes the following information:

- Three-generation pedigree using standardized symbols
- Health history of each family member
- Reproductive history
- Ethnic background of family members
- Documentation of variations in growth and development of family members
- Individual's and family's understanding of causes of health problems that occur in more than one family member
- Identification of questions that family members have about potential genetic risk factors in their family
- Identification of communication of genetic health information within the family

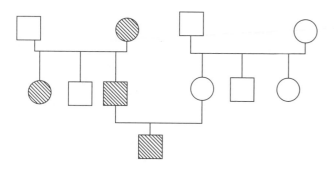

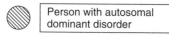

Person with autosomal dominant disorder

Figure 17–1 Autosomal dominant family pedigree.

Nurse's Role in Assessment

When a genetic risk is identified, the nurse, along with others in the health care team, has a responsibility to help the family understand that the risk is present and to help family members make decisions about management or surveillance. Where the risk exists for the future offspring of a couple, the option of prenatal diagnosis may be available. For example, in a family where both partners are carriers of cystic fibrosis, each future child would have a 25 percent chance of inheriting the condition. The nurse should be aware that the family has a number of options:

- Decide against having any more children
- Have a pregnancy with no form of genetic testing
- Have a pregnancy and have prenatal genetic diagnosis with an option to terminate an affected fetus
- Have a pregnancy using donor gamete
- Adopt a child
- Have a pregnancy using preimplantation genetic diagnosis to select only embryos that will not develop cystic fibrosis

In every case, the nurse's role is to support the family to make the decision that is most appropriate for its particular circumstances, culture, and beliefs (*AGNC Code of Ethics*, 2003). This can be difficult if the nurse's personal values conflict with the family's, but it is unethical for the nurse to try to influence the patient because of personal views. There may be conflicting opinions within the family, and the nurse may then play a part in enabling family members to express their views. Genetic testing is discussed with an individual or with the person's family if the testing can offer useful information to the person. In clinical genetics, more than one family member may be involved in decision making, and nurses should respect each person's autonomy.

> ❝When a nurse identifies a family history of cancer, the family should be asked whether they would like to learn more about their risks by seeing a genetic or familial cancer specialist. ❞

Preconception Education

It is ideal if a family has the opportunity to discuss difficult genetic decisions prior to a pregnancy. During a pregnancy, the emotional ties to the existing fetus may make decision making even more difficult for the parents. Preconception Counseling enables the couple to think about their options without time pressures.

Preconception Counseling (Iowa Interventions Project, 2000) is an intervention that includes providing information and support to individuals prior to pregnancy to promote health and reduce risks. Part of this intervention is the identification of a health risk profile that includes family history, prescription drug use, ethnic background, occupational and household exposures, diet, specific genetic disorders, and habits such as smoking, alcohol consumption, or street drug use. When a nurse identifies information that may present a risk for health problems in future offspring, the nurse should ask whether the woman or family would consider a more extensive evaluation from a genetic specialist. See Box 17–1 for an example of preconception education.

In addition to identifying inherited conditions, Preconception Counseling includes education regarding other risk factors that could change the outcome of a pregnancy. Prior to starting a pregnancy, this education includes explaining the importance of

---

Box 17–1

Jay and Sara are college students who are planning to be married. Both are of Ashkenazi Jewish ancestry. Although both have heard about Tay-Sachs disease and the availability of carrier testing, neither has had the carrier test. When Sara visited the student health office, she talked with the nurse about her fears that she may not be able to have healthy babies. She knew that Tay-Sachs disease, a degenerative neurological condition, is more common in Ashkenazi Jewish families and that no treatment will alter the course of the disease. Sara was interested in learning more about what a carrier test is, and the nurse offered to refer Sara to a genetics specialist. The nurse also reviewed Sara's health history and discussed the importance of taking a daily multivitamin that contains folic acid.

taking an adequate amount of folic acid, one of the B vitamins. Use of folic acid supplements has led to a decrease in the number of babies born with neural tube defects (NTDs) (MRC Vitamin Study Research Group, 1991). NTDs are congenital abnormalities that result from failure of closure of the neural tube by about the 4th week of gestation. These include anencephaly, spina bifida, and encephalocele. The background population risk for NTDs is approximately 1:1000. The risk for this condition varies according to ethnic background, with higher rates among British and Irish populations (Jorde, Carey, Bamshad, & White, 1999). A combination of genetic and environmental factors is believed to contribute to the risk for NTDs. Read more about NTDs in Box 17–2.

Risk Assessment in Adult-Onset Diseases

Genetic history taking and technologies are now being used as a risk assessment tools for adults, in relation to more common diseases such as cancer and coronary heart disease. The basic risk assessment is based on the genetic family pedigree, but additional genetic or biochemical tests may be used to clarify the risk to the individual. To ensure that the privacy of individual relatives is maintained, consent is required from living relatives to access their medical records and confirm relevant medical history. Family members who are seeking information can then be advised with regard to their risks and options for clinical screening and follow-up. One example is the assessment of risk for cancer when there is a strong family history of cancer. There is ample research evidence that individuals who find through counseling and testing that they do have an increased risk of cancer may experience psychological difficulties. They may feel that cancer is inevitable, whatever the numerical risk (Lynch & Lynch, 1994). Some persons may desire to have genetic testing even though there is no indication that the presence of cancer in their family is due to an inherited gene mutation. For these people, they may regard the test as an additional means of reassurance (Richards, 1993). The nurse needs to explore the family's feelings of grief and anxiety about the future, as well as its beliefs about the inheritance pattern. The nurse should then provide explanations that enable the family to put the information into its own specific context.

Increasingly, women with a family history of breast and/or ovarian cancer are seeking to reduce their risks of these conditions. This may be especially so in women whose own mothers have died at a relatively young age from breast and/or ovarian cancers (Loescher, 2003). All women have a risk of breast cancer (a lifetime risk of about 1 in 11 in the U.S. population), and they are offered mammography screening according to the standards of care or regional health policy. For women with a genetic family history that is consistent with familial breast and ovarian cancer, earlier and more frequent screening will be discussed by genetic and familial cancer specialists.

Two *autosomal* dominantly inherited conditions account for many familial cases of colorectal cancer. One is familial adenomatous polyposis (FAP). This condition is due to a mutation in the APC gene. The mutation causes the growth of multiple polyps inside the colon (usually at least 100), predisposing to adenocarcinoma of the colon or rectum. Individuals who are at risk are offered annual colonoscopic screening to detect and remove polyps, commencing at 10 to 12 years. However, the removal of individual polyps usually becomes unfeasible and the eventual treatment is colectomy, often in the late teens or early adulthood. This reduces cancer risk, but upper gastrointestinal tract endoscopy is still required, as some of those affected may develop polyps in the upper GI tract.

Another autosomal dominantly inherited familial colorectal cancer is hereditary nonpolyposis colon cancer (HNPCC). Families thought to have a HNPCC mutation are offered screening by colonoscopy from

---

Box 17–2

In 1992 the U.S. Public Health Service recommended that all women capable of becoming pregnant take 0.4 mg/400 mcg of folic acid daily. This is the amount of folic acid in most multivitamins. A daily intake of folic acid does not completely rule out the possibility that a baby will have a neural tube defect (NTD). However, for a couple with no prior history of NTDs, following the daily folic acid recommendations will reduce the chance for a NTD from the general population risk of 1 percent to about 0.5 to 0.7 percent (Centers for Disease Control,1992).

about 25 years of age. Additionally, screening for endometrial, stomach, and urinary tract cancer may be advised if cancers in those organs have been a feature of the family history or if there is a proven HNPCC mutation in the family. When a nurse identifies a family history of cancer, the family should be asked whether they would like to learn more about their risks by seeing a genetic or familial cancer specialist.

Discovery of health problems in more than one family member should be accompanied by a discussion with the family regarding its understanding of risks for potentially inherited disorders. Individuals and families may wish to be referred to an advanced practice genetics nurse, genetic counselor, or medical genetics specialist for a more comprehensive risk assessment and to learn about appropriate surveillance, health promotion, or diagnostic options.

Identification of risks based on one's family history is an important nursing responsibility. The ability to obtain a genetic family history requires sensitivity to the beliefs that people have about the causes of diseases within their family. Nurses assist individuals and families to obtain accurate information regarding genetic risks and treatment options when they identify family members' concerns and when they facilitate referrals for more comprehensive genetic evaluation and counseling.

ACUTE ILLNESS

As many genetic diseases result in inherent physical health problems, patients with a genetic condition often require acute medical or surgical care. For example, a child born with Down syndrome will require nursing care before, during, and after surgery for a congenital heart defect. An individual with cystic fibrosis or Duchenne muscular dystrophy will almost inevitably need treatment for acute respiratory infection at some stage in life. Of course, the individual with a genetic condition may also require acute health care for medical conditions that are not specifically connected with the genetic disease. In either case, attention to the patient's special needs brought on by the genetic condition is integral to good nursing care.

BENEFITS, NEGATIVE OUTCOMES, AND LIMITATIONS OF GENETIC TESTING

Genetic testing can be performed for several purposes, including prenatal diagnosis, detection of *carrier* status, predictive testing for familial disorders, and presymptomatic testing (Burke, 2002). The specific potential benefits, risks, and limitations of the tests are unique to each test. Nurses who participate in discussions about genetic testing must maintain current knowledge about these tests, as this information changes as new technology for testing and new interpretations of results become available. However, there are several general principles that apply to genetic tests.

Potential benefits of having a genetic test include the opportunity to learn whether one has, or has an increased likelihood of developing, an inherited disease. The test can lead to relief from worry about uncertainty about one's future health risks for a specific disease, and the results may be useful in making reproductive or disease management decisions.

Genetic tests also have negative outcomes, including the implications of genetic test results for disease risks of other biological relatives. It is important to remember that results of genetic tests are private and cannot be disclosed to other family members without the person's consent. Disclosure of one's test results to relatives can be difficult, and individuals undergoing genetic testing may need help from nurses and other health care providers in planning how to explain this information to relatives. Emotional distress over the results of the genetic test (either that one has a gene mutation or one does not) can occur. Moreover, persons undergoing genetic testing may be concerned about the potential for insurance or employment discrimination based on their genetic test results. Genetic tests also have limitations, and these will vary according to the specific test. For some tests, not all persons who want the test may qualify. This occurs when their family history does not suggest that the disease has a major genetic component. For some tests, it is possible that a result may be difficult to interpret and the person being tested may not know whether he or she is at increased risk to develop the disease. These are complex issues, and nurses who participate in genetic testing should become thoroughly prepared to provide education and assess understanding of the potential benefits, risks, and limitations of genetic testing (Burke, 2002; Scanlon & Fibison, 1995; Williams & Lea, 2002).

A clinical example illustrates the identification of a genetic condition in a patient who is admitted to the hospital for surgery. Maxine is a 34-year-old woman admitted for a cholecystectomy. The nurse who admits her obtains a genetic family history and records this in a three-generation pedigree, using the standardized symbols. He learns Maxine is worried about her children, particularly her daughter, who relies on her heavily. She has a 10-year-old son and a 6-year-old daughter. The daughter has hypotonia and attends a school for children with special educational needs. Maxine's parents are caring for the children, but as her mother has bilateral cataracts, this is not ideal. Maxine reports that she was in hospital for 8 days after the Cesarean section for her daughter, as they "couldn't wake her up properly." The anesthetist reads through her previous notes and is alerted to the fact that she did not respond well to the anesthetic agent during her Cesarean section. This and the history of cataracts in her mother indicate a possible diagnosis of myotonic dystrophy, an autosomal dominant genetic disorder. Maxine is offered a genetic test to determine whether she has myotonic dystrophy, and surgery is delayed for several days. The test result confirms that Maxine has myotonic dystrophy, and regional anesthesia is suggested as a safer option for Maxine (Rosenbaum & Miller, 2002). Prior to surgery she has an ECG, as patients with myotonic dystrophy are predisposed to cardiac arrhythmias.

Her children are tested and, as expected from the history, her daughter also has myotonic dystrophy. Her son is unaffected. For this family, the diagnosis has come as a shock, and the family needs time to adjust. An initial suggestion to discuss the risk of myotonic dystrophy with Maxine's brother is met with a refusal. The brother, Billy, has had a number of difficult events in his lifetime and Maxine does not want to worry him. However, after several months passed, Maxine decided that Billy should have the same right to be tested as she had. She is concerned that he might have an accident and his doctor would be unaware of the risks of anesthetic. She tells him and gives him a fact sheet provided by the genetic nurse, containing basic information about myotonic dystrophy, the nurse's contact details, and information about the local muscular dystrophy support group.

In this clinical example, collection of a family history revealed clinical data that were consistent with a genetic diagnosis. The family history also revealed clinical features of the diagnosis that were present in several family members. In addition to assisting with achieving an accurate diagnosis, the surgical nurse also recognized that the information was confidential and that Maxine was not ready to disclose the information to her brother. Through providing the intervention of Family Support (Iowa Interventions Project, 2000), the nurse continued to respect the family's values while also assisting Maxine to consider how disclosure of her diagnosis would be beneficial to her brother. Throughout the time the surgical nurse cared for Maxine, he also protected the privacy of Maxine's medical information and did not disclose this information to others, including family, until Maxine was ready to do so. Consideration of the impact of genetic information in an acute care situation encompasses addressing management of acute care problems as well as considering the impact of the diagnosis on each family member.

CHRONIC ILLNESS

Health problems with a major genetic component may improve, with appropriate treatment, or they may remain stable. Many conditions, however, lead to increasing loss of health and function throughout the person's life span. These genetic conditions require increasingly more complex care from health care providers and the family. In the chronic phase of a genetic condition, individuals and the family not only must come to terms with the permanent changes that come with the onset of symptoms of the illness (Rolland, 1994) but also must adapt their family routines and roles and locate needed resources to meet increasingly complex health care needs. One challenge that families face is making decisions about telling members of the family about the disorder and making decisions about predictive genetic testing. This can become even more complicated when more than one member of the family has the condition.

These issues are illustrated by using the example of Huntington disease (HD). HD is an inherited, progressive, neurodegenerative disorder characterized by involuntary motor movements, dementia, mood disturbances, and affective disorders. Although the onset can occur in childhood through old age, the average age at diagnosis is in one's middle 30s. This condition is inherited in an autosomal dominant manner. This means that each offspring of a person with HD has a 50 percent (1 in 2) chance of inheriting the gene that has the mutation associated with HD. The genetic mutation for HD has been identified, and adults who have a parent or grandparent with HD may have

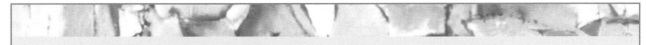

Brenda is a 34-year-old woman who recently learned that her ancestors had Huntington disease. Brenda's mother died in an automobile accident, and at a family gathering after her mother's services, an elderly aunt commented that it was a blessing that Brenda's mother did not develop the family disease. Brenda asked for more information, and her Aunt Helen said that several people on Brenda's mother's side, including her maternal grandmother, had died of HD. Brenda spoke with her father, who could not add much information, as Brenda's mother had moved away from her family as soon as she finished high school. Brenda talked with her brother, Steve, and they decided to seek predictive genetic testing to determine whether they had inherited the gene mutation for HD. Both Brenda and Steve agreed that they would not ask their other sister, Judy, as they believed she would not be interested in the information and it would only upset her.

predictive testing. In some families, older relatives have not lived near the family, or were placed in a long-term care facility, so younger family members may not know about the disease. One of the issues that family members face is the decision about when to tell family members about the disorder.

Families have their own traditions regarding sharing medical information. Some families are quite open, whereas others maintain the secrecy of medical information. In some families where there is a person with HD, parents may not pass the information on to offspring out of a need to protect them or out of a sense of shame because HD may have been misdiagnosed as alcoholism and dementia (Williams & Sobel, in press). In one study of families of persons with HD, most parents felt that the maturity of their children and their ability to comprehend the information were important. When families have not worked through the stages of grief associated with HD, other coping mechanisms such as denial may be important (Skirton, 1998).

Family discussion about HD includes not only the features of the disorder but also the implications of its inheritance. Family members may assume that people who most resemble the parent with HD are more likely to develop the condition. This process of *preselection* may influence the person's self-image and overall functioning (Kessler, 1988). Furthermore, when the family's beliefs are consistent with the person's actual risk, it can be difficult for people in the family to revise their ideas when the results of a genetic test reveal that the preselected person does not have the mutation for HD. There are many reasons for the difficulty in revising one's personal beliefs about disease risk. For example, siblings may have assumed that if one member of the family will develop the disease, others will be spared.

Predictive testing is the term that is used to refer to DNA testing to identify genetic mutations in persons who are at risk for a specific inherited disorder but do not have symptoms of the condition. Predictive testing is not possible for all inherited conditions.

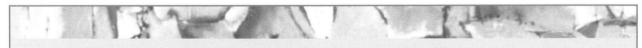

Fear of losing insurance is one reason that people at risk for specific inherited diseases decide not to have genetic testing. Although discrimination based on genetic information about a person is difficult to prove, some members of the public are concerned about this issue. The majority of states in the United States have passed some form of legislation addressing discrimination on the basis of genetic information and the privacy of this information. Nurses should be familiar with the statutes in the states in which they practice. In addition, the national Health Insurance Portability and Accountability Act (HIPAA) specifically bans certain uses of genetic information in identifying insurance eligibility. However, the act does not place limits on rates that insurance companies can require (Clayton, 2003).

However, if a gene mutation is commonly found in a disorder, as is the case with HD, or if a gene mutation is known to present in a person's family, then the test can identify whether a person is likely to develop the condition. Discussions about the potential benefits, risks, and limitations of genetic testing are usually conducted in a genetic testing clinical setting with genetics specialists. Maintaining the confidentiality of each family member's decision is critical and is consistent with the ethical principle of privacy. Family members may prefer to maintain privacy regarding their decision about predictive testing. This may reflect an attempt to avoid disagreements within the family or an attempt to protect others in the family from sadness or worry. People who have had predictive HD testing may also be reluctant to share this information with their primary care provider. This reflects a fear that any notation in their medical record may be accessed by an employer or insurance provider, leading to loss of employment or insurance.

Although laws have been passed in many states to prohibit insurance or employment discrimination based on a person's *genotype*, some individuals continue to be concerned that revealing their genotype may place them at risk for discrimination (Burgess, Adam, Bloch, & Hayden, 1997).

HD is just one example of an inherited disorder affecting multiple systems and requiring nursing interventions for both the individual and the family. In addition to the care required by the person with the condition, family members are coping with their own risks to develop the disease and, in some cases, deciding whether they want to have predictive testing. Despite these concerns, many family members attempt to maintain a sense of normalcy within the context of life with a chronic inherited condition. Respecting and supporting family efforts to maintain activities aimed at enjoying customary routines, in spite of limitations associated with the illness, is an important component of nursing care for the family.

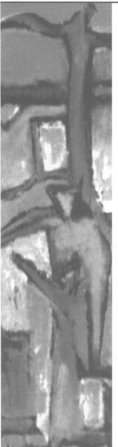

RESEARCH BRIEF

Purpose
The purpose of this study was to describe the concerns and psychosocial impact of predictive testing for Huntington disease on support persons, including members of the family.

Methods
Nineteen persons who had accompanied a person at risk for HD through the predictive genetic testing process (one was not a family member) responded to open-ended questions in a semi-structured interview. The 35- to 45-minute interviews were transcribed and the transcripts were analyzed for common themes.

Results
Family members attempted to provide constructive support to the person undergoing the testing. However, many were distressed about the implications of the test results for their own future responsibilities for their family member. Some family members had attempted to assume caregiver responsibilities. Others requested more specific information about HD and what they could expect to happen in the future.

Nursing Implications
This study identifies the importance for family members who accompany relatives through a predictive genetic testing process to receive information and emotional support from nurses and other health care providers. Family members need information and support not only during but also following the predictive testing process.

Source: Williams, J. K., Schutte, D. L., Holkup, P. A., Evers, C., & Muilenburg, A. (2000). Psychosocial impact of predictive testing for Huntington disease on support persons. *Neuropsychiatric Genetics, American Journal of Medical Genetics, 96*(3), 353–359.

END OF LIFE

Some genetic disorders shorten a person's life. End-of-life care for these families must include sensitivity to issues that arise when the condition is a genetic one.

Infants

One issue that a nurse should be aware of is the feeling of guilt that parents may experience when their newborn infant has a genetic condition that is life threatening. In some cases, infants with genetic disorders are born at the end of their lives. An example is an infant with Trisomy 18. Caused by the presence of an extra 18th chromosome in each of the cells in a baby's body, this condition is characterized by multiple, serious anomalies in major organs and systems. With supportive care, some infants with Trisomy 18 can survive beyond the usual life span. However, the majority of infants with this condition do not survive beyond their first birthday, and half die within the first month of life (Jorde et al., 1999). Although this condition is caused by a failure of chromosomes to separate during meiosis, parents may be troubled by feelings that they may have somehow caused the condition to occur in their infant. Parents should have the opportunity to meet with genetic specialists to discuss their questions about the cause and potential recurrence of this condition in their family.

Assisting parents with preparing for the loss of their baby is a nursing responsibility, and many of the activities that are useful for other parents losing children to non-genetic conditions will be appropriate. Examples of nursing activities in Grief Work Facilitation (Iowa Interventions Project, 2000) include the following:

- Encouraging parents to discuss their views about discontinuing life support
- Creating a private personalized environment for baptism if that is the parents' request
- Respecting parents' wishes regarding holding the infant through the end of the infant's life
- Creating keepsakes for the family

It is important that nurses avoid making comments that may be perceived as hurtful by parents or that indicate a lack of respect for the importance this baby had in the family's life. Comments such as "It's best to let your baby go" or "You can always try again" may not reflect the parents' feelings and limit the abilities of the nurse to provide individualized care.

Adolescents and Young Adults

End-of-life care is also important for families of teenagers or young adults who have a progressive genetic disorder. Duchenne muscular dystrophy (DMD) is a genetic condition that causes loss of muscle function, leading to death in the teen or early adult years due to cardiac or respiratory failure (Jorde et al., 1999). With new treatments, life expectancy may lengthen, but as yet no treatments have been found that alter the outcome of the disease. This is an X-linked recessive disorder, meaning that the mother may be a carrier of

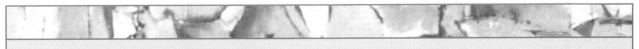

Jorge and Maria are the parents of twins; John in a normal newborn, and Joseph has multiple anomalies. He is found to have Trisomy 18. Maria delivered the babies at 34 weeks of gestation, and the infants are in the neonatal intensive care unit. Several physicians examined Joseph, and they have discussed Joseph's prognosis with the parents. Maria and Jorge have a 6-year-old daughter. Maria had hoped to have a large family, but she has had difficulty becoming pregnant. After discussing Joseph's prognosis with their family and their pastor, they decide not to request surgery for Joseph. They ask that the hospital chaplain baptize their baby, and the nurse offers to make a photographic record. They tell her that they do not want any photos, but they do accept her offer of the small shell that the chaplain used as the container for the water used in the baptism. Because of his serious congenital anomalies, Joseph is not expected to live for more than a few days. The nurse asks Maria if she would like to hold Joseph, and Maria accepts the nurse's offer, requesting that the nurse stay with her when she holds her baby. Jorge goes home to be with their daughter, telling the nurse that he cannot bear to stay. Maria held Joseph several times throughout the next 24 hours, and on the fifth day of life, he died.

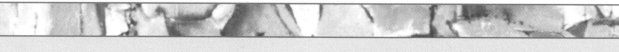

Barry is a 17-year-old boy who has Duchenne muscular dystrophy. He is the second of three children: his older sister Shelley is 19 and their younger brother Bradley is 12. Bradley also has DMD. Barry has been confined to a wheelchair since he was 11 years old. He now is having difficulty breathing, and his physician has talked with Barry and his parents about whether Barry wants to be put on a ventilator. Barry and his parents decide they do not want this option. The nurse in the neuromuscular disease management program has known Barry since he was 4 years old, and she and Barry enjoy talking with each other. She asks Barry if there are any things he would like to ask her. As they talk, Barry tells her about some items that he would like certain friends to have after he has died. Barry told the nurse that it was too hard to talk with his mom about these thoughts.

the gene mutation. In some families, there may be more than one boy with this condition.

Nurses and physicians are beginning to understand how to address family concerns about this disorder, especially regarding whether to request ventilator support when the person with DMD can no longer maintain respirations on his own. One nurse learned that parents wanted to discuss this decision but were hesitant to ask their health care providers; physicians also were hesitant to ask parents and teens about their wishes (Trout, 1997). The viewpoint of the teenaged boy or young adult with DMD also needs to be considered when decisions regarding life support, such as the use of a ventilator, are being considered. Families who have made a decision regarding end-of-life care need support from health care providers in documenting and communicating these decisions to health care providers who do not know the family.

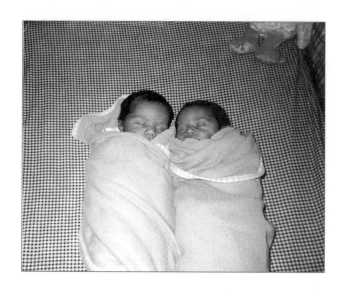

NURSING IMPLICATIONS

Understanding of how genetic factors influence health, risk for illness, and response to treatments will continue to emerge from research on the human genome. Nurses must be able to use this information to address health care needs of individuals and their families.

66 Application of genetic knowledge to nursing practice relies on a well-informed nursing workforce. Educational resources, including Web-based resources, are available to educators to promote integration of genetic concepts into nursing education. 99

Education

Application of genetic knowledge to nursing practice relies on a well-informed nursing workforce. Educational resources, including Web-based resources, are available to educators to promote integration of genetic concepts into nursing education. Although the scope of content will vary according to levels of nursing education, all nurses should receive education to enable them to (1) participate in collecting and obtaining genetic history information, (2) offer genetic information and provide explanations of genetic resources, (3) participate in the informed consent and informed decision-making process, (4) participate in the management of persons and families with conditions with a genetic component, and (5) evaluate and monitor the impact of genetic conditions, testing, and treatments on the person and the family (ISONG, 1998; Lea, Jenkins, & Francomano, 1998). This will require nurse educators who are knowledgeable regarding genetic issues that affect health and illness, as well as collaboration with genetics experts who specialize in the care of persons with genetically linked diseases. The detailed list of core competencies for all health care providers is a useful guideline for educators (NCHPEG, 2000).

Practice

Genetic factors that place people at risk for disease or affect their responses to treatments influence the health of individuals and members of their families. Nurses who understand the contributions of genetic factors will be able to use this knowledge in their practice, regardless of population or care setting. Core competencies (NCHPEG, 2000) for health professionals provide common guidelines for health professionals to integrate genetics into their practices.

Nurses must include knowledge of genetics in their patient and family assessments. Whenever a nurse meets a patient or family, the nurse can begin integrating genetics knowledge into the assessment process by being prepared to analyze the response to the assessment question: "Tell me about the health of your family members." Excellent resources to assist nurses to focus their genetic risk assessment questions can be found in current nursing journal articles, in educational materials, and in ongoing in-service opportunities. For example, the monograph "Genetic Issues for Perinatal Nurses," published by the March of Dimes (Williams & Lea, 2002), contains a step-by-step description of the family genetic risk assessment process. An example of in-service activities that focus on supporting integration of genetic knowledge into nursing practice is the genomics education program that is ongoing for over 5000 nurses who are employed at the Mayo Clinic (Pestka, 2004). These are just two examples of strategies to introduce and sustain implementation of genetics concepts into nursing practice.

One implication of genetic discovery for families is the need for nurses to continue to become aware of cultural values that may differ from their own and that will influence the decisions families make about genetic health topics. Traditions that reflect Western values—such as assuming that individuals, rather than family leaders, make health care decisions—will

require continued attention by all care providers. Although these beliefs may not be reflected in formal health care policies or procedures, they influence behaviors. Nurses who are aware of the values and beliefs of the families of their patients who are from another culture may alter practices that are offensive or inappropriate for these families.

Research

Research with families regarding genetic issues is very limited. However, researchers are beginning to develop a research-based body of knowledge in several important areas. Experiences of siblings of children with Down syndrome have been documented (Van Riper, 2000). Concerns such as sibling participation in long-term care planning for a family member with a condition that limits health or functional ability are as yet unreported. This is a topic for which additional family-focused research is needed.

Family needs regarding providing care to family members with HD are identified in the United States and in the United Kingdom (Rehak et al., 2003; Skirton & Glendinning, 1997). In the United Kingdom, this data led to the development of home health services that are consistent with family needs. The views of family members who accompany persons at risk for HD through predictive genetic testing also identified a need for information and caregiving support (Williams, Schutte, Holkup, Evers, & Muilenburg, 2000).

Research is needed in several important areas, including understanding the processes and factors that influence disclosure of genetic test results within families. Early research in this area suggests that disclosure is difficult when a person is the first in the family to be tested, and disclosure can be influenced by many variables such as gender, emotional closeness to the relative, and family patterns of sharing of medical information (Hamilton, 2003; Smith, West, Croyle, & Botkin, 1999). The impact of this disclosure on family members' understanding of genetic risks and on their own health promotion or disease prevention behaviors is, as yet, unknown.

Although the body of genetic nursing literature contains many descriptions of genetic conditions, nursing interventions with persons with genetic conditions, and integration of new genetic knowledge into clinical care, little of the clinical literature is concerned with family issues. Outcomes of nursing

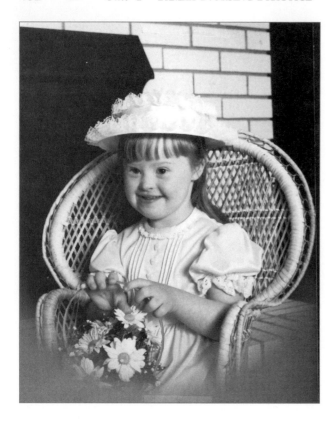

interventions, such as Family Therapy (Iowa Interventions Project, 2000) following the receipt of genetic risk information, have not yet been examined and reported. As noted throughout the chapter, communication of genetic information, coping with risk for illness among family members who are biologically related, and maximizing the abilities of the family to meet the health care needs of persons within the family are all topics for which research-based knowledge is not yet developed.

Health Policy

The impact of genetic discovery on family nursing has had several policy implications. One is the need to include knowledge required to support basic genetic competencies on licensure and on credentialing examinations. The American Academy of Nursing supports inclusion of genetic competencies for professional nurses (Lea, 2002), and in the United Kingdom the Department of Health is supporting work to define the basic competencies in genetics required for nurses at the point of their initial general professional registration (Genomics Policy Unit, 2003).

Continued efforts to strengthen legislation that prohibits discrimination based on one's genetic family history are essential. Nurses should support legislators who develop these laws but should also assist members of communities and employers to avoid situations where persons with a family history of an inherited condition are disadvantaged.

SUMMARY

Virtually all disease has a genetic component, as genes influence the body's response to all environmental agents, including microorganisms. This chapter focused on the effects of genetic diseases that are directly attributable to a mutation in one gene or to a chromosomal abnormality rather than on those that occur as a result of complex gene/environment interactions.

In many cases, biological relatives will share genetic risks—risks of inheriting a condition or passing it to their offspring. Although in some cases genetic testing has enabled those at risk to be identified before birth or before the onset of the disease, the options for testing also raise difficult issues for families and may cause internal conflict for individuals and disruption to the family. Ethics is a subject that cannot be confined to any specialty but should be entwined into the fabric of each nurse's professional practice. When dealing with families, specific ethical dilemmas resulting from the conflicts of interest between family members may arise; nurses cannot solve these dilemmas alone but should contribute constructively to the discussion.

Genetic disease may affect individuals at all stages of the life span, and nurses from all fields of health care are involved in caring for families who are dealing with the effects of genetic disease. Nurses must have a basic knowledge of genetics and inherited diseases, but they must also possess the skills to support the family through periods of adjustment and decision making. Acknowledging the family's experience of the genetic condition and their lay beliefs is essential to the nursing process.

CASE STUDY ➤

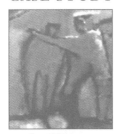

Mohammed and Alicia Ahmed are a couple in their late 20s. They live in a large city, and Mohammed develops software for a large corporation. Alicia is a primary-school teacher. In her first pregnancy, Alicia had some bleeding and miscarried at 9 weeks. No cause was found for the miscarriage, but Mohammed and Alicia felt that it was "just one of those things." Alicia had no problems becoming pregnant again and after the first 9 weeks was able to relax and really enjoy her pregnancy. She felt so lucky not to have any morning sickness and had a normal delivery. Mohammed was thrilled to be present at the birth of his daughter, Melissah.

Melissah did not pass her newborn hearing screening test, and after further investigation, she was found to have profound neurosensory deafness. Alicia and Mohammed were devastated. Their initial reaction was disbelief, but over the following weeks they began to wonder what had caused the problem. The pediatrician arranged for the couple to be seen by the genetics advanced practice nurse. She took a family history, finding out that there was no history of deafness in the family. However, when she drew the family tree, she learned that Alicia and Mohammed were second cousins. She explained that Melissah's hearing loss was likely caused by a recessive gene mutation carried by each parent. Carriers of a recessive gene mutation also have one normal copy of the gene; they usually have no signs of the condition. A baby may inherit a faulty copy of the same gene from both parents and therefore have no normal copy of that gene. The chance of any future child having the hearing loss was 1 in 4 for each pregnancy. The APN was most concerned about offering the family support as they tried to deal with a range of difficult emotions connected with this information.

Alicia and Mohammed expressed guilt at having caused their daughter's deafness. Although individuals have no control over which genes are passed on to the offspring, guilt is a common reaction in parents. The chance of a child inheriting a recessive condition is slightly higher if the parents are biological relatives related before marriage, and their consanguinity just added to their guilt. They felt that if they had not married each other, there would have been no problem. The couple came from a traditional Pakistani family, where large families are the norm, and they had planned on having a larger family. These plans were thrown into confusion, as they wondered whether they should risk having other children with hearing loss.

The genetics APN spent time with the couple over several months, listening to their concerns. It was particularly important not to offer advice, as each couple needs to come to the decision that is right for them in their particular circumstances. Overwhelming support from their families helped them. Melissah made progress after she was fitted with an implanted device to help her hearing. Gradually, the couple was able to accept that they had no direct influence on the situation with Melissah. However, they decided that they could not bear the guilt if the same thing should happen to another child. Prenatal diagnosis was not an option for them, as they strongly believed it would be wrong to start a pregnancy and then take the child's life. The family receives ongoing help from the pediatric nurse involved in the auditory clinic. They can contact the genetic APN if they wish to have further discussion in the future about any genetic aspects of the condition.

Discussion Questions

1. Mohammed and Alicia do not want to consider prenatal testing for any future pregnancies. It is customary for this information to be shared with parents of a child with a genetic condition. Should this information be offered to this couple?

2. Alicia tells the nurse that she is not able to talk with her husband's parents about Melissah's hearing loss, as they blame her for the problem. How would you respond to Alicia?

3. Some parents with deafness prefer to have children who also have profound hearing loss. How would you respond to Mohammed and Alicia if they were hearing impaired and wanted to have only hearing-impaired children?

References

AGNC code of ethics. (2003). Retrieved from http://www.agnc.co.uk/code_of_ethics.htm

American Association of Colleges of Nursing. (1998). *The essentials of baccalaureate nursing education for professional nursing practice.* Washington, DC: American Association of Colleges of Nursing.

Bennett, R. L. (1999). *The practical guide to the genetic family history.* New York: Wiley-Liss.

Bowe, K. (1995). Phenylketonuria: An update for pediatric community health nurses. *Pediatric Nursing, 21*(2), 191–194.

Burgess, M. M., Adam, S., Bloch, M., & Hayden, M. R. (1997). Dilemmas of anonymous predictive testing for Huntington disease: Privacy vs. optimal care. *American Journal of Human Genetics, 71*(2), 197–201.

Burke, W. (2002). Genetic testing. *New England Journal of Medicine, 347,* 1867–1875.

Burnham, J. B. (1986). *Family therapy.* London: Routledge.

Centers for Disease Control and Prevention. (1992, September 11). Recommendations for the use of folic acid to reduce the number of cases of spina bifida and other neural tube defects. *Morbidity and Mortality Weekly Report, 41*(RR-14).

Clayton, E. W. (2003). Ethical, legal, and social implications of genomic medicine. *New England Journal of Medicine, 349,* 4462–4469.

Cole, T. R. P., & Sleightholme, H. V. (2000). ABC of colorectal cancer. The role of clinical genetics in management. *British Medical Journal, 321,* 943–946.

Collins, F. S., Green, E. D., Guttmacher, A. E., & Guyer, M. S. (2003). A vision for the future of genomics research: A blueprint for the genomic era. *Nature, 422*(6934), 835–847.

Dallos, R., & Draper, R. (2000). *Introduction to family therapy.* Maidenhead: Open University Press.

Feetham, S. L. (1999). Families and the genetic revolution: Implications for primary healthcare, education, and research. *Family, Systems & Health, 17*(1), 27–43.

Finney Rutten, L. J., & Iannotti, R. J. (2003). Health beliefs, salience of breast cancer family history, and involvement with breast cancer issues: Adherence to annual mammography screening recommendations. *Cancer Detection and Prevention, 27*(5), 353–359.

Genomics Policy Unit. (2003). *Fit for practice in the genetics era: Defining what nurses, midwives and health visitors should know and be able to do in relation to genetics.* Report compiled by the Genomics Policy Unit, University of Glamorgan, and Medical Genetics Service for Wales, University Hospital of Wales.

GNCC. (2003). *Welcome to GNCC Online.* Retrieved December 28, 2003, from http://www.gncc@geneticnurse.org

Grant, S. S. (2000). Prenatal genetic screening. *Online Journal of Issues in Nursing, 5*(3).

Hamilton, R. (2003). *Experiencing predictive genetic testing: A grounded theory study of families.* Unpublished dissertation, University of Wisconsin, Madison.

Harper, P. S. (1998). *Practical genetic counselling* (5th ed.). Oxford: Butterworth Heinemann.

Hodgson, E. V., & Maher, E. R. (1999). *A practical guide to human cancer genetics* (2nd ed.). Cambridge: Cambridge University Press.

Iowa Interventions Project. (2000). In J. C. McCloskey & G. M. Bulechek (Eds.), *Nursing interventions classification (NIC)* (3rd ed.). St Louis: Mosby.

ISONG, International Society of Nurses in Genetics. (1998). *Statement on the scope and standards of genetics clinical nursing practice.* Washington, DC: American Nurses Association.

Janz, N. K., Wren, P. A., Schottenfeld, D., & Guire, K. E. (2003). Colorectal cancer screening attitudes and behavior: A population-based study. *Preventive Medicine, 37*(6), 627–634.

Jenkins, J., & Collins, F. S. (2003). Are you genetically literate? *American Journal of Nursing, 103*(4), 13.

Jorde, L., Carey, J., Bamshad, M., & White, R. (1999). *Medical genetics* (2nd ed.). St. Louis: Mosby.

Kessler, S. (1988). Invited essay on the psychological aspect of genetic testing V. Preselection: A family coping mechanism. *American Journal of Medical Genetics, 31,* 617–621.

Knebel, A., & Hudgings, C. (2002). End-of-life issues in genetic disorders: Literature and research directions. *Genetics in Medicine, 4*(5), 366–372.

Kruglanski, A. W. (1989). *Lay epistemics and human knowledge.* New York: Plenum Press.

Lau, R. (1997). Cognitive representations of health and illness. In D. Gochman (Ed.), *Handbook of health behavior research* (Vol. 1, pp. 51–70). New York: Plenum.

Lau, R. R., & Hartmann, K. A. (1983). Common sense representations of common illnesses. *Health Psychology, 2,* 167–185.

Lea, D. H. (2002). American Academy of Nursing position statement: Integrating genetics competencies into baccalaureate and advanced nursing education. *Nursing Outlook, 50*(4), 167.

Lea, D. H., Jenkins, J. F, Francomano, C. A. (1998). *Genetics in clinical practice: New directions for nursing and health care.* Sudbury, MA: Jones & Bartlett.

Leventhal, E. A., & Crouch, M. (1997). Are there differences in perceptions of illness across the lifespan? In K. J. Petrie & J. A. Weinman (Eds.), *Perceptions of health and illness.* Amsterdam: Harwood Academic Publishers.

Leventhal, H., Benyamini, Y., Brownlee, S., Diefenbach, M., Leventhal, E. A., Patrick-Miller, L., & Robitaille, C. (1997). Illness representations: Theoretical foundations. In K. J. Petrie & J. A. Weinman (Eds.), *Perceptions of health and illness.* Amsterdam: Harwood Academic Publishers.

Loescher, L. (2003). Cancer worry in women with hereditary risk factors for breast cancer. *Oncology Nursing Forum, 39*(5), 767–772.

Lynch, J., & Lynch, H. (1994). Genetic counseling and HNPCC. *Anticancer Research, 14,* 1651–1656.

Manetti, L., Pierro, A., Kruglanski, A., Taris, T., & Benzinovic, P. (2002). A cross-cultural study of the need for cognitive closure scale: Comparing its structure in Croatia, Italy, the USA, and the Netherlands. *British Journal of Social Psychology, 41,* 139–156.

Miki, Y., Swensen, J., Shattuck-Eidens, D., Fatreal, P. A., Harshman, K., Tavtigian, S., et al. (1994). A strong candidate for the breast and ovarian cancer susceptibility gene, BRCA1. *Science, 266,* 66–71.

Miller, S. M. (1995). Monitoring versus blunting styles of coping with cancer influence the information patients want and need about their disease. Implications for cancer screening and management. *Cancer, 76*(2), 167–177.

MRC Vitamin Study Research Group. (1991). Prevention of neural tube defects. *Lancet, 338,* 131–137.

NCHPEG, National Coalition for Health Professional Education in Genetics. (2000). *Core competencies in genetics essential for all health-care professionals.* Retrieved December 7, 2000, from *http://www.nchpeg.org/news-box/corecompetencies000.html*

NCHPEG, National Coalition for Health Professional Education in Genetics. (2003, Spring). *The genetic family history: A newsletter for health professionals.* Retrieved February 6, 2004, from *http://www.nchpeg.org/newsletter/inpracticespr03.pdf*

Oncology Nursing Society. (2003). *Genetics and cancer care: A guide for oncology nurses.* Retrieved November 26, 2003, from *www.ons.org/xp6/ONS/Clinical.xml/GeneticsToolkit.xml*

Pestka, E. L. (2004, January). *Genomics education for nurses in practice.* Poster session presented at the annual meeting of the National Coalition for Health Professional Education in Genetics, Bethesda, MD.

Rees, C. E., & Bath, P. A. (2000). The psychometric properties of the Miller Behavioural Style Scale with adult daughters of women with early breast cancer: A literature review and empirical study. *Journal of Advanced Nursing, 32*(2), 366–374.

Rehak, D., Schutte, D., Williams, J., McGonigal-Kenney, M., Pehler, S., Jarmon, L., & Paulsen, J. (2003, November). *Caregiving in families experiencing Huntington disease.* Poster session presented at the annual meeting of the International Society of Nurses in Genetics, Los Angeles, CA.

Richards, M. P. M. (1993). The new genetics: Some issues for social scientists. *Sociology of Health and Illness, 15*, 567–586.

Rolland, J. (1994). *Families, illness, & disability: An integrative treatment model.* New York: Basic Books.

Rosenbaum, H. K., & Miller, J. D. (2002). Malignant hyperthermia and myotonic disorders. *Anesthesiology Clinics of North America, 20*(3), 623–664.

Rothbaum, F., Rosen, K., Ujiie, T., & Uchida, N. (2002). Family systems theory, attachment theory, and culture. *Family Process, 41*(3), 328–350.

Scanlon, C., & Fibison, W. (1995). *Managing genetic information: Implications for nursing practice.* Washington, DC: American Nurses Association.

Skirton, H. (1998). Telling the children. In A. Clarke (Ed.), *The genetic testing of children* (pp. 103–112). Oxford, UK: Bios.

Skirton, H. (2001). The client's perspective of genetic counseling—A grounded theory study. *Journal of Genetic Counseling, 10*(4), 311–327.

Skirton, H., & Eiser, C. (2003). Discovering and addressing the client's lay construct of genetic disease: An important aspect of genetic healthcare? *Research and Theory for Nursing Practice: An International Journal, 17*(4), 339–352.

Skirton, H., & Glendinning, N. (1997). Using research to develop care for patients with Huntington's disease. *British Journal of Nursing, 6*(2), 83–90.

Skirton, H., & Patch, C. (2002). *Genetics for healthcare professionals: A lifestage approach.* Oxford: Bios.

Smith, K. R., West, J. A., Croyle, R. T., & Botkin, J. R. (1999). Familial context of genetic testing for cancer susceptibility: Moderating effect of siblings' test results on psychological distress one to two weeks after BRCA1 mutation testing. *Cancer Epidemiology, Biomarkers & Prevention, 8*, 385–392.

Trout, C. (1997). *Concerns about death of teens with DMD.* Unpublished master's project, University of Iowa.

Van Riper, M. (2000). Family variables associated with well-being in siblings of children with Down syndrome. *Journal of Family Nursing, 6*(3), 267–286.

Webster, D. M., & Kruglanski, A. W. (1994). Individual differences in need for cognitive closure. *Journal of Personality and Social Psychology, 67*, 1049–1062.

Williams, J. K., & Lea, D. H. (2002). *Genetic issues for perinatal nurses* (2nd ed.). White Plains, NY: March of Dimes Birth Defects Foundation.

Williams, J. K., Schutte, D. L., Holkup, P. A., Evers, C., & Muilenburg, A. (2000). Psychosocial impact of predictive testing for Huntington disease on support persons. *Neuropsychiatric Genetics, American Journal of Medical Genetics, 96*(3), 353–359.

Williams, J. K., & Sobel, S. (in press). Genetic conditions: The example of Huntington disease. In S. Miller, S. McDaniel, J. Rolland, & S. Feetham (Eds.), *Individuals, families, and the new genetics.*

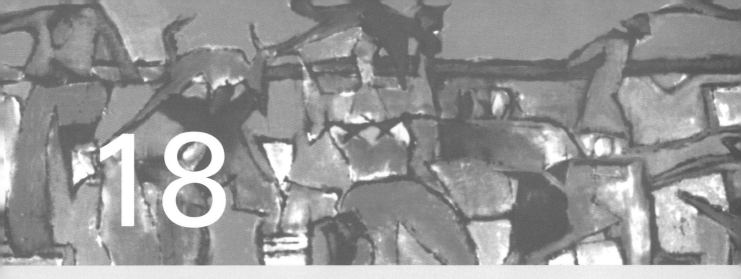

18

International Family Nursing

Susan Elliott, PhD, RNC, FNP, WHNP

CRITICAL CONCEPTS

- Professional registered and advanced practice nurses cross international borders to practice, consult, educate, and conduct nursing research.

- Although multiple nations are integrating family theories into nursing education and practice, no one family nursing theory is universal in application to all global cultures.

- Cultural awareness, sensitivity, and adaptation are essential to successful international experiences. No nurse can be competent in the care of all culturally diverse patients.

- Health and well-being are ultimately defined by the client, family, community, or culture. Health practices are influenced by poverty, gender inequality, lack of adequate food supply or appropriate intake, lack of pure water supply, poor sanitation, the sociopolitical environment, the level of illiteracy/education, and spiritual beliefs and rituals.

- Community-based health care is a proven international nursing practice model and research agenda.

- The nurse should not enter a cultural experience with a predetermined definition, theory, and action care plan but rather should enter the encounter with an openness to begin learning by listening and observing.

- Nurses are at risk if they practice with the false assumptions and expectations that all clients from a given culture will respond in the same manner.

- Unless the patient, family, community, and culture unite in common health-promoting beliefs and practices, the health of the family is in jeopardy.

- As women are the primary global lay and professional caregivers, nurses are encouraged to empower women by seeking organizational support of programs that enhance women's confidence and decision-making abilities, aid in improving women's access to health care, and develop women's health partnerships and community-based health workers.

INTRODUCTION

Nurses are the primary providers of global health care, especially to underserved families living in rural and isolated areas (Vonderheid & Al-Gasseer, 2002; Youssef & Tornquist, 1997). Influenced by the love of travel, a spiritual calling, challenging new career opportunities, a desire to serve in unique and diverse settings, or financial enticements, nurses are now crossing international borders in record numbers (see Box 18–1). Wherever and whatever the scope of the nursing practice, care of the family and community, as well as the individual, has long been fundamental to who nurses are and what nurses do. In 1933, Harmer wrote: "The patient can never be rightly understood or adequately cared for considered apart from his family and community relationships . . . the nurse is therefore concerned not only with the care of the individual patient but with the family, the community, and the health of the people" (Harmer, 1933, p. 5).

In addition to the United States, nations who formally promote family nursing theories are limited. Examples include Japan, Finland, Sweden, Korea, Iceland, Chile, Portugal, and Canada. As is discussed later in this chapter, this list expands when the definition of family includes community. However, with international nursing migration at an all-time high, it should be presumed that the majority of nurses coming from Third World nations to work in the United States have not been formally educated in family nursing theory (Flynn & Aiken, 2002).

The purpose of this chapter is to introduce issues common to providing family nursing care in culturally diverse international settings, to discuss issues that impact global health and well-being, and to discuss community-based health care as a proven international family nursing practice model. The purpose is not to discuss each family theory from an international perspective. It is to discuss international issues to be considered when applying family theories in international environments. "Nurses" and "nursing" refer to professional registered nurses and advanced practice nurses.

Nursing care promotes family health. The World Health Organization (WHO) defines health not only as the absence of disease or deformity but also as living at the highest standard of well-being possible (Toebes, 1999). International nursing involves all nurses caring for the global community, Westernized nurses caring for patients from and in Third World communities, and Third World nurses advancing in the care of their own. The WHO encourages member nations to have nurse and nurse-midwife involvement in all levels of health policy decision making, in the expansion of nurse and midwifery practice roles and services, in the expansion of resources for nursing education and research, and in the accountability for such actions to the WHO (Thompson, 2002; Vonderheid & Al-Gasseer, 2002). Utilizing the wide range of entry-level education, practice role labels, and requirements, the WHO (2002) identifies the following common attributes of global nursing practice:

Box 18–1   INTERNATIONAL FAMILY NURSING OPPORTUNITIES

Many private organizations and national governments require a minimum bachelor of science degree for employment and/or to obtain registered nurse credentials. The following is a sample of global career and service opportunities for nurses.

- American Embassy and Department of State staff
- World Health Organization
- Private corporation employee health
- Cruise ship staff
- Government consultations in health policy, nursing education, conflict resolution
- Faculty for nursing schools and universities
- Peace Corps
- Career assignment or volunteer service through faith-based and nonprofit organizations such as World Vision, Mercy and Truth, Empowering Lives International, Doctors Without Borders, and Nazarene Compassionate Ministries
- Student nurse international experience

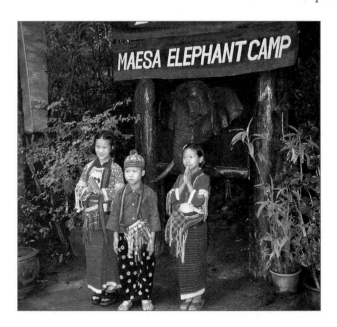

- Caring for, supporting, and comforting clients
- Continuously assessing and monitoring health needs and responses to interventions
- Advocacy and education of clients and communities
- Identifying care gaps and developing appropriate responses
- Delivering and coordinating health services across the care spectrum

Table 18–1 identifies leading global health concerns that require nursing prevention and intervention. Infectious diseases, most certainly HIV/AIDS, malaria, upper respiratory, and diarrhea-causing diseases, as well as maternal hemorrhage and infection, continue to disproportionately affect developing nations. Chronic disease, such as cardiovascular disease, diabetes, obesity, and cancer, is now recognized as a global health crisis (Joint WHO/FAO Expert Consultation, 2003). Health conditions are influenced not only by pathophysiological processes but also by poverty, illiteracy, gender inequality, war and conflict, unstable and disinterested governmental systems, and environmental concerns that include inadequate nutrition, safe water sources, and sanitation (Organisation [sic] for Economic Co-operation and Development, 2003). Common to undeveloped nations is the lack of interest in, and/or infrastructure for, promotion of health and disease prevention. The lack of access to health care is then compounded by the active recruitment of Third World nurses to high-paying positions in the United States, England, Germany, Australia, and other developed nations. International nursing migration divides family and friends while widening the gap in the existing crisis health care systems.

> 66 Health conditions are influenced not only by pathophysiological processes but also by poverty, illiteracy, gender inequality, war and conflict, unstable and disinterested governmental systems, and environmental concerns that include inadequate nutrition, safe water sources, and sanitation (Organisation [sic] for Economic Co-operation and Development, 2003). 99

NURSING EDUCATION

A growing number of domestic schools of nursing and universities are enhancing international health content in their core curriculum, offering their students international experiences and/or establishing new international health specialty options. Point Loma Nazarene University (San Diego, California) offers their undergraduate nursing students experiences in Romania, India, and Mexico. California State University (Los Angeles, California) includes an optional international health experience in their graduate International Health Family Nurse Practitioner program. Azusa Pacific University (Azusa, California) now offers a Ph.D. in International Health Nursing.

These learning opportunities are consistent with the goals, objectives, and nursing competencies of the American Association of Colleges of Nursing (1998, 2003), the National Organization of Nurse Practitioner Faculties (2004), the World Health Organization, and the International Council of Nursing (Goodyear, 2003). All promote cultural sensitivity in evidence-based research and practice, supported by a growing body of scholarly nursing journals publishing international data and practice guidelines. Such learning opportunities also promote language acquisition, helping to meet the national standards for culturally and linguistically appropriate services in health care (Department of Health and Human Services, 2000).

Based on a survey of 100 schools of nursing, da Gloria Miotto Wright, Godue, Manfredi, and Korniewicz (1998) recommended that the following international health content be included in nursing curriculums:

1. Social, political, economic, health, and demographic trends that influence the design and

Table 18-1 | **GLOBAL LEADING CAUSES OF DEATH, BOTH SEXES**

RANK	0-4 YR.	5-14 YR.	15-29 YR.	30-44 YR.	45-59 YR.	>60 YR.
1	Lower respiratory infections 2,134,248	Childhood cluster diseases 200,139	HIV/AIDS 855,406	HIV/AIDS 1,249,048	Ischemic heart disease 931,267	Ischemic heart disease 5,694,495
2	Diarrheal diseases 1,315,412	Road traffic injuries 118,212	Tuberculosis 354,692	Cerebrovascular accidents 368,501	Cardiovascular disease 573,065	Cardiovascular disease 4,312,376
3	Childhood cluster diseases 1,108,666	Drowning 113,614	Tuberculosis 238,021	Road traffic injuries 302,922	Tuberculosis 413,851	Chronic obstructive pulmonary diseases 2,285,834
4	Low birth weight 1,025,488	Lower respiratory infections 112,739	Self-inflicted injuries 216,661	Ischemic heart disease 224,986	HIV/AIDS 322,996	Lower respiratory infections 1,225,643
5	Malaria 905,838	Diarrheal diseases 88,430	Interpersonal violence 188,451	Self-inflected injuries 215,263	Trachea, bronchus, lung cancers 275,895	Trachea, bronchus, lung cancers 886,787
6	Birth asphyxia and birth trauma 787,179	Malaria 76,257	War injuries 95,015	Interpersonal violence 146,751	Cirrhosis of liver 226,975	Hypertensive heart disease 754,495
7	HIV/AIDS 419,480	HIV/AIDS 46,022	Drowning 78,639	Cerebrovascular accidents 145,965	Lower respiratory infections 226,105	Diabetes mellitus 612,725

(continued on page 461)

8	Congenital heart anomalies 281,751	War injuries 43,671	Lower respiratory infections 65,153	Cirrhosis of liver 135,072	Road traffic injuries 212,040	Tuberculosis 536,303
9	Protein-energy malnutrition 172,530	Tuberculosis 36,362	Poisonings 61,865	Lower respiratory infections 102,431	Diarrheal diseases 210,994	Stomach cancer 529,461
10	STDs excluding HIV 142,176	Tropical cluster diseases 31,845	Fires 61,341	Liver cancer 84,279	Chronic obstructive pulmonary disease 181,458	Colon and rectal cancers 441,961

Note: Because of poor reporting policies and strategies in many nations, the above statistics are considered to be lower than reality. In addition to those listed, the top 10 causes of global female morbidity and mortality include breast cancer, maternal hemorrhage, uterine cancer, and fires. For males, causes include meningitis, unipolar and bipolar depressive disorders, alcohol abuse, and falls. Because the majority of vehicle-related deaths are not accidents, the WHO uses the term "road traffic injuries."

Source: World Health Organization. (2000). *Injury: A leading cause of the global burden of disease.* Geneva: Author.

HISTORICAL PERSPECTIVES

International and missionary nursing were formally established by Florence Nightingale. Nightingale stated, "On February 7, 1837, God spoke to me and called me to His service" (Florence Nightingale Museum, 1999). She would later cross borders and serve in an international environment, establishing a foundation for modern nursing to serve around the world. For the next 100 years, missionary nurses were the primary crossers of international borders in the care of global populations and in the establishment of nursing education programs for indigenous peoples (Elliott, 2000).

The International Council of Nursing (ICN) was formed in 1889, and today ICN has 125 member nations. ICN defines nursing as encompassing "autonomous and collaborative care of individuals of all ages, families, groups and communities, sick or well and in all settings. Nursing includes the promotion of health, prevention of illness, and the care of ill, disabled and dying people. Advocacy, promotion of a safe environment, research, participation in shaping health policy and in patient and health systems management, and education are also key nursing roles" (International Council of Nursing, 2002). In an effort to ensure global safe professional nursing care, ICN recently published *ICN Framework of Competencies for the Generalist Nurse* in February 2003 (International Council of Nursing, 2004).

implementation of a health care system at both national and international levels

2. A strategic plan with international health curriculum and activities, with faculty interested in working in teams to create partnership and collaborative strategies
3. An interdisciplinary approach to the international health curriculum with national and international conditions or trends and technical cooperation among countries and through international organizations
4. A vision of international health as a leadership tool for nurses in national and international communities (da Gloria Miotto Wright et al., 1998)

COMMON THEORETICAL PERSPECTIVES

Scholarly nurses highly value theories as central to defining the concept and actions of nurses. In the international practice arena, it readily becomes evident that no one theory, nor Western interpretation of a theory, is applicable to all cultures and peoples. For example, family developmental theory assumes progression from single adult to marriage, to young parenthood, to families with adolescents, to launching of the children, to later life (Wong, Perry, & Hockenberry, 2002). This theory does not acknowledge the many global family systems that do not include an adolescent phase or the launching of children to independent living. For instance, Masasi and

African tribes have rituals that initiate children into adulthood at puberty. Asian communities often expect multigenerational families to continue living within the same household.

Defining the family, a dynamic process in the United States, is a global challenge. To understand the definition of family within the culture under his or her care, the nurse must move beyond theories to a higher level of knowledge known as *belief systems* and *worldviews*. This process utilizes *synchronic* and *diachronic* patterns of knowledge acquisition. Synchronic family knowledge involves learning how persons, families, and systems operate and what functions they serve. Diachronic family knowledge investigates and values the history, the personal lived experience of individuals within the family (Heibert, 1994). The nurse should not enter a cultural experience with a predetermined definition, theory, and action care plan but rather should enter the encounter with an openness to begin learning by listening and observing.

Orientation and perception of health, illness, and disease must also be considered when applying a theoretical model. Western health care is biomedically based and is the foundation of nursing education in developed nations. Illness and altered health are primarily deemed to have a pathological origin, and professionally trained health care personnel treat patients with medications and technology. Entering global cultures with a biomedical agenda is comparable to colonialism of old. Other health practices may be displaced, communication is often formal, the attitude can be authoritarian and deemed confrontational,

COMMUNITY AS FAMILY

The African's primary allegiance is to the tribe. One's existence is not in being an individual or in being a member of a family. It is in being a member of a tribe. Africans introduce themselves by stating both their name and tribal identity. John Mbili stated, "Whatever happens to the individual happens to the whole group, and whatever happens to the whole group happens to the individual" (Corduan, 1998). Therefore, most tribes see all extended family and community adults as parents of the tribe's children. Every child refers to every woman in the community as mother and to every man as father. All adults have a voice and role in raising every child. Although women are the traditional primary health care givers within the tribe, the health and well-being of the tribe are at risk because each adult ultimately remains free of obligation to maintain any care or responsibility for any one child. This is dramatically evident in the present sub-Saharan AIDS epidemic. Grandmothers try to care, but with so many tribal members dying and with the ultimate lack of responsibility, there are a crisis number of abandoned AIDS orphans across the African continent. These children cluster together in effort to create a new sense of tribe. Unfortunately, they lack the role models, education, and skills to move out of a poor-health existence.

the viewpoint is *etic* (the outsider's), and knowledge and truth demand objective and scientific data (Heibert, 1994; Shaffer, 1990).

As the Western model was found to be inadequate and inappropriate for cultural care, anticolonialism emerged to create dialogue for consensus and to hear the *emic* (insider's) voice (Heibert, 1994). Social science emerged. Sociocultural care seeks to know the client's subjective reasoning for the illness (de Villiers & Tjale, 2000) while offering the promise of prevention and cure developed within Western health care systems. Messias (2001) stated, "[N]urses and nursing students must engage in constructive challenges to the dominance of Western biomedicine as the framework for social decision-making about health and illness. They must be willing to examine critically the underlying values of medical services, public health, professionalism, community development, and consumer participation" (p. 11).

CULTURAL AWARENESS AND SENSITIVITY

The ability to challenge the Western biomedical model as applicable to the present client and family under the nurse's care requires cultural awareness and cultural sensitivity. Culture is the environmental influence that forms each individual's beliefs and values, sense of identity, self-worth, and behavioral guidelines (Cortis, 2003). As culture molds the individual, it also influences family roles, structures, actions, responses, challenges, and adaptations (Mercer, 1989). The family functions within what was taught to the parents

about health, illness, disease, roles, rituals, relationships, power structures, decision making, and coping (Denham, 2003). Therefore, cultural awareness and sensitivity are requirements for safe and effective family nursing care (de Villiers & Tjale, 2000). Leininger, transcultural nursing theorist, developed distinct definitions of nursing within culture, care, and diversity, which should be studied for application in direct care and policy development (Leininger, 1996). See Table 18–2.

Nursing educators, hospital administrators, governmental policy makers, and insurance carriers have written, mandated, and taught about cultural awareness, sensitivity, and competency. *Cultural awareness* begins with self-reflection as to one's own nationality, race, ethnicity, cultural norms and practices, values, and beliefs regarding health and well-being. Awareness encourages nurses to analyze and interpret how the beliefs and practices learned within their own home, culture, environment, and faith are or are not in harmony with those taught in nursing schools and practiced in health care services. Awareness is an ongoing process, which may create a level of cultural conflict. Adaptation and conflict resolution are discussed later in this chapter.

Cultural sensitivity is the awareness of others. It entails an understanding that others may view health and well-being beliefs and practices differently. Sensitivity endeavors to capture an essence of the importance of the differences to the client (Sawyer et al., 1995). Cultural sensitivity does not require the nurse to understand the difference. It does require compassion and respect for the client and accommodation

Table 18–2 LEININGER'S CULTURAL CARE THEORY DEFINITIONS

- Culture: the lifeways of a particular group with its values, beliefs, norms, patterns, and practices that are learned, shared, and transmitted intergenerationally
- Care: the abstract and manifest phenomena and expressions related to assisting, supporting, enabling, and facilitating ways to help others with evident or anticipated needs in order to improve health, a human condition, or a lifeway
- Cultural care diversity: refers to cultural variability or differences in care meanings, patterns, values, symbols, and lifeways among and between cultures
- Cultural and social structure dimensions: refers to the dynamic, holistic, and interrelated patterns or features of culture (or subculture) related to religion (spirituality), kinship (social), political (and legal), economic, education, technology, cultural values, language, and ethnohistorical factors of different cultures

Source: Leininger, M. (1996). Cultural care theory, research, and practice. *Nursing Science Quarterly, 9*(2), 71–78.

to the belief and/or practice whenever possible. Determining when and how to accommodate particular beliefs and practices requires informed critical thinking on the part of the nurse.

Many health care agencies now mandate cultural competency. Comments such as "We are convinced that nurses will be able to provide culturally competent and contextually meaningful care for clients from a wide variety of cultural backgrounds" (Andrews & Boyle, 2003, p. IX) support this goal. Based on research of culturally diverse nursing students in the classroom, Rew, Becker, Cookston, Khosropour, and Martinez (2003) conceptualized cultural competency as awareness (the affective dimension), sensitivity (the attitudinal dimension), knowledge (the cognitive dimension), and skill (the behavioral dimension). The authors define awareness as analysis of how personal beliefs, attitudes, and actions are influenced by one's cultural background. Cultural sensitivity is determining to value another's culture. Knowledge is the gaining of facts about the new culture. Lastly, skill is practice integration of actions, those that do not compromise the nurse's beliefs and yet demonstrate respect for what is important to the other person (Rew et al., 2003).

Westernized nurses, for example, place great value in informing patients of all components of their diagnosis and care plan and in maintaining patient confidentiality. Although this may be the desire of many patients, it is not the standard in global communities and families. Patients of various cultures are known to not want full disclosure (Purnell & Paulanka, 2003). While on a short-term mission caring for families in the mountains of Guatemala, a nurse practitioner strived to educate an older woman of her vaginal cancer and

need for transport to the city hospital. The only multilingual female translator was a 15-year-old (not the ideal person), and she refused to deliver the message to the woman. It was discovered that this culture strictly prohibits a younger person from delivering bad news to an older person. To do so would bring shame and disciplinary action to the 15-year-old. The community leaders met and decided it was better for an older man to inform this woman of her condition. The community determined what she would know and how she would be informed (Elliott, 1992).

Nurses are expected to be culturally aware and culturally sensitive in the nursing care of all clients seen within their routine practice role and specialty. However, no nurse can be expected to be competent in the care of all cultures. The wide array of tribes, languages, nations, practices, peoples, families, and cultures proves too vast to know and understand. Leininger stated, "People are born, live, become ill, and die within a cultural belief and practice system, but are dependent upon human care for growth and survival . . . the ultimate goal [for nursing practice] is culturally congruent care" (Leininger, 1988, p. 155). Culturally congruent care promotes nurses' decisions and actions as to what within the culture should be preserved, what may be accommodated, and what beliefs and practices require repatterning and change (Leininger, 1988). This begins with listening to each patient's voice. The patient's voice may be that of the family.

Hearing the Client's Voice

Culturally sensitive nursing care begins with the nurse hearing the client's voice (Sawyer et al., 1995).

Routine nursing assessment of onset, location, duration, characteristics, aggravating factors, and relieving factors is important yet sterile. The influence and importance of how the client and the family view the presenting symptoms is sometimes lost in such detail. Therefore, it is essential that the nurse establish, and make every effort to maintain, an open and respectful nurse-client dialogue in an effort to learn the client's perception of health and health needs (Martin & Henry, 1989).

Hearing the client's voice is enhanced by obtaining cultural knowledge prior to the encounter, an essential component of international nursing. Cultural knowledge is sought from reliable sources and it provides the nurse with generalizations about the culture (Cortis, 2003). Generalizations are not stereotyping but rather a beginning point of reference. For example, smoking is a major health concern in European countries, and the family nurse should inquire whether the patient from Europe smokes. In contrast, stereotyping is conclusory and sets the nurse up for failure. In stereotyping, the nurse assumes that because the patient is from Europe, he/she must be a smoker. Nurses are at risk if they practice with the false assumptions and expectations that all clients from a given culture will respond in the same manner.

Kleinman (1980) developed eight simple yet insightful questions to help clarify generalizations and to help health care providers hear the client and understand the patient's personal meaning attributed to the illness or condition. These are listed in Table 18–3. In order to learn the family's perception, the nurse might ask: "Has anyone else in your family had this problem? What do your family members believe caused the problem or could treat the problem? Who in your family is most concerned about the problem? How can your family be helpful to you in dealing with this problem?" (Campbell, McDaniel, & Cole-Kelly, 2003). Prior cultural knowledge allows the nurse to rephrase questions into the appropriate context.

The patient and family answers to these questions are often in conflict with those of the Western health care provider. While the Western provider seeks to identify the pathological cause of illness, the sociocultural explanation of the illness or disease often addresses the balance or equilibrium between the body and the environment. Belief in the influences of God/a god, spirits, ancestors, and sorcery as causers of the presenting symptoms or situation is common (de Villiers & Tjale, 2000). American's tend to view spirituality as one small, often insignificant, dimension of the client and state of health. This is not the case around the world. Many international cultures do not believe in the germ theory. To these cultures, health is a spiritual issue, and these cultures turn to traditional healers, witch doctors, ancestor worship, or the worship of multiple gods deemed to oversee health, marriage selection, fertility, harvest yield, and so on (see Box 18–2). Nurses should be mindful of the client's perspective so that they can work with the family to achieve the following:

- Reduce health risks
- Maintain optimal levels of wellness
- Develop routines and achieve goals that enhance the processes of becoming, health, and well-being
- Accommodate changes that maximize health potentials
- Support family members through normative and nonnormative life experiences

---

Table 18–3 **CULTURAL ASSESSMENT: EIGHT QUESTIONS TO ASK YOURSELF AND THEN YOUR CLIENT**

1. What do you think caused your illness?
2. Why do you think your illness started when it did?
3. What do you think your illness does to you?
4. How severe is your illness?
5. What are the chief problems your illness has caused you?
6. What do you fear most about your illness?
7. What kind of treatment do you think you should receive?
8. How do you hope to benefit from treatment?

Source: Kleinman, A. (1980). *Patients and healers in the context of culture.* Berkley, CA: University of California Press.

Box 18–2 CULTURAL PRACTICES: THE USE OF TRADITIONAL HEALERS AND THE ROLE OF THE FAMILY IN CARE

The following examples demonstrate the use of traditional healers, those referred to as *curanderos*, indigenous healers, herbalists, bonesetters, lay midwives, or witch doctors in various nations. For instance, witch doctors are those who for centuries have utilized human body parts and poisons to bring about healing or punishment. Another example that is common to many cultures is ancestor worship. Ancestor worship endeavors to restore health, bring income, and ensure a high yield of crops by honoring and satisfying the spirits of the dead through sacrifices of food, animals, and children. Family beliefs and practices influence the use of traditional healers and the acceptance or rejection of Western medical practices. In every patient encounter, the nurse should consider that although the patient may have migrated to a developed, Westernized environment, centuries-old beliefs and practices are not left behind (D'Avanzo & Geissler, 2003; Elliott, 2000). The level of family involvement in patient care is no doubt influenced by the global nursing shortage.

- Afghanistan—Illness is considered a sign of spiritual weakness, and therefore the appearance of health is very important to the males of the society. They do not seek care. Families are responsible for providing all hospital care, including food, supplies, and comfort (Amowitz, 2003).
- Algeria—Magical-religious beliefs are very important. People believe in protection from the "evil eye," the source of illness, by wearing amulets "inscribed with Koranic verses and putting the Fatma hand (a hand with five fingers) on a chain around the neck" (Khelladi, 2003).
- Belgium—A strong user of biomedical medicine, the 75 percent Roman Catholic population does believe that a pilgrimage may cure cancer. Extended families are restricted from caring for their own in hospitals. Husbands and wives may help each other with laundry and bathing (McLeod, 2003).
- Bolivia—Traditional healers are known as *kallawayas*. Open for business in the village market, these healers rely on llama fetuses, charms, and plant amulets (Bender, 2003).
- Burkina Faso—Hospitals are viewed as a place to die. There are two levels of indigenous healers. The *tradipraticians* primarily strive to alleviate symptoms. The witches and wizards cast spells. These healers are in awe of the hospital staff and will not enter hospital doors (Ledru & Dahourou, 2003).
- Cambodia—This is one of many cultures that believes in *yin* (cold) and *yang* (hot). "*Yin* (representing females, negative forces, the soul, the earth, the moon, the night, water, cold, and darkness) and *yang* (representing males, positive forces, day, fire, heat, expansion, and daylight) must be in absolute equilibrium for optimum health" (Touch, 2003). Illness is the result of an imbalance of yin and yang, caused by food and environment or by supernatural evil spirits, demons, gods, or spells (Touch, 2003).
- Haiti—Haiti is considered the poorest nation in the Western Hemisphere. As of January 1, 2004, the official religion was voodoo. Voodoo combines a belief in God and a belief in magic. Illness caused by magic can be healed only by magic. Voodoo utilizes the shaman, the herbalist, the midwife, the bonesetter, and the injectionist. Honored as the sources of wellness and illness are the spirits of African ancestors, deceased family members, and Biblical figures. Members of a family, a common term for relatives and friends, unite to care for each other during illness (Colin & Paperwalla, 2003).
- Indonesia—Birth and death rituals and patterns of behavior are governed by the *adat*, the way of the ancestors. Blessings are received by walking past a graveyard. The community, as well as the family, has a voice in caring for the sick (Aditama, 2003).
- Lebanon—Although most citizens understand biomedical health care, they continue to view illness as the result of jealous acquaintances who have cast the "evil eye" on them. Family is expected to stay with relatives in the hospital. Their primary responsibility is to serve coffee or candy to visitors (Adib & Mikkey, 2003).
- Mexico—Common to many Latin nations, the *curandero* practices *curanderismo* within his or her local community. Curanderismo, formed from ancient Aztecan, Mayan, and Incan rituals, believes that illness is a punishment from the gods for sin. The Spanish and Catholic influence sees health as chance or God's

(continued on page 467)

will. Treatments include prayer, candles, herbs, and comforting reassurance. Although physicians are held in high regard, the decision of the male in the family has authority over the physician in determining patient care. Family members are involved in direct care as long as a female does not have to touch male genitalia (Dumonteil & Leon, 2003; Padilla, Gomez, Biggerstaff, & Mehler, 2001).

- Swaziland and South Africa—Traditional healers are used first; patients go to biomedical healers only when there is no cure. The two main subgroups of healers are *iNyangas* (those who treat STDs, HIV, and other medical conditions with plants) and sangomas (those who call on ancestors and other spirits for healing). Traditional healers do practice in the hospital. Families are responsible for providing meals and direct care of relatives in the hospital. Following death, the body is taken to the family kraal (home) in order to inform the ancestors of the death (Dube & Guli, 2003; Giarelli & Jacobs, 2003; Hospersa Nurses Forum, 2000).

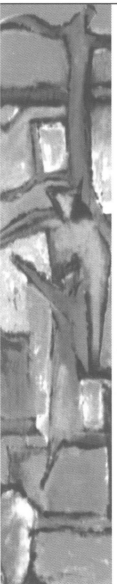

RESEARCH BRIEF

Purpose
Identify the perceptions of, and patient referrals to, traditional healers, faith healers, and alternative medical providers of registered nurses living in the Northern Province of South Africa.

Methodology
Survey of 102 registered nurses.

Results
Referrals by registered nurses to these providers were low and done in response to the client's interest, not as a last resort. Patient education stressed the potential harmful effects of seeking these healers, and only faith healers were considered to offer any benefits to the client.

Nursing Implications
Nurses should attempt to learn about traditional healers practicing within the local community, and nursing assessment should include asking patients and families about the use of traditional healers.

Source: Peltzer, K. (2000, August). *Attitudes of nurses toward traditional healing, faith healing, and alternative medicine in the RSA.* Presented at the University of South Africa Global Health Conference, Pretoria, South Africa.

Purpose
Identify the rate of use of *curanderismo* (Latin traditional healing) by Hispanic patients living in Denver, Colorado.

Methodology
Survey of 405 patients seen at the Denver Health Medical Center.

Results
One hundred eighteen (29.1 percent) had been to a *curandero* (Latin traditional healer) in their lifetime, and 48 (40.7 percent) had been to such a healer within the last 12 months. Ninety-six (81.4 percent) had not informed their physician, whereas 86 (72.9 percent) believed they had benefited from the treatment of the curandero.

(continued on page 468)

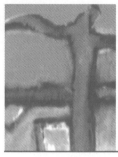

(Continued)

Nursing Implications
Migration to a new country does not terminate long-standing cultural beliefs or practices, and traditional healers are available in Westernized nations. Nursing assessment should include asking about the use of traditional healers.

Source: Padilla, R., Gomez, V., Biggerstaff, S., & Mehler, P. (2001). Use of *curanderismo* in a public health care system. *Archives of Internal Medicine, 161,* 1336–1340.

- Enable family members to obtain information, resources, education, counseling, or other forms of support that enhance health routines (Denham, 2003)

COMMUNITY-BASED HEALTH CARE

A proven and expanding demonstration of nurses listening to client (individuals, families, and communities) voices is community-based health care (CBHC), a global family care model. CBHC entails nurses acting on what they learned by listening and then, as caregivers and educators, training lay workers in the direct care of their own community and family. Missionary nurse Carolyn Myatt (2000) stated that CBHC is "empowering people to solve their own problems by use of methods and technologies appropriate to the *indigenous culture* and society which leads to 'ownership of and responsibility for' a health care delivery system within the community they themselves manage and sustain." Unless the patient, family, community, and culture unite in common health-promoting beliefs and practices, the health of the family is in jeopardy.

> ❝Unless the patient, family, community, and culture unite in common health-promoting beliefs and practices, the health of the family is in jeopardy.❞

Nurses have been at the forefront of primary health care in communities since the 1978 Declaration of Alma Ata. This declaration called for the action of governments, health care providers, and world communities to promote and provide health education, food supply and nutrition, safe water and sanitation, maternal and child health programs, immunizations, prevention and control of locally endemic diseases, treatment of common disease and injuries, and provision of essential drugs (International Conference on Primary Health Care, 1978; Mosby, 1990). CBHC promotes accessibility to health care by offering "personal, sociocultural, economic, and system-related factors that enable individuals, families, and communities to have timely, needed, necessary, continuous, and satisfactory health services" (Gulzar, 1999, p. 17).

CBHC in India, for example, began through a faith-based central hospital and basic nursing education program. By 1987 the hospital staff was providing care through 10 community-based clinics. Today this CBHC program extends to 140 villages and affects the health of over 150,000 family members. Each village is visited twice a month by a team of nurses and doctors. Nurse-trained village health workers provide continuous community care through well-child and immunization clinics, nutritional rehabilitation programs, HIV/AIDS education and antenatal clinics, and the management of all well-mother deliveries (Noah, 2003).

Another success story is in Papua New Guinea. Here CBHC includes nurses training traditional birth attendants in family planning, pure water supply education, better crop-growing projects, and chicken- and rabbit-raising projects for protein sources. Such a significant improvement in female and neonatal

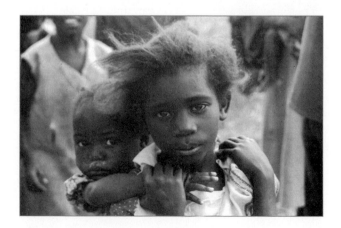

morbidity and mortality took place that the CBHC program was adopted by the island's government as policy for the entire national health care system. This recognition and policy change led to adoption of the same CBHC design by the Solomon Islands (Myatt, 2000; Nazarene Compassionate Ministries, 2002).

Nigeria's CBHC program, established after an advanced practice nurse worked for years within a village awaiting community leaders' willingness to want a community health committee, is now improving family health by having nurses train traditional birth attendants (Stevenson, 2002). The training curriculum and process began by interviewing 51 untrained midwives. They were given a voice and they expressed a willingness to learn. The nurse teaches those who serve the local family and community about the menstrual cycle, antenatal care, management of well labor and birth, basic high-risk management, process of patient transfer, breast-feeding, newborn care, HIV/AIDS, and family planning (Stevenson, 2002). Instruction includes aseptic techniques (prevention of blood-borne contamination and newborn tetanus), proper dosing and use of herbs, cord care, and signs and symptoms of life-threatening illnesses such as malaria (Irinoye, Adeyemo, & Elujoba, 2001).

In Swaziland, the community also chooses who will care for them. The community decides whom to send for the 3-month training. In commitment to the community, training is not held during the important harvest season. While the community-selected representative is attending the course, all local community families unite in care of the children and the household. The majority of the over 3000 attendees to date are women, thus elevating their status within the community. Traditional healers are also part of this select group. Curriculum includes prenatal care, nutrition, HIV/AIDS, pure water supply, sanitation, and the importance of not using the same contaminated razor blade or knife on multiple persons during traditional healing and ritualistic practices (Elliott, 2000).

Demonstrated in all programs is an emphasis on prenatal and women's health care, which is proven to be central to the care and well-being of the entire family. The greater understanding a woman has regarding the importance of nutrition and breast-feeding, consequences of substance abuse and high-risk lifestyle, family planning, pure water, and well-child care (Feachem, 2001), the greater impact she has on the health promotion and disease prevention in her immediate family and community. As women are the primary global lay and professional caregivers, nurses are encouraged to empower women by seeking organizational support of programs that enhance women's confidence and decision-making abilities, aid in improving women's access to health care, and develop women's health partnerships and community-based health workers (Messias, 2001).

CBHC programs in India, Papua New Guinea, and Nigeria were developed and expanded by American nurses serving internationally as missionary nurses for the Church of the Nazarene. Swaziland's CBHC program was developed by an indigenous nurse who had previously been educated by missionary nurses. Orchard and Karmaliani (1999) promote nurses as community development specialists needed in developing countries to aid in the following:

- Altering cultural practices that have a negative impact on health
- Promoting those practices that have a positive impact on health
- Providing health education that both promotes healthy lifestyles and prepares community members to lead and sustain their own community-based health care system

Missionary nursing is only one practice methodology through which nurses can improve the health of families and communities.

CBHC programs that do not promote change usually fail because of the lack of community voice throughout the process. The Western approach to health care is to enter a family/community/culture with a predetermined need and plan of interaction. Examples of Western approach model designs include the community-oriented primary care cycle (Goldberg, 2003) and a British community pediatric team model (Gregg & Appleton, 1999). Lacking in both model designs is preplanning interaction with the people. When the community is not granted an early and continuous voice, programs are not as successful. In general, successful CBHC is dependent on hearing the voice of the family and the community during all stages of program assessment, development, implementation, ongoing management, and evaluation. To further enhance the effectiveness of CBHC and further document the role of family nursing in CBHC, more nursing research is needed.

> **❝CBHC is dependent on hearing the voice of the family and the community during all stages of program assessment, development, implementation, ongoing management, and evaluation.❞**

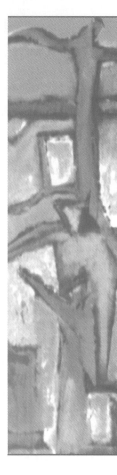

RESEARCH BRIEF

Purpose

To share the lessons learned about how Native American families "view and manage the care of children with chronic conditions" from the Indian Family Stories Project, a community-based program with Native American youth, families, and community representatives.

Method

Participatory action research, listening to the needs of the community through open-ended interviews.

Results

To improve the care of their children with asthma, the families asked health care providers to be trained in and show respect of (1) traditional Native American beliefs and practices, (2) the role of the Native American extended family in the care of the children, and (3) normal Native American cultural patterns of communication. The Community Asthma Action Plan and the Cultural Education Action Plan were developed and successfully implemented.

Nursing Implications

"The philosophy of the research team needs to be congruent with the cultural and community context" (Garwick & Auger, 2003). Continuity and follow-through by the research team builds trust in the community and partnerships that yield success in meeting the action plan goals.

Source: Garwick, A., & Auger, S. (2003). Participatory action research: The Indian Family Stories Project. *Nursing Outlook, 51*(6), 261–266.

COMMUNITY-BASED HEALTH CARE IN AMERICA: A MODEL FOR THE PREVENTION OF HIV/AIDS IN INTERNATIONAL COMMUNITIES

This community-based health care model for the prevention of HIV/AIDS in international communities now living in rural America was designed by a family nurse practitioner faculty member and two graduate family nurse practitioner students. The model demonstrates how multiple issues are important and interrelated in the spread of HIV/AIDS and how each must be addressed in the CBHC program. The issues were identified during Elliott's training of HIV/AIDS home-care workers across Zambia in 2002 and from the students' assessments of their home nations, China and the Philippines. In Zambia, representatives of various tribes were asked in training sessions to identify which culturally accepted practices put individuals and family members at risk of HIV contamination. Identified causal factors included the following:

- Marriage succession—Mandatory marrying of the widow to her dead husband's brother, regardless of the number of wives he already has.
- Death rituals—Mandatory shaving of a corpse's head and the head of each remaining family member with the same contaminated razor blade.
- Poverty and illiteracy—Prostitution for survival. A saying on the streets is "It is better to die of AIDS tomorrow than of starvation today."

(continued on page 471)

- Traditional healers—Utilizing the same contaminated knife for ritualized female genital mutilation, circumcision, or body cuts to drive out evil spirits.

American nurses should consider the issues identified in Africa in clustered communities living in the United States. Migration to a Western culture with new national laws does not end long-held cultural beliefs and practices.

Source: Elliott, S., Galindo, J., & Luu, S. (2003). *International clients in rural America: The impact of cultural worldview and practices in HIV/AIDS prevention and intervention.* Presented March 28, 2003, at HIV Prevention in Rural Communities: Sharing Successful Strategies III, Bloomington, IN.

CULTURAL ADAPTATION

The success of CBHC, or of any family nursing care model in a new culture, requires cultural encounters, which can be interesting, rewarding, and very challenging. These encounters are enhanced when the nurse crosses borders to live and work within a new cultural environment. In that situation, the nurse is isolated from his or her personal cultural norms, values, practices, and resources. Practicing within the home nation challenges the nurse for an 8- to 12-hour shift. Practicing in a new host nation challenges the nurse not only in the service environment but also through all activities of daily living.

In the new international setting, the nurse must relearn, if not come to reunderstand and revalue, new units of intervention, which define identity, health care promotion, disease prevention, and healing. A new process of prioritizing family needs, resources, and actions is required (Long, 2000). Long (2000) described three units of intervention as relationship to self, relationship to others, and relationship to the environment. Relationship to self includes hygiene and personal caregiving, risk behaviors, identity, worth, and efficacy. Relationship to others is the interaction within the family and community. Components include the population group, caregiving agencies and organizations, and the nurse. Relationship to the environment addresses the patterns of exposure to harm, economic structures and employment, and all cultural practices, values, and beliefs.

Anthropologists Spradley and Phillips (1972) utilized *The Cultural Readjustment Rating Questionnaire* to rate the adaptation of Peace Corps and international students in their stress-related adjustment to a new international environment. The readjustment

CASE STUDY ➤

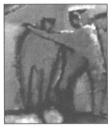

Three young American nurses met in a small African nation ready for volunteer service within a mission hospital. The hospital bedded 250 patients with a medical staff of about five physicians. The nationals spoke both their tribal language and British English, and the nursing roles and titles were defined by the British system. As the bachelor-degreed nurses were educated in the American Western health care system, an immediate practice and autonomy paradigm shift was required for them to practice independently in this new country. These nurses faced challenges of catching babies without midwifery skills, suturing without experience, diagnosing and treating tropical ailments without the necessary education, and striving to understand the role of the witch doctor within the hospital system. The change crisis was enhanced by the fact that they were assigned to supervisory positions within an unknown health care system.

Two of the nurses adapted well through active interaction with the nationals and other missionaries. These nurses served their committed time and continued to have other international service experiences. The third nurse did not fare so well. The cultural crisis and progressive culture shock led to her returning home within 2 months, and she required several years of psychotherapy before her recovery was complete. It was reported that she never left the United States again (Elliott, 1979).

questionnaire items listed in Table 18–4 demonstrate various conditions and situations the international nurse of today will face. The authors state, "Cultural practices of every sort are reported to induce stress: toilet training, puberty rites, residential change, polygamous households, belief in malevolent gods, competition, and discontinuities between childhood socialization and adult roles" (Spradley & Phillips, 1972, p. 518). There were two unexpected findings of this study. The first was that neither previous intercul-

tural experience nor a similar cultural background to the new culture influenced the appraisal and adaptation process needed within the new environment. Second, knowing the language alone also did not prove significant in cultural adaptation. It remained necessary to understand the cultural definitions of the words and the issues (Spradley & Phillips, 1972). See the following case study for an illustration of nurses working abroad and trying to learn new units of intervention.

Table 18–4　CULTURAL READJUSTMENT ITEMS

1. The type of food eaten
2. The type of clothes worn
3. How punctual people are
4. Ideas about what offends people
5. The language spoken
6. How ambitious people are
7. Personal cleanliness of most people
8. The general pace of life
9. The amount of privacy I would have
10. My own financial state
11. Type of recreation and leisure time activities
12. How parents treat their children
13. The sense of closeness and obligation felt among family members
14. The amount of body contact such as touching and standing close
15. The subjects that should not be discussed in normal conversation
16. The number of people of my own race
17. The degree of friendliness and intimacy between unmarried women and men
18. How free and independent women seem to be
19. Sleeping practices such as amount of time, time of day, and sleeping arrangement
20. General standard of living
21. Ideas about friendship—the way people act and feel toward friends
22. The number of people of my religious faith
23. How formal and informal people are
24. My own opportunities for social contacts
25. The degree to which my good intentions are misunderstood by others
26. The number of people who live in the community
27. Ideas about what is funny
28. Ideas about what is sad
29. How much friendliness and hospitality people express
30. The amount of reserve people show in their relationships to others
31. Eating practices such as amount of food, type of eating, and ways of eating
32. Type of transportation used
33. The way people take care of material possessions

Source: Spradley, J., & Phillips, M. (1972). Culture and stress: A quantitative analysis. *American Anthropologist, 74*(3), 518–529.

CASE STUDY ➤

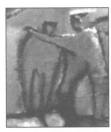

A 22-year-old Hispanic male student traveled to a South American country for 10 days with a group of nursing students from an American university. Before traveling, the students participated in an 8-hour cultural knowledge and sensitivity seminar. Within 3 days of arrival in the host nation, the student began to lash out in violent words and threatening body language. He became disruptive to the group process and cried easily. The student was removed from the immediate setting and given the opportunity to express what about the culture he found distressing. It was discovered that he was a member of a wealthy family and this was his first experience of seeing "his own" in such states of poverty. He was highly offended and embarrassed by what he saw. The group leader and two host nation leaders spent hours discussing different perspectives of poverty with him. What he saw as poverty was seen as wealth by the *nationals*. The student learned that poverty does not equate to stupidity. With a fresh perspective, he reentered the team of student nurses and functioned well. He returned home the following week expressing a new respect of and compassion for "his own" (Elliott, 1995).

The risk of *cultural maladaptation* and *culture shock* is an ever-present reality for international health care workers. Unresolved culture shock may result not only in ineffective and nonproductive nursing care of the new clients but also in the nurse experiencing depression, psychosis, withdrawal, abnormal and disruptive behaviors, menstrual irregularities, eating disorders, insomnia, stress-induced cardiac and hormonal crisis, and/or suicide. Whether the international nurse is leaving Western civilization to serve in a Third World country or the reverse, mechanisms for support during cultural adaptation are essential for the health and well-being of the nurse. The following case study demonstrates cultural conflict and the need for support during the crisis.

Stages of Culture Shock

The stages of culture shock are common throughout literature and international service preparation materials. Initial shock and adjustment are common for any nurse traveling to and arriving in a new country. Fellow travelers, as well as local customs authorities and weather changes, all may cause the nurse to question the decision of international service. With prior knowledge and arrangements made and a welcoming committee present, early adjustment often proceeds without significant physical and emotional distress (Jones, 2001).

After recuperation from jet lag, the physical symptoms associated with crossing multiple time zones within a short period of time (World Health Organization, 2003), the first days and weeks in a new host country are often described as the "honeymoon" phase. This is the euphoria experienced by the temporary traveler to a region. What one sees and hears is interesting because it is superficial. Unfortunately, this phase is easily shattered by random and often unexpected, unexplained new lived experiences.

True conflict begins when the new culture does not conform to the expectations of the nurse (Spradley & Phillips, 1972). Progressive negative attitudes and emotions toward the people and the culture ensue. The very people who could serve to help the nurse adjust become threatening. "The first step in critical contextualization is to study the culture phenomenologically. If at this point the [nurse] shows any criticism of the customary beliefs and practices, the people will not talk about them for fear of being condemned" (Heibert, 1994, pp. 88, 89).

This lack of trust, as well as anger, hostility, and mutual isolation, continues unless active and dynamic intervention takes place. Ideally, the family nurse serving internationally will maintain a home support system with whom the nurse can discuss the areas of conflict. However, this alone is inadequate. Those at home have no insight into the reality of what the nurse is experiencing. Therefore, the nurse should immediately seek supportive host nationals or others from the home nation also living in the host county. Establishing friendships and mentorship relationships to instruct, guide, and assist in the transition helps prevent culture shock in the nurse and will provide the intervention necessary to halt the cycle of isolation. These friendships can help the nurse understand and respect the value of the new culture to the people.

Through successful prevention, intervention, and motivation, individuals often recover from culture shock. As the nurse adapts to new activities of daily living and establishes honored relationships, a sense of well-being and a sense of humor return. As the nurse grows more knowledgeable about local demographics, the role of the nurse and traditional healers, family structures and the family voice for health care communication and decision making, resources and existing programs that support family health, and patterns for nursing care, the nurse becomes more comfortable.

True *cultural integration* or *enculturation* is a rewarding yet slowly progressing process. Ideally, those who serve internationally should learn and observe for at least 2 years before making comments or recommendations for change. During this time, nationals watch to see whether the nurse can be trusted. Even if the family nurse enters the experience informed about the culture and health care beliefs, it is only through the lived experience of patient care and interaction that the belief begins to have meaning for the nurse. Missionaries report having been deeply embedded within a culture for over 30 years, only to leave with just a basic understanding of the true meaning and worldview behind a belief or practice that is so important to the indigenous people.

Eventually the international nurse returns home to experience some degree of reverse culture shock. Home is not the same. Family dynamics changed. People aged. Even television images of reality changed. Professionally, nursing and biomedical knowledge and truths were challenged and revised. Health care policies and equipment were not stagnant. Common reverse culture shock sources include new awareness of the vast amount of medical waste in Western countries, the gross expenditures for health care services, the inequality of services provided at home versus abroad, and the limited autonomy and role of the nurse within the United States.

SUMMARY

Crossing borders to care for families, communities, and diverse cultures offers professional nurses unique practice, consultation, education, and research opportunities. It also introduces nurses to unique challenges, which can become great rewards. This chapter has discussed the following critical issues, all of which are important to the success or failure of family nursing care in international settings. Whatever the final definition of family may be, international borders are open to nurses who are willing to cross.

- Family nurses need to acquire knowledge about global disease and illness endemic to the new host nation and then listen to family beliefs about the cause of the illness.
- Cultural awareness, sensitivity, and adaptation are essential to meeting the needs of the individual, the family, the community, the culture, and the nurse.
- Realities that influence health, well-being, and nursing care within a culture include poverty, gender inequality, lack of adequate food supply or intake, lack of pure water supply, poor sanitation, the sociopolitical environment, degree of population illiteracy, and population spiritual beliefs and practices.
- A proven family nursing practice model and research need is community-based health care (CBHC). CBHC listens to the voice of the community throughout all stages of project assessment, development, implementation, and evaluation. Through participatory action research, the needs of the community are met and the role of the family nurse is validated.
- Nurses are the primary global health care providers, and global families need more nurses.

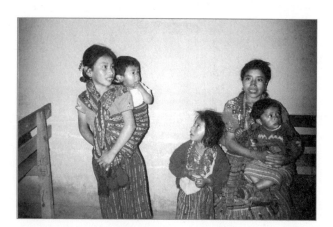

References

Abid, S., & Mikkey, F. (2003). Lebanon. In C. D'Avanzo & E. Geissler (Eds.), *Pocket guide to cultural health assessment* (3rd ed., pp. 443–449). St. Louis: Mosby.

Aditama, T. (2003). Indonesia. In C. D'Avanzo & E. Geissler (Eds.), *Pocket guide to cultural health assessment* (3rd ed., pp. 358–361). St. Louis: Mosby.

American Association of Colleges of Nursing. (1998). *The essentials of baccalaureate education for professional nursing practice.* Washington, DC: American Association of Colleges of Nursing.

American Association of Colleges of Nursing. (2003). *Working paper on the role of the clinical nurse leader.* Washington, DC: American Association of Colleges of Nursing.

Amowitz, L. (2003). Afghanistan. In C. D'Avanzo & E. Geissler (Eds.), *Pocket guide to cultural health assessment* (3rd ed., pp. 1–6). St. Louis: Mosby.

Andrews, M., & Boyle, J. (2003). *Transcultural concepts in nursing care* (4th ed.). Philadelphia: Lippincott.

Bender, D. (2003). Bolivia. In C. D'Avanzo & E. Geissler (Eds.), *Pocket guide to cultural health assessment* (3rd ed., pp. 91–97). St. Louis: Mosby.

Campbell, T., McDaniel, S., & Cole-Kelly, K. (2003). Family issues in health care. In R. Taylor (Ed.), *Family medicine: Principles and practice* (6th ed., pp. 24–32). New York: Springer.

Colin, J., & Paperwalla, G. (2003). People of Haitian heritage. In L. Purnell & B. Paulanka (Eds.), *Transcultural health care: A culturally competent approach* (2nd ed., pp. 72–117) [CD-ROM]. Philadelphia: FA Davis.

Corduan, W. (1998). *Neighboring faiths*. Downer's Grove, IL: InterVarsity Press.

Cortis, J. (2003). Culture, values and racism: Application to nursing. *International Nursing Review, 50*(1), 55–64.

da Gloria Miotto Wright, M., Godue, C., Manfredi, M., & Korniewicz, D. (1998). Nursing education and international health in the US, Latin America, and the Caribbean. *IMAGE: Journal of Nursing Scholarship, 30*(1), 31–36.

D'Avanzo, C., & Geissler, E. (2003). *Pocket guide to cultural health assessment* (3rd ed.). St. Louis: Mosby.

Denham, S. (2003). *Family health: A framework for nursing*. Philadelphia: FA Davis.

Department of Health and Human Services. (2000). *A practical guide for implementing the recommended national standards for culturally and linguistically appropriate services in health care*. Washington, DC: Department of Health and Human Services.

de Villiers, L., & Tjale, A. (2000, November). Rendering culturally congruent and safe care in culturally diverse settings. *Africa Journal of Nursing and Midwifery*, 21–24.

Dube, E., & Guli, N. (2003). Swaziland. In C. D'Avanzo & E. Geissler (Eds.), *Pocket guide to cultural health assessment* (3rd ed., pp. 741–744). St. Louis: Mosby.

Dumonteil, E., & Leon, M. (2003). Mexico. In C. D'Avanzo & E. Geissler (Eds.), *Pocket guide to cultural health assessment* (3rd ed., pp. 520–525). St. Louis: Mosby.

Elliott, S. (1979). Lived experience, Swaziland.

Elliott, S. (1992). Lived experience, Guatemala.

Elliott, S. (1995). Lived experience, Venezuela.

Elliott, S. (2000). *Missionary nurse Dorothy Davis Cook, 1940–1972: "Mother of Swazi nurses."* Doctoral dissertation, University of San Diego, San Diego, CA.

Elliott, S., Galindo, J., & Luu, S. (2003). *International clients in rural America: The impact of cultural worldview and practices in HIV/AIDS prevention and intervention*. Presented March 28, 2003, at HIV Prevention in Rural Communities: Sharing Successful Strategies III. Bloomington, IN.

Fadiman, A. (1997). *The spirit catches you and you fall down*. New York: Farrar, Straus, & Giroux.

Feachem, R. (2001). The roles of government. In C. Koop, C. Pearson, & M. Schwarz (Eds.), *Critical issues in global health*. San Francisco: Jossey-Bass.

Florence Nightingale Museum. 2 Lambeth Palace Road, London SE1 7EW. September 3, 1999.

Flynn, L., & Aiken, L. (2002). Does international nurse recruitment influence practice values in U.S. hospitals? *Journal of Nursing Scholarship, 34*(1), 67–73.

Friedman, M., Bowden, V., & Jones, E. (2003). *Family nursing research, theory, and practice* (5th ed.). Upper Saddle River, NJ: Prentice Hall.

Galanti, G. (1997). *Caring for patients from different cultures*. Philadelphia: University of Pennsylvania Press.

Garwick, A., & Auger, S. (2003). Participatory action research: The Indian Family Stories Project. *Nursing Outlook, 51*(6), 261–266.

Giarelli, E., & Jacobs, L. (2003). Traditional healing and HIV-AIDS in KwaZulu-Natal, South Africa. *American Journal of Nursing, 103*(10), 36–47.

Goldberg, B. (2003). Population-based health care. In R. Taylor (Ed.), *Family medicine: Principles and practice* (6th ed., pp. 41–46). New York: Springer.

Goodyear, R. (2003, January 27). *International health and issues related to nursing education and practice*. California State University, Los Angeles Faculty Development.

Gregg, J., & Appleton, R. (1999). Community child health: An essential specialist service for the millennium. *The Lancet, 354*, su28–30.

Gulzar, L. (1999). Access to health care. *Image: Journal of Nursing Scholarship, 31*(1), 13–19.

Harmer, B. (1933). *Textbook of the principles and practice of nursing* (p. 5). New York: The Macmillan Co.

Hartley, L. (2002). Examination of primary care characteristics in a community-based clinic. *Journal of Nursing Scholarship, 34*(4), 377–382.

Heibert, P. (1994). *Anthropological reflections on missiological issues*. Grand Rapids, MI: Baker Books.

Hospersa Nurses Forum. (2000). Traditional healing. *Nursing Today, 3*(3), 15.

International Conference on Primary Health Care. (1978). *Declaration of Alma Ata*. Geneva: World Health Organization.

International Council of Nursing. Retrieved September 16, 2002, from *http://www.icn.ch/definition.htm*

International Council of Nursing. (2003). *ICN offers guidance on global nurse competencies*. Retrieved January 30, 2004, from *http://www.icn.ch/PRO5_03.htm*

Irinoye, O., Adeyemo, A., & Elujoba, A. (2001). Care of women during pregnancy and labour [sic] by traditional birth attendants in Ile-Ife, Nigeria. *Africa Journal of Nursing and Midwifery, 3*(2), 14–18.

Joint WHO/FAO Expert Consultation. (2003). *Diet, nutrition and the prevention of chronic diseases*. Geneva: World Health Organization.

Jones, N. (2001). *The rough guide to travel health*. London: Penguin Group.

Khelladi, H. (2003). Algeria. In C. D'Avanzo & E. Geissler (Eds.), *Pocket guide to cultural health assessment* (3rd ed., pp. 13–20). St. Louis: Mosby.

Kleinman, A. (1980). *Patients and healers in the context of culture*. Berkley, CA: University of California Press.

Ledru, E., & Dahourou, G. (2003). Burkina Faso. In C. D'Avanzo & E. Geissler (Eds.), *Pocket guide to cultural health assessment* (3rd ed., pp. 126–133). St. Louis: Mosby.

Leininger, M. (1988). Leininger's theory of nursing: Cultural care diversity and universality. *Nursing Science Quarterly, 1*(4), 152–160.

Leininger, M. (1996). Cultural care theory, research, and practice. *Nursing Science Quarterly, 9*(2), 71–78.

Long, W. (2000). *Health, healing, and God's kingdom*. Harrisonburg, VA: R.R. Donnelly & Co.

Lutzen, K. (2000). A global perspective on domestic and international tensions in knowledge development. *Journal of Nursing Scholarship, 32*(4), 335–337.

Martin, M., & Henry, M. (1989). Cultural relativity and poverty. *Public Health Nursing, 6*(1), 28–33.

McAllister, C., Green, B., Terry, M., Herman, V., & Mulvey, L. (2003). Parents, practitioners, and researchers: Community-based participatory research with Early Head Start. *American Journal of Public Health, 93*(10), 1672–1679.

McLeod, M. (2003). Belgium. In C. D'Avanzo & E. Geissler (Eds.), *Pocket guide to cultural health assessment* (3rd ed., pp. 72–80). St. Louis: Mosby.

Mercer, R. (1989). Theoretical perspectives on the family. In C. Gillis (Ed.), *Toward a science of family nursing*. Menlo Park, CA: Addison-Wesley.

Messias, D. (2001). Globalization, nursing, and health for all. *Journal of Nursing Scholarship, 33*(1), 9–11.

Minkler, M., Blackwell, A., Thompson, M., & Tamir, H. (2003).

Community-based participatory research: Implications for public health funding. *American Journal of Public Health, 93*(8), 1210–1213.

Mosby, W. (1990). Principles of community health. In D. Ewert (Ed.), *A new agenda for medical missions*. Brunswick, GA: MAP International.

Myatt, C. (2000, September). *A new health challenge in Papua New Guinea: Community-based health care*. Presented at Nazarene Health Care Fellowship Global Health Conference, Guatemala City, Guatemala.

National Organization of Nurse Practitioner Faculties. (2004, April 21–25). Conference in San Diego, CA.

Nazarene Compassionate Ministries. (2002, Winter). *NCM today* (pp. 3–4). Kansas City, MO: Church of the Nazarene.

Noah, A. (2003). *Reynolds Memorial Hospital, Washim: A profile*. Unpublished. Received September 15, 2003.

Orchard, C., & Karmaliani, R. (1999). Community development specialists in nursing in developing countries. *Image: Journal of Nursing Scholarship, 31*(3), 295–298.

Organisation [sic] for Economic Co-operation and Development. (2003). *Poverty and health*. Geneva: World Health Organization.

Padilla, R., Gomez, V., Biggerstaff, S., & Mehler, P. (2001). Use of *curanderismo* in a public health care system. *Archives of Internal Medicine, 161*, 1336–1340.

Peltzer, K. (2000, August). *Attitudes of nurses toward traditional healing, faith healing, and alternative medicine in the RSA*. Presented at the University of South Africa Global Health Conference, Pretoria, South Africa.

Purnell, L., & Paulanka, B. (2003). *Transcultural health care: A culturally competent approach* (2nd ed.). Philadelphia: FA Davis.

Rew, L., Becker, H., Cookston, J., Khosropour, S., & Martinez, S. (2003). Measuring cultural awareness in nursing students. *Journal of Nursing Education, 42*(6), 249–257.

Sawyer, L., Regeu, H., Proctor, S., Nelson, M., Messias, D., Barnes, D., & Meleis, A. (1995). Matching versus cultural competence in research: Methodological considerations. *Research in Nursing and Health, 18*, 557–567.

Shaffer, R. (1990). Community-based health development. In D. M. Ewert (Ed.), *A new agenda for medical missions* (pp. 40–48). Brunswick, GA: MAP International.

Spradley, J., & Phillips, M. (1972). Culture and stress: A quantitative analysis. *American Anthropologist, 74*(3), 518–529.

Stevenson, C. (2002). *Community-based health care in Nigeria*. Presented October 28, 2002, at California State University, Los Angeles School of Nursing, Los Angeles, CA.

Thompson, J. (2002). The WHO Global Advisory Group on Nursing and Midwifery. *Journal of Nursing Scholarship, 34*(2), 111–113.

Toebes, B. (1999). Towards an improved understanding of the international human right to health. *Human Rights Quarterly, 21*, 661–679.

Touch, C. (2003). Cambodia. In C. D'Avanzo & E. Geissler (Eds.), *Pocket guide to cultural health assessment* (3rd ed., pp. 143–149). St. Louis: Mosby.

Vonderheid, S., & Al-Gasseer, N. (2002). World Health Organization and global health policy. *Journal of Nursing Scholarship, 34*(2), 109–110.

Wong, D., Perry, S., & Hockenberry, M. (2002). *Maternal child nursing care* (2nd ed.). St. Louis: Mosby.

World Health Organization. (2000). *Injury: A leading cause of the global burden of disease*. Geneva: Author.

World Health Organization. (2002). *Strategic directions for strengthening nursing and midwifery services*. Geneva: Author.

World Health Organization. (2003). *International travel and health*. Geneva: Author.

Youssef, E., & Tornquist, E. (1997). *Nursing practice around the world*. Geneva: World Health Organization.

Bibliography

Fadiman, A. (1997). *The spirit catches you and you fall down*. New York: Farrar, Straus, & Giroux.

Koop, C. E., Pearson, C., & Schwarz, M. R. (2001). *Critical issues in global health*. San Francisco: Jossey-Bass.

World Health Organization. (2003). *International travel and health*. Geneva: Author.

World Health Organization. (2002). *Traditional medicine strategy*. Retrieved from *http://www.who.int/medicines/library/trm/trm_strat_eng.pdf*

Futures of Families and Family Nursing

CHAPTER 19
The Futures of Families, Health, and Family Nursing

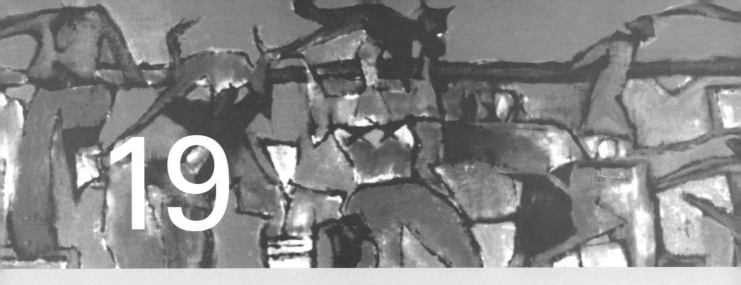

19

The Futures of Families, Health, and Family Nursing

Shirley May Harmon Hanson RN, PMHNP, PhD, FAAN, CFLE, LMFT

CRITICAL CONCEPTS

- American families are ever changing, and these changes affect the health care system and family nursing.

- Some people believe that the traditional family is outmoded and cannot cope with the realities of everyday life. Other people believe that increasing alienation necessitates a sense of family and community and that families are working harder to create this in their own lives.

- Present and future demographics demonstrate trends in the United States that help to predict areas of new developments in nursing and the

  health care field, such as increased cultural diversity, higher divorce rates, rise in health disparities, expanding numbers of family forms, swelling aging population, and resurgence of modern technology in taking care of people.

- Changes and trends in other parts of the world parallel what is happening in the United States.

- The future of family nursing research, education, practice, and policy must evolve to keep pace with demographic, social, and technological changes in the world.

INTRODUCTION

American families and health care changed dramatically during the 20th century, and these drastic changes appear to be accelerating in the 21st century. Nuclear families consisting of mother, father, and their joint biological children are no longer the principal family structure; they are now just one of a multitude of well-recognized family forms. Indeed, Coontz (1998) noted that no normative family structural form exists in contemporary society; the dominance of a traditional familial structure has been a fictional notion throughout most of American history. Today we recognize that there are a variety of family forms, each of which is tenable and each of which has its own unique characteristics, qualities, and values. As family structures have become more diverse, the complexity of preparing health care providers for family care has intensified.

The purpose of this final chapter is to look to the future—to the extent that we can in these changing times—of families and health, and what this might mean for family nursing practice during the early years of this century. The chapter will also address the factors that influence family nursing and the future of family nursing theory, practice, research, education, and social policy.

The evolving development and implementation of nursing care of families is based on the assumption that families are the basic unit of society. This orientation will continue into the future, despite life-altering world events, evolving family demographics and value systems, fluctuating definitions of "family," changing health care delivery systems, and conflicting ideas about nursing education and practice.

CHANGING FAMILIES

American families have generally been romanticized as the foundation of emotional relationships and security. Some believe that families as a unit are in great jeopardy because of all the changes over time. Yet others see these changes as part of an evolutionary process. For example, Coontz (1998) and Dunphy (2001) reminded us that families have always been in a state of flux and often in crisis, and they noted that idealizing families of previous decades discounts the strengths that families have developed over time in coping with a changing society.

In contrast, Popenoe (1996, 1999) and Popenoe and Whitehead (1999) asserted that American families are in decline and that action must be taken immediately

to strengthen the institution of the family. Dreman (1997a) continued this when he summarized this age-old dilemma pertaining to the future of families:

> *Is there life for the family in the 21st century? Who will prevail—the optimists or the pessimists? The pessimists claim that family life in its present form is doomed. This gloomy forecast is attributable to increased demands from the workplace, rampant technological advancement and the pursuit of personal achievement at the expense of interpersonal needs and values. The pessimists among us feel that the traditional family is outmoded and no longer capable of coping with the realities of contemporary living. The optimists claim the opposite, that is, that increasing alienation and emphasis on the occupational sphere necessitates a sense of family, community, and belonging as a haven from work-related stress. (p. xi)*

Whitehead (1992) and Doherty (1992, 2001) provided broad overviews of where family life has been and may be going. They wrote that the last 50 years of American family life experienced three distinct cultural periods. The first was called *traditional familism* or *institutional family*. This period extended from the mid-1940s to the mid-1960s and was characterized by the dominance of married couples with children, a high birth rate, a low divorce rate, and a high degree of marital stability. The period was marked by a robust economy, a rising standard of living, and an expanding middle class. Culturally, it was defined by conformity to social norms, the ideology of separate spheres for men and women, and idealization of family life. The television emblem of postwar family life was, and still is, *Ozzie and Harriet*. The chief family value for this period was responsibility.

The second period was called the period of *individualism* or the *psychological family*. This period extended from the mid-1960s to the mid-1980s and was characterized by greater demographic diversity, a decline in the birth rate, an accelerating divorce rate, individual and social experimentation, the breakdown of the separate spheres ideology, the creation of a singles "lifestyle," idealization of career and work life, and the search for meaning in life through self-expression. The emblematic television shows of this period were the *Mary Tyler Moore Show* in the 1970s and *L.A. Law* in the 1980s. Both programs treated work relationships and workplace as the primary realm of intimacy, nurturing, and fulfillment. The chief family value for this period was satisfaction.

The third period, which is where we are now, was termed the period of *new familism* or the *pluralistic family* and has resulted largely from the fact that the baby boomers have reached adulthood and parenthood. This period is characterized by a leveling off of divorce rates, a leveling off of workforce participation among women, and the highest number of births since 1964. Socially, it is less uptight than the first period but more uptight than the second period. It appears to be shifting away from expressive individualism and a fascination with self toward a greater attachment to family and commitment to others. We are beginning to see couples place happiness and well-being of the family above their individual desires or ambitions. A growing number of men and women are cutting back on work to devote more time to children. Women's career plans are including the time to actively participate in raising young children. These new families have greatly influenced the media culture, through TV programs such as *Murphy Brown*, *Thirtysomething*, and *Life Goes On* and the later programs such as *Home Improvement* and *Everybody Loves Raymond*. Flexibility and diversity are the hallmarks of this new period.

If a new familistic ethos is emerging, it is good news for children. There are many positive aspects to the social and cultural changes of the past 25 years: greater choice for adults, greater freedom and opportunities for women, and greater tolerance for difference and diversity. The quality of the family of the future depends on whether family ethic and policies can be established that will help develop and maintain healthy bonds between family members in different living arrangements and between families and their communities.

FUTURE OF AMERICAN FAMILIES

At the beginning of the 21st century, profound structural and demographic changes are occurring in family life (Dreman, 1997a, pp. 3–4). The traditional two-parent nuclear family is viewed by many as a relic of the past. These changes are reflected in major changes in divorce, marriage, fertility, and longevity rates, as well as increasing rates of female employment, accompanied by changes in family structures, lifestyles, and the family life cycle. Accelerating rates of stress and violence in the family reflect strain between work and the family, evolving gender conflicts, ambiguity in parental roles of the biological versus the socializing parent in the case of stepparents, or parenting roles as a result of high-tech reproduction techniques. At the same time of rapid social, industrial, and technological

change, family values of community, belonging, and family-related status are often usurped by individualism, autonomy, and the pursuit of career-related prestige.

Many family scholars synthesized data from a variety of sources to describe recent and futuristic changes in the composition, economic stability, and diversity of American families (Teachman, Tedrow, & Crowder, 2000; Bianchi & Casper, 2000; Bumpass & Lu, 2000; Casper & Bianchi, 2002; U.S. Bureau of the Census, 2003a, 2003b). According to these sources, the declining prevalence of early marriage, increasing level of marital dissolution, and growing tendency to never marry, especially among some racial and ethnic groups, reflect changes in the relative economic prospects of men and women. They concluded that marriage is becoming less valued as a source of economic stability. These developments indicate that relatively more children are born outside of marriage, spend at least part of their childhood in a single-parent household, and endure multiple changes in family composition. Concurrently, sharp changes in the economic stability of families, characterized most notably by a growing importance of women's income and increasing economic inequality among American families, have been taking place, creating challenging issues for all families and for both genders.

If present trends endure to the year 2050, the overall population of the United States will have grown to over 400 million people (see Figure 19–1). The largest growth will be in the nation's Hispanic and elderly populations. A large part of the increase will occur through immigration alone, with cities and states on the East and West Coasts receiving a disproportionate share of these immigrants. Average household size will decline. The median age of the population will increase.

Family Trends in the United States

Several other family scholars have speculated on what they deem are some of the general and specific family trends that will influence American families in the future (Coltrane & Collins, 2001; Cox, 2002).

Aging Population in the United States

The aging of Americans is the first general but major family trend. From 1950 to 2000 the total resident population of the United States increased from about 150 million to 281 million. This rate of increase

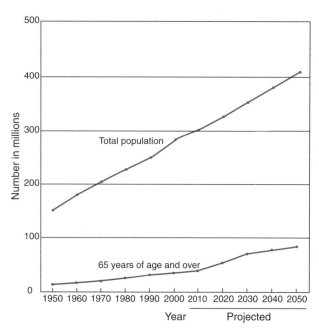

Figure 19–1 Total and elderly population: United States, 1950–2050. Adapted from National Center for Health Statistics. (2003). *Health, United States, 2003: Chartbook on trends in the health of Americans* (DHHS Publication No. 2003-1232, p. 22). Washington, DC: U.S. Government Printing Office.

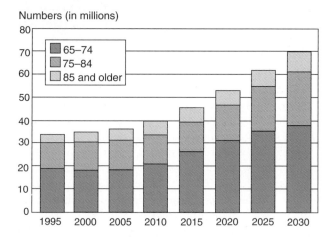

Figure 19–2 Projection of the elderly population by age, 1995–2030. From U.S. Bureau of the Census. (1993). *Population projections of the United States by age, sex, race, and Hispanic origin: 1995 to 2050.* Current Population Reports (Series P-25, No. 1130). Washington, DC: U.S. Government Printing Office.

Found in: The Institute for the Future. (2003). *Health and Health 2010. The forecast, the challenge* (2nd ed., p. 254). San Francisco: Jossey-Bass.

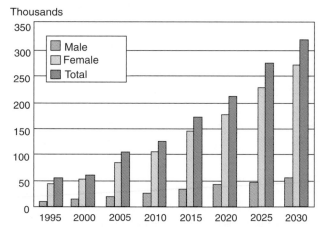

Figure 19–3 Centenarians in the United States, 1995–2030. From U.S. Bureau of the Census. (1993). *Population projections of the United States by age, sex, race, and Hispanic origin: 1995 to 2050.* Current Population Reports (Series P-25, No. 1130). Washington, DC: U.S. Government Printing Office.

Found in: The Institute for the Future. (2003). Health and Health 2010. The forecast, the challenge (2nd ed., p. 254). San Francisco: Jossey-Bass.

represents an average annual growth rate of 1 percent. During the same time, the elderly population of 65 years and older grew twice as rapidly and increased from 12 million to 35 million people. Over the next 50 years, the elderly population will continue to increase more rapidly than the total population. This aging of the population has important consequences for the health care system (National Center for Health Statistics, 2003). As the elderly fraction of the population increases, more services will be required for the treatment and management of chronic and acute health conditions. Providing health care services needed by Americans of all ages will be a major challenge in the 21st century (Figure 19–2).

Of particular significance is the projected growth in the "oldest old," the population aged 85 and above. The health and income status of this age group will be compromised, raising questions about the funding of health, social service, and long-term care (LTC) needs of this population. In 2000, 4.2 million people reached age 85. By 2010, the number of people aged 85 and older will increase to 5.7 million. By 2030, the number of people aged 85 and older will have grown to 8.5 million (Figure 19–3). As more families will have members that are elderly, family nurses will be chal-

lenged to address the needs of the aging family. Spouses will live longer together. Elderly children will be taking care of elderly parents, and, in some cases, elderly parents will be taking care of elderly children. Given the current health care system, Medicare will be stretched to the limits; therefore, managing resources will be a significant part of family nursing in the future.

Racial and Ethnic Changes in the United States

The changing ethnicity in America is the second general and major trend that creates greater challenges in promoting health in families. A decade ago, Wisensale noted "that the United States was evolving into a multiracial, multicultural, and multilingual society . . . in short, we as a nation are changing color" (1992, p. 420). Between 1995 and 2050, it is estimated that the proportion of Caucasians in the total population will decrease from 74 percent to 53 percent. In Figure 19–4, we see fewer Caucasians and a lot more of everything else. The proportion of Hispanics, African-Americans, and Asians will increase respectively 10 to 24 percent, 12 to 13 percent, and 3 to 8 percent. Only Native Americans will stay constant (see Figure 19–4). Minority families tend to be economically disadvantaged and have less access to health care, which is evident in many health outcomes such as teenage pregnancy rates, low-birth-weight newborns, high incidence of alcohol and drug abuse, and high incidence of family violence (Cox, 2002).

Although the population of all races will grow, some will grow faster than others. Hispanics in particular will increase dramatically, and their political power is sure to grow as well. Figure 19–5 shows how diversity differs according to the region of the country. Figure 19–6 demonstrates the changing ethnic composition of American families by state in 2010. Family nurses will be challenged more than ever to provide culturally competent family care. As many of the tools and assessments are geared toward Caucasian white middle-class Americans, new family assessments tools will become even more necessary. Recruitment of

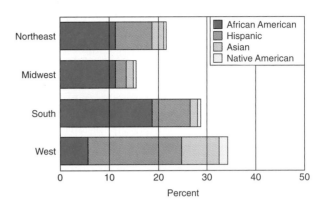

Figure 19–5 Diversity and regionality of the U.S. population, 2010. From The Institute for the Future. (2003). *Health and health care 2010: The forecast, the challenge.* San Francisco: Jossey-Bass/Wiley; U.S. Census Bureau, *Statistical Abstract, 2000.*

Found in: The Institute for the Future. (2003). *Health and Health 2010. The forecast, the challenge* (2nd ed., p. 20). San Francisco: Jossey-Bass.

culturally diverse family nurses will be a must for the academic arena.

Specific Family Trends

The following specific projections and trends for the future of families provide an important lens through which to view the future (Bianchi & Casper, 2000; Casper & Bianchi, 2002; Bumpass & Lu, 2000; The

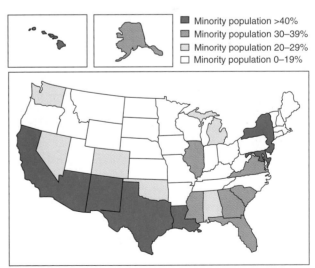

Figure 19–6 Changing ethnic composition of American families: 2010. Adapted from Coltrane, S., & Collins, R. (2001). *Sociology of marriage and the family: Gender, love, and property* (p. 571). Belmont, CA: Wadsworth/Thomson Learning.

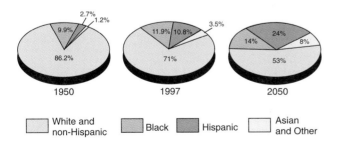

Figure 19–4 U.S. racial and ethnic composition, 1950–2050. Adapted from Cox, F. D. (2002). *Human intimacy: Marriage, the family and its meaning* (p. i). Belmont, CA: Wadsworth/Thomson Learning.

Institute for the Future, 2003; U.S. Bureau of the Census, 2003a, 2003b; World Future Society, 2004). Box 19–1 depicts some other selected family trends for the future of America.

Marriage rates remain high in the United States and are among the highest of all developed nations in the world. But there was a slight decline in the rate of marriage following WWII largely because of the trend to postpone marriage and the increase in the rates of cohabitation. On the whole, Americans will continue to believe in the institution of marriage, despite the fact that marriages continue to dissolve due to abandonment, separation, divorce, or death of a spouse. Family nurses are challenged to include the family, when there are such varied family forms. The issue of the Health Insurance Portability and Accountability Act (HIPAA) makes working with families complex in many ways, but it does require the patient to identify who can be included in their medical information. The real concern in all these situations is for the children. There are more children born to single mothers, to cohabiting parents, and in families that end in divorce. In all of these situations, the children may be affected by unstable relationships and poverty.

Divorce rates during the 1970s and 1980s increased

Box 19–1 SELECTED FAMILY TRENDS AND QUESTIONS FOR THE FUTURE

- *The marriage rate* has been dropping, although the decline has been leveling out in the last few years. The age at marriage has been going up sharply. Most women do not marry until their late 20s, and the trend may reach the point at which a majority will not marry until after 30. Men have always married later than women have, but their age at marriage has been rising more slowly than that of women. How far can these trends go? Will the average woman marry a man her own age? Will people ordinarily be getting married in their 30s or 40s? Will we reach the point at which most people never marry?

- *Premarital sexual experience* has increased, and it now occurs for a large majority of both men and women. Women's sexual behavior has tended to converge with that of men, both in premarital and extramarital sex. Does this mean that marriage as a sexual relationship is being displaced?

- *The divorce rate* has risen to a level at which half of all marriages are expected to end in divorce. In the last two decades, however, the divorce rate has remained stable and even dropped a little. Will it stay at this high level? Or is this just a temporary resting point in a curve whose shape has been uphill for more than a century? On the other hand, are there social conditions that could reverse its direction and bring the divorce rate back down again?

- *The remarriage rate* has been running parallel to the marriage rate. Divorced people tend to get remarried at about the same rate as they married in the first place, so divorces are not fatal to the family system. At the same time, marriages are popular because people are having more of them. Nevertheless, as the marriage rate has been dropping, the remarriage rate has been falling off somewhat too. Has the pattern leveled out, with most people going through several marriages in succession? Or are we in transition to a situation in which most people are going to be either unmarried or permanently divorced, and the marrieds-plus-remarrieds will become a declining majority?

- *Family violence*, including spouse abuse, child abuse, and elder abuse, has come into the spotlight. The amount of abuse that is *officially reported* has gone up sharply in recent years, but it is likely that previously a great deal of family violence was not reported. Can it be that this family conflict is an indication of forces that are in the long run tearing the family apart?

- *The birth rate* has been dropping over the long term but rising in the past few years. For decades it has hovered around replacement level, with two children born for every woman. The *age of childbearing* has also been rising, which parallels the later age of marriage. Women who put off marrying until their late 20s and early 30s are delaying having children for another few years after that. How far can this go? There has been a biological upper limit on women's childbearing by the late 40s; as women get married later, their number of years of childbearing is reduced. This may mean that birth rates will drop in the future. What is there to keep the birth rate from falling all the way to zero?

(continued on page 485)

There are a number of side effects of the falling birth rate:

- Nonmarital births are increasingly common. Most of the increase is due to unmarried women over the age of 20 giving birth. In the black population, where the marriage rate is especially low, the proportion of births that are nonmarital has risen to well over half.
- *The average household size* has gotten smaller. Few families have large numbers of children. On the other hand, there are many singles and childless couples. At the upper end of the age spectrum, we see an increasing number of senior citizens, with a preponderance of widows among the oldest. The mom-and-dad-and-kids family has become a minority.
- *The ethnic composition of families* has been changing in the United States. The trend toward declining birth rates is strongest in the white population, composed of ethnic groups of European origin. With their birth rates near replacement level, recent growth in U.S. population has been due primarily to immigration, especially to groups from Asia and Latin America. Immigrant ethnic groups tend to have more-traditional family structures and higher birth rates.

Adapted from Coltrane, S., & Collins, R. (2001). *Sociology of marriage and the family: Gender, love, and property* (5th ed., p. 570). Belmont, CA: Wadsworth/Thomson Learning.

rapidly. More than 50 percent of all marriages are said to end in divorce. In recent years, there has been a slight trend downward thought to be due to the increase in age at first marriage, which lowers the risk of divorce. Divorce will continue to be the typical way the majority of marriages end.

Birth rates are down after the baby boom following WWII. Children's overall share of the population has declined and will continue to decline in the foreseeable future as fertility rates stay low and baby boomers age. Delays in first marriage often mean that couples delay having their first child. The birth rate among never-married women is rising and will likely continue to rise; unmarried motherhood currently accounts for almost one-third of all births in the United States. Fertility rates will likely stay below replacement (2.0) for the general population, although there is a significant variation in fertility rates across socioeconomic, racial, and ethnic groups. Migration families have high fertility and will help keep population replacement up in the United States. The majority of children that are being born in America are to immigrant women. This trend again emphasizes the need for family nurses to be culturally competent.

The proportion of married women (with or without children) employed in the workforce has increased rapidly in the past 40 years, with the greatest growth among married women with preschool children. The combined necessity of the economy and increased higher education for women resulting in occupational skills will continue the upward trend in maternal employment. Mothers in two-parent households carry increasing economic responsibilities. Working moth-

ers are here to stay. Given that women will continue to be stretched and will continue to experience role overload and strain, family nurses must incorporate the knowledge of family roles and concepts of role negotiation, role sharing, and how to change expectations surrounding roles.

The future of families is one of diversity of family forms and new roles for its members. There is little evidence that any force will move families back toward the supposed "idyllic nuclear family" of the 1950s (Coontz, 1998). Families and intimate relations will continue to evolve. For example, continuous changes in relationships appear in single-parent families, gay and lesbian partnerships, interracial marriages, and multigenerational families (new extended family). Diversity includes both cohabitation and living as a single. Chapter 5 in this textbook—Family Structure, Function, and Process—is an elaboration of the diverse family structure, function, and process.

The future of families will call for increased kinds of and changing marital roles. Twenty years ago, it was predicted by many that household equality was quickly approaching. However, it appears that working women simply added a second "shift" to their lifestyles. The home and child care are still considered the province and responsibility of women. Although more men are involved in housework and child care, more men have also abandoned their families and failed to provide court-ordered child support after divorce. Role options in families will continue to become more flexible, but at the same time, families will probably continue to have a gender-based division of labor.

Box 19–2

Some of the growing key multigenerational challenges for caregiving are the following:
1. The average American has more parents than children.
2. A growing percentage of elders have children who themselves are over 65.
3. Most married couples aged 51 to 61 have living parents, children, and grandchildren.
4. Increasing numbers of elders live in quadruple-generation families.
5. Age-related health problems are affecting both the health care receivers and providers.

Source: The Institute for the Future. (2003). *Health and health care 2010: The forecast, the challenge.* San Francisco: Jossey-Bass/Wiley.

More middle-generation adults face caregiving for children and caregiving for elders at the same time. They find themselves in the "sandwich generation" between prolonged dependency of adult children remaining or returning to the home of origin and elderly parents and grandparents entering into their homes on a somewhat permanent basis (see Box 19–2). It is also estimated that more and more of our nation's children will be raised or partially raised by their grandparents (Cox, 2002).

The increase in the number of elderly, accompanied by the decline in the fertility rates and decreased mortality, has a direct impact on families. The fastest-growing population group is individuals older than 85 years of age, who are more likely to be frail and dependent and possess multiple health needs. The availability of kin to provide family care becomes a major issue for families. Families will be managing care of family members from a distance, via phone, e-mail, and fax technology (Kinsella, 1996; Kaakinen, 1999). What the future may hold is that the oldest of the old will be cared for by their children in their 80s or grandchildren in their 60s (Kaakinen, 1999; Dreman, 1997b).

Families will have more complicated family histories and kinship relationships resulting from divorce, remarriage, and serial relationships. Society will need to come up with a whole new vocabulary on how to relate to the complexity of relationships in modern families.

The U.S. population will be better educated in the future. For example, in 2005 fifty-five percent of people aged 25 years and older will have the equivalent of one year of college (The Institute for the Future, 2003) (Figure 19–7).

In the year 2010, 50 percent of the population will have a family income of $53,000 or more in constant 1999 dollars. Income disparity, a critical factor in determining health, will increase (The Institute for the Future, 2003, p. 21) (Figure 19–8). Because the average per capita income in America will increase in real dollars, the good news is that higher income is generally associated with improved health. The disturbing news is that the gap between the richest 25 percent and the poorest 25 percent of the population is widening. When income disparity among the population widens, the overall health status of the population worsens. This negative consequence on the nation's overall health status will remain a significant social and health issue well into the future.

Genetic technology will definitely be a part of our future. Today, we are moving rapidly toward a future when the knowledge of our genetic makeup and its

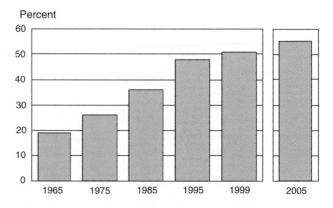

Figure 19–7 Percentage of people age 25 and older who have attended college. From U.S. Census Bureau, *Statistical Abstract, 2000.*

Found in: The Institute for the Future. (2003). *Health and Health 2010. The forecast, the challenge* (2nd ed., p. 94). San Francisco: Jossey-Bass.

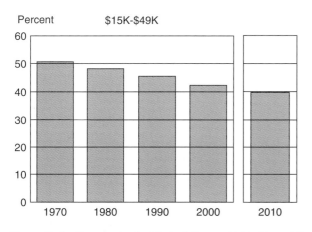

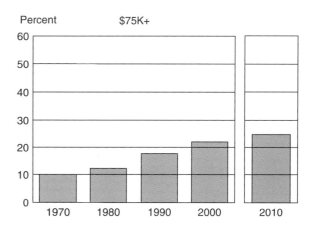

Figure 19–8 Income in the United States, 2010. From The Institute for the Future. (2003). *Health and health care 2010: The forecast, the challenge.* San Francisco: Jossey-Bass/Wiley; U.S. Census Bureau, *Money Income in the United States, 1999.* Found in: The Institute for the Future. (2003). *Health and Health 2010. The forecast, the challenge* (2nd ed., p. 22). San Francisco: Jossey-Bass.

implications for our individual futures will radically transform the world around us. What are the social, legal, political, and ethical issues arising for the future from recent advanced discoveries made in genetic research (Williams, Tripp-Reimer, Schutte, & Barnette, 2004)? See Chapter 17 in this book for a discussion of genomics and family nursing across the life span.

People born today in the United States will have to be very resilient as they move into the future. Many people can expect to live in 11 different family configurations over their lifetime. To understand this analogy, individuals need to conceptualize what constitutes a family in a broad sense of the word. First, they will be born to biological parents, and many live in a nuclear intact two-parent family. Second, their parents may get divorced and they will live in a single-parent family. Third, their custodial parent may remarry and their family structure becomes a step family or remarried family. Fourth, their remarried parents may divorce, so they go back to a single-parent family. Fifth, our hypothetical people grow up, leave home, and become single adults in their own households. Sixth, most young people will cohabitate with one or more partners before they marry. Seventh, they will finally marry and now live in a nuclear family, most often with children. Eighth, they themselves will divorce and now head their own single-parent family. Ninth, they may remarry a second time and form a stepparent or remarried family. Tenth, a second divorce is common and they will become a single-parent family or just a single-adult family again.

Finally, many people will live single throughout the rest of their lives. Many other variations may occur depending on sexual orientation, ethnicity, faith system, or country of origin. This pattern of family exposure appears to be more characteristic of Western countries, although it is quickly happening in other parts of the world as well. Families of the future must be able to define themselves broadly and be able to adapt quickly to the changing internal and external environment around them.

WORLD DEMOGRAPHIC TRENDS

Thus far, the focus of family demographic trends has been American families. It is impossible to view U.S. families without looking at two major global trends as well: population and aging. In the book *Which World? Scenarios for the 21st Century*, Hammond (1998) presented low, medium, and high population projections from 1995 for the year 2050 (see Table 19–1). These projections include what Hammond termed industrialized regions, transitional regions, and developing regions. It is clear that global concerns are shared by all. This planet has surpassed a population of 6 billion, with the United States constituting only 5 percent of the world's population.

The International Conference on Population and Development (ICPD+5) believes that population concerns are at the heart of sustainable development strategies. The United Nations projected that the world population will not level off until it reaches 9 billion in 2050 (247 children are born each minute

**Table 19–1   WORLD POPULATION PROJECTIONS, 2050
(IN MILLIONS)**

	1995	2050		
		LOW	MEDIUM	HIGH
Industrial Regions				
North America	297	301	384	452
Europe	383	293	346	389
Japan	125	96	110	122
Transitional Regions				
Russia	148	97	114	142
Eastern Europe	152	110	131	156
Developing Regions				
Latin America	471	643	802	991
China	1,220	1,198	1,517	1,765
Southeast Asia	511	664	827	1,010
India[a]	929	1,231	1,533	1,885
Sub-Saharan Africa	586	1,518	1,783	2,089
North Africa and Middle East	348	650	785	930
World Total[b]	*5,687*	*7,662*	*9,367*	*11,156*

[a]The corresponding numbers for South Asia as a whole are 1,225 for 1995 and 1,786, 2,194,
  and 2,665 (low, medium, and high projections, respectively) for 2050.
[b]The regional numbers do not add up to the world total because a number of countries have
  been omitted to simplify.
Source: Hanson, S. M. H. (Ed.). (2001). *Family health care nursing: Theory, practice, and research*
  (2nd ed.). Philadelphia: FA Davis.

in the world). (Contact http://www.unfpa.org for more information on the ICPD's plan of action.) Riche (1998), former head of the U.S. Census Bureau, reported the facts on aging, fertility, the new healthy living, and population change. Figure 19–9 shows the soaring world population trends from 1800 to 2050 and emphasizes that this growth takes place primarily in poor nations. Figure 19–10 shows the world population by billions with an emphasis on the contributions of China and India.

The second major world demographic change after population growth pertains to the aging of the world population. Figure 19–11 shows a comparison of the global aging patterns over time among continents. The graying of the world appears to be affecting industrialized countries due to their advanced medical technology and standards of living. In North America the current life expectancy is 77 years; it is 69 years in Latin America and the Caribbean, 73 in Europe, 66 in Asia, and 51 in Africa. By 2030 the number of Americans over 65 will nearly double from 39 to 69 million and the elderly will constitute 20 percent of the population. This aging trend brings up all kinds of resource and ethical issues for countries around the world (Box 19–3).

HEALTH OF AMERICAN FAMILIES

Thus far in this chapter, changing families and the futures of American families have been addressed from

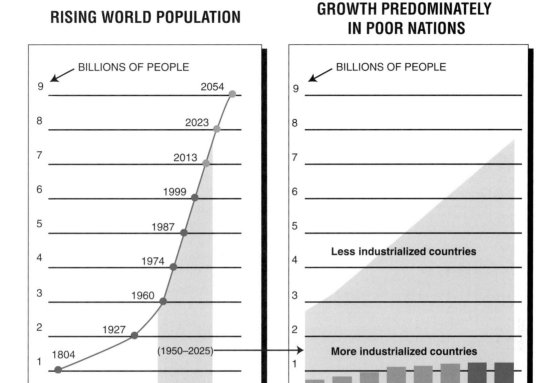

Reference: United Nations Population Division

In 1804 the world's population reached the 1 billion mark. It took 123 years to reach 2 billion whereas it took only 12 years to go from 5 to 6 billion. Due to a decline in the fertility rate and the aging of the population, the world's population will level off at 10 billion (approx.) by the year 2200.

Because the growth rates of less industrialized countries have been significantly higher than those of more industrialized countries, in the past 50 years, the net gain in the world's population has taken place in the world's poorest areas.

Note:

More industrialized countries and areas include North America, Europe, Japan, Australia, and New Zealand.

Less industrialized countries and areas include All of Africa, all of Asia except Japan, the Transcaucasian and Central Asian countries of the former Soviet Union, all of Latin America and the Caribbean, and all of Oceania except Australia and New Zealand.

Figure 19–9 Soaring world population and growth nations. From Hanson, S. M. H. (Ed.). (2001). *Family health care nursing: Theory, practice, and research* (2nd ed.). Philadelphia: FA Davis; United Nations Population Division.

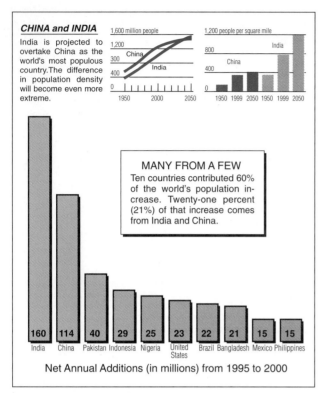

Figure 19–10   World populations by billions. From Hanson, S. M. H. (Ed.). (2001). *Family health care nursing: Theory, practice, and research* (2nd ed.). Philadelphia: FA Davis; United Nations Population Division.

the standpoint of aging, race and ethnicity, marriage and divorce, birth rates, and family caregiving, as well as some of the challenges that go along with these trends. World demographic trends were also summa-

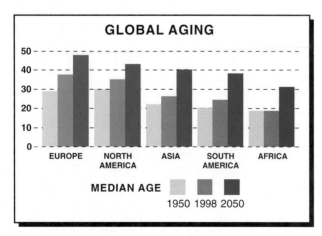

Figure 19–11   Global aging. From Hanson, S. M. H. (Ed.). (2001). *Family health care nursing: Theory, practice, and research* (2nd ed.). Philadelphia: FA Davis; United Nations Population Division.

rized. Next, the health of American families will be examined, and we will look at how this might relate to families in the future. The actual health status of the American public has implications for when, where, and how family nurses go about their practice.

Healthy People

Healthy People was the initial family social policy program established by the federal government in 1979 that developed national health targets and new health policies (U.S. Department of Health, Education and Welfare, 1979). The five challenging goals set forth by this Surgeon General's report were to reduce mortality among various age groups: infants, children, adolescents, young adults, and adults. Through the combined efforts of the nation's public health agencies, most of the goals were accomplished by 1990. *Healthy People 2000* (U.S. Department of Health, Education and Welfare, 1979) was then developed with objectives for the next 10 years built upon the prior success of the first Surgeon General's report, and this was the product of unprecedented collaboration among government, voluntary, and professional organizations, businesses, and individuals. The framework for *Healthy People 2000* consisted of three broad goals: increase the span of healthy life for Americans, reduce health disparities among Americans, and achieve access to preventive services for all Americans. This broad approach to health promotion, health protection, and prevention services provided direction for individuals to change personal behaviors and for organizations and communities to support good health through health promotion policies.

The U.S. Department of Health and Human Services developed newer proposals titled *Healthy People 2010 Objectives* (1998) and *Healthy People 2010: Understanding and Improving Health* (2000), which are the programs in place for the period from 2000 to 2010. See Figure 19–12 for the model underlying these programs. See Table 19–2 and Table 19–3 for the 28 focus areas and the 10 leading health indicators developed for the Healthy People in Healthy Communities program. These new proposals were different from earlier programs because of advancement in preventive therapies, vaccines and pharmaceuticals, assistive technologies, and computerized systems that have changed the face of health care and how it is practiced. New relationships were defined between public health departments and health care delivery organizations. With demographic changes in the United States reflecting an older and more racially

Box 19–3   IF WE COULD SHRINK THE EARTH

If we could shrink the Earth's population to a village of precisely 100 people, with all the existing human ratios remaining the same, that village would resemble the following:

- 57 would be Asians.
- 21 would be Europeans.
- 14 would be from the Western Hemisphere, both north and south.
- 8 would be Africans.
- 52 would be female.
- 48 would be male.
- 70 would be nonwhite.
- 30 would be white.
- 70 would be non-Christian.
- 30 would be Christian.

- 89 would be heterosexual.
- 11 would be homosexual.
- 6 would possess 59 percent of the entire world's wealth, and all 6 would be from the United States.
- 80 would live in substandard housing.
- 70 would be unable to read.
- 50 would suffer from malnutrition.
- 1 would be near death; 1 would be near birth.
- 1 (yes, only 1) would have a college education.
- 1 would own a computer.

Note: Although these statistics have been challenged by some (www.snopes2.com/science/stats/populate.htm), when one considers our world from such a compressed perspective, the need for acceptance, understanding, and education becomes glaringly apparent.

diverse population, these new facts created new demands on existing public health and overall health care systems. Other global forces—including war and terrorism, food supplies, emerging infectious diseases, and environmental interdependence—presented new public health challenges. The two major goals of these latest government mandates were to (1) increase quality and years of healthy life and (2) eliminate health disparities. Each goal contains numerous objectives and the ways in which these objectives can be reached.

Table 19–2   HEALTHY PEOPLE 2010: 28 FOCUS AREAS

1. Access to Quality Health Services	14. Immunization and Infectious Diseases
2. Arthritis, Osteoporosis, and Chronic Back Conditions	15. Injury and Violence Prevention
3. Cancer	16. Maternal, Infant, and Child Health
4. Chronic Kidney Disease	17. Medical Product Safety
5. Diabetes	18. Mental Health and Mental Disorders
6. Disability and Secondary Conditions	19. Nutrition and "Obesity"
7. Educational and Community-Based Programs	20. Occupational Safety and Health
8. Environmental Health	21. Oral Health
9. Family Planning	22. Physical Activity and Fitness
10. Food Safety	23. Public Health Infrastructure
11. Health Communication	24. Respiratory Diseases
12. Heart Disease and Stroke	25. Sexually Transmitted Diseases
13. HIV	26. Substance Abuse
	27. Tobacco Use
	28. Vision and Hearing

Source: Healthy People in Healthy Communities. Retrieved from http://www. healthypeople.gov/publications/HealthyCommunities2001/healthycom01hk.pdf

Table 19–3   **TEN LEADING HEALTH INDICATORS: HEALTHY PEOPLE IN HEALTHY COMMUNITIES**

In a Snapshot…

HEALTHY PEOPLE 2010 identifies a set of health priorities that reflect 10 major public health concerns in the United States. These 10 Leading Health Indicators are intended to help everyone more easily understand the importance of health promotion and disease prevention. Motivating individuals to act on just one of the indicators can have a profound effect on increasing the quality and years of healthy life and on eliminating health disparities— for the individual, as well as the community overall.

SUBJECT TOPIC	PUBLIC HEALTH CHALLENGE
Physical Activity	Promote regular physical activity.
Overweight and Obesity	Promote healthier weight and good nutrition.
Tobacco Use	Prevent and reduce tobacco use.
Substance Abuse	Prevent and reduce substance abuse.
Responsible Sexual Behavior	Promote responsible sexual behavior.
Mental Health	Promote mental health and well-being.
Injury and Violence	Promote safety and reduce violence.
Environmental Quality	Promote healthy environments.
Immunization	Prevent infectious disease through immunization.
Access to Health Care	Increase access to quality health care.

Source: Healthy People in Healthy Communities: A community planning guide using Healthy People
2010. Retrieved from http://www.healthypeople.gov/publications/
HealthyCommunities2001/healthycom01hk.pdf

The major premise is that the health of individuals cannot be separated from the health of larger communities. Therefore, the vision became "healthy people in healthy communities." More information about this program can be found on the Healthy People 2010 home page at http://health.gov/healthypeople. Box 19–4 (*Healthy People 2010*) is the United State's contribution to the World Health Organization's (WHO) "Health for All" strategy. The United States hopes to provide models for world policy and strategies for populations' health improvement.

Health Parameters

One way of evaluating a country's health is to have specific health parameters that tell part of that story. Life expectancy is one measure often used to gauge the overall health of a population. During the 20th century, life expectancy at birth increased from 48 to 74 years for men and from 51 to almost 80 years for women. Improvements in nutrition, housing, hygiene, and medical care contributed to decreases in death

rates throughout the life span. Life expectancy after age 65 also increased during the last century. Improved access to health care, advances in medicine, healthier lifestyles, and better health before age 65 are factors underlying decreased death rates among the elderly. Although the overall trend in life expectancy for the United States has been upward throughout the 20th century, the gain in years of life expectancy for women generally exceeded that for men (Figure 19–13).

Chronic health conditions causing limitation of activity among working-age adults by age in the United States from 1999 to 2001 were studied by health surveys that measured limitation of activity (Figure 19–14) (National Center for Health Statistics, 2003). Because the aging population is growing and older people have most of the chronic conditions, a large percentage of health care resources will be used in the treatment of various chronic conditions. Among younger and older working adults, arthritis and other musculoskeletal conditions were the most frequent conditions. Among persons 18 to 44, mental illness

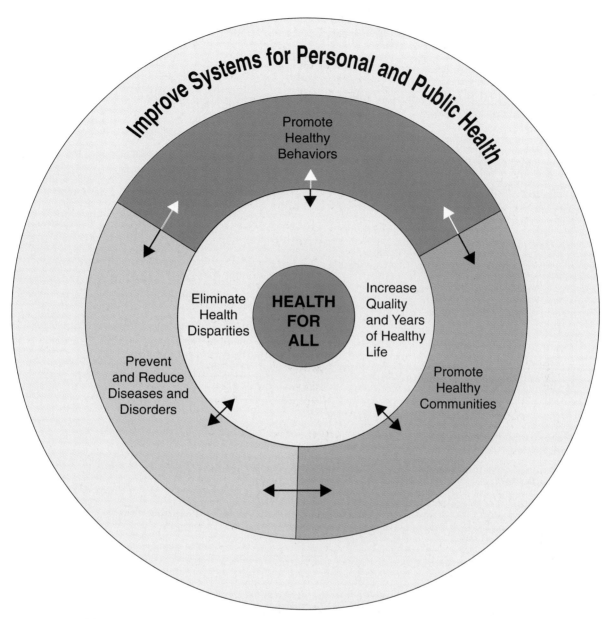

Figure 19–12 Healthy People 2010—Healthy People in Healthy Communities. From U.S. Department of Health and Human Services, Office of Public Health and Science. (1998). *Healthy people 2010 objectives: Draft for public comment.* Washington, DC: U.S. Government Printing Office; U.S. Department of Health and Human Services, Office of Public Health and Science. (2000). *Healthy people 2010: Understanding and improving health* (2nd ed.). Washington, DC: U.S. Government Printing Office.

was the second most prevalent cause of activity limitation. Among older working-age adults (45 to 64 years), heart disease was the second most frequently mentioned condition.

Mortality rates are another measure of the nation's health status. These rates are usually broken down by age groups. Mortality among teens and young adults (15 to 24 years of age) declined by almost 40 percent over the past 50 years (National Center for Health Statistics, 2003). The leading causes of death in 2000 were related to either injury or chronic disease, in contrast to 1950, when the leading cause of death was infectious diseases. Unintentional injury (e.g., motor vehicle–related injuries) was the leading cause of death for teens and young adults over the past 50 years, but these injuries have declined during this period.

Box 19–4 HEALTHY PEOPLE 2010

Goals

1. Increase quality and years of healthy life
2. Eliminate health disparities

Objectives

Promote Healthy Behaviors

1. Physical activity and fitness
2. Nutrition
3. Tobacco use

Promote Healthy and Safe Communities

1. Educational and community-based programs
2. Environmental health
3. Food safety
4. Injury/violence prevention
   a. Injuries that cut across intent
   b. Unintentional injuries
   c. Violence and abuse
5. Occupational safety and health
6. Oral health

Improve Systems for Personal and Public Health

1. Access to quality health services
   a. Preventive care
   b. Primary care

   c. Emergency services
   d. Long-term care and rehabilitative services
2. Family planning
3. Maternal, infant, and child health
4. Medical product safety
5. Public health infrastructure
6. Health communication

Prevent and Reduce Diseases and Disorders

1. Arthritis, osteoporosis, and chronic back conditions
2. Cancer
3. Diabetes
4. Disability and secondary conditions
5. Heart disease and stroke
6. HIV
7. Immunization and infectious diseases
8. Mental health and mental disorders
9. Respiratory diseases
10. Sexually transmitted diseases
11. Substance abuse

Source: U.S. Department of Health and Human Services, Office of Public Health and Science. (1998). *Healthy people 2010 objectives: Draft for public comment.* Washington, DC: U.S. Government Printing Office; U.S. Department of Health and Human Services. (2000). *Healthy People 2010: Understanding and improving health* (2nd ed.). Washington, DC: U.S. Government Printing Office.

Homicide and suicide were the second and third leading causes of death in this age group in 2000. Whereas homicide declined between 1960 and 1995, suicide nearly tripled. Firearm-related deaths accounted for nearly three-fifths of suicides and four-fifths of homicides among teens and young adults in 2000. Males are substantially at higher risk of homicide and suicide. Black males were 8 times more vulnerable to death by homicide than white males.

Since 1950, mortality among adults 24 to 44 declined by more than 40 percent (Figure 19–15) (National Center for Health Statistics, 2003). In 2000, unintentional injury, cancer, and heart disease—the three leading causes of death among persons 25 to 44 years of age—accounted for one-half of all deaths in this age group. The next two leading causes of

death in this age group were suicide and human immunodeficiency virus (HIV). HIV disease death rates among persons 25 to 44 vary by sex and race. The risk is higher for males than for females and higher for blacks/Hispanics than for other racial groups.

Death rates for adults 45 to 64 declined over the past 50 years (National Center for Health Statistics, 2003). In 2000 cancer, heart disease, stroke, diabetes, and chronic lower respiratory diseases together accounted for 70 percent of all deaths in this age group. Men had a higher death rate than women did, and adults with a high-school education or less had a death rate more than twice the rate for high-school graduates or those with additional education.

Three-quarters of all deaths in the United States occur among persons 65 years of age and over

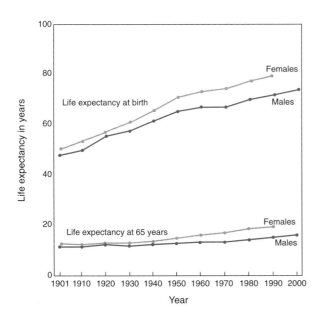

Figure 19–13 Expectancy at birth and at 65 years of age by sex: United States, 1901–2000. Adapted from National Center for Health Statistics. (2003). *Health, United States, 2003: Chartbook on trends in the health of Americans* (DHHS Publication No. 2003-1232, p. 47). Washington, DC: U.S. Government Printing Office.

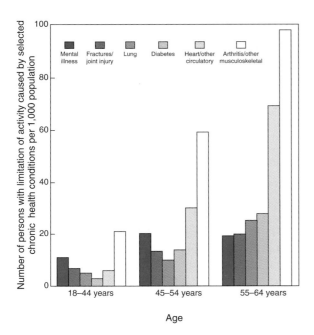

Figure 19–14 Selected chronic health conditions causing limitation of activity among working-age adults by age: United States, 1999–2001. Adapted from National Center for Health Statistics. (2003). *Health, United States, 2003: Chartbook on trends in the health of Americans* (DHHS Publication No. 2003-1232, p. 43). Washington, DC: U.S. Government Printing Office.

(National Center for Health Statistics, 2003). The leading causes of death in this age group are heart disease, cancer, stroke, chronic lower respiratory diseases (including influenza/pneumonia), and diabetes, which account for three-fourths of the deaths.

An important shift in the burden of disease in the future is related to the huge impact of chronic disease around the world. The World Health Organization (WHO) defined "burden of disease" as a combination of untimely death and disability (The Institute for the Future, 2003, p. 22). The organization's study revealed that the burden of conditions such as depression, alcohol dependence, or schizophrenia has been seriously underestimated by traditional approaches using only mortality and morbidity figures. Because an illness causes both death and disability, predictions are that mental illness, especially unipolar depression, will have a larger impact than cancer by the year 2010. The burden of disease is shifting from diseases caused by infectious organisms to disorders with behavioral causes (smoking and alcohol abuse). It is estimated that lifestyle behaviors alone contribute to 50 percent of an individual's health status (see Figure 19–16). Much more needs to be done to implement effective health management and disease prevention programs. The current focus on wellness is a phenomenon more often seen in higher socioeconomic classes in society, which already tend to have better health status anyway.

FACTORS INFLUENCING FAMILIES AND FAMILY NURSING

There are many factors that influence families and family nursing. Many of these were addressed in the review of U.S., world, and family demographics and trends earlier in this chapter. A discussion of some additional factors follows.

Terrorism and War

Terrorism and war are having profound effects on individuals, families, communities, and the health care system. In the aftermath of the terrorist attacks on New York City and Washington, D.C., in 2002, immense changes took place in the American psyche followed by vigorous action in this country's effort to protect itself and to confront terrorism. Other major acts of violence in this country also affect families and family health, such as the 1995 bombing of the Alfred P. Murrah Federal Building in Oklahoma City and the 1999 shootings at Columbine High School in

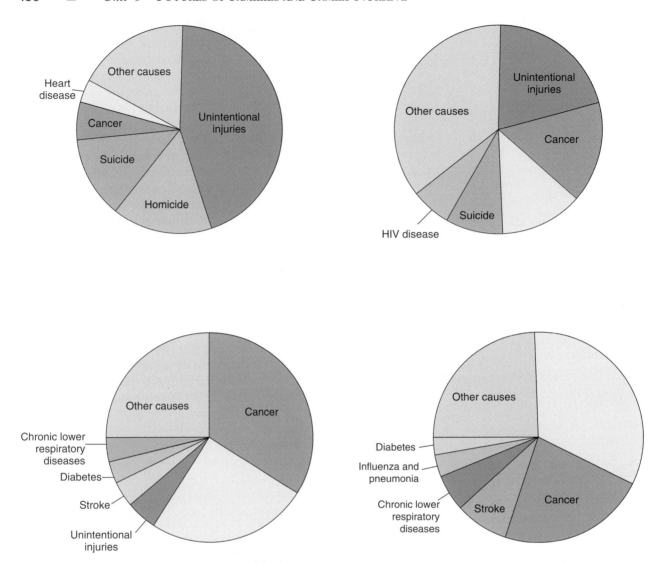

'Figure 19–15   Percentages of leading causes of death among persons 15 to 24 years, 25 to 44 years, 45 to 64 years, and 65 and over: United States, 2000. Adapted from National Center for Health Statistics. (2003). *Health, United States, 2003: Chartbook on trends in the health of Americans* (DHHS Publication No. 2003-1232, pp. 50–57). Washington, DC: U.S. Government Printing Office.

Littleton, Colorado (http://nimh.nih/gov/publicat/ violence.cfm). The National Strategy for Homeland Security and the Homeland Security Act of 2002 were established to mobilize and organize the homeland against terrorist attacks (http://www.dhs.gov/). All of the frightening current events and their meaning for our future have increased the number of people writing and conducting family-related research. For example, there are ongoing studies on terrorism and children (Myers-Walls, 2004), coping when a family member has been called to war (Whealin & Pivar, 2004), post-traumatic stress disorder (Whealin & Pivar, 2004), adaptation in military families (Pittman,

Kerpelman, & McFadyen, 2004), and building strong communities for military families (Martin, Mancini, Bowen, Mancini, & Orthner, 2004).

Terrorism, war, and violence are an important and timely topic and have major ramifications for families and the health care system, family nurses in particular. Nurses serve in many capacities and in different settings that deal with the action and aftermath of these violent world events. For example, nurses serve in the military on the front line of duty, nurses care for victims and sometimes perpetrators of acute physical and mental trauma, nurses help patients to rehabilitate, and nurses work with the families who are

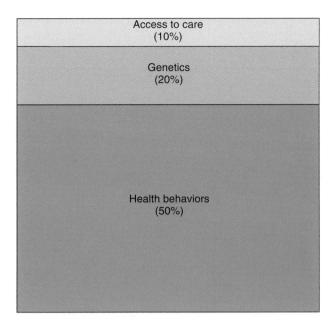

Figure 19–16 Determinants of health. From The Institute for the Future. (2003). *Health and health care 2010: The forecast, the challenge*. San Francisco: Jossey-Bass/Wiley; Centers for Disease Control and Prevention.
Found in: The Institute for the Future. (2003). *Health and Health 2010. The forecast, the challenge* (2nd ed., p. 23). San Francisco: Jossey-Bass.

afflicted by these activities. No health care professional, community, or organization is excluded from working with people who live with the stress of current world events and the human condition. Nurses need to be educated to learn how families adapt to these stressors and to learn successful ways to intervene in such family events.

Health Care Workforce: Future Supply and Demand

The Institute for the Future (2003) studied the health care workforce to predict future supply and demand of a variety of health care workers (p. 95). The researchers stated that there has been little fundamental change in the way health professionals are organized and the way they interact with each other. There has been little change in the way that physicians practice medicine, and physicians remain central figures in American health care. Although nurse practitioners (NPs), physicians' assistants (PAs), and other providers possess skills well suited to the demands of an environment with a greater focus on cost containment and managing health behaviors, their roles are limited by their small numbers and the political control exercised by the medical profession.

The nursing profession is the most qualified to respond to current changes in the health needs of families. Nursing education focuses more on behavioral and preventive aspects of health care than does that of physicians. Registered nurses (RNs) are the largest single group of health providers in the United States, numbering over 2.2 million. Hospitals continue to employ two-thirds of all RNs even though there is more health care taking place in ambulatory care settings, nursing homes, subacute nursing facilities, and community health clinics. In 1996 it was projected that there was an adequate supply of RNs to meet the needs of the future. These projections were incorrect because they did not consider the impact of the dwindling number of applicants to schools of nursing, the aging population of the nurse workforce, and the exodus of nurses from acute care settings because of poor working conditions (The Institute for the Future, 2003, p. 103.) By 2001, the existing and projected shortage of nurses was viewed as a national disaster, and it still is a major concern among health care leaders.

Multiple factors account for the present and future shortage of RNs overall, and the major impact has fallen on hospitals—on the acute care nursing units in the emergency department and in the operating room. Stress, irregular working hours, declining working conditions, low morale, and frustration at providing suboptimal care have amplified the shortage. Burnout has become commonplace. Table 19–4 summarizes the projected RN requirements by employment settings for the years 2000 to 2010. Figure 19–17 shows the projected supply of RNs for the years 2000 to 2020 (Cooper, Laud, & Dietrich, 1998). In the fast-paced health care settings, nurses are challenged to practice family nursing. It is easy to only deal with the ill individual and not venture into family nursing. As the shortage continues, nurses will be stretched even thinner, thus endangering the practice of family nursing. Illness is clearly a family affair, and families should be included in the care.

Religion

Religious institutions have a major impact on families and the health practices of families. Many of the traditions of family life are closely tied to religious ceremonies, including weddings, births, passing into adulthood, and healing rituals. Families have passed these practices from generation to generation. In addition, many families find it helpful to use spiritual sources for strength, meaning, and assistance when they are experiencing hardship, using such strategies

| Table 19–4 | PROJECTED RN REQUIREMENTS BY EMPLOYMENT SETTING, 2000–2010 | | | | | | |

	TOTAL	HOSPITALS	NURSING HOMES	AMBULATORY CARE	PUBLIC/ COMMUNITY HEALTH	NURSING EDUCATION	OTHER
2000	1,969,000	1,231,800	128,200	134,200	364,300	37,800	72,500
2005	2,095,000	1,305,200	138,000	142,600	387,200	41,500	80,200
2010	2,232,000	1,386,100	152,600	150,700	411,000	45,500	87,400

Source: Projections by Division of Nursing, Bureau of Health Professionals, Health Resources and Services Administration, U.S. Department of Health and Human Services, March 1996. Found in: The Institute for the Future. (2003). *Health and Health 2010. The forecast, the challenge* (2nd ed., p. 104). San Francisco: Jossey-Bass.

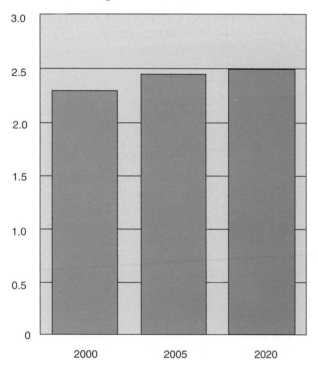

Millions of registered nurses

Figure 19–17   Projected supply of RNs, 2000–2020. From Projections by Division of Nursing, Bureau of Health Professionals, Health Resources and Services Administration, U.S. Department of Health and Human Services, March 1996.

Found in: The Institute for the Future. (2003). *Health and Health 2010. The forecast, the challenge* (2nd ed., p. 104). San Francisco: Jossey-Bass.

as prayer, becoming more involved in religious activities, and developing greater faith (Anderson & Evison, 2004). Further, religion has been recognized as playing an important role in the mental health of individuals and families, in their outlook on life, and in their lifestyle (Fong & Sandhu, 1993). Family nurses need to be aware of families' cultural and religious beliefs and practices. Because of the diversity of religious practices within even small communities today, nurses will encounter various spiritual customs that may influence families' responses to health care practices. Nurses need to study ways to promote spiritual dimensions of health and not just refer patients to someone else. Nurses are central to helping patients make sense of the meaning of their illness and mobilizing actions to assist patients in spiritual distress, especially in light of increased chronic health conditions and palliative end-of-life care. Religion and faith have a major impact on individual and family lives. The present wars around the world have underscored how people of different faiths and value systems have difficulty understanding and respecting another person's belief system.

Sexuality

Human sexuality is another element affecting families today. During the sexual revolution of the late 1960s and 1970s brought about by the development of the birth control pill, premarital sexual behavior became more common and cohabitation became an accepted form of family life. Births to unmarried women increased dramatically over the past decade. For example, births to unmarried women between the ages of 15 and 44 increased so much that they now account for approximately one-third of all live births in the United States (U.S. Bureau of the Census, 2003a). Today, the threat of acquired immune deficiency syndrome (AIDS) has heightened awareness of the danger of random sexual activity.

One of the leading issues of this decade has been in the area of same-gender marriages. Gay and lesbian couples have long sought ways to become joined in matrimony. They have based their arguments on equal rights for all Americans. This topic has divided the community into liberal and conservative camps. See Chapter 6 (Families, Nursing, and Social Policy) for more discussion of this issue and the nursing implications for practice.

Health Care Technology

As a result of advances in technology, the complexity of health care practices has increased significantly in the past two decades. Ongoing technological development will continue to result in rapid changes in health care. Family nurses will be challenged to provide personalized care with high-touch delivery to family members as a balance to the dehumanization that can occur with highly technical patient care.

Changes in technology have not only increased the complexity of health care but also changed the nature of nursing practice in acute care settings and in the home. Today, patients stay in the hospital for much shorter periods of time and return to their homes while still requiring care. Thus, the family must either provide the care or ensure that appropriate providers come into the home for follow-up care. In addition, the use of computers is changing practice. For example, minimum data sets have been created to track delivery of care with the result that data on assessments, interventions, referrals, follow-up, and so forth are now providing ongoing information.

The use of video technology and satellite telecommunication systems is no longer new. One of the major uses today is for health education, both basic education and continuing education. Nurses in rural areas receive continuing education and are able to pursue advanced degrees through educational video networks. Patient care via telecommunications systems is becoming more common, primarily through consultation with experts over interactive video.

Genetics

Genetics is the central science for health care in the future. In a guest editorial for the *Journal of Family Nursing,* Feetham (1999, pp. 3–9) summarized the need for a nursing paradigm that requires nurses to understand and incorporate human genetics in their practice. Because this is such an important topic for the future of family nursing, a new chapter written for this book by Williams and Skirton was devoted to this topic (see Chapter 17).

The burgeoning genetic knowledge is a result of the Human Genome Project (HGP), which began in the mid-1980s as an international research program led by the U.S. Department of Energy (DOE) and the National Institutes of Health (NIH). This science will help make possible the identification of individuals at risk for disease and the diagnosis and treatment of disease, none of which was conceivable until recently. These findings result in unique challenges for families, requiring health professionals to understand how discoveries in molecular genetics will increase their ability to interpret the clinical symptoms of patients and inform their clinical management. Nurses must understand the trajectory of these genetic discoveries and that the knowledge of risk may change over time. This knowledge has major implications for all health professionals working with individuals and their families. Genetic discoveries help health scientists treat primary dysfunction or disease progression rather than just treating symptoms.

Nurses need to be aware of the research and to stay current in their areas of specialization. Genetics is an area where family nurses can provide significant leadership. The paucity of attention to family systems and family relationships in the collection and dissemination of genetic information places family members and families at increased risk. It is documented that most health professionals do not practice within the context of the family (Feetham, 1999). Nurses need to assist families and know that family relationships may be affected as a result of the process of genetic risk identification. Families expect nurses to interpret public, clinical, and scientific literature, and that includes new cutting-edge research from molecular genetics. Nurses can help by encouraging individuals to consider how genetic testing and results may affect family relationships.

Nurses need to be aware that HGP discoveries have significant ethical, legal, and social implications. The National Coalition for Health Professional Education in Genetics (NCHPEG) promotes health professional education and access to information about advancements in human genetics (www.nchpeg.org). Nurses should help provide leadership to the genetic revolution, and family nursing had a particularly strong role in this revolution.

Ethnic Diversity

During most of the 20th century, the minority American population was the African-American population, and they composed a relatively stable proportion (13 to 15 percent). Between 1960 and 1990 the minority population tripled in size to compose 25 percent of the U.S. population (Coltrane & Collins, 2001). By the year 2010, minorities will increase to 33 percent of the nation's people, with Hispanics the most numerous. It will soon become a misnomer to label such groups as "minority" as the numbers change. By 2010, 19 states will be composed of more than one-third minority children. That means that early in the 21st century, a substantial proportion of people in the United States will belong to these ethnic groups. This changing ethnic diversity has impact on the structure, function, and process of American families, the health care system, and particularly family nursing. Not only will nurses be working with a larger variety of ethnic groups, but also they will need to become more culturally competent. Hopefully the number of culturally diverse health care providers will grow in the future, which will help make health care culturally relevant and sensitive.

Health Care Reform

Health care reform is a major issue in America today. Some of the questions being asked include the following:

- Does every person have the right to health care?
- What does universal access to health care really mean?
- How will individuals pay for their health insurance?
- If not individuals, who should pay for health care?
- Should there be a standard benefit health insurance package that individuals have a right to?

The rising costs of health care have made it impossible to ignore these issues any longer. Nearly all the states, as well as the federal government, are examining health care. Managed care has become the primary mode of organizing health care delivery. In a managed care system, insurance companies contract with selected health care providers to furnish a comprehensive set of health care services to individuals who are enrolled in an insurance program with a predetermined monthly premium (The Institute for the Future, 2003). Participants in managed care systems generally have a primary care provider who manages their care. There are financial incentives for patients to use the providers and facilities associated with the managed care plans in which they are enrolled. As managed care plans are emerging and shifting, variations in the mode of operation are also occurring, including which health care providers are to be included and what services will be covered.

The roles of public health departments, which have been the primary providers of health care to poor families in many areas of the country, are also changing. In some instances, public clinics are becoming part of managed care health plans. Many of these decisions are being made at the community level. It is critical that nurses participate in the decision making and advocate the role of nursing in future health care systems.

Nurses who receive third-party reimbursement must continue to be visionary in guiding their practice to ensure their inclusion in managed care plans. As primary care providers, family nurses who practice with an understanding of the dynamics of families will provide more-effective nursing care. Although the number of nurses graduating with advanced degrees has increased markedly during the past 20 years, there are still insufficient numbers of primary care nurses and nurses with a sound foundation in family nursing practice.

In order to have an impact on health care delivery, nurses need to become active at every level of the political system and advocate for family issues. Voting is no longer enough. Nurses must get to know the political candidates and elected officials in their cities, districts, and states, attend campaign events, write letters on health care issues from a nursing perspective, offer assistance in analyzing issues related to health care reform, and volunteer to serve on local or state commissions or boards related to health. The challenge today is to establish health care systems in which nurses are provided opportunities to work with families as well as with individuals.

With the rising cost of health care and attempts to get these costs under control, budgets are under constant scrutiny. It is essential that family nurses demonstrate, through practice and research, the benefits of family health care. Families respond positively to nurses practicing with a family nursing perspective (Gillis & Knafl, 1999). Additional studies are needed to examine the effectiveness of family nursing practice. Nurses must help families meet the developmental and situational transitions in life. In the 21st century, we can no longer afford to overlook the family's role in health protection and promotion. The health care system must view families as a significant influence on health care outcomes, and it is our job to help the system view them that way.

Nurses also have another critical role in the face of health care reform. The changes in health care that are on the horizon mean that families must become better-educated consumers of health care services. More than ever, families will need to become adept at participating in the decisions that will affect their health. Nurses need to acquire the knowledge and skills to empower families through participating in community organizations, coalition building, and other political activities.

FUTURE OF FAMILY NURSING: THEORY, PRACTICE, RESEARCH, EDUCATION, AND SOCIAL POLICY

What are the implications of the changes in U.S. and world demographics, the health care system, and factors that influence families and family nursing to the future of family nursing theory, practice, research, education, and social policy? And what is the state of family nursing today in regard to these five areas of practice?

Family Nursing Theory

Family nursing theory is an evolving area of study within the nursing profession. As mentioned in the theoretical chapter of this textbook (Chapter 3), family nursing theory has drawn from the family social science theories, family therapy theories, and nursing models/theories. The trend to use integrated (eclectic) models from within and outside of nursing will continue. There is a need to further develop hybrid family nursing models drawn from these three genres of family nursing theory and to reconceptualize and test their efficacy in family nursing.

Family Nursing Practice

Family nursing practice has been an evolving specialty area within nursing (Hanson, 2001) and will continue to affect health care significantly in the future, especially with the current focus on health care reform in the United States. Whereas 10 years ago family nursing was considered an emerging specialty, the recent trend has been to integrate the family as client into all the traditional nursing specialties (i.e., medical/surgical nursing, pediatric nursing, community health nursing). The barriers that confront the practice of family nursing (see Chapter 8, Family Nursing Assessment and Intervention) need to be addressed in the new health care delivery systems. As health care is moved into family homes and the community, nurses will be called upon to serve families as a unit of care. This community-based family nursing care will be affected by the trends such as caring for large numbers of aging and especially the oldest of the old patients, serving populations of diverse ethnic backgrounds, using more high technology to care for patients, and adjusting to the continuous changes and reforms in the health care industry.

Research

Most family nursing research has traditionally focused on individuals rather than families as a unit of analysis (Houck & Kodadek, 2001) (see Chapter 4, "Research in Families and Family Nursing"). Research pertaining to families and mental health is further advanced than research on families and physical health. Recently nursing has awakened to the connection between family dynamics and health and illness. More recent research studies reported in family nursing (Hinshaw, Feetham, & Shaver, 1999) focused on the science of nursing research of families from three perspectives: research in normative family transitions, research in nonnormative family transitions, and family policy (Gillis & Knafl, 1999; McCubbin, 1999; Feetham & Meister, 1999). It is clear that further family-centered nursing research needs to be conducted by scholars in family nursing. Further research should be conducted on the implications of world changes on family structure, function, and process. Nurses are in key positions to study the aging population, study diverse populations, and test practice theories with specialized populations. What we need are (1) meta-studies across phenomena, (2) research priorities for studying family trends supported by funding, (3) replication studies, and (4) intervention studies. See Chapter 4 of this textbook.

Education

Family nursing education needs to continue to include more family-focused study in nursing curricula. Earlier studies in family nursing education (Hanson,

2001; Hanson & Heims, 1992; Hanson, Heims, & Julian, 1992; Wright & Bell, 1989) reported the following: (1) more family content is being included in undergraduate and graduate nursing curricula, but it could be made more explicit, (2) an eclectic approach to family assessment is taught rather than the use of specific models, and (3) many clinical experiences are still focused on individuals rather than on families as a whole. A recent trend in the United States has been to integrate family-centered content into other traditional course work rather than create or preserve exclusive family nursing courses in the curriculum, and this is most notable in master's programs where nurse practitioner training has moved to disease management of individuals. This trend may be cause for concern because integration of content usually results in dilution or loss of family nursing content. In order for family nursing to be practiced in hospital and community-based settings, more nurses need to be educated specifically in family nursing.

Social Policy

Nursing theory, practice, research, and education all have ramifications for the development of family social policy. As professionals, nurses participate in the development of legislation and governmental policy. Legislative and legal actions that have a direct/indirect impact on families and health are called *family social policy*. The range of social policy decisions that affect families is vast and includes health care access and coverage, low-income housing, social security, taxes, welfare, food stamps, pension plans, affirmative action, and education. Although all governmental policies affect families, the United States has little overall, official, explicit family policy (Feetham & Meister, 1999; Gebbie & Gebbie, 2001). Feetham and Meister (1999) reported on the state of the family nursing research and the degree to which the science corresponded with family policy. They concluded that although a lot of research is being done, few of the results find their way into family social policy. See Chapter 6 in this textbook (Families, Nursing, and Social Policy) for more elaboration on this topic.

SUMMARY

This century has been characterized by an increasingly technological and global society, transcending the boundaries of the traditional nuclear family and demanding increasing instrumental and emotional investment in the work sphere (Dreman, 1997b). Changing gender roles, decreased marriage and fertility rates, increased divorce rates, ambiguity in parental roles, "high-tech" reproductive methods, family violence, and other evolving phenomena have resulted in a breakdown in the traditional family infrastructure that has served as a basis for the education, nurturance, and identity of its members. Individualism, autonomy, and the pursuit of career-related status may usurp traditional family values such as community, belonging, and family-related status, as society "progresses" along the inevitable pathways of increasing modernization. Strong and healthy families are needed to provide the stability, belonging, and sense of community necessary to a society characterized by flux, alienation, and individualism, and family nursing can do its part in making that happen. The prevailing theme seems to be that a sense of family roots and belonging may complement rather than undermine a person's search for autonomy by diminishing the existential anxiety precipitated by a changing and sometimes incomprehensible world. Family stability promotes flexibility in the face of change and family and communal belonging, as well as promoting healthy autonomy and interpersonal nurturance and connectedness contributing to individuality and achievement. Work and domestic realms are complementary rather than antagonistic spheres of influence and can cross-fertilize and contribute to optimal performance in each domain.

The movement of family health care nursing requires nurses to expand beyond traditional nursing and traditional families. A more integrated approach allows family nurses to practice more comprehensively by incorporating the four areas of family as context, family as client, family as system, and family as a component of society. Family health care nursing is challenging and rewarding and represents the future practice of all nurses. To some degree, all nurses should become futurists. A good futurist characterizes society, accounts for present situations, generates a coherent image of the future, and provides a road map or description of how to get there. A continuum of time defines the past, present, and future. No facts exist about the future; rather we have past facts, present options, and projected possibilities for the future. The future represents freedom, power, and hope. Join us in defining the future of families and family nursing in this first decade of the new millennium.

SQ STUDY QUESTIONS

1. What do you see as the future for families in the United States and around the world? Describe the rationale for your response.

2. What are the specific family demographic trends in the United States?

3. Name some world demographic changes that you are aware of.

4. Why are religion, sexuality, health care technology, and genetics important for family health care nursing? What are some other factors that you can think of?

5. Why and how is family nursing theory, practice, research, education, and social policy important for the future of family health care nursing?

6. Imagine that you are looking into a crystal ball. Make one prediction for the future of families and one for family nursing.

7. In what ways can nurses affect family social policy legislation at the federal and state levels?

8. What role will you play in the future of family health care nursing?

References

Anderson, H., & Evison, I. S. (Eds.). (2004). *The family handbook: The family, religion and culture.* Westminster: John Knox Press.

Bianchi, S. M., & Casper, L. M. (2000). American families. *Population Bulletin, 55*(4), 1–44.

Bumpass, L. L. & Lu, H. (2000). Trends in Cohabitation and Implications For Children's Family Contexts in the United States. *Population Studies, 54*(1), 29–41.

Calhoun, A. W. (1960). *A social history of the American family.* New York: Barnes & Noble.

Casper, L. M., & Bianchi, S. M. (2002). *Continuity and change in the American family.* Thousand Oaks, CA: Sage.

Coltrane, S., & Collins, R. (2001). *Sociology of marriage and the family: Gender, love, and property* (5th ed.). Belmont, CA: Wadsworth/Thomson Learning.

Coontz, S. (1998). *The way we really are: Coming to terms with America's changing families.* New York: Basic Books.

Cooper, R. A., Laud, P., & Dietrich, C. L. (1998). Current and projected workforce of nonphysician clinicians. *Journal of the American Medical Association, 280*(9), 788–794.

Cox, F. D. (2002). *Human intimacy: Marriage, the family and its meaning* (9th ed.). Belmont, CA: Wadsworth/Thomson Learning.

Doherty, W. J. (1992). Private lives, public values: The new pluralism. *Psychology Today, 25*(3), 32, 37, 82.

Doherty, W. J. (1997). *Intentional family.* New York: Addison Wesley.

Doherty, W. J. (2001). *Take back your marriage: Sticking together in a world that pulls us apart.* New York: Guilford.

Dreman, S. (1997a). On the threshold of a new era: An introduction. In S. Dreman (Ed.), *The family on the threshold of the 21st century: Trends and implications* (pp. 3–17). Mahwah, New Jersey: Lawrence Erlbaum Associates, Publishers.

Dreman, S. (1997b). Is the family viable? Some thoughts and implications for the third millennium. In S. Dreman (Ed.), *The family on the threshold of the 21st century: Trends and implications* (pp. 283–294). Mahwah, New Jersey: Lawrence Erlbaum Associates, Publishers.

Dunphy, L. H. (2001). Families on the brink, on the edge. In P. L. Munhall, P. L. & V. M. Fitzsimons, *The emergence of family into the 21st century* (pp. 3–15). Boston: Jones and Bartlett Publishers/National League for Nursing Press.

Feetham, S. L. (1999). The future in family nursing is genetics and it is now. *Journal of Family Nursing, 5*(1), 3–9.

Feetham, S. L. & Meister, S. B. (1999). Nursing research of families: State of the science and correspondence with policy. In A. S. Hinshaw, S. L. Feetham, & J. L. F. Shaver (Eds.), *Handbook of clinical nursing research* (pp. 251–273). Thousand Oaks, CA: Sage Publications.

Fong, L., & Sandhu, D. (1993). Religion and the family in a global context. In K. Altergott, (Ed.), *One world. Many families.* Minneapolis: National Council on Family Relations.

Fuchs, V. R., & Garber, A. M. (2003). Health and medical care. In H. J. Aaron, J. M. Linsay, & P. S. Nivola (Eds.), *Agenda for the nation* (pp. 145–182). Washington, DC: Brookings Institution Press.

Gebbie, K., & Gebbie, E. (2001). Families, nursing and social policy. In S. M. H. Hanson's *Family health care nursing: Theory, practice and research* (2nd ed., pp. 364–385). Philadelphia: FA Davis.

Gillis, C. L., & Knafl, K. A. (1999). Nursing care of families in non-normative transitions: The state of science and practice. In A. S. Hinshaw, S. L. Feetham, & J. L. F. Shaver (Eds.) *Handbook of clinical nursing research* (pp. 231–250). Thousand Oaks, CA: Sage Publications.

Hammond, A. (1998). *Which world? Scenarios for the 21st century.* Washington, DC: Island Press/Shearwater Books.

Hanson, S. M. H. (2001). Families and family nursing in the new millennium. In S. M. H. Hanson (Ed.), *Family health care nursing: Theory, practice, and research* (2nd ed.). Philadelphia: FA Davis.

Hanson, S. M. H., & Heims, M. L. (1992). Family nursing curricula in U.W. schools of nursing. *Journal of Nursing Education, 31*(7), 305–308.

Hanson, S. M. H., Heims, M. L., & Julian, D. J. (1992). Education for family health care professionals: Nursing as a paradigm. *Family Relations, 41,* 49–53.

Hinshaw, A. S., Feetham, S. L., & Shaver, J. L. F. (Eds.). (1999). *Handbook of clinical nursing research.* Thousand Oaks, CA: Sage Publications.

Houck, G. M., & Kodadek, S. (2001). Research in families and family nursing. In S. M. H. Hanson (Ed.), *Family health care nursing: Theory, practice and research* (2nd ed.). Philadelphia: FA Davis.

Kaakinen, J. (1999). Aging families and environment. In C. Dempsey & R. Butkus (Eds.), *All creation is groaning: An interdisciplinary vision for life in a sacred universe.* Collegeville, MN: Liturgical Press.

Kinsella, K. (1996). Aging and the family: Present and future demographic issues. In T. Blieszner, & V. Bedford (Eds.),

Aging and the family: Theory and research. Westport, CT: Praeger.

Martin, J. A., Mancini, D. L., Bowen, G. L., Mancini, J. A., & Orthner, D. (2004). *NCFR policy brief: Building strong communities for military families*. Minneapolis: National Council on Family Relations.

McCubbin, M. (1999). Normative family transitions and health outcomes. In A. S. Hinshaw, S. L. Feetham, & J. L. F. Shaver (Eds.), *Handbook of clinical nursing research* (pp. 201–250). Thousand Oaks, CA: Sage Publications.

McCubbin, M. A., & McCubbin, H. I. (1993). Families coping with illness: The resiliency model of family stress adjustment, and adaptation. In C. B. Danielson, B. Hamel-Bissell, & P. Winstead-Fry (Eds.), *Families, health & illness: Perspectives on coping in intervention* (pp. 21–65). St. Louis: Mosby.

McCubbin, H. I., McCubbin, M. A., Thompson, A. I., & Thompson, E. A. (1998). Resiliency in ethnic families: A conceptual model for predicting family adjustment and adaptation. In H. I. McCubbin, E. A. Thompson, A. I. Thompson, U. J. E. Fromer (Eds.), *Resiliency in Native American and immigrant families* (pp. 3–48). Thousand Oaks: Sage.

Myers-Walls, J. A. (2004). Terrorism and children. Retrieved April 8, 2004, from http://www.ces.purdue.edu.terrorism/

Myers-Walls, J. A. (in press). Children as victims of war and terrorism. *Journal of Aggression, Maltreatment, & Trauma, 8*(1/2/3).

National Center for Health Statistics. (2001). *Healthy people 2000 final review*. Hyattsville, MD: Public Health Service.

National Center for Health Statistics. (2003). *Health, United States, 2003: Chartbook on trends in the health of Americans* (DHHS Publication No. 2003-1232). Washington, DC: U.S. Government Printing Office.

National Center for Post Traumatic Stress Disorder (PTSD). (2004). *A national center for PTSD fact sheet*. Retrieved April 8, 2004, from http://www.ncptsd.org/war/familycoping.htm

Pittman, J. F., Kerpelman, J. L., & McFadyen, J. M. (2004). Internal and external adaptation in army families: Lessons from operations Desert Child and Desert Storm. *Family Relations, 53*(3), 249–260.

Popenoe, D. (1999). *Life without father: Compelling new evidence that fatherhood and marriage are indispensable for the good of children and society*. Cambridge, MA: Harvard University Press.

Popenoe, D., Elshtain, J. B., & Blankenhorn, D. (1996). *Promises to keep*. Lanham, MD: Rowman & Littlefield.

Popenoe, D., & Whitehead, B. D. (1999). *Should we live together: What young adults need to know about cohabitation before marriage*. New Brunswick, NJ: The National Marriage Project, Rutgers, The State University of New Jersey.

Riche, M. F. (1998). *From pyramids to pillars: The new demographic reality*. Washington, DC: Communications Consortium Media Center.

Teachman, J. D., Tedrow, L. M., & Crowder, K. D. (2000). The changing demography of America's families. Understanding families into the new millennium: A decade in review [Special issue]. *Journal of Marriage and the Family, 62*(4), 1234–1268.

The Institute for the Future. (2003). *Health and health care 2010: The forecast, the challenge*. San Francisco: Jossey-Bass/Wiley.

U.S. Bureau of the Census. (2003a). *Statistical abstracts of the United States. 2003*. Washington, DC: U.S. Government Printing Office.

U.S. Bureau of the Census. (2003b). *Households, by type: 1940 to present*. Washington, DC: U.S. Government Printing Office. Retrieved July 2004 from http://www.census.gov/population/www/socdemo/hh-fam.html

U.S. Department of Health, Education and Welfare. (1979). *Healthy people: The Surgeon General's report on health promotion and disease prevention*. DHEW Publication No. 79-55071. Washington, DC: U.S. Government Printing Office.

U.S. Department of Health and Human Services, Office of Public Health and Science. (1998). *Healthy people 2010 objectives: Draft for public comment*. Washington, DC: US Government Printing Office.

U.S. Department of Health and Human Services. (2000). *Healthy people 2010: Understanding and improving health* (2nd ed.). Washington, DC: U.S. Government Printing Office.

Whealin, J., & Pivar, I. (2004). Coping when a family member has been called to war. Retrieved April 8, 2004, from http://www.ncptsd.org/war/familycoping.htm

Whitehead, B. D. (1992). A new familism? *Family Affairs, 5*, 1–2.

Williams, J. K., Tripp-Reimer, T., Schutte, D., & Barnette, J. J. (2004). Advancing genetic nursing knowledge. *Nursing Outlook, 52*(2), 73–79.

Wisensale, S. K. (1992). Toward the 21st century: Family change and public policy. *Family Relations, 41*, 417–422.

World Future Society. (2004). *Forecasts for the next 25 years*. Bethesda, MD: World Future Society.

Wright, L., & Bell, J. (1989). A survey of family nursing education in Canadian universities. *The Canadian Journal of Nursing Research, 21*(3), 59–74.

Bibliography

Allen, W. D., & Eiklenborg, L. (2003). *Vision 2003: Contemporary family issues*. Minneapolis: National Council on Family Relations.

Bender, D. L., & Leone, B.. (Eds.). (2001). *America beyond 2001: Opposing viewpoints*. San Diego: Greenhaven Press, Inc.

Bomar, P. J. (2004). *Promoting health in families: Applying family research and theory to nursing practice*. Philadelphia: Saunders/ Elsevier.

Bomar, P. J. (2004). Family health promotion and family nursing in the new millennium. In P. J. Bomar (Ed.), *Promoting health in families: Applying family research and theory to nursing practice*. Philadelphia: Saunders/Elsevier.

Central Intelligence Agency. (2004). *The world factbook 2004*. Dulles, VA: Brassey's.

Cherlin, A. J. (2000). How is the 1996 Welfare Reform Law affecting poor families? In A. J. Cherlin (Ed.), *Public and private families: A reader* (2nd ed.). New York: McGraw-Hill.

Coleman, M., & Ganong, L. (2003). *Points & counterpoints: Controversial relationship and family issues in the 21st Century*. Los Angeles: Roxbury Publishing Company.

Council on Families in America. (1995). *Marriage in America: A report to the nation*. New York: Institute for American Values.

Edelman, M. W. (1998). *The state of America's children: A report from The Children's Defense Fund (State of America's children yearbook 2000)*. Washington, DC: Children's Defense Fund.

Eshleman, J. R. (2003). *The family* (10th ed.). Boston: Pearson Education.

Farley, R. (1996). *The new American reality: Who we are, how we got here, where we are going*. New York: Russell Sage Foundation.

Federal Interagency Forum on Child and Family Statistics. (2002). *America's children key national indicators of well-being, 2003*. Washington, DC: U.S. Government Printing Office.

Feetham, S. L. (1999). Families and the genetic revolution: Implications for primary healthcare, education, and research. *Families, Systems & Health, 17*(1) 27–43.

Fields, J., & Casper, L. M. (2001). America's families and living arrangements, 2000. *Current Population Reports, Series P20-537*. Washington, DC: U.S. Census Bureau.

Galvin, K. (2004). The family of the future: What do we face? In A. L. Vengelisti (Ed.) *Handbook of family communication*. Mahwah, NJ: Lawrence Erlbaum Associates.

Glenn, N. (1997). *Closed hearts, closed minds: The textbook story of marriage*. New York: Institute for American Values.

Goldscheider, F., Hogan, D., & Bures, R. (2001). A century (plus) of parenthood: Changes in living with children, 1980–1990. *History of the Family, 6*, 477–494.

Institute of Medicine. (2001). *Crossing the quality chasm: A new health system for the 21st century.* Washington, DC: National Academy Press.

Kirschling, J. M., Gilliss, C. L., Krentz, L., Camburn, C. D., Clough, R. S., Duncan, M. T., Hendricks, J., Howard, J. K. H., Roberts, C., Smith-Young, J., Tice, K. S., & Young, T. (1994). "Success" in family nursing: Experts describe phenomena. *Nursing and Health Care, 15,* 186–189.

Lamanna, M. A., & Riedmann, A. (2003). *Marriages and families: Making choices in a diverse society* (8th ed.). Belmont, CA: Wadsworth/Thomson Learning.

Markley, O. W., & McCuan, W. R. (Eds.) (1996). *America beyond 2001: Opposing viewpoints.* San Diego: Greenhaven Press, Inc.

McKenry, P. C., & Price, S. J. (Eds.) (2000). *Families & change: Coping with stressful events and transitions.* Thousand Oaks, CA: Sage Publications.

Milardo, R. M. (2000). Understanding families into the new millennium: A decade in review. *Journal of Marriage and the Family, 62*(4).

Munhall, P. L., & Fitzsimons, V. M. (2001). *The emergence of family into the 21st century.* Boston: Jones and Bartlett Publishers/National League for Nursing Press.

Pesut, D. J. (1997). Facilitating futures thinking. *Nursing Outlook. 45,* 155

Popenoe, D., & Whitehead, B. D. (1999). *Should we live together? What young adults need to know about cohabitation before marriage.* New Brunswick, NJ: The National Marriage Project, Rutgers University.

Porter-O'Grady, T. (2001). Profound change: 21st century nursing. *Nursing Outlook, 49*(4), 182–186.

Price, S. J., McKenry, P. C., & Murphy, M. J. (2000). *Families across time: A life course perspective.* Los Angeles: Roxbury Publishing Company.

Seccombe, K., & Warner, R. L. (2004). *Marriages and families: Relationships in social context.* Belmont, CA: Thomson/Wadsworth.

Thornton, A., & Young-DeMarco, L. (2001). Four decades of trends in attitudes toward family issues in the United States: The 1960s through the 1990s. *Journal of Marriage and the Family, 63*(4), 1009–1037.

University of Washington School of Nursing. (2003). *Connections: The Future of Nursing. 14*(1). Seattle: Author.

Waite, L. J., Bachrach, C. A., Hinden, M, Thomson, E., & Thornton, A. T. (2000). *The ties that bind: Perspectives on marriage and cohabitation.* New York: Aldine de Gruyter.

Waite, L. J., & Gallagher, M. (2000). *The case for marriage: Why married people are happier, healthier and better off financially.* Garden City, New York: Doubleday.

Wilcox, B. L. (1997). Genetic technology: The brave new world? *Family Futures, 1*(4), 4–5.

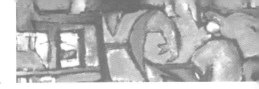

APPENDIX A
RESOURCE LIST
FOR FAMILY NURSING

Academy for Adolescent Health
http://www.healthyteens.com/

Administration for Children and Families (ACF)
370 L'Enfant Promenade SW
Washington, DC 20447
(202) 619–0257
http://www.acf.hhs.gov

Administration on Aging
U.S. Department of Health and Human Services
1 Massachusetts Avenue, Suites 4100 & 5100
Washington, DC 20201
(202) 619–0724
http://www.aoa.gov

Administration on Children and Families
Switzer Building, Room 330
C Street SW
Washington, DC 20201
(202) 205–8347
FAX: (202) 205–9721

Adolescent Health Resources
http://www.cdc.gov/HealthyYouth/

African American Family Services Resource Center
2616 Nicollet Avenue South
Minneapolis, MN 55408
(612) 871–7878
FAX: (612) 871–2567
http://www.aafs.net

Agency for Health Care Policy and Research (AHCPR)
Public Health Service
Executive Office Center, Suite 501
2101 E. Jefferson St
Rockville, MD 28052
http://www.ahcpr.gov

Agency for Healthcare Research and Quality (AHRQ)
540 Gaither Road
Rockville, MD 20850

(301) 427–1364
http://www.ahrq.gov
http://www.ahrq.gov/consumer/espanoix.htm

Aging America Resource Guide
http://www.agingusa.com/

AIDS Caregivers Support Network
2536 Alki Avenue SW, #138
Seattle, WA 98116
(206) 937–3368
http://www.wolfenet.com

AIDS Healthcare Foundation
6255 W. Sunset Boulevard
21st Floor
Los Angeles, CA 90028
(323) 860–5200
http://www.aidshealth.org

Alcoholics Anonymous (AA): General Service Office
P.O. Box 459 Grand Central Station
New York, NY 10163
(212) 870–3400
http://www.alcoholicsanonymous

Allergy & Asthma Network Mothers of Asthmatics (AANMA)
http://www.aanma.org/

Alliance for Children and Families
http://www.alliance1.org/

Alliance of Genetic Support Groups
http://geneticalliance.org

Alterations in Family Processes Care Plan
http://www.mcentral.com/careplans/plans/fp.html

Alternatives to Marriage Project
http://www.unmarried.org/

Alzheimer's Association
http://www.StandByYou.org

Alzheimer's Disease and Related Disorders Association (ADRDA)
919 N. Michigan Ave, Suite 1000
Chicago, IL 60611-1676
(800) 272–3900
http://www.alzheimers.org

America Saves
http://www.americasaves.org/

American Academy of Child & Adolescent Psychiatry
http://www.aacap.org/publications/factsfam/index.htm
This site contains information on a range of topics for families with children with illnesses.

American Academy of Nursing (AAN)
(202) 651–7238
FAX: (202) 554–2641
E-mail: aan@ana.org

American Academy of Pediatrics
http://www.aap.org

American Alliance of Health, Physical Exercise, Recreation and Dance
http://www.aahperd.org

American Association for Marriage and Family Therapy
112 South Alfred Street
Alexandria, VA 22314-3061
(703) 838–9808
FAX: (703) 838–9805
http://www.aamft.org

American Association of Homes for the Aging
901 E. Street NW, Suite 500
Washington, DC 20036
(202) 233–4000

American Association of Retired Persons (AARP)
601 E. Street NW
Washington, DC 20049
(202) 434–2777
http://www.aarp.org

American Association of Suicidology
4201 Connecticut Avenue NW
Suite 408
Washington, DC 20008
(202) 237–2280
http://www.suicidology.org

American Association of Therapeutic Humor
http://www.aath.org/

American Brain Tumor Association
http://neurosurgery.mgh.harvard.edu/abta/

American Cancer Society
1599 Clifton Road
Atlanta, GA 30329–4251
(800) ACS-2345
http://www.cancer.org

American Diabetes Association
ATTN: National Call Center
1701 North Beauregard St.
Alexandria, VA 22311
(800) 342–2383
http://www.diabetes.org

American Family Society
P.O. Box 80
Rockville, MD 20851

American Family Therapy Academy (AFTA)
1608 20th Street NW, 4th Floor
Washington, DC 20009
(202) 333–3690
FAX: (202) 333–3692
E-mail: afta@afta.org
http://www.afta.org

American Health Care Association
1200 15th Street NW
Washington, DC 20005
(202) 833–2050
http://www.ahca.org

American Heart Association
National Center
7272 Greenville Avenue
Dallas, TX 75231
(800) AHA-USA1
(800) 242–8721
http://www.americanheart.org

American Lung Association
61 Broadway, 6th Floor
New York, NY 10006
(212) 315–8700
http://www.lungusa.org

American Medical Association
http://www.ama-assn.org

American Nurses Association
600 Maryland Avenue SW
Suite 100 West
Washington, DC 20024
(202) 651–7000
(800) 274-4ANA(4262)
FAX: (202) 651–7001
http://nursingworld.org
http://www.ana.org
Other affiliates of ANA at same address:
American Nurses Credentialing Center (ANCC):
ancc@ana.org
American Nurses Foundation (ANF): anf@ana.org
American Academy of Nursing (AAN): aan@ana.org

American Nurses Credentialing Center (ANCC)
(202) 651–7000 or (800) 284-CERT(2378)
E-mail: ancc@ana.org

American Nurses Foundation (ANF)
(202) 651–7227
FAX: (202) 651–7354
E-mail: anf@ana.org
http://www.anfonline.org

American Obesity Association
http://www.obesity.org/subs/childhood/

American Pain Society
4700 W. Lake Avenue
Glenview, IL 60025
(847) 375–4715
http://www.ampainsoc.org

American Parkinson Disease Association
1250 Hylan Blvd
Staten Island, NY 10305
(800) 223–2732

American Psychiatric Nurses Association
1555 Wilson Boulevard, Suite 515
Arlington, VA 22209
(703) 243–2443
FAX: (703) 243–3390
E-mail: inform@apna.org

American Public Health Association
http://www.apha.org

American Stroke Association
National Center
7272 Greenville Avenue

Dallas, TX 75231
(800) 4-STROKE
(800) 478–7653
http://www.americanheart.org

Annie E. Casey Foundation
http://www.aecf.org

Arthritis Foundation
1330 West Peachtree Street
Atlanta, GA 30309
(404) 872–7100
http://www.arthritis.org

Asian and Pacific Islander American Health Forum
(APIAHF)
450 Sutter Street, Suite 600
San Francisco, CA 94108
(415) 954–9988
FAX: (415) 954–9999
http://www.apiahf.org

Assets Approach to Promoting Healthy Child Development
http://www.search-institute.org

Association of African American People's Legal
Council
PO Box 20053
Detroit, MI 48220

Association of Critical Care Nurses
101 Columbia
Aliso Viejo, CA 92656
(949) 362–2000
(800) 899–2226
http://www.aacn.org

Association of Jewish Family and Children's Agencies
557 Cranburg Road, Suite 2
East Brunswick, NJ 08816-5419
(800) 634–7346
FAX: (732) 432–7127
http://www.ajfca.org

Association of Women's Health, Obstetric, and
Neonatal Nurses (AWHONN)
700 14th Street NW, Suite 600
Washington, DC 20005-2019
http://www.awhonn.org

Bandaides and Blackboards
http://funrsc.fairfield.edu/jfleitas/contents.html

Bright Futures at Georgetown University
http://www.brightfutures.org

Brownson's guide to nursing organizations
http://diannebrownson.tripod.com/passages.html

Calgary Family Assessment Model
http://www.uic.edu/nursing/genetics/Lecture/
Family/Calgary%20Family%20Framework/CFAM/
cfam1.htm

Cancer Topics—Information presented by the National
Cancer Institute and National Institutes of Health
http://cancer.gov/cancerinformation

Center for Family Resources
384 Clinton Street
Hempstead, NY 10550

Center for Food Safety and Applied Nutrition
Food and Drug Administration (FDA)
200 C Street SW
Washington, DC 20204
(202) 205–5615
FAX: (202) 205–5532

Center for Loss & Life Transition
http://www.centerforloss.com

Center for Mental Health Services
Substance Abuse and Mental Health Services Administration (SAMHSA)
Parklawn Building, Room 18C-07
5600 Fishers Lane
Rockville, MD 20857
(301) 443–7790
FAX: (301) 443–7912
http://www.mentalhealth.org

Center for Practice and Technology
Agency for Health Care Policy and Research
6010 Executive Boulevard, Suite 300
Rockville, MD 20852
(301) 594–4015
FAX: (301) 594–4027

Center for Substance Abuse Prevention
Substance Abuse and Mental Health Services Administration
Rockwall II Building, Room 950
5600 Fishers Lane

Rockville, MD 20857
(301) 443–9931
FAX: (301) 443–6394

Centers for Disease Control and Prevention
1600 Clifton Rd
Atlanta, GA 30333
(404) 639–3311
http://www.cdc.gov/
This site provides current information about specific
chronic diseases and conditions, data statistics, conferences, and other helpful links.

Centers for Medicare and Medicaid Services (CMS)
Center for Medicaid and State Operation
7500 Security Boulevard
Baltimore, MD 21244
(410) 786–3000
http://cms.hhs.gov/medicaid
http://cms.hhs.gov.medicaid/statemap.asp

Center for Medicare Management
7500 Security Boulevard
Baltimore, MD 21244
(800) 633–4227
TTY: (877) 486–2048
http://www.medicare.gov

Child Abuse and Neglect Programs
200 Independence Ave. SW
Washington, DC 20201
http://www.acf.dhhs.gov/index.htm

Child Abuse Resources
http://www.nlm.nih.gov/medlineplus/childabuse.html

Child Care and Development Fund
200 Independence Ave. SW
Washington, DC 20201
http://www.acf.dhhs.gov/index.htm

Child Support Enforcement Program
200 Independence Ave. SW
Washington, DC 20201
http://www.acf.dhhs.gov/index.htm

Child Trends
4301 Connecticut Ave. NW, Suite 350
Washington, DC 20008
(202) 572–6000
http://www.childtrends.org

Child Welfare League of America
440 First Street NW, Third Floor
Washington, DC 20001–2085
(202) 638–2952
FAX: (202) 638–4004
http://www.cwla.org/cwla/index.html

Child Welfare Services
200 Independence Ave. SW
Washington, DC 20201
http://www.acf.dhhs.gov/index.htm

Childhood Asthma
http://www.aaaai.org/patients/publicedmat/tips/
childhoodasthma.stm

Children and Youth Health
http://www.cyh.sa.gov.au

Children with Disabilities
http://www.childrenwithdisabilities.ncjrs.org
This site provides access to a wide range of federal,
state, local, and national resources for families with
children with disabilities.

Children's Defense Fund
25 E Street NW
Washington, DC 20001
(202) 628–8787
E-mail: cdfinfo@childrensdefense.org
http://www.childrensdefense.org/

Children's Health Insurance Program (CHIP)
Health Care Financing Administration
7500 Security Boulevard
Baltimore, MD 21244
(410) 786–3000
http://www.hcfa.gov/init/children.htm

Children's Health
http://kidshealth.org

Chronic Care: Robert Wood Johnson
http://www.improvingchroniccare.org/index.html
This is a site sponsored by the Robert Wood Johnson
Foundation supporting a model of health care that
would improve chronic illness care.

Cohabitation Nation
http://www.cohabitationnation.com/

Combined Health Information Database
http://chid.nih.gov/
The Combined Health Information Database is a
bibliographic database produced by several U.S.
federal government agencies. It contains health information and health education resources.

Commission on Family and Medical Leave Act
http://www.dol.gov/dol/esa/public/regs/compli-
ance/whd/fmla/family.htm

Common Thread
http://www.commonthread.org/
Day-to-day experience of being a seriously ill or
disabled child

Couple Communication Program
http://www.couplecommunication.com/

Crisis, Grief and Healing—Men and Women
http://www.webhealing.com

Department of Health and Human Services
200 Independence Ave. SW
Washington, DC 20201
http://www.os.dhhs.gov

Depression & Bipolar Support Alliance
730 N. Franklin Street, Suite 501
Chicago, IL 60610-7204
(312) 988–1150
FAX: (312) 642–7243
http://www.DBSAlliance.org

Depression After Delivery, Inc.
91 East Somerset Street
Raritan, NJ 00869
http://www.depressionafterdelivery.com

Diversity Rx
Diversity Rx is a clearinghouse of information on
the World Wide Web on how to meet the language
and cultural needs of minorities, immigrants, refugees,
and other diverse populations seeking health care.
"Diversity Rx is sponsored by The National
Conference of State Legislatures, Resources for Cross
Cultural Health Care, and the Henry J. Kaiser Family
Foundation."
http://www.diversityrx.org

Division of Adolescent and School Health
National Center for Chronic Disease Prevention and
Health Promotion
Centers for Disease Control and Prevention
4770 Buford Highway NE, Mailstop K-29
Atlanta, GA 30341–3724
(770) 488–3254
FAX: (770) 488–3110

Division of Health Promotion Statistics
National Center for Health Statistics
Centers for Disease Control and Prevention
6525 Belcrest Road, Room 770
Hyattsville, MD 20782
(301) 436–3548
FAX: (301) 436–8459

Division of Prevention Research and Analytic Methods
Epidemiology Program Office
Centers for Disease Control and Prevention
Mailstop D01
Atlanta, GA 30333
(404) 639–4455
FAX: (404) 639–4463

Division of Public Health
Public Health Program Practice Office
Centers for Disease Control and Prevention
4770 Buford Highway NE, Mailstop K-29
Atlanta, GA 30341–3742
(770) 488–2469
FAX: (770) 488–2489

Dogpile Search Engine
http://www.dogpile.com/

Dougy Center National Center for Grieving Children
and Families
http://www.grievingchild.org

Down Syndrome WWW Page
http://www.nas.com/downsyn

eCollege
Web-based educational instruction
http://www.realeducation.com/

Elders
http://www.aoa.dhhs.gov/elderpage.html#ea

ElderWeb
http://www.elderweb.com

Emergency Nurses Association
915 Lee Street
Des Plains, IL 60016–6569
(800) 900–9659
http://www.ena.org

End of Life: Improving Care of Dying Children
http://www4.nationalacademies.org/news.nsf/isbn/03
09084377?OpenDocument

Families USA
http://www.familiesusa.org/site/PageServer

Family & Society Studies Worldwide Database—Free
30-day trial
http://www.nisc.com/

Family Caregiving
http://www.caregiver.com

Family Health and Social Services Center
Southeast Asian Health Coalition
26 Queen Street
Worcester, MA 01610
(508) 860–7700
FAX: (508) 860–7990
http://www.fchw.org

Family Index Database—Information on the study of
families
http://ncfr.famindx.com

Family Power Tools
http://familytools.cjb.net/

Family Preservation and Family Support
200 Independence Ave. SW
Washington, DC 20201
http://www.acf.dhhs.gov/index.htm

Family Resources Coalition
200 South Michigan Avenue, Suite 1520
Chicago, IL 60604

Family Reunion Planning
http://www.family-reunion.com/reunion.htm

Family Trends
http://www.infoplease.lycos.com/ipa/A0001548.
html

Family Violence Prevention Fund
http://www.igc.org/fund/

Fatherhood
http://aspe.hhs.gov/fathers/fhoodini.htm

Federal Interagency Forum on Child and Family
http://www.childstats/gov/
This site provides data about health, behavior, and social environment.

Focus on the Family
http://www.family.org/

Food and Drug Administration
Parklawn Building, Room 15A-08
5600 Fishers Lane, MS HFY-40
Rockville, MD 20857
(301) 443–5470
FAX: (301) 443–2446
http://www.fda.gov

Foster Care/Adoption Assistance/Independent Living
200 Independence Ave. SW
Washington, DC 20201
http://www.acf.dhhs.gov/index.htm

Futuristic Book Store
http://www.wfs.org/wfs

General Accounting Office
http://www.gao.gov

Genetics Education Center
http://www.kumc.edu/gec/

GeroWeb
http://www.iog.wayne.edu/GeroWebd/GeroWeb.html

Global Health Council
http://www.health.gov/nhic/NHICScripts/Entry.cfm?HRCode=HR1699

Global RN discussion list
School of Nursing
University of California
San Francisco
http://nurseweb.ucsf.edu/www/globalrn.htm

Gottman Institute
http://www.gottman.com/

Grandparent Raising Grandchildren
http://www.firstgov.gov/Topics/Grandparents.shtml

Grief Watch—Resources for bereaved families and professional caregivers
http://www.griefwatch.com

GROWW—Chat room for bereaved people
http://www.groww.com

Head Start
200 Independence Ave. SW
Washington, DC 20201
http://www.acf.dhhs.gov/index.htm

Health Canada
http://www.hc-sc.gc.ca/

Health Finder
Lay health information in English and Spanish
http://www.healthfinder.gov/

Health Resources and Services Administration (HRSA)
Parklawn Building, Room 14–33
5600 Fishers Lane
Rockville, MD 20857
(888) 275–4772
(301) 443–2460
FAX: (301) 443–9270
http://www.hrsa.gov

HealthGate
http://www.healthgate.com

Healthy People 2010
http://www.health.gov/healthypeople/

HealthyPlace.com
A community of people providing mental health information, support, and the opportunity to share experiences helpful to others
http://www.concernedcounseling.com

Housing and Urban Development
451 Seventh St. SW
Washington, DC 20410
http://www.hud.gov/index.html

Human Development and Family Life Bulletin
http://www.hec.ohio-state.edu/famlife/bulletin/bull-main.htm

Human Genome Project Information
http://www.ornl.gov/TechResources/Human_Genome/home.html

Human Rights Campaign
919 18th Street NW
Washington, DC 20006
(202) 628–4160
FAX: (202) 347–5323
http://www.hrc.org/

Incest Survivors Anonymous
P.O. Box 17245
Long Beach, CA 90807
(562) 428–5599
http://www.lafn.org/medical/isa/home.html

Indian Health Services (HIS)
The Reyes Building
801 Thompson Avenue, Suite 400
Rockville, MD 20852-1627
(301) 443–3593
http://www.ihs.gov

Institute for Family-Centered Care
http://www.familycenteredcare.org

Institute for Urban Family Health
http://www.institute2000.org/

Institute of Medicine
500 Fifth Street NW
Washington, DC 20001
(202) 334–2352
FAX: (202) 334–1412
E-mail: iomwww@nas.edu

Institution for American Values
1841 Broadway, Suite 211
New York, NY 10023
(212) 246–3942
FAX: (212) 541–6665
E-mail: iav@worldnet.att.net

Interagency Forum on Child and Family Statistics
http://www.childstats.gov

International Childbirth Education Association (ICEA)
PO Box 20048
Minneapolis, MN 55420
http://www.icea.org

International Council of Nurses
http://www.icn.ch

International Council of Nurses International Nurse Practitioner/Advanced Practice Nursing Network

http://icn.ch/networks_ap.htm
International Lactation Consultant Association (ILCA)
1500 Sunday Drive, Suite 102
Raleigh, NC 27607
http://www.ilca.org

International Society of Nurses in Genetics
http://www.kumc.edu/gec/prof/isong.html

Kids Count
Annie E. Casey Foundation
701 St. Paul St.
Baltimore, MD 21202
(410) 547–6600
http://www.aecf.org/kidscount

Kids Health
http://www.kidshealth.org/parent/index.html

La Leche League International
1400 N. Meacham Road
Schaumburg, IL 60173–4048
http://www.lalecheleague.org

Lesbian, Gay, and Bisexual Concerns (American Psychological Association)
http://www.apa.org/pi/lgbc/

Life Innovations, Inc.
http://www.prepare-enrich.com/

Marital Health
http://healthway.hypermart.net/marriag8.htm

Marriage and Parenting
http://www.drheller.com/parenting.html

Mastering Stress—eTherapy, a series of questionnaires aimed at helping people deal with stress
http://www.masteringstress.com

Maternal and Child Health Bureau
Health Resources and Services Administration
5600 Fishers Lane
Rockville, MD 20857

Medicaid
Health Care Financing Administration
7500 Security Boulevard
Baltimore, MD 21244
(410) 786–3000

http://www.hcfa.gov/medicaid/medicaid.htm
Medicare
Health Care Financing Administration
7500 Security Boulevard
Baltimore, MD 21244
(410) 786–3000
http://www.hcfa.gov/medicare/medicare.htm

Men's Health Network
http://www.menshealthnetwork.org/library

Mended Hearts
7272 Greenville Avenue
Dallas, TX 75231–4596
Information line: (888) HEART99 or (888) 432–7899
National office: (214) 706–1442
http://www.mendedhearts.org

Merck Manual
http://www.merck.com/mrkshared/mmanual_home2/
home.jsp
This is a searchable site with basic information on specific conditions as well as many articles that would be
helpful for families managing chronic illness.

Military Family Resource Center
CS4, Suite 302, Room 309
1745 Jefferson Davis Hwy.
Arlington, VA 22202–3424
(703) 602–4964
DSN: 332–4964
FAX: (703) 602–0189
DSN FAX: 332–0189
http://www.mfrc-dodqol.org

Mirasol—At a cost of $29,600, a 40-day intensive pro-
gram for eating disorders
http://www.edrecovery.com

Motherhood Web directory:
http://hometown.aol.com/Solhouse5/index.html

National Alliance for Caregiving
http://www.caregiving.org

National Alliance for Hispanic Health
1501 16th Street NW
Washington, DC 20036–1401
(202) 387–5000
FAX: (202) 797–4353
http://www.hispnichealth.org

National Alliance for the Mentally Ill (NAMI)
Colonial Place Three
2107 Wilson Boulevard, Suite 300
Arlington, VA 22201
(800) 950–NAMI
http://www.nami.org

National Asian Pacific Center on Aging
1511 Third Avenue, Suite 914
Seattle, WA 98101
(206) 624–1221
http://www.ncoa.org/lcao/members/napca.htm

National Association for Children of Alcoholics
11426 Rockville Pike
Suite 301
Rockville, MD 20852
(888) 554–2627
http://www.nacoa.org

National Association for Hispanic Elderly
234 East Colorado Blvd., Suite 300
Pasadena, CA 91101
(626) 564–1988
http://www.nih.gov/nia/related/aoaresrc/dir/127.htm

National Association of Adult Day Care
180 East 4050 South
Murray, UT 84107
(801) 262–9167

National Association of Area Agencies on Aging
(202) 296–8130

National Association of Home Health Agencies
426 C Street NE, Suite 200
Washington, DC 20002
(202) 547–1717

National Campaign to Prevent Teen Pregnancy
http://www.teenpregnancy.org/Default.asp?bhcp=1

National Cancer Institute
National Institutes of Health
Building 31, Room 10A49
31 Center Drive, MSC 2580
Bethesda, MD 20892–2580
(301) 496–9569
FAX: (301) 496–9931
http://cancer.gov/clinicaltrials
Information about new anticancer drugs and treat-
ments

National Caucus for the Black Aged
1424 K Street NW, Suite 500
Washington, DC 20006
(202) 797–8227

National Center for Chronic Disease Prevention and
Health Promotion
Centers for Disease Control and Prevention
4770 Buford Highway NE, Mailstop K10
Atlanta, GA 30341–3724
(770) 488–5000
FAX: (770) 488–5966

National Center for Complementary and Alternative
Medicine (NCCAM) Clearinghouse
P.O. Box 7923
Gaithersburg, MD 20898
(888) 644–6226
(301) 519–3153
http://nccam.nih.gov

National Center for Cultural Competence
http://www.ama-assn.org/ama/pub/category/1981.
html

National Center for Elder Abuse
http://www.elderabusecenter.org

National Center for Grieving Children and Families
http://www.dougy.org or http://www.griefnet.org
Dougy Center is a national support center. Griefnet
offers 30 e-mail support groups and two Websites, a
directory of resources, newsletters, and more.

National Center for Health Statistics
U.S. Department of Health and Human Services
Centers for Disease Control and Prevention
Hyattsville, MD 20782
(301) 458–4000
http://www.cdc.gov/nchs

National Center for HIV, STD, and TB Prevention
Centers for Disease Control and Prevention
1600 Clifton Road NE, Mailstop E-07
Atlanta, GA 30333
(404) 639–8008
FAX: (404) 639–8600

National Center for Infectious Diseases
Centers for Disease Control and Prevention
1600 Clifton Road NE, Mailstop C-12
Atlanta, GA 30333
(404) 639–3401

FAX: (404) 639–3039
National Center for Injury Prevention and Control
Division of Violence Prevention
Centers for Disease Control and Prevention
4770 Buford Highway NE, Mailstop K60
Atlanta, GA 30341–3724
(770) 488–4276
FAX: (404) 488–4349
E-mail: FIVPINFO@cdc.gov

National Centers for Chronic Disease Prevention and
Health Promotion
Centers for Disease Control and Prevention
4770 Buford Highway NE, Mailstop K40
Atlanta, GA 30341–3724
(770) 488–5403
FAX: (770) 488–5971

National Child Abuse Hotline
(800) 422–4453

National Child Care Information Center
http://www.nccic.org/

National Clearinghouse for Alcohol and Drug Information
P.O. Box 2345
Rockville, MD 20847
(800) 729–6686
http://www.ncadi.samhsa.gov

National Clearinghouse on Child Abuse & Neglect
P.O. Box 1182
Washington, DC 20013
(800) FYI-3366
E-mail: nccanch@calib.com
http://nccanch.acf.hhs.gov/

National Clearinghouse on Families and Youth
(NCFY)
P.O. Box 13505
Silver Spring, MD 20911–3505
Voice/TTY: (301) 608–8098
FAX: (301) 608–8721
http://www.ncfy.com

National Coalition for Health Professional Education
in Genetics (NCHPEG)
http://www.nchpeg.org

National Coalition for the Homeless
http://nch.ari.net/

National Coalition of Hispanic Health Human Services Organizations
1501 Sixteenth St. NW
Washington, DC 20036
(202) 387–5000

National Committee to Prevent Child Abuse
332 S. Michigan Avenue, Suite 950
Chicago, IL 60604
(312) 663–3520
http://www.childabuse.org

National Council on Aging
http://www.ncoa.org

National Council on Family Relations
3989 Central Ave. NE, #550
Minneapolis, MN 55421
(763) 781–9331
(888) 781–9331
FAX: (763) 781–9348
E-mail: info@ncfr.com
http://www.ncfr.org

National Council on the Aging
409 Third Street SW, Suite 202
Washington, DC 20024
http://www.ncoa.org

National Domestic Violence Hotline
(800) 799-SAFE

National Down Syndrome Society
http://www.ndss.org

National Foundation for Depressive Illness, Inc.
P.O. Box 2257
New York, NY 10116
(800) 239–1265
http://www.depression.org

National Gay and Lesbian Task Force
1700 Kalorama Road NW
Washington, DC 20009–2624
(202) 332–6483
FAX: (202) 332–0207
TTY: (202) 332–6219
http://www.ngltf.org/

National Gerontological Nursing Association
7250 Parkway Drive, Suite 510
Hanover, MD 21706
National Health Information Center (NHIC)

P.O. Box 1133
Washington, DC 20013–1133
(301) 565–4167
(800) 336–4797
FAX: (301) 984–4256
http://nhic-nt.health.org/

National Heart, Lung and Blood Institute
National Institutes of Health
31 Center Drive, MSC 2486
Bethesda, MD 20892–2486
(301) 496–5437
FAX: (301) 480–4907
http://www.nhlbi.nih.gov

National Hispanic Prenatal Hotline
(800) 504–7081

National Hospice & Palliative Care Organization
1700 Diagonal Road, Suite 625
Arlington, VA 22314
(703) 837–1233
http://www.nhpco.org

National Hospice Organization
301 Maple Avenue W, Suite 506
Vienna, VA 22180
(703) 938–4449

National Immunization Program
Centers for Disease Control and Prevention
1600 Clifton Road NE, Mailstop E-05
Atlanta, GA 30333
(404) 639–8200
FAX: (404) 639–8626

National Indian Council on Aging
10501 Montgomery Blvd. NE, Suite 210
Albuquerque, NM 87110
(505) 292–2001
http://www.omhrc.gov/mhr2/orgs/88O0655.htm

National Information Center on Health Services Research and Health Care Technology (NICHSR)
National Library of Medicine
8600 Rockville Pike, Room 4S-410
Mailstop 20
Bethesda, MD 20894
(301) 496–0176
FAX: (301) 402–3193
http://www.nlm.nif.gov/nichsr/nichsr.html
National Institute of Arthritis and Musculoskeletal and Skin Diseases

National Institutes of Health
Natcher Building
45 Center Drive
Bethesda, MD 20892–6600
(301) 594–5014
FAX: (301) 402–2406

National Institute of Child Health and Human
Development
PO Box 3006
Rockville, MD 20847
(800) 370–2943
http://www.nichd.nih.gov

National Institute of Dental Research
National Institutes of Health
Building 45, Room 3 AN-44B
45 Center Drive, Mailstop 6401
Bethesda, MD 20892–6401
(301) 594–5391
FAX: (301) 480–8254

National Institute of Diabetes and Digestive and
Kidney Diseases
National Institutes of Health
Building 45, Room 6AN38J
9000 Rockville Pike
Bethesda, MD 20892
(301) 594–8867
FAX: (301) 480–4237

National Institute of Mental Health (NIMH)
Office of Communications
6001 Executive Boulevard, Room 8184, MSC 9663
Bethesda, MD 20892–9663
(301) 443–4513
(866) 615-NIMH (toll-free)
FAX: (301) 443–5158
E-mail: nimhinfo@nih.gov
http://www.nimh.nih.gov

National Institute of Nursing Research
http://ninr.nih.gov/ninr/

National Institute of Occupational Safety and Health
Centers for Disease Control and Prevention
200 Independence Ave. SW, Room 733G
Washington, DC 20201
(202) 401–0721
FAX: (202) 260–4464
National Institute on Aging
Building 31, Room 5C27

31 Center Drive, MSC 2292
Bethesda, MD 20892
(301) 496–1752
http://www.nia.nih.gov

National Institutes of Health (NIH)
Building 1, Room 260
9000 Rockville Pike
Bethesda, MD 20892
(301) 496–1508
FAX: (301) 402–2517
(301) 496–6614
FAX: (301) 480–9654
http://www.nih.gov/
http://health.nih.gov
Website sponsored by the National Institutes of
Health that provides health information for families
dealing with common diseases, conditions, and illnesses.

National Kidney Foundation
30 East 33rd Street, Suite 1100
New York, NY 10016
(800) 622–9010
(212) 889–2210
http://www.kidney.org

National Mental Health Association (NMHA)
2001 N. Beauregard Street, 12th floor
Alexandria, VA 22311
(800) 969–6942
http://www.nmha.org

National Multiple Sclerosis Society
205 East 42nd Street
New York, NY 10017
(212) 986–3240

National Organization for Women
1000 16th Street NW, Suite 700
Washington, DC 20036
(202) 331–0066
FAX: (202) 785–8576
TTY: (202) 331–9002
http://www.now.org/

National Park and Recreation Association
http://www.nrpa.org/

National Partnership for Women & Families
http://www.nationalpartnership.org/
National Resource Center on Homelessness and
Mental Illness (NRCHMI)

Policy Research Associates, Inc.
345 Delaware Avenue
Delmar, NY 12054
(800) 444–7415
FAX: (518) 439–7612
http://www.nrchmi.samhsa.gov

National Self-Help Clearinghouse
Graduate School and University Center of the City
University of New York
365 5th Avenue, Suite 3300
New York, NY 10016
(212) 817–1822
E-mail: info@selfhelpweb.org

National Student Nurses Association
http://www.nsna.org/

National Women's Health Information Center
http://www.4women.org

Navajo Family Health Resource Network
P.O. Box 1869
Window Rock, AZ 86515
(520) 928–5092
FAX: (520) 928–5099
http://www.navajofamilyhealth.org/index.html

Neuman Systems Model
http://www.neumansystemsmodel.com

No Kidding! The international social club for child-free and childless couples and singles
Box 2802
Vancouver, BC, Canada V6B 3X2
www.nokidding.net

Nursing Care Assessment Satellite Training (NCAST)
University of Washington
Box 357920
Seattle, WA 98195–7920
http://www.ncast.org

Nutrition: American Dietetic Association
http://www.eatright.org/nuresources.html

Office for Civil Rights Temporary Assistance for Needy Families (TANF)—Welfare Reform Page
http://www.hhs.gov/ocr/tanfintro.htm
Office of Clinical Standards and Quality Health Care
Health Care Financing Administration

S1-13-23 South Building
C3-24-07 South Building
&500 Security Boulevard
Baltimore, MD 21244–1850

Office of Disease Prevention and Health Promotion
Office of Public Health and Science
U.S. Department of Health and Human Services
1101 Wootton Parkway, Suite LL100
Rockville, MD 20852
(240) 453–8280
FAX: (240) 453–8282
http://odphp.osophs.dhhs.gov/

Office of Minority Health Resource Center
PO Box 37337
Washington, DC 20013–7337
(800) 444–6472
FAX: (301) 589–0884
http://www.omhrc.gov

Office of Policy and External Affairs
Agency for Toxic Substances and Disease Registry
1600 Clifton Road, NE, Mailstop E60
Atlanta, GA 30333
(404) 639–0500
FAX: (404) 639–0522

Office of Policy, Planning, and Evaluation
National Institute of Environmental Health Sciences
National Institutes of Health
Building 101, Room B250
PO Box 12233, Mail Drop B2-08
111 Alexander Drive
Research Triangle Park, NC 27709
(919) 541–3484
FAX: (919) 541–4737

Office of Population Affairs
Suite 200 West
4350 East West Highway
Bethesda, MD 20814
(301) 594–7608
FAX: (301) 594–5980

Office of Women's Health
712E HHH Building
200 Independence Avenue SW
Washington, DC 20201
(202) 690–7650
Office on Disability and Health
National Center for Environmental Health

Centers for Disease Control and Prevention
4770 Buford Highway NE, Mailstop F029
Atlanta, GA 30341–3724
(770) 488–7094
FAX: (770) 488–7075

Office on Smoking and Health
National Center for Chronic Disease Prevention and
Health Promotion
Centers for Disease Control and Prevention
4770 Buford Highway NE, Mailstop K50
Atlanta, GA 30341–3724
(770) 488–5797
FAX: (770) 488–5767

Older Women's League
1325 G Street NW
Lower Level B
Washington, DC 20005

ONCOLINK—The University of Pennsylvania
Cancer Center
Offers a wide variety of information about cancer and
treatments
http://cancer.med.upenn.edu/

Parents and Child with Disabilities
http://www2.state.id.us/dhw/ecic/HW/illnessChil-
dren.htm
This is a clearinghouse site with a plethora of information that would be particularly useful to parents
with a child with a newly diagnosed chronic illness.

Parents Anonymous
6733 South Sepulveda Blvd., #270
Los Angeles, CA 90048
(800) 352–0386
http://www.parentsanonymous.org

Parents without Partners
1650 South Dixie Highway, Suite 510
Boca Raton, FL 33432
(561) 391–8833
E-mail: pwp@jti.net
http://www.parentswithoutpartners.org/

Parents, Friends, and Families of Lesbians and Gays
(PFLAG)
1101 14th Street NW, Suite 1030
Washington, DC 20005
(202) 638–4200

FAX: (202) 638–0243
http://www.pflag.org/pflag.html

Pharmacy information
http://www.drugstore.com

Phone directory searches (by city, type of business,
name)
http://www.infobel.com/teldir/default.asp

Physical Activity and Health Branch
Division of Nutrition and Physical Activity
National Center for Chronic Disease Prevention and
Health Promotion
4770 Buford Highway NE, Mailstop K-47
Atlanta, GA 30341–3724
(770) 488–5513
FAX: (770) 488–5486

Population Council
One Dag Hammarskjold Plaza
New York, NY 10017
(212) 339–0500
http://www.popcouncil.org

Population Reference Bureau
1875 Connecticut Ave. NW, Suite 520
Washington, DC 20009
(202) 483–1100
http://www.prb.org

President's Council on Physical Fitness and Sports
731-H Hubert Humphrey Building
200 Independence Avenue, SW
Washington, DC 20201
(202) 690–5148
FAX: (202) 690–5211

Program Support Center (PSC)
Director of Customer Relations
5600 Fishers Lane, Room 17A-39
Rockville, MD 20857
(301) 443–1494
http://www.psc.gov

Public Broadcasting System—See video "Shattering
the Silences"
http://www.pbs.org/shattering

Public Health Program Practice Office
Centers for Disease Control and Prevention

4770 Buford Highway NE, Mailstop K-36
Atlanta, GA 30341–3724
(770) 488–2402
FAX: (770) 488–2428

RAND Center for the Study of Aging
http://www.rand.org/labor/aging/

Resources for Nurses and Families
http://pegasus.cc.ucf.edu/~wink

Rural Information Center
10301 Baltimore Avenue, Room 304
Beltsville, MD 20705–2351
(800) 633–7701
FAX: (301) 504–5181
TTY/TDD: (301) 504–6858
http://www.nal.usda.gov/ric

RxAssist
http://www.rxassist.org
This website offers health care providers the information they need to access pharmacy assistance programs for their patients and families.

SeniorNet—Bringing wisdom to the information age
http://www.seniornet.org/php/

Shape Up America
http://www.shapeup.org/general/

Sigma Theta Tau International
550 West North Street
Indianapolis, IN 46202
(317) 634–8171
(888) 634–7575 (U.S./Canada)
(800) 634–7575.1 (International)
FAX: (317) 634–8188
E-mail: research@stti.iupui.edu
http://www.nursingsociety.org

Smokefree
http://www.smokefree.gov/

Society for Education and Research in Psychiatric Nursing (SERPN)
1211 Locust Street
Philadelphia, PA 19107
(800) 826–2950
FAX: (215) 545–8107

E-mail: info@ispn-psych.org
Stand for Children
http://www.stand.org/

Substance Abuse and Mental Health Services Administration
Parklawn Building, Room 12C-26
5600 Fishers Lane
Rockville, MD 20857
(301) 443–6067
FAX: (301) 594–6159

Temporary Assistance for Needy Families
200 Independence Ave. SW
Washington, DC 20201
http://www.acf.dhhs.gov/index.htm

Tools for Coping with Life Stressors
http://www.coping.org/

U.S. Census Bureau
4700 Silver Hill Road
Washington, DC 20233
http://www.census.gov

U.S. Census Bureau—United States Census 2000
http://www.census.gov/main/www/cen2000.html

U.S. Department of Housing and Urban Development
451 7th Street SW
Washington, DC 20410
(202) 708–1712
TTY: (202) 708–1455
http://www.hud.gov

UNICEF House
3 United Nations Plaza
New York, NY 10017
(212) 326–7000
FAX: (887) 326–7465
http://www.unicef.org

United Ostomy Association
2001 West Beverly Blvd.
Los Angeles, CA 90057
(213) 413–5510

Urban Institute
http://www.urban.org/

Veterans Administration
810 Vermont Avenue NW
Washington, DC 20420
(202) 233–4000
http://www.va.gov

Visiting Nurses Association of America
3801 East Florida Avenue, Suite 900
Denver, CO 80210
(800) 426–2547
http://www.vnaa.org

WebMD—Contact for medical information
http://www.webmd.com

Welfare to Work Challenge
200 Independence Ave. SW
Washington, DC 20201
http://www.acf.dhhs.gov/index.htm

Whole Nurse
http://www.wholenurse.com/nursing.htm

WidowNet—Information, bibliographies, and other
resources for widows and widowers
http://www.fortnet.org/WidowNet/

Women Organized Against Rape
1233 Locust Street, Suite 202
Philadelphia, PA 19107
Phone hotline: (215) 985–3333
FAX: (215) 985–9111
E-mail: info@woar.org

Women's Policy Research
http://www.iwpr.org
The Institute for Women's Policy Research provides

data, press releases, and research articles about public
policy issues that focus on women and families.
Work and Family Information Center
The Conference Board
845 Third Avenue
New York, NY 10022

World Future Society (WFS)
7910 Woodmont Ave, Suite 450
Bethesda, MD 20814
(800) 989–8274
http://www.wfs.org/wfs

World Health Organization
Avenue Appia 20
1211 Geneva 27
Switzerland
(+ 41 22) 791 2111
FAX: (+41 22) 791 3111
http://www.who.int/en/

Young Widows and Widowers—Newsletter and other
grief information especially helpful to widows with
children
http://www.youngwidowsandwidowers.com

YoungWidow.org—Online support groups for young
widows and widowers
http://www.ywbb.org/index.shtml

Youth Programs
200 Independence Ave. SW
Washington, DC 20201
(301) 443–2170
FAX: (301) 443–1797
http://www.acf.dhhs.gov/index.htm

APPENDIX B
GLOSSARY

Ableism: Prejudice against those without full physical capabilities.

Acculturation: A process in which gradual changes are produced by the influence of one culture on another so that the two cultures become more similar.

Acute myocardial infarction: An occluded coronary artery results in prolonged myocardial ischemia that leads to irreversible injury and necrosis of a portion of the heart muscle. The location of the infarction depends on which coronary artery is occluded.

Adaptation: A process of managing the demands of stressors through the use of resources, coping, decision-making, and problem-solving strategies. A family's necessity to adjust to its external and internal environments.

Adaptive Model of Family Health: In this model, families are adaptive if they have the ability to change and grow and possess the capacity to rebound quickly after a crisis.

Affective function: The ways family members relate to one another and those outside the immediate family boundaries.

Aggregate of people: A group of people with similar characteristics, such as all people who are homeless or all people diagnosed with a particular disease.

Alienation: Feeling separate from larger social groups to the extent that the individual suffers emotional pain.

Ambiguous loss: A grief reaction to a vague situation; that is, the family member is physically absent but psychologically present (e.g., hospitalized family member) or the family member is physically present but psychologically absent (e.g., as noted with head injury, Alzheimer's disease).

Anticipatory loss: A wide range of intense emotional grief reactions in response to an expected or threatened loss over the course of the chronic illness.

Assessment: A continuously evolving process of data collection in which the nurse, drawing on the past and the present, is able to predict or plan the future.

Assimilationist: To assimilate means to lose individual identity (cultural, racial, sexual traits) in order to align more closely with social norms. A common example of assimilation is the experience of immigrants who do not pass their native language on to their children.

Attachment: An enduring emotional tie between persons that develops and grows over time that is not transient or easily abandoned. Attachment is specific and unique to the involved individuals. Attachment implies love, tenderness, and affection. Involved individuals seek proximity to each other and yearn to be in each other's presence. Attachment relationships can withstand anger, frustration, and periods of separation.

Baby boom: The period after the end of World War II when fertility rates in the United States (and some other countries) were exceptionally high. Demographers usually define as "baby boomers" everyone born in the 19 years from 1946 through 1964.

Beliefs systems: A domain of reality, traditions, or paradigms. Application of the assumptions of the worldview into actions. Where challenges to the worldview are tested as new theory or outside information is introduced.

Biological family: Family relationships defined by genetic connection.

Bisexual: This term is often used by people whose sexual objects of choice include both men and women.

Blaming the victim: Instead of considering greater social structures and their impact on the world, society blames those who suffer. For example, low-income housing projects are required to have removed all lead-based paints. However, many have not done this, and so many children still suffer from poisoning that comes from eating the chips (which are sweet). Families are then targeted by public health officials with public service campaigns to teach their kids about the danger. If the kids then get sick, the parents are blamed, not the tardy landlord.

Burden of disease: The World Health Organization defined "burden of disease" as a combination of untimely death and disability.

Centenarian: A person who is 100 years old or older.

Change Theory: This theory underscores the paradoxical relationship between persistence (stability) and change in a family system. Changes in the family's structure occur as compensation for outside influences on the family system and paradoxically have the purpose of maintaining stability within the family.

Child abuse or neglect: "Abuse" is a comprehensive term that includes physical, emotional, and sexual harm; "neglect" is not providing for a child's basic physical, educational, or emotional needs.

Childbearing cycle: The period of time beginning with the pre-conceptual period when a parent considers getting pregnant and including the prenatal period of pregnancy, the labor and birth, and the postpartum period during which the woman's body returns to the normal pre-pregnancy physiological state and family adaptation to a new member takes place.

Chosen family: Family relationships defined by anything besides genetics: love, sex, affection, money, housing, and so on.

Chronic illness: A disease or condition that has existed for 3 months or longer, does not resolve spontaneously, and is rarely cured. It can affect physical, emotional, intellectual, social, or spiritual functioning.

Client story: Refers to the problem the family is currently experiencing.

Clinical Family Health Model: Examined from this perspective, a family is healthy if its members are free from physical, mental, and social dysfunction.

Closed family system: A family that functions in isolation from other social systems and social institutions.

Cohabitation: Two adults living together in a sexual relationship who have not married in a religious or civil ceremony are said to be cohabiting.

Cohabiting families: Heterosexual couples who choose to live together outside of the marriage covenant, a phenomenon that has become increasingly common over the last two decades.

Cohort: For demographers, a group of people defined by experiencing an event during the same time period. Examples are the people born from 1950 to 1954, everyone who married from 1980 to 1989, or those who graduated from college in 2002.

Coming out: The informal process gay people go through in revealing their identity to their family, friends, and coworkers.

Community as client: A broad interpretation of the unit of service that addresses the entire community's needs.

Concepts: Concepts are mental images or abstract representations of phenomena. They are the building blocks of theory that represent the main ideas expressed by the theory, sometimes termed "variables." They exist on a continuum from empirical (concrete) to abstract. Examples of concrete concepts are gender and age; examples of abstract concepts are family and health.

Conceptual model or framework: The terms "model" and "framework" are sometimes used interchangeably to mean a set of interrelated concepts that symbolically represent and convey a mental image of a phenomenon. They are more abstract and more comprehensive than a theory. They integrate concepts into a meaningful configuration or pattern. They are less predictive than a theory and only symbolize that there is a relationship among the concepts in the framework. For example, nursing models are not considered stringent enough to be theories because they are not predictive.

Confluence: The process of combining activities to promote togetherness; it fosters family unity and closeness.

Contemporary families: Families that may take one of several different forms including single parent (biological, adoptive, step), intact nuclear (biological, adoptive), intergenerational, extended without parent, same-sex, cohabiting or domestic partnerships, and institutions (foster care, group homes, residential or treatment centers).

Contingency contract: A contract with a health professional or other support person that includes the process of setting a goal and identifying costs and rewards of goal attainment. The purpose of the contingency contract is to reinforce behaviors needed to reach a goal.

Contract: A binding agreement between two or more parties.

Correlational family studies: Studies that assess the relationships among characteristics of families, family relations, and individual family members. The purpose of this research design is to examine specific relationships between two or more variables of interest.

Cue logic: The process of clustering data into meaningful groups so that the relationships between the issues can be identified.

Cultural awareness: Self-reflection of one's own

nationality, race, ethnicity, and cultural norms as well as practices, values, and beliefs related to health and well-being.

Cultural integration or enculturation: A lifelong process of learning about and coming to understand another culture's worldviews or beliefs demonstrated in the culture's common behaviors and practices.

Cultural maladaptation: Unresolved culture shock, remaining in a dysfunctional state, which has negative impact on the individual and surrounding environment.

Cultural shock: A progressive-stage risk common to experiencing a new cultural environment or situation.

Culture: Sets of shared worldviews and adaptive behaviors derived from simultaneous membership in a variety of contexts, such as ecological setting (rural, urban, suburban), religious background, nationality and ethnicity, social class, gender-related experiences, minority status, occupation, political leanings, migratory patterns and stage of acculturation, or values derived from belonging to the same generation, partaking of a single historical moment, or holding a particular ideology.

Data: Pieces of information collected in a study to answer research questions.

Demography: The statistical study of human populations, especially with reference to size and density, distribution, and vital statistics; the factors that cause populations to grow, move, or change, such as fertility, migration, and mortality; and the consequences of those changes. Family demographers describe and explain changes in marriage, divorce, remarriage, and cohabitation; fertility and child rearing; and other family roles. They also describe how these changes affect the number and composition of families in a population and the consequences of those changes for individuals, families, and societies.

Descriptive analysis: Basically describes the sample and the characteristics assessed. For example, families may be described in terms of parental marital status, family income level, education level of the partners or spouses, and number of children.

Descriptive research: Distinguished from exploratory research by its specification of variables about families that it seeks to describe or assess in a population.

Desired outcomes: These are developed for each presenting present state. To determine whether the outcome is being achieved or not, the nurse identi-

fies tests or measures that will provide information about the resolution of the problems. Nurses make decisions about which nursing interventions are most appropriate for the family.

Developmental Model of Health and Nursing (DMHN): This has a goal of collaborating and increasing the capacity of families and individuals in health promotion in everyday life situations. In this interaction model, the nurses' role changes at each phase of the health promotion process, thereby empowering clients toward improving their health status.

Developmental task: Psychological and social tasks associated with growth and change or transition. Specifically, the developmental tasks of pregnancy are those associated with transition to parenthood and the psychosocial assimilation of the expected baby into the life of the mother and father.

Developmental Theory: According to developmental theory, human beings have specific tasks at specific periods in their life span, and successful achievement of the tasks at one stage of life leads to happiness and success with later tasks. Failure to achieve tasks leads to unhappiness, disapproval, and difficulty in achieving later tasks.

Developmental transitions: Predictable changes that occur in an expected time line congruent with movement through the eight family stages.

Deviant: As a necessary result of social norms, those people or things that do not fit are "deviant." The term was originally from the field of statistics, describing the data that lay outside of the bell curve.

Diachronic: A system of knowledge that involves seeking to know and understand a person's history through their reality.

Disability: A substantial limitation on a person's ability to participate in a major life activity (such as work, schooling, self-care, recreation).

Disease prevention: Activities that protect the population from actual or potential diseases and disabilities and their consequences.

Diseases and pathological conditions: Abnormal patterns of physical, social-emotional, or family processes.

Do Not Resuscitate (DNR): Refers to do-not-resuscitate orders, explicit orders that are written by a physician directing care providers not to revive or sustain the vital functions of persons in respiratory or cardiac arrest.

Ecomap: A diagrammatic assessment procedure (drawing) that portrays the family's relationships to other systems in the community in which the family is imbedded (e.g., work, school, church).

Emic: An insider's view and subjective understanding of his or her own world or condition.

Empowerment: The process of providing information and resources to help others to reach a goal.

Epidemiology: The study of the distribution of states of health and the causes of deviations from health in populations and the application of this study to control the health problems.

Essentialism: Reducing the cause of a characteristic or behavior to one cause. Biological essentialism explains everything as the product of genes or blood.

Ethclass: The intersection of social class and ethnicity. This intersection produces identifiable dispositions and behavioral patterns in families.

Ethnic groups: Different from race, ethnic groups are those people with shared cultural practices and characteristics such as food, clothing, religion, music, and the like, in any combination.

Ethnicity: A group's sense of "peoplehood" based on a combination of race, religion, ancestral history, and nationality.

Ethnography: A systematic process of observing, detailing, describing, documenting, and analyzing patterns of a culture to understand the patterns of people in their familiar environment.

Etic: An outsider's objective analysis of another person's views, understanding, or reality.

Eudaimonistic Family Health Model: Professionals who use this model as their philosophy of practice focus on efforts to maximize the family's well-being and to support the entire family and individual members in reaching their highest potential.

Evaluation: Evaluation is the appraisal of the changes experienced by the client in relation to goal achievement and realization of expected outcomes.

Experimental designs: Allow the researcher to control or manipulate causal or independent variables and to assign families randomly to treatment and control groups. Experiments are designed to allow the inference of a functional or causal relationship between causal factors (independent variables or treatments) and individual or family outcomes (dependent variable).

Exploratory studies: Are conducted when little is known about a phenomenon of interest. The purpose of exploratory research is to generate ideas, insights, or understandings about family phenomena that are not well understood.

Face-to-face interviews: Entail an interviewer asking a respondent questions and recording the answers.

Familism: A social pattern in which the family assumes a position of ascendance over individual interests.

Family: Most official statistics use the U.S. Census Bureau definition: two or more persons living together who are related by blood, marriage, or adoption. Note that this differs from the usual meaning in conversation—close relatives, whether they are living together or not.

Family-centered care: A system-wide approach to family health care. The delivery of safe, quality health care while recognizing, focusing on, and adapting to both the physical and psychosocial needs of the client, patient, and family.

Family child health nursing: Using nursing actions that consider the relationship between family tasks and health care and their effects on family well-being and children's health.

Family coping: The family's efforts to strengthen the family as a unit, maintain the well-being of its members, and use family and community resources to manage stress and hardship.

Family Cycle of Health and Illness: This model depicts the dynamic movement of the family through seven phases of wellness and illness in family life. Phases include (1) family health promotion and risk reduction, (2) family vulnerability and symptoms of illness, (3) sick role assumed and family illness appraisal, (4) contact with the health care system and diagnosis of the problem/illness, (5) family acute response to illness, (6) adaptation to illness and recovery, and if a terminal illness, (7) death of a member and family reorganization.

Family functioning: The individual and cooperative processes used by developing persons to dynamically engage one another and their diverse environments over the life course. Family purposes are important for optimizing family outcomes. Functions are usually described as affective functions, family socialization and social placement functions, health care functions, reproductive functions, and economic functions.

Family health: A dynamic, changing relative state of well-being that includes the biological, psychological, spiritual, sociological, and cultural factors of individual members and the whole family system.

Family Health Model: In this approach, Sharon Denham views family health as a process over time of family member interactions and health-related behaviors. The model assumes that family health involves all members who reside within a household and includes their interactions with one another and their environments.

Family health promotion: Achieving maximum family well-being throughout the family life course.

Family households: Households maintained by a family householder, including any unrelated people who reside there.

Family Interaction Model: Used by family child health nurses to facilitate and teach healthful activities for growth in families, prevent injury and disease, and treat disease and illness conditions.

Family Interactional Theory: In this theory, the family is viewed as a unit made up of interacting personalities. It examines internal family dynamics, including communication processes, roles, decision making and problem solving, and socialization patterns. The major emphasis is on family roles.

Family intervention research: Typically involves an experimental design by which one group of families receives or participates in an intervention and another group does not participate or receives a different intervention.

Family Leave Act: On February 5, 1993, President Clinton signed the 1993 Family Leave Act, which requires employers with more than 50 workers to provide up to 12 weeks of unpaid leave to employees at a child's birth or adoption or to care for members of their families who are ill.

Family Life-Cycle Theory: A descriptive developmental theory about the tasks and processes for families. Stages are based on the age of the oldest child of a nuclear family. The most common family life-cycle theory by Duvall has been criticized for not being applicable to nontraditional families. Similar theories for divorced and blended families have been proposed.

Family process: The ongoing interaction between family members through which they accomplish their instrumental and expressive tasks. The nursing process considers the family, not the individual, as the unit of care.

Family-related research: Research that focuses on relationships between selected family members, using data reported from individuals.

Family research: Research that focuses on the family unit as a whole.

Family roles: Formal (overt or explicit) and informal (covert or implicit) clusters of behavior associated with family membership. Roles may be assigned or individually assumed and are used by the family to maintain its homeostasis.

Family social science theories: These are a set of theories about how families work that are based in the social science theories, especially sociology.

Family spirituality: Involves transcendence, meaning, and compassion for others and provides the basis for harmony, communication, and wholeness among family members.

Family stages: Nurses anticipate the family reorganization necessary to accommodate the growth and development of family members.

Family Stress Theory: The family stress model explores how families adapt to events that are perceived as stressful and have the potential to be disruptive to families, thereby resulting in crisis.

Family Systems Theory: In the systems theory, families are viewed as an organized whole, and individuals in the family are interdependent and interactive. Every family system has features designed to maintain stability or homeostasis, although these features may be adaptive or maladaptive. At the same time, the family changes constantly in response to stresses and strains from the external environment, as well as from the internal family environment.

Family Systems Therapy Theory: Murray Bowen developed this theoretical approach to families in 1978. Family systems theory begins with the assumption that anxiety is an inevitable, omnipresent part of life. Chronic anxiety is the basic cause of dysfunction in individuals and in families.

Family tasks: (1) To secure shelter, food, and clothing; (2) to develop emotionally healthy individuals who can manage crisis and experience nonmonetary achievement; (3) to ensure each individual's socialization in school, work, spiritual, and community life; (4) to contribute to the next generation by giving birth, adopting a child, or foster-caring for a child; and (5) to promote the health of family members and care for them during illness.

Family therapy theories: Family therapy models are influenced by general systems theory and are practice-oriented. These models are concerned with what can be done to facilitate change in "dysfunctional" families: they are both descriptive and prescriptive. That is, they not only describe and explain observations made in practice but also suggest treatment or intervention strategies.

Family transitions: Events that signal a reorganization of family roles and tasks. They may be developmental or situational.

Family values: A family's system of ideas, attitudes, and beliefs about the worth or priority of entities, or ideas that bind together the members of a family in a common culture.

Fertility rates: Fertility rates are the number of births to women in a defined population during a year, divided by the number of persons in the population (alternately expressed per thousand persons, per thousand women, or per thousand women ages 15 to 49, the prime years for childbearing). Age-specific fertility rates are limited to women in a particular age group, for example, the number of births to women ages 25 to 29 per thousand women in that age group. The total fertility rate is the number of births that a typical woman in the population would have during her whole life if age-specific rates were to stay the same throughout her life.

Fictive kin: A concept from anthropology along the lines of chosen family but carrying the implication that the fictive kin is not "real."

Frame: The lens or different perspective that nurses use to gather, cluster, and interpret data gathered in the client story.

Framework of Systemic Organization: Marie-Louise Friedemann's theory is built on the view of the family as client. The family is described as a social system that has the expressed goal of transmitting culture to its members.

Functional aspect of family: Family unit composed of intimate, interactive, and interdependent persons who share some values, goals, resources, responsibilities, decisions, and commitment over time.

Functional kin: When fictive kin become fully integrated as a family.

Gay: Someone who practices homosexuality or chooses a queer lifestyle; having a sexual attraction for persons of the same sex. "Gay man" may be used to refer to males, whereas "lesbian" may be used to refer to females.

Gender: Socially and culturally defined roles for males and females. Gender speaks to the way in which different sexes behave. Femininity encompasses long hair, makeup, and soft speech; masculinity includes athletic prowess, aggressiveness, and never wearing dresses. Femininity is usually associated with females and masculinity with males. However, none of these behaviors is biologically driven; there is no gene in women telling them to curl their hair. Females and males in practice combine many masculine and feminine traits in their daily lives.

Genogram: A format for diagramming a family that illustrates family structure. Other information on the drawing may include family constellation, health history, and family relationships. Sometimes called a family tree.

GLBT: Gay, lesbian, bisexual, and transgendered.

Grounded theory: A theory that is generated or constructed from data provided by families; thus, the specific theory is connected closely with the data and is said to be "grounded" in data.

Head Start: A national program that provides comprehensive developmental services for low-income, preschool children ages 3 to 5 as well as social services for their families. Education, socio-emotional development, physical and mental health, and nutrition are all components.

Health patterns: The family's and family members' understandings and behaviors associated not merely with the absence of disease and incapacitation but with optimal physical, mental, and social well-being.

Healthy People: The name given to the family social policy program initiated by the federal government in 1979 and still in use to this day, which has resulted in national health targets and new health policies.

Hermeneutic phenomenology: An approach to the study of shared family meanings and family concerns.

Heterosexism: Prejudice against people who are not heterosexual/straight.

Homophobia: Fear of homosexuals (e.g., gay, lesbian, bisexuals, and transgendered).

Homosexual: This term was invented at the beginning of the 20th century by psychoanalysts studying people who found themselves attracted to their same sex. Because of the term's use as a disease category, it is generally not used within the communities it refers to. See **GLBT**.

Household: Consists of all the people who occupy a housing unit, which could be a house, apartment, or other group of rooms.

Human Becoming Theory: This theory was developed by Rose Marie Parse in 1992. The concept of family and who makes up the family is continually becoming and evolving. The role of the nurses is to use therapeutic communication to invite each member of the family to uncover his or her understanding of the meaning of the experience, learn what the meaning of the experience is for each other, and discuss the meaning of the experience for the family as a whole.

Human Genome Project: The Human Genome Project (HGP) began in the mid-1980s as an international research program led in the United States by the Department of Energy (DOE) and the National Institutes of Health (NIH). Its purpose was to map human genes in order to diagnose and treat disease, as well as to identify individuals at risk for disease.

Hypothesis: A hypothesis is a statement that postulates some sort of relationship between concepts and propositions that is crucial to a theory. It is a way of stating an expected relationship between concepts.

Illness patterns: Behaviors and processes families go through to manage a condition or disease and the medical treatments that become a part of their daily lives.

Illness transitions: Transitions through acute, chronic, and end-of-life phases.

Immigrants: Persons who have moved to the United States from another country intending to stay a long time. Tourists, students, and those here for short-term business assignments are not usually counted as immigrants until they decide to stay long-term. Census statistics cannot differentiate between those intending to stay and those here temporarily, so many reports refer generally to the "foreign-born," all current residents born in another country.

Implementation: The fourth step of the nursing process; it involves carrying out or putting into effect the care plan developed during the planning phase.

Indigenous culture/people: Those living in a region during the time of conquest or colonialism who, irrespective of their legal status, continue to live and function within their native political, social, economic, and cultural subsystem.

Interactional Family Therapy Model: This approach views the family as a system of interactive or interlocking behaviors or communication processing.

Interracial: Families or people of more than one race.

Interval-scale measurement: Interval scales have equal numerical distances between intervals while following rules of mutually exclusive categories, exhaustive categories, and rank ordering (e.g., temperature).

In vitro fertilization (IVF): Embryos are generated outside of the body and transferred (at least two) after successful fertilization with sperm.

Judgment: The decision the nurse makes to evaluate client progress toward the desired outcomes.

Keystone issue: The primary problem that the client and family are presently experiencing.

Labeling: Labeling theory suggests that we give people labels (loser, woman, black, Latina, cop, addict) in order to categorize and so know how to interact with them. If someone is simply a *woman*, she loses the complexity of her humanity.

Labor force participation: Economic statistics define the labor force as everyone who either works for pay (including people who have their own business or farm) or is unemployed but actively looking for work.

Lesbian: Equivalent to "homosexual," lesbian is a preferred term for women whose sexual object of choice is other women.

Life expectancy: The average number of years of life remaining for members of a defined population, assuming that current age-specific mortality rates apply throughout their lives. Life expectancy is usually calculated from birth but can also be expressed, for example, as the average number of years of life remaining at age 65. If age-specific mortality rates continue to improve, then most people born in the year 2004 will in fact live longer than the life expectancy calculated in 2004 using age-specific mortality rates prevailing in 2004.

Limitation: Inability to perform without assistance an important life activity, or the need for an assistive device to see, hear, or move around.

Longitudinal research designs: Research questions that are concerned with continuity, naturally occurring change, and predictability over time, in which the same families are studied over time.

Meals on Wheels: Community programs that deliver food to homebound people.

Measurement: The process of linking theoretical ideas or concepts to empirical indicators or variables. The assignment of numbers to individuals, objects, events, or situations according to specified rules; the process of using an instrument to measure a particular attribute, assigning numbers to the attributes, and using the data for statistical analysis. Measurement can be a part of the assessment process.

Medicaid: Medicaid is a jointly funded, federal-state health insurance program for certain low-income and needy people.

Medicare: The nation's largest health insurance program, covering people age 65 and over, those who have permanent kidney failure, and certain people with disabilities.

Mode of data collection: Refers, in part, to whether

the nature of the data is individual, relational, or transactional.

Morbidity: The number of persons with an illness, divided by the number of persons in a defined population. Morbidity rates can refer either to prevalence (those who are sick on a particular day) or to incidence (the number of new cases of a disease in a population that occur during a time period, such as 1 month or 1 year).

Mortality: The number of deaths in the population in a given time or place and/or the proportion of deaths to the population.

Mortality rate: The number of deaths during a period of time, usually 1 year, in a defined population, divided by the number of persons in that population at a specific time (typically, the middle of the year). Mortality rates are usually expressed per 1000 people or per 100,000 people. Age-specific mortality rates refer to particular age groups, for example, the number of deaths of 15- to 19-year-olds in a year per 1000 people in that age group. Cause-specific mortality rates refer to deaths attributed to particular causes, for example, the number of deaths due to melanoma in 1 year per 100,000 people.

Narrative inquiry: This form of inquiry analyzes the narratives or created structures of the stories, on the assumption that family members, as narrators telling their stories, select, order, and prioritize events based on their meaning for the individuals involved.

Nationals: Population living in their own home nation.

Neuman Systems Model: Betty Neuman developed this model in 1983. She viewed the family as a system composed of family member subsystems. The family's primary goal is to maintain its stability by preserving the integrity of its structure.

Nominal-scale measurement: Nominal scales are the lowest level of measurement used when data can be organized into categories that are exclusive and exhaustive, but the categories cannot be compared (e.g., gender, race, nursing diagnoses).

Non-family household: A residence where the householder lives alone or a household shared by people who are not related.

Nonmarital fertility: The nonmarital fertility rate is the number of births to unmarried women in a particular year, divided by the number of unmarried women. The nonmarital fertility ratio is the percentage of all births that are to unmarried women. Other terms for nonmarital include "illegitimate" or "out-of-wedlock."

Norm: Culturally expected behavior, appearance, or structure.

Normalization: An ongoing process of actively accommodating the child's evolving physical, emotional, and social needs.

Normative: Those forces that structure members of society to fit norms.

Normative (on-time) illnesses: Common, expected, and predictable illnesses (e.g., arthritis for couples over the age of 70 years).

Nuclear family: Family with parents and children only; extended family is the nuclear family plus other blood-related kin or relationships formed by a marriage tie.

Nurse/client contract: An agreement between the nurse and client (family) to work together to attain goals that are determined by the client.

Nursing diagnosis: A clinical judgment about individual family or a community response to actual and potential health problems or life processes. Nursing diagnoses provide the basis for selection of nursing interventions to achieve outcomes for which the nurse is accountable.

Nursing process: An orderly, systematic manner of determining the client's problems, making plans to solve them, initiating the plan or assigning others to implement it, and evaluating the extent to which the plan was effective in resolving the problems identified.

Obesity: Persons with a body mass index (BMI) of 30 or more are classified by the World Health Organization as obese. Those with a BMI of 25 to 29.9 are classified as overweight. BMI is calculated as weight (in kilograms) divided by height (in meters) squared.

Observational methods: Systematic procedures for observing behavior and recording what happens.

Open family system: A family that encourages interchanges between the family and the multiple systems existing in the outside world.

Ordinal-scale measurement: Ordinal scales yield data that can be ranked, but intervals between the ranked data are not necessarily equal (e.g., levels of coping).

Outcome Present-State Testing Clinical Reasoning Model (OPT): A dynamic systematic clinical reasoning process that emphasizes the outcome of care.

Parent vigilance: Families spend hours at the bedside "watching over their children."

Parish nurse: A nursing role where the responsibilities of the community or family nurse are combined with spiritual counseling from a holistic perspective to improve the well-being of parishioners and families.

Partner: An alternative to the terms "girlfriend," "boyfriend," or "spouse." Often used within gay, lesbian, bisexual, and transgendered communities.

Pedophilia: Adult sex with children.

Percutaneous transluminal coronary angioplasty (PTCA): Procedure performed by an interventional cardiologist to improve revascularization and perfusion of oxygenated blood to the heart muscle. During the procedure, a catheter with a balloon tip is passed into the stenotic coronary artery. When the balloon tip is positioned over the coronary lesion, multiple balloon inflations of variable pressure and duration are used to improve the diameter of the stenotic arterial segment.

Permeability of family boundaries: The status of a family boundary that selectively allows access or admittance to some influences but not others. Family boundaries are permeable to the extent that some influences are allowed admittance whereas others are excluded. Totally closed boundaries do not allow outside forces to influence the family system, whereas totally open boundaries allow all influences to affect the family. Boundaries of the family are healthy to the extent that their permeability allows needed influences to be admitted while destructive influences are prohibited or screened out.

Planning: The third step of the nursing diagnosis. It involves the selection or design of nursing interventions in consultation and collaboration with the client, which facilitates the achievement of the desired objectives. It is the process by which objectives are determined, interventions are chosen, and the care plan is written.

Postpartum period: Defined medically as the six weeks during which the mother's body returns to the pre-pregnant physiological state. Psychological changes may take longer.

Poverty: The official poverty measure since 1962 has been defined as an income level three times the cost of a basic diet defined by the U.S. Department of Agriculture. The income levels are adjusted for families of different sizes and are updated each year to reflect increases in consumer prices. In 2003, the poverty line for a family of two adults and two children was $18,660.

Present state: Represents the current health status of the client/family that includes the most relevant or pressing issues confronting the family client.

Prevention: (1) Primary: focuses on preventing the occurrence of health problems; (2) secondary: designed to identify and treat health problems early; (3) tertiary: aimed at correcting health problems and preventing further deterioration.

Primary prevention: Actions designed to prevent a disease from occurring; reduces the probability of a specific illness occurring and includes active protection against unnecessary stressors or threats.

Propositions: Propositions are statements about the relationship among two or more concepts. An example is that the family unit interacts with the health of the individual members of the family.

Public health nursing: The synthesis of nursing knowledge and practice and the science and practice of public health, implemented via systematic use of the nursing process and other processes, designed to promote health and prevent illness in population groups. The focus of care is the aggregate. The goal of care is the promotion of health and the prevention of illness.

Qualitative analysis: Organization and interpretation of nonnumeric data for the purpose of discovering important underlying dimensions and patterns of relationships.

Qualitative approaches: Sample phenomena and the data are texts or transcripts of interview discourse.

Qualitative data: Information collected in narrative (nonnumeric) form such as the transcript of an unstructured interview.

Quantitative analysis: Manipulation of numerical data through statistical procedures for the purpose of describing phenomena or assessing the magnitude and reliability of relationships among them.

Quantitative approaches: Quantitative approaches to family nursing research typically sample populations of children, parents, and/or families.

Quantitative data: Information collected in numerical form.

Queer: At one time a slur against gay, lesbian, bisexual, or transgendered people, "queer" has been reclaimed as a term to describe sexual orientation and to reflect the continuum of sexual practices and tastes.

Questionnaires: Surveys that can be mailed to respondents or administered in a group or family setting; the respondents mark the answers themselves with complete anonymity.

Race: Seemingly straightforward, the concept of race has a complicated history. An examination of the census records over this century reveals that the categories have expanded from Irish, Italian,

Northern European, Negro, and Octoroon to white, non-white Hispanic, Asian and Pacific Islander, American Indian (sometimes by tribe), African-American, Caribbean-American, and so on. All of these people have been in this country throughout the century, but their racial category recognition has changed. Sociologists now define "race" as a group of people with shared physical characteristics.

Ratio-scale measurement: Ratio scales are the highest level of measurement that meets the rules of other forms of measure: mutually exclusive categories, exhaustive categories, rank ordering, equal spacing between intervals, a continuum of values, and an absolute zero (e.g., weight).

Reflection: A strategy that nurses use to review and learn from clients to enhance and expand their practice base.

Reliability: Essentially refers to the dependability and consistency of a measure.

Reliability of measurement: Reliability of measurement is crucial to obtaining meaningful data about families.

Resiliency Model of Family Stress, Adjustment, and Adaptation: This model explores how families process stressful or threatening life events through evaluation and assessment of the stressor and through the use of problem-solving and coping skills in the process of achieving homeostasis.

Risk: The probability that individuals in the community will be affected by a health problem.

Role: Relatively homogeneous sets of behaviors that are normatively and culturally defined and expected of individuals based on developmental stages, gender, social expectations, and social positions.

Role-Performance Family Health Model: This view of family health is based on the idea that family health is the ability of family members to perform their routine roles and achieve developmental tasks.

Roy's Adaptation Model: This model was developed by Sister Callista Roy in 1976. This model describes and explains how adaptation occurs in family and offers insight into ways to assist families to adapt to health issues.

Same-sex families: Male or gay partners and female or lesbian partners who often cohabitate but may choose to live separately due to reasons such as social acceptance or employment that results in long-distance relationships.

Sample: The term "sampling" pertains to who or what is selected to be studied. More specifically, the term "sample" refers to a subset or part of a whole, and "sampling" refers to how the sample or subgroup is chosen.

Sandwich generation: "Sandwich generation" is a colloquial term that refers to the middle generation of adults who are between prolonged dependency of adult children remaining or returning to the home of origin and elderly parents and grandparents requiring care by their adult children.

Secondary analysis: Involves using previously collected data or secondary data sources to answer questions not asked by the original investigator or to ask similar questions in new ways.

Secondary data sources: Include data sets from completed projects on related topics, family and social archives, large-scale surveys, and public records.

Secondary prevention: Early diagnosis and prompt treatment; includes activities such as screening for disease.

Selective reduction: The procedure of removing (aborting) unwanted fetuses in multiple pregnancies.

Self-care Deficit Theory: Dorothea Orem's theory depicts the family as the basic conditioning unit, in which the individual learns culture, roles, and responsibilities. The specific focus is on the role of family in helping its individual family members achieve self-care.

Self-reports: Data collection by self-report consists of asking people questions directly through questionnaires, face-to-face interviews, or telephone interviews. Also called **survey method.**

Sex: The reproductive structure of human bodies. Although sex is generally thought to include only males (penis, scrotum, chest hair, facial hair, etc.) and females (vagina, uterus, breasts), 1 in every 2000 live births is "intersexed." These infants are born with a mixture of female and male traits. Most are then surgically "assigned" to one or the other sex. This term describes only biology, not behavior.

Sexism: Prejudice against a sex. Generally applied to an expectation that women are not as qualified or competent as men are.

Sexual orientation: The object (person) toward whom sexual desire is directed; the object with whom one wants to explore sexuality.

Sexuality: The sexual acts that give an individual pleasure.

Single family: Family in which the head of the household has never been or is not currently married.

Single-parent family: A family with one or more children, with only one parent living with and caring for the children. The parents of the children may be divorced or separated, one parent may have died, or the parents may never have married. Families with one parent temporarily living away (e.g., for work or a military deployment) are not usually included in statistics on single-parent families. Other adults (including grandparents or a cohabiting partner) may live in the same household.

Situational transitions: Include changes in personal relationships, roles and status, the environment, physical and mental capabilities, and the loss of possessions.

Social class: A large group of people with relatively similar incomes, amount of wealth, education, life conditions, life chances, and lifestyles. Synonymous with socioeconomic status.

Social support: The amount of help actually received, satisfaction with that help, and the person's network providing that help. Help received may be in the form of instrumental or physical aid, information, emotional support, or the appraisal of one's role performance.

Solidarity: Strong shared group identity that leads to promotion of that group and its causes. Class solidarity would include working for unions in order to secure or better the lives of those within the working class.

Stent: Small device, often consisting of stainless steel woven mesh, inserted into a diseased coronary artery to provide structural support to the coronary artery that has been newly reopened by a percutaneous transluminal coronary angioplasty.

Stereotype: Exaggerated, often extreme, expectations of certain people that keep people from recognizing difference and humanity. For example, the stereotypical nurse is a white woman, when in truth many men of color work in the field. Denying them recognition makes their successful functioning difficult.

Stigma: Derived from the Christian tradition wherein people evidencing blood on their palms or feet such as Christ did when nailed to the cross are said to have "stigmata." A stigma is a social marker that labels people negatively, as deviants. Stigmas may include race, physical disability, sex, sexual orientation, clothing, tattoos, and religion.

Straight: A colloquial term for heterosexual people.

Structural Family Therapy: This systems-oriented model uses spatial and organizational metaphors to describe problems and develop solutions. The family is viewed as an open sociocultural system that is continually faced with demands for change, both from within and from outside the family.

Structural-Functional Theory: The family is considered a small group that has features common to all small groups. The family is viewed as a social system. This theory assumes that social systems carry out functions that serve individuals and society. The individuals in the family act in accordance with a set of internalized norms and values, which are learned primarily through socialization.

Structure: An ordered set of relationships among family subsystems and between the family and other social systems.

Survey method: Data collection method that consists of asking people questions directly or through questionnaires, face-to-face interviews, or telephone interviews. Also called **self-reports.**

Synchronic: A system of knowledge that seeks to understand how systems and structures of reality function.

Tertiary prevention: Activities aimed at correcting health problems and preventing further deterioration; also focuses on preventing recurrences of the problem.

Theory: Theories are abstract general ideas, composed of concepts and the relationships among concepts. They are abstract general ideas that are subject to rules of organization. They are selected and organized as abstract representations of phenomena. They are sets of statements that tentatively describe, explain, or predict relationships among concepts. Examples of theories are family systems theory and family development theory.

Theory of Goal Attainment: Imogene King developed this theory in 1981. It is derived from systems theory. She defined "family" as a small group of individuals bound together for the socialization of the members. The family was the vehicle for transmitting values and norms of behavior across the life span.

Theory of Unitary Human Beings: This is an abstract theory based on general systems theory and draws on many fields of study, including anthropology, sociology, astronomy, religion, philosophy, history, and mythology. The family is a constant open-system energy field that is ever changing in its interactions with the environment.

Traditional family: A family is perceived to be the norm or mainstream, usually two parents with consanguineously related children where roles and power are related to gender.

Transgender: Different from transsexuals, transgendered people feel more comfortable displaying or living in a particular gender, which may be different from their sex—for example, a woman who binds her breasts and wears men's suits or a man who wears makeup and dresses. Transgendered people are not necessarily gay. A transgendered man may still desire women. However, as a result of social and historical forces, transgendered people are included with others who have suffered oppression for expressing themselves "differently," such as gays, lesbians, and bisexuals.

Transition points: Individual members and the family grow and change phases.

Transsexuals: Transsexuals are those people who have undergone some form of physical change (hormones, surgery, or both) in order to achieve a body to suit the gender they prefer. For example, a transsexual biological female who feels more "real" as a man will take on masculine attributes as well as male hormones and might undergo a radical mastectomy and construction of male genitalia.

Triangulation: The use of two or more research methods in a single study.

Validity: Refers to the appropriateness of the specific use of a given measure; it answers the question "Did the instrument actually measure what it was meant to measure?"

Vertical diffusion: A dynamic that occurs when one family member initiates health behavior changes and thereby influences another member to make similar changes.

Welfare reform: 1996's Personal Responsibility and Work Opportunity Reconciliation Act. An effort to "reform" welfare and its purported abuses.

Worldviews: Highest level of knowledge and views of reality within a cultural subgroup; that which gives a sense of order and meaning.

Xenophobia: Fear of outsiders (e.g., people from a different country, community, town, social group).

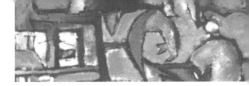

APPENDIX C
FAMILY SYSTEMS STRESSOR-STRENGTH INVENTORY (FS³I)
Shirley May Harmon Hanson • Karen B. Mischke

Instructions for Administration

The Family Systems Stressor-Strength Inventory (FS³I) is an assessment and measurement instrument intended for use with families (see Chapter 8). It focuses on identifying stressful situations occurring in families and the strengths families use to maintain healthy family functioning. Each family member is asked to complete the instrument on an individual form before an interview with the clinician. Questions can be read to members unable to read.

After completion of the instrument, the clinician evaluates the family on each of the stressful situations (general and specific) and the strengths they possess. This evaluation is recorded on the family member form.

The clinician records the individual family member's score and the clinician perception score on the Quantitative Summary. A different color code is used for each family member. The clinician also completes the Qualitative Summary, synthesizing the information gleaned from all participants. Clinicians can use the Family Care Plan to prioritize diagnoses, set goals, develop prevention and intervention activities, and evaluate outcomes.

Family Name _____ Date _____

Family Member(s) Completing Assessment _____

Ethnic Background(s) _____

Religious Background(s) _____

Referral Source _____

Interviewer _____

	Family Members	Relationship in Family	Age	Marital Status	Education (highest degree)	Occupation
1.	_____	_____	_____	_____	_____	_____
2.	_____	_____	_____	_____	_____	_____
3.	_____	_____	_____	_____	_____	_____
4.	_____	_____	_____	_____	_____	_____
5.	_____	_____	_____	_____	_____	_____
6.	_____	_____	_____	_____	_____	_____

Family's current reasons for seeking assistance:

_____

_____

_____

Source: Hanson, S. M. H. (2001). *Family health care nursing: Theory, practice, and research* (2nd ed.), pp. 425–437. Philadelphia: F. A. Davis.

Part I: Family Systems Stressors (General)

DIRECTIONS: Each of 25 situations/stressors listed here deals with some aspect of normal family life. They have the potential for creating stress within families or between families and the world in which they live. We are interested in your overall impression of how these situations affect your family life. Please circle a number (0 through 5) that best describes the amount of stress or tension they create for you.

STRESSORS	FAMILY PERCEPTION SCORE					CLINICIAN PERCEPTION
	DOES NOT APPLY	LITTLE STRESS	MEDIUM STRESS		HIGH STRESS	SCORE
1. Family member(s) feel unappreciated	0	1	2	3	4	5	_____
2. Guilt for not accomplishing more	0	1	2	3	4	5	_____
3. Insufficient "me" time	0	1	2	3	4	5	_____
4. Self-Image/self-esteem/ feelings of unattractiveness	0	1	2	3	4	5	_____
5. Perfectionism	0	1	2	3	4	5	_____
6. Dieting	0	1	2	3	4	5	_____
7. Health/Illness	0	1	2	3	4	5	_____
8. Communication with children	0	1	2	3	4	5	_____
9. Housekeeping standards	0	1	2	3	4	5	_____
10. Insufficient couple time	0	1	2	3	4	5	_____
11. Insufficient family playtime	0	1	2	3	4	5	_____
12. Children's behavior/ discipline/sibling fighting	0	1	2	3	4	5	_____
13. Television	0	1	2	3	4	5	_____
14. Overscheduled family calendar	0	1	2	3	4	5	_____
15. Lack of shared responsibility in the family	0	1	2	3	4	5	_____
16. Moving	0	1	2	3	4	5	_____
17. Spousal relationship (communication, friendship, sex)	0	1	2	3	4	5	_____
18. Holidays	0	1	2	3	4	5	_____
19. In-laws	0	1	2	3	4	5	_____
20. Teen behaviors (communication, music, friends, school)	0	1	2	3	4	5	_____
21. New baby	0	1	2	3	4	5	_____
22. Economics/finances/ budgets	0	1	2	3	4	5	_____
23. Unhappiness with work situation	0	1	2	3	4	5	_____
24. Overvolunteerism	0	1	2	3	4	5	_____
25. Neighbors	0	1	2	3	4	5	

Additional Stressors: _____

_____

Family Remarks: _____

_____

Clinician: Clarification of stressful situations/concerns with family members.

Prioritize in order of importance to family members: _____

_____

Part II: Family Systems Stressors (Specific)

DIRECTIONS: The following 12 questions are designed to provide information about your specific stress-producing situation/problem or area of concern influencing your family's health. Please circle a number (1 through 5) that best describes the influence this situation has on your family's life and how well you perceive your family's overall functioning.

The specific stress-producing situation/problem or area of concern at this time is: _____

_____

_____

STRESSORS	FAMILY PERCEPTION SCORE			CLINICIAN PERCEPTION SCORE
	LITTLE	MEDIUM	HIGH	SCORE
1. To what extent is your family bothered by this problem or stressful situation? (e.g., effects on family interactions, communication among members, emotional and social relationships) .1	2	3	4 5	_____

Family Remarks: _____

_____

Clinician Remarks: _____

_____

2. How much of an effect does this stresssful situation have on your family's usual pattern of living? (e.g., effects on lifestyle patterns and family developmental task) 1	2	3	4 5	_____

Family Remarks: _____

_____

Clinician Remarks: _____

_____

3. How much has this situation affected your family's ability to work together as a family unit? (e.g., alteration in family roles, completion of family tasks, following through with responsibilities) 1	2	3	4 5	_____

Family Remarks: _____

_____

Clinician Remarks: _____

_____

Has your family ever experienced a similar concern in the past?
1. YES   If YES, complete question 4
2. NO   If NO, complete question 5

STRESSORS	FAMILY PERCEPTION SCORE			CLINICIAN PERCEPTION
	LITTLE	MEDIUM	HIGH	SCORE

4. How successful was your family in dealing with this situation/problem/concern in the past? (e.g., workable coping strategies developed, adaptive measures useful, situation improved) . . . . .1　　2　　3　　4　　5　　_____

Family Remarks: _____

Clinician Remarks: _____

5. How strongly do you feel this current situation/ problem/concern will affect your family's future? (e.g., anticipated consequences) . . . . .1　　2　　3　　4　　5　　_____

Family Remarks: _____

Clinician Remarks: _____

6. To what extent are family members able to help themselves in this present situation/problem/ concern? (e.g., self-assistive efforts, family expectations, spiritual influence, family resources) . . . . .1　　2　　3　　4　　5　　_____

Family Remarks: _____

Clinician Remarks: _____

7. To what extent do you expect others to help your family with this situation/problem/ concern? (e.g., what roles would helpers play; how available are extra-family resources) . . . . .1　　2　　3　　4　　5　　_____

Family Remarks: _____

Clinician Remarks: _____

STRESSORS	POOR	SATISFACTORY	EXCELLENT	SCORE

8. How would you rate the way your family functions overall? (e.g., how your family members relate to each other and to larger family and community) . . . . .1　　2　　3　　4　　　　5　　_____

Family Remarks: _____

Clinician Remarks: _____

STRESSORS	FAMILY PERCEPTION SCORE			CLINICIAN PERCEPTION SCORE
	POOR	SATISFACTORY	EXCELLENT	SCORE

9. How would you rate the overall physical health status of each family member by name? (Include yourself as a family member; record additional names on back.)

a. _____	1	2	3	4	5	_____
b. _____	1	2	3	4	5	_____
c. _____	1	2	3	4	5	_____
d. _____	1	2	3	4	5	_____
e. _____	1	2	3	4	5	_____

10. How would you rate the overall physical health status of your family as a whole? 1   2   3   4   5   _____

Family Remarks: _____

Clinician Remarks: _____

11. How would you rate the overall mental health status of each family member by name? (Include yourself as a family member; record additional names on back.)

a. _____	1	2	3	4	5	_____
b. _____	1	2	3	4	5	_____
c. _____	1	2	3	4	5	_____
d. _____	1	2	3	4	5	_____
e. _____	1	2	3	4	5	_____

12. How would you rate the overall mental health status of your family as a whole? 1   2   3   4   5   _____

Family Remarks: _____

Clinician Remarks: _____

Part III: Family Systems Strengths

DIRECTIONS: Each of the 16 traits/attributes listed below deals with some aspect of family life and its overall functioning. Each one contributes to the health and well-being of family members as individuals and to the family as a whole. Please circle a number (0 through 5) that best describes the extent to which the trait applies to your family.

	DOES NOT APPLY	FAMILY PERCEPTION SCORE				CLINICIAN PERCEPTION
MY FAMILY:		SELDOM	USUALLY		ALWAYS	SCORE
1. Communicates and listens to one another 0		1	2	3	4	5	_____

Family Remarks: _____

Clinician Remarks: _____

2. Affirms and supports one another 0		1	2	3	4	5	_____

Family Remarks: _____

Clinician Remarks: _____

3. Teaches respect for others 0		1	2	3	4	5	_____

Family Remarks: _____

Clinician Remarks: _____

4. Develops a sense of trust in members 0		1	2	3	4	5	_____

Family Remarks: _____

Clinician Remarks: _____

5. Displays a sense of play and humor 0		1	2	3	4	5	_____

Family Remarks: _____

Clinician Remarks: _____

MY FAMILY:	DOES NOT APPLY	FAMILY PERCEPTION SCORE				CLINICIAN PERCEPTION SCORE
		SELDOM	USUALLY		ALWAYS	

6. Exhibits a sense of shared responsibility 0   1   2   3   4   5   _____

Family Remarks: _____

Clinician Remarks: _____

7. Teaches a sense of right and wrong 0   1   2   3   4   5   _____

Family Remarks: _____

Clinician Remarks: _____

8. Has a strong sense of family in which rituals and traditions abound 0   1   2   3   4   5   _____

Family Remarks: _____

Clinician Remarks: _____

9. Has a balance of interaction among members 0   1   2   3   4   5   _____

Family Remarks: _____

Clinician Remarks: _____

10. Has a shared religious core 0   1   2   3   4   5   _____

Family Remarks: _____

Clinician Remarks: _____

11. Respects the privacy of one another 0   1   2   3   4   5   _____

Family Remarks: _____

Clinician Remarks: _____

12. Values service to others 0   1   2   3   4   5   _____

Family Remarks: _____

Clinician Remarks: _____

My Family:	Does Not Apply	Family Perception Score				Clinician Perception Score
		Seldom	Usually		Always	

13. Fosters family table time and
    conversation 0   1   2   3   4   5   _____

Family Remarks: _____

Clinician Remarks: _____

14. Shares leisure time .0   1   2   3   4   5   _____

Family Remarks: _____

Clinician Remarks: _____

15. Admits to and seeks help with problems . . .0   1   2   3   4   5   _____

Family Remarks: _____

Clinician Remarks: _____

16a. How would yor rate the overall
    strengths that exist in your family? 0   1   2   3   4   5   _____

Family Remarks: _____

Clinician Remarks: _____

16b. Additional Family Strengths: _____

16c. Clinician: Clarification of family strengths with individual members: _____

Family Systems Stressor-Strength inventory (FS³I) Scoring Summary
Section 1: Family Perception Scores

Instructions For Administration

The Family Systems Stressor-Strength Inventory (FS³I) Scoring Summary is divided into two sections: Section 1, Family Perception Scores, and Section 2, Clinician Perception Scores. These two sections are further divided into three parts: Part I, Family Systems Stressors (General); Part II, Family Systems Stressors (Specific); and Part III, Family Systems Strengths. Each part contains a Quantitative Summary and a Qualitative Summary.

Quantifiable family and clinician perception scores are both graphed on the Quantitative Summary. Each family member has a designated color code. Family and clinician remarks are both recorded on the Quantitative Summary. Quantitative Summary scores, when graphed, suggest a level for initiation of prevention/intervention modes: Primary, Secondary, and Tertiary. Qualitative Summary information, when synthesized, contributes to the development and channeling of the Family Care Plan.

Part 1 Family Systems Stressors (General)

Add acores from questions 1 to 25 and calculate an overall numerical score for Family Systems Stressors (General). Ratings are from 1 (most positive) to 5 (most negative). The Does Not Apply (0) responses are omitted from the calculations. Total scores range from 25 to 125.
Family Systems Stressor Score (General)
$(_{25}) \times 1 =$
Graph score on Quantitative Summary, Family Systems Stressors (General), Family Member Perception Score. Color-code to differentiate family members.
Record additional stressors and family remarks in Part I, Qualitative Summary: Family and Clinician Remarks.

Part II Family Systems Stressors (Specific)

Add scores from questions 1 through 8, 10, and 12 and calculate a numerical score for Family Systems Stressors (Specific). Ratings are from 1 (most positive) to 5 (most negative). Questions 4, 6, 7, 8, 10 and 12 are reverse scored.* Total scores range from 10 through 50.

Family Systems Stressor Score (Specific)
$(_{10}) \times 1 =$
Graph score on Quantitative Summary, Family Systems Stressors (Specific) Family Member Perception Score. Color-code to differentiate family members.
Summarize data from questions 9 and 11 (reverse scored) and record family remarks in Part II, Qualitative Summary: Family and Clinician Remarks.

Part III Family Systems Strengths

Add scores from questions 1 through 16 and calculate a numerical score for Family Systems Strengths. Ratings are from 1 (seldom) to 5 (always). The Does Not Apply (0) responses are omitted from the calculations. Total Scores range from 16 to 80.
$(_{16}) \times 1 =$
Graph score on Quantitative Summary: Family Systems Strengths, Family Member Perception Score. Record additional family strengths and family remarks in Part III, Qualitative Summary: Family and Clinician Remarks.

Source: Mischke-Berkey, K., & Henson, S. M. H. (1991). *Pocket guide to family assessment and intervention.* St. Louis: Mosby.
*Reverse scoring:
Question answered as (1) is scored 5 points.
Question answered as (2) is scored 4 points.
Question answered as (3) is scored 3 points.
Question answered as (4) is scored 2 points.
Question answered as (5) is scored 1 point.

Section 2: Clinician Perception Scores

Part I Family Systems Stressors (General)*

Add scores from questions 1 through 25 and calculate an overall numerical score for Family Systems Stressors (General). Ratings are from 1 (most positive) to 5 (most negative). The Does Not Apply (0) responses are omitted from the calculations. Total scores range from 25 to 125.

Family systems Stressor Score (General)

$(_{25}) \times 1 =$

Graph score on Quantitative Summary, Family Systems Stressors (General) Clinician Perception Score.

Record clinicians' clarification of general stressors in Part I, Qualitative Summary: Family and Clinician Remarks.

Part II Family Systems Stressors (Specific)

Add scores from questions 1 through 8, 10, 12 and calculate a numerical score for Family Systems Stressors (Specific). Ratings are from 1 (most positive) to 5 (most negative). Questions 4, 6, 7, 8, 10, 12 are reverse scored.* Total scores range from 10 to 50.

Family Systems Stressor Score (Specific)

$(_{10}) \times 1 =$

Graph score on Quantitative Summary, Family Systems Stressors (Specific), Clinician Perception Score.

Summarized data from questions 9 and 11 (reverse order) and record clinician remarks in Part II, Qualitative Summary: Family and Clinician Remarks.

Part III Family Systems Strengths

Add scores from questions 1 through 16 and calculate a numerical score for Family Systems Strengths. Ratings are from 1 (seldom) to 5 (always).

The Does Not Apply (0) responses are omitted from the calculations. Total scores range from 16 to 80.

$(_{16}) \times 1 =$

Graph score on Quantitative Summary, Family Systems Strengths, Clinician Perception Score.

Record clinicians' clarification of family strengths in Part III, Qualitative Summary: Family and Clinician Remarks.

---

*Reverse scoring:

Question answered as (1) is scored 5 points.
Question answered as (2) is scored 4 points.
Question answered as (3) is scored 3 points.
Question answered as (4) is scored 2 points.
Question answered as (5) is scored 1 point.

Quantitative Summary of Family Systems Stressors: General and Specific Family and Clinician Perception Scores

DIRECTIONS: Graph the scores from each family member inventory by placing an "X" at the appropriate location. (Use first name initial for each different entry and different color code for each family member.)

	Family Systems Stressors (General)			Family Systems Stressors (Specific)	
Scores for Wellness and Stability	Family Member Perception Score	Clinician Perception Score	Scores for Wellness and Stability	Family Member Perception Score	Clinician Perception Score
5.0			5.0		
4.8			4.8		
4.6			4.6		
4.4			4.4		
4.2			4.2		
4.0			4.0		
3.8			3.8		
3.6			3.6		
3.4			3.4		
3.2			3.2		
3.0			3.0		
2.8			2.8		
2.6			2.6		
2.4			2.4		
2.2			2.2		
2.0			2.0		
1.8			1.8		
1.6			1.6		
1.4			1.4		
1.2			1.2		
1.0			1.0		

*PRIMARY Prevention/Intervention Mode: Flexible Line   1.0–2.3
*SECONDARY Prevention/Intervention Mode: Normal Line   2.4–3.6
*TERTIARY Prevention/Intervention Mode: Resistance Lines   3.7–5.0

*Breakdowns of numerical scores for stressor penetration are suggested values.

Family Systems Strengths
Family and Clinician Perception Scores

DIRECTIONS: Graph the scores from the inventory by placing an "X" at the appropriate location and connect with a line. (Use first name initial for each different entry and different color code for each family member.)

SUM OF STRENGTHS AVAILABLE FOR PREVENTION/ INTERVENTION MODE	FAMILY SYSTEMS STRENGTHS	
	FAMILY MEMBER PERCEPTION SCORE	CLINICIAN PERCEPTION SCORE
5.0		
4.8		
4.6		
4.4		
4.2		
4.0		
3.8		
3.6		
3.4		
3.2		
3.0		
2.8		
2.6		
2.4		
2.2		
2.0		
1.8		
1.6		
1.4		
1.2		
1.0		

*PRIMARY Prevention/Intervention Mode: Flexible Line   1.0-2.3
*SECONDARY Prevention/Intervention Mode: Normal Line   2.4-3.6
*TERTIARY Prevention/Intervention Mode: Resistance Lines   3.7-5.0

*Breakdowns of numerical scores for stressor penetration are suggested values.

Qualitative Summary Family and Clinician Remarks
Part I: Family systems Stressors (General)

Summarize general stressors and remarks of family and clinician. Prioritize stressors according to importance to family members.

_____
_____
_____
_____

Part II: Family Systems Stressors (Specific)

A. Summarize specific stressors and remarks of family and clinician.

_____
_____
_____

B. Summarize differences (if discrepancies exist) between how family members and clinicians view effects of stressful situation on family.

_____
_____
_____

C. Summarize overall family functioning.

_____
_____
_____

D. Summarize overall significant physical health status for family members.

_____
_____
_____

E. Summarize overall significant mental health status for family members.

_____
_____
_____

Part III: Family Systems Strengths

Summarize family systems strengths and family and clinician remarks that facilitate family health and stability.

_____
_____
_____

Family Care Plan*

| Diagnosis General & Specific Family System Stressors | Family Systems Strengths Supporting Family Care Plan | Goals Family & Clinician | Prevention/Intervention Mode | | Outcomes Evaluation and Replanning |
			Primary, Secondary, or Tertiary	Prevention/ Intervention Activities	

*Prioritize the three most significant diagnoses.

APPENDIX D
THE FRIEDMAN FAMILY ASSESSMENT MODEL (SHORT FORM)

The following form is shortened for ease in assessing the O' Shea family (Appendix C) and other families. If you are not sure what data should be covered in each of the assessment areas below, please refer to Appendix A for the long form, where more detailed questions/areas are presented, or refer to the related chapters where both content and assessment areas are addressed.

Before using the following guidelines in completing family assessments, two words of caution are noted: First, not all areas included below will be germane for each of the families visited. The guidelines are comprehensive and allow depth when probing is necessary. The student should not feel that every subarea needs be covered when the broad area of inquiry poses no problems to the family or concern to the health worker. Second, by virtue of the interdependence of the family system, one will find unavoidable redundancy. For the sake of efficiency, the assessor should try not to repeat data, but to refer the reader back to sections where this information has already been described.

Identifying Data

1. **Family Name**
2. **Address and Phone**
3. **Family Composition: The Family Genogram** (See Figure 8-1).
4. **Type of Family Form**
5. **Cultural (Ethnic) Background**
6. **Religious Identification**
7. **Social Class Status**
8. **Social Class Mobility**

Developmental Stage And History Of Family

9. **Family's Present Developmental Stage**
10. **Extent of Family Developmental Tasks Fulfillment**
11. **Nuclear Family History**
12. **History of Family of Origin of Both Parents**

Environmental Data

13. **Characteristics of Home**
14. **Characteristics of Neighborhood and Larger Community**
15. **Family's Geographical Mobility**
16. **Family's Associations and Transactions with Community**

Family Structure

17. **Communication Patterns**
    Extent of Functional and Dysfunctional Communication (types of recurring patterns)
    Extent of Emotional (Affective) Messages and How Expressed
    Characteristics of Communication Within Family Subsystems
    Extent of Congruent and Incongruent Messages
    Types of Dysfunctional Communication Processes Seen in Family
    Areas of Closed Communication
    Familial and Contextual Variables Affecting Communication
18. **Power Structure**
    Power Outcomes
    Decision-making Process
    Power Bases
    Variables Affecting Family Power
    Overall Family System and Subsystem Power (Family Power Continuum Placement)
19. **Role Structure**
    Formal Role Structure
    Informal Role Structure
    Analysis of Role Models (optional)
    Variables Affecting Role Structure
20. **Family Values**
    Compare the family ot American core values or family's reference group values and/or identify important family values and their importance (priority) in family.
    Congruence Between the Family's Values and the Family's Reference Group or Wider Community

Source: Friedman, M. M., Bowden, V. R., Jones, E. G. (2003). *Family nursing: Research, theory, and practice, 5th ed.* p 593–594.

Disparity in Value Systems
Presence of Value Conflicts in Family
Effect of the Above Values and Value Conflicts on Health Status of Family

Family Functions

21. **Affective Function**
    Mutual Nurturance, Closeness, and Identification
    Family attachment diagram, Figure 14-2, is helpful here.
    Separateness and Connectedness
    Family's Need-Response Patterns
22. **Socialization Function**
    Family Child-rearing Practices
    Adaptability of Child-rearing Practices for Family Form and Family's Situation
    Who Is (Are) Socializing Agent(s) for Child(ren)?
    Value of Children in Family
    Cultural Beliefs that Influence Family's Child-rearing Patterns
    Social Class Influence on Child-Rearing Patterns
    Estimation About Whether Family Is at Risk for Child-rearing Problems and if So, Indication of High-Risk Factors
    Adequacy of Home Environment for Children's Needs to Play
23. **Health Care Function**
    Family's Health Beliefs, Values, and Behavior
    Family's Definitions of Health-Illness and Its Level of Knowledge
    Family's Perceived Health Status and Illness Susceptibility
    Family's Dietary Practices
    Adequacy of family diet (recommended 3-day food history record).
    Function of mealtimes and attitudes toward food and mealtimes.
    Shopping (and its planning) practices.

Person(s) responsible for planning, shopping, and preparation of meals.
Sleep and Rest Habits
Physical Activity and Recreation Practices
Family's Therapeutic and Recreational Drug, Alcohol and Tobacco Practices
Family's Role in Self-care Practice
Medically Based Preventive Measures (physicals, eye and hearing tests, immunizations, dental care)
Complementary and Alternative Therapies
Family Health History (both general and specific diseases— environmentally and genetically related)
Health Care Services Received
Feelings and Perceptions Regarding Health Services
Emergency Health Services
Source of Payments for Health and Other Services
Logistics of Receiving Care

Family Stress, Coping, And Adaptation

24. **Family Stressors, Strengths, and Perceptions**
    Stressors Family Is Experiencing
    Strengths That Counterbalance Stressors
    Family's Definition of the Situation
25. **Family Coping Strategies**
    How the Family Is Reacting to the Stressors
    Extent of Family's Use of Internal Coping Strategies (past/present)
    Extent of Family's Use of External Coping Strategies (past/present)
    Dysfunctional Coping Strategies Utilized (past/present; extent of use)
26. **Family Adaptation**
    Overall Family Adaptation
    Estimation of Whether Family Is in Crisis
27. **Tracking Stressors, Coping, and Adaptation Over Time**

INDEX

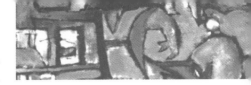

INDEX OF NAMES

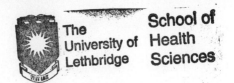

The
University of
Lethbridge

School of
Health
Sciences